Physiology and Biochemistry of the Domestic Fowl

Physiology and Biochemistry of the Domestic Fowl

Volume 5

Edited by

B. M. Freeman
Houghton Poultry Research Station,
Houghton, Huntingdon,
England

1984

ACADEMIC PRESS

(Harcourt Brace Jovanovich, Publishers)

London Orlando San Diego San Francisco New York
Toronto Montreal Sydney Tokyo São Paulo

ACADEMIC PRESS INC. (LONDON) LTD.
24–28 Oval Road
London, NW1 7DX

United States Edition Published by
ACADEMIC PRESS INC.
(Harcourt Brace Jovanovich Inc.)
Orlando, Florida 32887

British Library Cataloguing in Publication Data

Physiology and biochemistry of the domestic fowl.
Vol. 5
1. Poultry
I. Freeman, B. M.
636.5 SF483

ISBN 0-12-267105-8
LCCCN 75-170757

Typeset and printed in the United Kingdom by W. & G. Baird Ltd. The Greystone Press, Caulside Drive, Antrim.

Contributors

A. R. Akester, Sub-department of Veterinary Anatomy, University of Cambridge, Tennis Court Road, Cambridge CB2 1QS, England.

M. E. Coates, National Institute for Research in Dairying, University of Reading, Shinfield, Reading, Berkshire RG2 9AT, England.

G. Cramb, Department of Physiology and Pharmacology, University of St. Andrews, St. Andrews, Fife KY16 9TS, Scotland.

F. J. Cunningham, Department of Physiology and Biochemistry, University of Reading, Reading, Berkshire RG6 2AJ, England.

C. G. Dacke, Physiology Department, Marischal College, University of Aberdeen, Aberdeen AB9 1AS, Scotland.

I. R. Falconer, School of Biological Sciences, University of New England, Armidale, New South Wales 2351, Australia.

B. M. Freeman, Houghton Poultry Research Station, Houghton, Huntingdon, Cambridgeshire PE17 2DA, England.

A. B. Gilbert, Agricultural and Food Research Council's Poultry Research Centre, Roslin, Midlothian EH25 9PS, Scotland.

D. G. Gilmour, Institut d'Embryologie du CNRS, 94130 Nogent-sur-Marne, France.

H. D. Griffin, Agricultural and Food Research Council's Poultry Research Centre, Roslin, Midlothian EH25 9PS, Scotland.

P. E. Lake, Agricultural and Food Research Council's Poultry Research Centre, Roslin, Midlothian EH25 9PS, Scotland.

D. R. Langslow, Chief Scientist's Team, Nature Conservancy Council, Godwin House, George Street, Huntingdon, Cambridgeshire PE18 6BU, England.

R. J. Levin, Department of Physiology, University of Sheffield, Sheffield S10 2TN, England.

L. N. Payne, Houghton Poultry Research Station, Houghton, Huntingdon, Cambridgeshire PE17 2DA, England.

M. M. Perry, Agricultural and Food Research Council's Poultry Research Centre, Roslin, Midlothian EH25 9PS, Scotland.

P. C. Powell, Houghton Poultry Research Station, Houghton, Huntingdon, Cambridgeshire PE17 2DA, England.

C. G. Scanes, Department of Animal Sciences, Rutgers – The State University, New Brunswick, New Jersey 08903, U.S.A.

A. Stockell Hartree, Agricultural and Food Research Council's Animal Research Station, Cambridge CB3 0JQ, England.

T. G. Taylor, School of Biochemical and Physiological Sciences, University of Southampton, Southampton SO9 3TU, England.

J. W. Wells, Agricultural and Food Research Council's Poultry Research Centre, Roslin, Midlothian EH25 9PS, Scotland.

Preface

With the publication of volume 5, the task of bringing the original three volumes of the series up to date has been completed. Sadly, the coverage is not quite as wide as I had wished, but I hope that the reader will be generous enough to overlook the fault and the fact that the availability of the material has meant that the organization of the individual volumes is not entirely satisfactory.

One innovation in this volume is the inclusion of an appendix giving biochemical and physiological data on the adult fowl. It is hoped that this may prove a useful and quick source of quantitative information that is discussed in the body of the book.

I am grateful to the staff of Academic Press, London for their expert assistance in producing the two volumes; particular mention must be made of Emily Wilkinson, Clio Timaeus and Diana Beaven.

Houghton

B. M. Freeman
October, 1983

FOR MARGARET

Contents

7. The Cardiovascular System

A. R. AKESTER

8. Blood Groups
D. G. GILMOUR

9. The Lymphoid System
L. N. PAYNE and P. C. POWELL

10. Steroid Hormone Production by the Ovary

J. W. WELLS and A. B. GILBERT

11. Yolk Formation

H. D. GRIFFIN, M. M. PERRY and A. B. GILBERT

12. The Male in Reproduction

P. E. LAKE

Appendix: Biochemical and Physiological Data

B. M. FREEMAN

Subject Index

Contents of Volume 4

1 Absorption from the Alimentary Tract

R. J. LEVIN

Department of Physiology, University of Sheffield, England

PHYSIOLOGY BIOCHEMISTRY DOMESTIC
FOWL, VOL. 5 ISBN 0–12–267105–8

I. Introduction

At the time of the original review* (Hudson, Levin and Smyth, 1971) it was one of the few that covered the whole field of absorptive function in the chicken. Since then a number of reviews on specific aspects of intestinal function in the chicken have become available. Because of the limitation on space, re-reviewing all the references analysed in these articles would serve little useful purpose. Thus, wherever possible, the reader is referred to existing reviews of the subject and usually only studies not included in them will be cited individually.

II. Methods

A. Isolated Enterocytes

The technique developed for preparing functionally isolated enterocytes

* This chapter is dedicated to the memory of Professor David Smyth (1908–1979) who initiated me into studying intestinal function.

(mucosal cells) from the small intestine of chickens (Kimmich, 1970) has been exploited extensively by its originator (Kimmich, 1975; Kimmich and Carter-Su, 1978; Kimmich and Randles, 1975; Carter-Su and Kimmich, 1980) to examine the mechanisms of sodium-dependent solute uptake and transfer. Other workers have employed the technique to study the metabolism of the isolated enterocytes (Porteus, 1979), the transfer of folic acid and folate (Eilam *et al.*, 1981) and the relation between Na^+-sensitive solute transfer and Na^+/K^+ pump activity (Sepulveda *et al.*, 1982). In this latter study the use of phenylmethyl sulphonyl fluoride, a protease inhibitor, was reported to improve the cell viability of the enterocyte.

B. Brush Border Membranes

Putkey *et al.* (1982) found that the usual methods of preparing mammalian brush border membranes proved unsatisfactory when applied to chicken intestine. They developed a new procedure that gave a 25–30% yield of brush borders when isolated from cockerel intestine.

III. Calcium

Calcium absorption and its control has been repeatedly and exhaustively reviewed (Hurwitz, 1976; Lawson and Emtage, 1974; Norman, 1979; De Luca, 1979; Murer and Hildmann, 1981; Kenny, 1982). Much of the work has utilized the chick intestine. The classical model formulated from these studies has been summarized by De Luca (1979). The active form of the vitamin, 1,25-dihydroxyvitamin D_3, probably enters the enterocyte by passive diffusion, where it binds with a cytosol receptor that is then translocated to the nucleus. The complex on binding to the nuclear chromatin initiates the production of calcium transport proteins via the usual gene transcription process and mRNA. These protein(s) appear at the brush border allowing the calcium to enter the enterocyte and be sequestered in vesicles or mitochondria. The calcium is then extruded into the interstitial fluid by a sodium-sensitive process at the baso-lateral membranes. The permeability of the enterocyte membrane is also increased by the vitamin allowing an increased influx (lumen-to-plasma) of calcium which is then pumped out. Unfortunately, numerous investigations have shown a number of weaknesses in this model. A recent review (Nemere and Norman, 1982) has examined in detail the more elaborate actions that vitamin D has on enterocyte membranes (see Section IIID).

A. Calcium-binding Protein (CaBP)

The physiological role of the calcium-binding protein in response to the stimulation of calcium absorption by vitamin D remains unanswered. Wasserman *et al.* (1974) commented that "the molecular role of the CaBP in the calcium translocation process remains unknown although theories and hypotheses are rampant". More recently, Kenny (1982) has summarized the evidence for and against the concept of a primary role of the CaBP as a carrier in calcium transport. While the amount of CaBP is changed in the same direction as calcium transport for a variety of responses, like response to vitamin D, age and egg laying, dietary manipulation and feeding extracts of *S. malacoxylon*, it does not rise in the chicken enterocytes until 7 h after the intracardiac injection of 1,25-dihydroxyvitamin D_3, even though calcium absorption is increased within 2 h (Spencer *et al.*, 1978). Spencer *et al.* (1978) suggested that the CaBP is a mechanism for sustaining but not initiating the increased calcium transport, because it buffers the free intracellular concentration of calcium in the enterocyte. Kenny (1982) agrees with this proposal. The greatest concentration of CaBP is in the duodenum, the concentration falling continuously to the ileum (Taylor and Wasserman, 1965). The cellular location of the protein is contentious. Taylor and Wasserman (1970) claimed that it was located in goblet cells and the microvillar region of enterocytes, but not at the basolateral membrane, cytoplasm or nucleus, while Morrissey *et al.* (1978a) claimed the exact opposite.

The duodenal CaBP shows a dose–response relationship in rachitic chicks (Bar and Wasserman, 1974) with the pro-hormone vitamin D_3. The hormonal form of the vitamin (1,25-dihydroxyvitamin D_3) initiates CaBP synthesis more rapidly (~ 2 h) that the pro-hormone form (Spencer *et al.*, 1976a). The amount of CaBP is dependent on the concentrations of dietary calcium and phosphorus.

B. Brush Border Studies

1. Calmodulin in Brush Borders

Calmodulin was found in isolated brush borders from chicken intestine in tight association with the cytoskeletal elements of the microvillar filament bundle (Howe *et al.*, 1980). It was speculated that it could be involved in the cyclic movements of the microvilli (Mooseker, 1976), control of enzymes in microvillus membrane, or as a possible carrier for Ca^{2+} in its vectorial movement across the enterocyte, or by acting as a Ca^{2+} "sink" in a region where other sinks (smooth endoplasmic reticulum, mitochondria) are absent.

2. Brush Border Preparations

Chick brush border membranes specially prepared for calcium transport studies (Wilson and Lawson, 1980) showed a fourfold difference between external and internal Ca^{2+} concentration. The majority of the ion was membrane bound to the interior of the vesicles as it could not be replaced with vesicle exposure to lanthanum. The vesicles possessed a high affinity binding site (5×10^{-5} M), more in the duodenum than ileum. Vitamin D increased the number of sites.

C. Studies with Embryonic Chicken Duodenum in Organ Culture

Corradino and Wasserman (1971) and Corradino (1973) showed that vitamin D_3 and its metabolites could induce CaBP in the cells of embryonic duodenum *in vitro*. Later Corradino, using the organ-cultured intestine, examined the inhibition of 1,25-dihydroxycalciferol by actinomycin D and α-amanitin (Corradino, 1973), the interactions of adenylate cyclase system and the vitamin D_3-mediated calcium absorption mechanism (Corradino, 1974), the direct inhibition of the vitamin D_3-mediated mechanism by diphenylhydantoin (Corradino, 1976) and by cadmium (Corradino, 1979).

D. Vitamin D and Intestinal Membrane

The lack of relationship between intestinal CaBP and $1,25(OH)_2D_3$-mediated stimulation of calcium transport (Spencer *et al.*, 1976; Morrissey *et al.*, 1978b) and the evidence that protein synthesis is not an obligatory step in initiating vitamin-D dependent calcium transport has caused an increase of studies on calcium absorption in relation to changes in membrane properties mediated by vitamin D. These have been reviewed by Nemere and Norman (1982). They conclude that the actions of the vitamin D on the enterocyte are pleiotropic. They review the many studies which show the effects on the glycocalyx, brush border and basolateral membranes involving complex changes in the membrane carbohydrates, lipids, and proteins. Alterations in the latter include not only those of calcium binding proteins but also of many enzymes and cytoskeletal proteins. The possible role of vesicular carriers was discussed (Golgi, lysosomal, and pinocytotic). No clear cut mechanism for calcium movement could be offered, but a model involving vesicular transport and/or protein carriers was suggested.

E. Effects of Glucocorticoids and Dietary Intake

Calcium absorption from ligated loops of duodenum, jejunum and ileum has been measured in chicks treated with betamethasone (25 μg kg^{-1} for 14 days) and diet-restricted birds with a growth rate equal to the glucocorticoid dosed animals. Absorption was depressed in the duodenum and jejunum by both conditions, but in the ileum, while betamethasone has little effect, dietary restriction doubled calcium absorption (Fox and Heath, 1981). This enhanced function was sufficient to restore the calcium absorption from the entire small intestine.

IV. Sugars

The digestion and absorption of carbohydrate by chicken intestine was reviewed by Levin (1976). The following section updates that publication.

A. Studies *In Vivo*

1. Kinetic Studies in Fed Animals

Ruano *et al.* (1974) measured the kinetics of galactose absorption in urethanized chickens and reported an "apparent K_m" of 16 mM and a J_{max} of 2 μmol cm^{-2} 10 min^{-1}. The data were uncorrected for unstirred layers and non-saturating components. Levin *et al.* (1983) developed a technique to obtain the kinetic parameters for the hexose active (saturable) electrogenic transfer of the jejunum and ileum *in vivo*. The "apparent K_m's" and J_{max}'s were corrected for the effects of unstirred layers (Levin, 1979, 1982; Gardner and Atkins, 1982) and non-saturating components. These corrected kinetic parameters were designated as the real K_m and J_{max}, to distinguish them from the apparent parameters and the "true K_m" and J_{max} of the actual transfer site (mechanism). The parameters obtained for glucose and galactose in the jejunum and ileum are shown in Table 1. The K_m is much greater than that found by Ruano *et al.* (1974), despite the corrections for non-saturating components.

The sites of absorption of dietary glucose and glucose liberated from starch were assessed in 7-week-old chickens using non-absorbed markers (Riesenfeld *et al.*, 1980). Most of the glucose was absorbed in the upper intestine, especially when the hexose was the major dietary carbohydrate. Glucose absorption from starch lagged behind that of dietary glucose, as only 60% of the starch was digested at the level of the lower jejunum. This indicates that the enzymatic breakdown of the carbohydrate is the rate-limiting factor in glucose absorption from starch diets.

Table 1

Real kinetic parameters for the electrogenic absorption of glucose and galactose in the jejunum and ileum of fed anaesthetized chickens[a]

	Glucose		Galactose	
	Real K_m (mM)	Real J_{max} (nmol $cm^{-2}s^{-1}$)	Real K_m (mM)	Real J_{max} (nmol $cm^{-2}s^{-1}$)
Jejunum	12 ± 2	1 ± 0·03	48 ± 8	1·8 ± 0·1
Ileum	3·7 ± 1·1	1·7 ± 0·11	13·3 ± 3·9	2·6 ± 0·15

[a]Results are given as means ± SEM for 7–12 chickens. From Levin and Mitchell (1982) and Levin *et al.* (1983).

2. *Dietary Influences*

Male chicks fed on an isocaloric carbohydrate-free diet had higher rates of duodenal glucose and fructose absorption *in vivo* and greater intestinal transfers of these two sugars *in vitro* compared with chicks fed on diets rich in carbohydrate (Gauthier *et al.*, 1979). Withdrawal of food for 3 days had marked effects on the real kinetic parameters for glucose and galactose active (electrogenic) absorption *in vivo*, in the jejunum and ileum of anaesthetized chickens (Levin and Mitchell, 1982). The kinetic parameters obtained are shown in Table 2. Compared with the fed values, the ileal K_m's for glucose and galactose were unchanged but the J_{max} for glucose was decreased significantly. In the jejunum, fasting induced decreases in the K_m's and increases in the J_{max}'s for both hexoses. One mechanistic interpretation of the K_m is that it is an index of the affinity of the absorption mechanism for its substrate. Thus the data suggest that fasting enhances the affinity of the absorption mechanisms for the hexoses. The topic has been discussed by Levin (1983).

Table 2

Real kinetic parameters for the electrogenic absorption of glucose and galactose in the jejunum and ileum of 3-day-fasted anaesthetized chickens[a]

	Glucose		Galactose	
	Real K_m	Real J_{max}	Real K_m	Real J_{max}
Jejunum	3·0 ± 1·0	1·2 ± 0·03	20 ± 5	2·3 ± 0·1
Ileum	1·5 ± 0·8	1·4 ± 0·04	21 ± 7	2·2 ± 0·2

[a]Results are given as means ± SEM for 7–10 chickens. From Levin and Mitchell (1982). Units for real K_m and J_{max} as in Table 1.

B. Effects of Inhibitors

Rings of everted intestine from broiler chicks fed aflatoxin for 3 weeks showed significant increases in the uptake of glucose per gram of intestine compared with intestine from birds given a normal diet without the toxin (Ruff and Wyatt, 1976). Unfortunately, the authors did not use pair fed controls, so the enhanced uptake may be due to the effects of semi-starvation influencing intestinal transfer function—see Levin (1976, 1983) for comment. The effects of four raw legumes, field beans, soybeans, bitter retch, and navy beans, were assessed on the intestinal absorption of galactose *in vivo* and on its transfer by intestinal rings incubated *in vitro*. Only the diets containing navy bean or soybean depressed the absorption *in vivo*, but all diets caused depressed transfers *in vitro* (Lasheras *et al.*, 1980). The reason for these effects is unknown.

Jejunal slices exposed to $HgCl_2$ had markedly reduced carrier mediated uptakes of D-glucose, but the diffusive entry was unaffected (Miller *et al.*, 1980). It was found that intestine from young chicks (2 days old) was more inhibited by the mercury salt than intestine from 21-day-old chicks.

Cytochalasin B inhibited the exit of 3-O-methylglucose across the basolateral membranes of isolated enterocytes, but had no action on its sodium-dependent active transport into the enterocyte across the brush border membrane (Kimmich and Randles, 1979). Diez de los Rios *et al.* (1980), however, could not find any effect with Cytochalasin B using segments of chicken intestine. They suggested that its lack of action was probably due to its failure to reach the basolateral membranes in the intact tissue strips.

C. Studies on Isolated Enterocytes

Kimmich and his co-workers have published a large number of papers using his preparation of isolated enterocytes to examine the brush border and basolateral systems for the transfer of sugars, especially in relation to the energetics and kinetics of sugar transport. There is an extensive review of these studies (Kimmich, 1981). Those interested in the details of the transport kinetics, driving forces, transport efficiency and Na^+-sugar coupling stoichiometry in chicken enterocytes should refer to this detailed and extensive discussion.

D. Effects of Age

The early studies were reviewed by Hudson *et al.* (1971) and Levin (1976). Hudson and Levin (1968) examined the transfer of glucose and galactose across everted intestine from newly hatched and 32-day-old chicks, using ten different parameters. Those utilizing serosal transfer were found to be poor measures of transfer function, because of the increasing thickness of the developing intestine trapping the transferred sugars in the gut wall. However, even the mucosal transfer per gram of intestine decreased with age (Levin, 1976). Scharrer (1972a) also found that the mid-jejunum from 7-week-old chickens transported less galactose than intestine from 2-week-old chickens. Raheja *et al.* (1977), apparently unaware of these previous studies, again examined the transfers of glucose and the non-metabolized glucalogue 3-O-methylglucose across everted jejunum from 7-day-old and 12-week-old chickens. Mucosal glucose uptake (per gram intestine), the serosal/mucosal concentration ratio for the glucalogue and the metabolism of glucose all decreased continuously over the developmental period, confirming the previous work. Although not directly examining the effects of age on hexose transfer, the studies of Miller *et al.*. (1980) on the effects of mercuric chloride on gut glucose transfer *in vitro* also showed that the glucose uptake per gram of tissue in control intestine from young chickens (2 days old) was much greater than that from the 21-day-old birds. Shehata *et al.* (1981) studied the development of the transport system for 3-O-methylglucose in jejunal slices and glucose for jejunal brush border membrane vesicles. Kinetic analysis showed low rates of transport in slices from embryos 2 days before hatching or newly hatched chicks, but they increased to a maximum 2 to 7 days after hatching. The rates then declined to adult values over the next 14 days. The "apparent K_m" did not change over the period. The picture was somewhat different with the vesicles, glucose transport was greater in 2-day vesicles than in 21-day vesicles, but the "apparent K_m" like the slices was unchanged. It is possible that the noted difference is due to actual differences in the transport processes for the dietary sugar (glucose) and the glucalogue (3-O-methylglucose) rather than for the preparation (see Levin, 1976 for references on glucose isocarriers).

Lerner *et al.* (1976) compared the *in vitro* influx (at a single concentration) of a range of substances into the jejunum and ileum of 1-day-old and 56-day-old chicks. Differential changes in uptake were noted.

E. Effect of pH

The influence of pH on the transfer of D-galactose across everted sacs of jejunum and ileum has been studied *in vitro*. Lowering the incubating buffer's pH to 6·4 increased the jejunal galactose transfer but left ileal transfer unaffected. At pH 5·4 jejunal transfer was inhibited (Scharrer, 1972b). Studies in rat had shown that jejunum and ileum responded differently *in vitro* to changes in incubating pH (Thompson *et al.*, 1970).

V. Amino Acids, Peptides and Proteins

Although there are some minor differences, the absorption of amino acids across the chicken small intestine is very similar to that observed in other species. The subject has been reviewed by Kan (1973), Boorman (1976) and Lerner (1971, 1978). The general field of amino acid transfer has been the focus of articles by Lerner (1978) and Munck (1981), who also discuss aspects of transfer across chicken intestine.

A. Amino Acid Absorption *In Vivo*: Jejunal and Ileal Kinetics

A new method to allow the kinetic characterization *in vivo* of the saturable absorption mechanisms for amino acids in the chicken jejunum and ileum has been developed by Levin *et al.* (1983). The technique allowed the estimation of the kinetic parameters of K_m and J_{max} for the absorption process corrected for unstirred layer effects and non-saturable processes. These were designated "real K_m" and J_{max} to distinguish them from the "apparent K_m" and J_{max} and the "true K_m" and J_{max} of the actual carrier site. The technique has allowed the first comparative evaluation of the absorption mechanisms *in vivo* for a number of amino acids unconfounded by artifacts induced by unstirred layers and non-saturating processes (see Levin, 1979 and Gardner and Atkins, 1982 for comment). The K_m's and J_{max}'s of the various amino acids for the jejunum and ileum are listed in Table 3. A possible mechanistic interpretation may be derived from the data. The affinity of all the transferring mechanisms for the amino acids appears higher in the ileum than in the jejunum while the J_{max} is either similar (histidine, methionine, AIB) or even greater (glycine and valine). These findings led the authors to conclude that the enterocytes of the

Table 3

The kinetic parameters of real K_m (mM) and J_{max} (pmol cm^{-2} s^{-1}) for saturable amino acid absorption processes in the jejunum and ileum *in vivo*[a]

Amino acid	Jejunum K_m	Jejunum J_{max}	Ileum K_m	Ileum J_{max}
Amino-isobutyric acid (AIB)	4·6 ± 0·9	46 ± 7	2·5 ± 0·2	56 ± 6
Glycine	4·2 ± 0·4	37 ± 5	2·7 ± 0·2	55 ± 6
Histidine	3·4 ± 0·7	132 ± 12	0·8 ± 0·2	129 ± 4
Methionine	4·9 ± 0·6	147 ± 14	1·9 ± 0·6	148 ± 5
Valine	3·2 ± 0·7	38 ± 7	1·5 ± 0·2	82 ± 13

[a]Results are given as means ± SEM for 6–10 chickens. From Levin and Mitchell (1982) and Levin *et al.* (1983).

chicken ileum are functionally equipped and anatomically well-sited to act as "scavengers" of the small intestine.

The importance of choice of base upon which to express absorption data was emphasized by the study of Mitchell and Levin (1981). They measured the maximum absorptive capacities (J_{max}) for glycine, valine and methionine in the ileum and jejunum obtained by the technique of Levin *et al.* (1983). These were calculated per unit surface area and per region (10 cm lengths). The J_{max} per cm^2 gave the ileal enterocytes a greater absorbing capacity than the jejunal ones for glycine and valine but not for methionine. When the J_{max}'s were calculated on a segment basis, however, those for glycine and valine for the two areas were not different, but for methionine the jejunal value was now some 1·9 times greater than the ileal.

B. Effects of Dietary Restriction

The effects of dietary restriction on the intestinal absorption of amino acids is a contentious issue, as the results have been conflicting (Munck, 1981; Levin and Mitchell, 1982; Levin 1983). Gous (1977) studied the uptakes *in vitro* of 2 mM L-arginine, glycine, L-lysine and L-phenylalanine into intestinal rings prepared from cockerels that had their food restricted so as to lose either 12, 19 or 27% of their body weight. Only in the case of L-arginine and L-lysine was the uptake increased by the restrictions.

A different approach was undertaken by Levin and Mitchell (1982) who investigated the effects of the complete withdrawal of food for 3 days on the kinetics of absorption of glycine, methionine, histidine, valine and α-amino isobutyric acid (AIB) in the jejunum and ileum of anaesthetized chickens. They found that of the possible nine changes in K_m and J_{max} that theoretically could occur (Table 4), five were observed to occur. In the ileum, the K_m and J_{max} for AIB, methionine, histidine and glycine were unchanged, but for valine, the K_m increased while the J_{max} remained unaltered. The changes that occurred in the jejunal transfer parameters were more complicated. Three groups were obvious, one where the K_m was unchanged but the J_{max} increased (glycine and AIB), one where the K_m decreased and the J_{max} was unchanged (methionine and histidine) and one where the K_m decreased but the J_{max} increased (valine). The differential changes in K_m and J_{max} for the amino acids indicate that fasting (and presumably dietary restriction) has specific actions on enterocyte absorption mechanisms rather than general effects. The use of real K_m and J_{max} to identify these adaptations in jejunum and ileum is well illustrated by the study. The mechanistic interpretation of the results would assume that the K_m is an index of the affinity changes of the system for the amino acids while the J_{max} is the index of its maximum transfer capacity.

Table 4
The nine possible theoretical ways that K_m and J_{max} can change (with regard to each other) for absorption mechanisms[a]

Type	K_m	J_{max}	Type	K_m	J_{max}
1	↓ Decrease	↓ Decrease	5	°No change	°No change
2	↑ Increase	↑ Increase	6	°No change	↑ Increase
3	↓ Decrease	↑ Increase	7	°No change	↓ Decrease
4	↑ Increase	↓ Decrease	8	↑ Increase	°No change
			9	↓ Decrease	°No change

[a]After Levin and Mitchell (1982).

C. Transport Pathways

Much research energy has been expended into unravelling the various transport pathways and their specificities for amino acids in the enterocytes. The studies have been described by Wiseman (1968, 1974) and lately by Munck (1981). The usual categories involved are transport mechanisms for neutral amino acids (±-aminomonocarboxylic acids), basic amino acids (cationic), acidic (anionic) amino acids and imino acids. These mechanisms are present in the enterocytes of chicken intestine (Kan, 1973; Lerner, 1971, 1978). Lerner (1978) has discussed the multiple transport systems proposed for the chicken, many of the studies coming from his own laboratory. In the case of the specificity of the neutral amino acid transferring system he proposed a complex system composed of some seven possible separate components gleaned from experimental inhibition studies (Lerner, 1971, 1978). A later analysis (Lerner and Messier, 1980) used a two site model to explain neutral amino acid transfer. Using segments of fasted chicken intestine, Lerner and Steinke (1977) reported a distinct Na^+-dependent transport system for glutamic acid and a diffusion mechanism.

D. Effect of Cyclic AMP

The influx of amino acids across the brush border is unaffected by cyclic AMP (Burrill *et al.*, 1974, 1976), although it increased the inhibitory effect of lysine on the transport of a neutral amino acid.

E. Peptide Absorption

The absorption of intact peptides into the enterocytes, with subsequent release of the peptide or the free amino acids into the blood, has been the subject of many studies (Matthews and Adibi, 1976), yet remarkably little investigation has been undertaken with chicken intestine. While Kan (1973) mentioned the possible importance in nutritional studies in fowls, he could only quote the study of Kushak *et al.* (1973) who found, as in other animals, that the uptake of amino acids in peptide form was faster than the uptake as free amino acids. The only other study appears to be that of Hunter and Chvapil (1981). They examined the absorption of ^{125}I-labelled peptides (sized into ranges by ultrafiltration) given by gavage to 3-day-old fasted chickens. Smaller peptides were cleared from the proximal jejunum faster than larger peptides and their digestion products were more completely incorporated into muscle protein. It was suggested that smaller peptides were of greater nutritional value to young chicks than larger peptides.

F. Colonic Amino Acid Transport

In most animals colonic epithelial cells are not involved in transepithelial movement of amino acids. In the chicken, however, the colon has a saturable uptake mechanism for methionine (Lerner *et al.*, 1975) and for leucine (Lind *et al.* 1980a).

G. Vitamin B_6 Antagonists

The role of vitamin B_6 in the mechanisms of absorption of amino acids by the enterocytes of the small intestine is uncertain. The conflicting results of the importance of the vitamin for amino acid absorption in different species has been discussed by Lerner (1978). The only study using chickens measured the absorption of glycine, leucine, and methionine in the mid-jejunum of 24-h fasted cockerels, large, multiple doses of the B_6 antagonist deoxypyridoxine either being injected or circulated in the lumen (Tasaki and Yokata, 1970). The results were inconclusive. Glycine absorption was unaffected, but leucine and methionine showed apparent decreases. The results were not statistically assessed, nor was absorption characterized by kinetic methods. R. J. Levin and M. A. Mitchell (unpublished) fed the B_6 antagonists isoniziad (30 mg kg^{-1} day^{-1}) or 4-deoxypyridoxine (same dose) for 10 days to female chickens and then assessed the absorption of methionine *in vivo* by their technique that allows the best estimates of the real kinetic parameters for the active electrogenic absorption of amino acids *in vivo* (see Section VA). The kinetic parameters for the control group were a real K_m of 7 ± 1·1 mM (mean ± SEM) and a J_{max} of 176 ± 19 (pmol cm^{-2} s^{-1}). Neither the parameters for the isoniazid fed group (real K_m = 5 ± 0·6, J_{max} = 182 ± 9 pmol cm^{-2} s^{-1}) nor those for the 4-deoxypyridoxine group (real K_m = 6·1 ± 0·9, J_{max} = 179 ± 10 pmol cm^{-2} s^{-1}) were significantly different. Thus, the daily feeding of two known vitamin B_6 antagonists for 10 days had no significant action on jejunal methionine active transfer mechanisms *in vivo*. As the enterocytes of chicken intestine have a replacement rate of about 2 days (Imondi and Bird, 1966), the 10 day regime of feeding the antagonists does not induce the generation of enterocytes with specific deficiencies in the active mechanism for methionine absorption.

VI. Salt and Water Transport

A. Coprodeum and Colon

A large literature has developed on the function and control of the cloaca (coprodeum), rectum (colon), and caeca. This has been described in numerous publications by Skadhauge (1973, 1976, 1978, 1981a,b), Thomas (1982) and Thomas and Skadhauge (1982). Because of the wealth of review material available, only the briefest of comment on coprodeum and colonic function will follow. Thomas (1982) has called the cloaca (coprodeum), colon (rectum), caeca and the caudal portion of the ileum the "integrative segment" of the lower bowel, because this is the part of the gut where ureteral urine can mix with intestinal fluids and be modified by the transporting epithelium of the various organs. The colonic–coprodeum segment can absorb 10–15% of water and 65% of the NaCl from the ureteral urine (Skadhauge, 1973). In the absence of a transmural osmotic difference the net Na^+ absorption drives a solute-linked water flow (Thomas and Skadhauge, 1979). Dietary NaCl intake can modify the Na^+ transport of the colon–coprodeum by 100% (Thomas and Skadhauge, 1979). Sodium depletion (by low sodium diets) enhances Na^+ absorption, apparently by increasing the amiloride-sensitive transport sites for sodium in the luminal membranes (Bindslev, 1979, 1981) of about 20% of the coprodeal cells. These cells also acquire a mitochondria-rich cytoplasm (Christensen and Bindslev, 1982). Diets containing high NaCl suppress the NaCl and solute-linked water absorption of the colon–coprodeum (Thomas and Skadhauge, 1979). Interestingly, the high NaCl diets induce a colonic glucose and amino acid stimulated Na^+ absorption, both *in vivo* and *in vitro* (Lind *et al.*, 1980a) and a secretion of K^+ and chloride. In the coprodeum, luminal glucose and amino acid have no effect or transport or water flux.

Assessment of the individual functions of the colon and coprodeum under *in vivo* conditions (Rice and Skadhauge, 1982a) using iso-osmotic perfusion revealed that the net colonic Na^+ flux (mucosa to serosa) was five times greater than that of the coprodeum. In the colon this was linked to a water flow, but no such movement was detected in the coprodeum. The coprodeum is thus functionally water tight (Bindslev, 1981), acting as a storage site for ureteral urine, while the colon can actively modify the water and electrolyte content of the urine and digesta. Previous studies using *in vitro* preparations of coprodeum (Chosniak *et al.*, 1977; Lind *et al.*, 1980a) suggested that coprodeal modification of urine could play an important role in electrolyte balance, but the *in vivo* studies show that its capacity is limited and small, concomitant with its "bladder" functions. Sodium loading in the domestic fowl causes a marked depression in net electrolyte and water absorption of both coprodeum and colon (Rice and Skadhauge, 1982b) and in their transmural potential differences. These results were consistent with previous data obtained with *in vitro* preparations. It is interesting to note that the colon–coprodeum of the hen could become important for studies to isolate the membrane components of the Na^+ entry transport system. As the tissue can be easily converted from an inactive to a highly active Na^+ absorber, it presents good advantages to the experimenter. However, binding studies with the amiloride analogue benzamil, a ligand for epithelial sodium channels, have shown that only a small fraction of its binding can represent the functional Na^+ entry sites (Cuthbert *et al.*, 1982).

B. Hormonal Control

Studies on the possible hormonal mechanisms that control the salt and water transport activity of the colon and coprodeum have focused on aldosterone (Thomas, 1982). Aldosterone injected into fowls fed on high Na^+ diets induces in the colon–coprodeum many of the properties associated with low-Na^+ adaptations and it was concluded that the hormone reproduced qualitatively all the *in vitro* effects of a low-Na^+ diet (Thomas *et al.*, 1980). Other factors to be investigated, such as cyclic AMP which induces a transient change in the electrical transport activity across the lower intestine, may be the cause of the inability of aldosterone to mimic all the *in vivo* actions of a low-Na^+ diet.

C. Small Intestine

In contrast to the numerous studies of the lower intestine, few studies have been undertaken since the last review on salt and water absorption by the small intestine (Hudson *et al.*, 1971). Hurwitz *et al.* (1970) used yttrium-91 (a non-absorbable marker) for assessing *in vivo* the absorption of water and ions along the intestine in laying fowls that had been loaded with or depleted of NaCl. The absorption of Na^+ and K^+ was most rapid in the jejunum and greater than in the rectum. In the ileum, Na^+ was absorbed but K^+ was secreted; low Na diets increased this ileal Na^+ absorption and K^+ secretion.

The net serosal fluid and sodium transport across everted sacs of jejunum obtained from 9-day and 28 to 35-day-old cockerels were studied *in vitro* by Morley *et al.* (1980). Both transports were significantly lower in older birds compared to younger birds. Salt loading had a significant 34% increase on the water transport in the older birds, but not on sodium transport. No effects on either salt or water transfer were apparent in the younger birds. The dietary salt manipulation greatly increased the plasma prolactin concentrations in the older birds (238%), but not in the younger ones. Morley *et al.* (1981) then assessed the effects of ovine prolactin on the transport of sodium and fluid across the everted sacs of jejunum from 9-day-old cockerels and by an *in vivo* balance technique. Prolactin injections for 7 days (100 μg day^{-1}) were found to reduce the transfer of sodium and fluid across both the jejunum and rectum. Arginine vasopressin, a possible contaminant in the prolactin preparation was ineffective on both issues when injected for 7 days (100 μg day^{-1}). The authors suggested that prolactin may play an important role in osmoregulation in the domestic fowl by reducing the permeability of the small intestine (and rectum?) to salt and water. Unfortunately, the actual concentration of prolactin induced by the dosing schedule were not measured, so that it is not clear whether the study involved physiological or pharmacological levels. It is also unfortunate that in all of the reported studies on sodium transfer, the transintestinal electrical potential difference was not measured. The changes in the driving force for the ionic movements in the various conditions thus remain undefined and will have to be reassessed in new experiments if the mechanisms are to be characterized fully.

Assessment of the leakiness or permeability of the duodenum in the layer hen (Warren) was made by Mongin and deLaage (1977) using solutions of varying osmolality and PEG-C^{14} as an index of fluid movements. They found that the duodenum possessed a low "reflection coefficient" (high solute permeability) equipping it for its function of secretion of Na^+ and Cl^- into the lumen.

VII. Caecal Functions

Caeca in the domestic fowl can reach lengths of up to 20 cm with a maximal diameter of 1·5 cm and are filled with yellow brown faeces, quite different from those of the cloaca. The functions attributed to the organ (water absorption, carbohydrate digestion, microbial synthesis of vitamins and their absorption and immunization) have been discussed by Hill (1971), Jayne-Williams and Fuller (1971), McNab (1973) and by Skadhauge (1981b). The latter author reviews in detail the functions and involvement of the caeca in relation to osmoregulation. Despite a number of studies, the overall importance of the caeca to the chicken is contentious. Hill (1971), for example, regards them as playing a minor role in the digestive process. Because a limited number of caecectomized chickens have been claimed to show a greater percentage of moisture in their faeces compared to normal birds (see Skadhauge, 1981b for references) it has been proposed that the caeca have a role in fluid resorption. The studies are far from conclusive. Skadhauge (1981b) argues that, as caecectomy alters the digestibility of dry matter and causes changes in renal handling of fluid, only a total water budget in normal and caecectomized birds will resolve the organ's function in relation to water balance. It should be remembered that caecal contents do not only derive from dietary and bacterial presence but that the chicken's own urine is able to enter (Koike and McFarland, 1966; Akester *et al.*, 1967), probably under the force of antiperistaltic waves. Rice and Skadhauge (1982a,b) investigated the electrolyte and water transport by the caeca *in vivo* in dehydrated, low-NaCl diet hens. When physiological concentrations of acetate (40 mM) and glucose (15 mM) were present in the lumen significant absorption of sodium chloride and water was induced. The authors argued that the enhanced absorption established the caeca as important sites in the reabsorption of water and electrolytes in the stressed hen (dehydration and low NaCl dietary intake). Thomas (1982) mentions unpublished studies that he has made on the ion movements across everted caecal sacs incubated *in vitro* with glucose. They showed a pronounced uptake of Na^+ (251 ± 27 μmol g(wet wt)$^{-1}$ h^{-1}), but had low levels of chloride uptake (29 ± 12 μmol g(wet wt)$^{-1}$ h^{-1} and K^+ secretion (37 ± 7 μmol g(wet wt)$^{-1}$ h^{-1}). He suggests that this Na^+ absorption is the possible driving force for any caecal water absorption.

VIII. Fats, Fatty Acids and Bile Acids

The chicken can absorb a high proportion of its energy requirement in the form of fat (Fedde *et al.*, 1960). The absorption of fats is by the same processes that occur in other monogastric species. Freeman (1976) examined these processes for the chicken and concluded that the major route of fat absorption was by micelles (Garrett and Young, 1975) although limited amounts could be absorbed by other routes (i.e. particulate fat absorption, diffusion). While earlier work indicated that the site of absorption was below the jejunum,

Hurwitz *et al.* (1973), using ^{14}C-labelled fatty acid and non-absorbed markers, reported evidence for identifying the jejunum as the major site of fat absorption in the chick and laying hen. Some absorption however, did occur in the ileum.

The sites of absorption and secretion of fatty acids and bile acids were examined in 16-month-old, laying hens, using the non-absorbed marker yttrium-91 (Hurwitz *et al.*, 1973). In the duodenum a large fatty acid secretion was observed, together with dihydroxycholanic bile acids. Absorption occurred along the length of the intestine, but the jejunal rate was greater than that of the ileum (unlike the case in the rat). Nearly 93% of the secreted bile acids were absorbed by the small intestine. Feeding raw soybean meal is known to markedly depress fat absorption in young chicks. Hurwitz and his co-workers undertook two studies to assess where the agent acted. A marked increase in secretion of bile constituents into the soybean fed chicks was observed and the soybean factor appeared to be interfering with the absorption of fatty acids and bile acids in the lower jejunum and ileum (Sklan *et al.*, 1973, 1975). During the first week after hatching the absorption of dietary corn oil and beef tallow was less than at days 8 to 15 after hatching (Carew et al., 1972). The loci for the differences in absorption between the two ages were not identified.

IX. Phosphate

A. Studies *In Vivo*

Hurwitz (1976) noted, in his review on phosphate absorption in the chicken, the paucity of studies that had been published. With diets containing normal calcium and phosphate, the major site of absorption is the upper jejunum, but there is a net (phosphate) secretion at the duodenum. With low calcium diets net absorption of phosphate was observed in the duodenum (Hurwitz and Bar, 1966, 1969). Vitamin D treatment of vitamin D-deficient chicks increased phosphate absorption *in vivo* (Hurwitz and Bar, 1972). Phosphate depleted chicks showed only a small increase in intestinal transport capacity, suggesting that this process is unlikely to be a major basis of phosphate absorption (Hurwitz, 1976).

B. Studies *In Vitro*

Everted jejunal sacs made from vitamin D_3-deficient or repleted chicks were used by Peterlik *et al.* (1981) to measure the movements of labelled phosphate across the mucosal and serosal boundaries. Vitamin D had no influence on the efflux of phosphate into the mucosa fluid nor on the exchange of phosphate on the serosal border. The entry into the enterocytes, however, involved a saturable, high affinity (K_m = 0·2 mM) active transport process whose V_{max} was increased 2·5 fold by vitamin D. As the K_m was unaltered it was assumed that the hormone had no effect on the "carrier" affinity. However, the active transport of phosphate is sodium dependent and vitamin D appeared to bring about a basic change in the properties of the system. Vitamin depleted gut showed an increasing affinity of the carrier for phosphate with increasing sodium concentration, but with vitamin D_3 repleted chicks the system now showed an increase in its J_{max}. Isolated brush border vesicles from the two vitamin conditions exhibited phosphate uptake that confirmed the existence of this Na^+-dependent phosphate transport system and the effects of the vitamin upon it. Matsumoto *et al.* (1980) reported similar findings. Peterlik *et al.* (1981) also found that vitamin D treatment affected the glucose transfer system in isolated brush-border vesicles from jejunum and ileum but not those from the duodenum. The V_{max} was enhanced and the K_m was lowered. The glucose transfer system and the phosphate system showed mutual inhibition in the vesicles, but a mechanistic explanation for the interaction was difficult to establish.

X. Iron

Using cannulated duodenal-jejunal loops in anaesthetized 6-week-old chickens, Marti *et al.* (1980) examined the mechanism of absorption of iron. They circulated ^{59}Fe dissolved in a calcium-free Ringer-Locke buffer (pH 6·2) with carrier Fe in concentrations ranging from 12·5 to 1555 μM $FeCl_3$. Large concentrations of glucose (55 mM), L-histidine (100 mM) and ascorbic acid (ten times the $FeCl_3$ concentrations) were also present in the buffer. The absorption of iron was a linear function of its luminal concentration up to 695 μM, but saturated at 1559 μM. Laying hens had a greater net transfer of iron compared with non-laying hens and adult males, but there was no difference between males and non-laying hens (Saiz *et al.*, 1980). Intramuscular oestrogen (or diethylstilboestrol) administered to male chickens for 3 days did not significantly influence iron absorption, although it depressed the haematocrit.

XI. Lead

Mykkänen and Wasserman (1981), using an isolated loop of intestine in anaesthetized 3-week-old cockerels, found that lead was rapidly taken up by the intestinal tissue but only slowly released to the bloodstream, unlike calcium which had a rapid accumulation and release to the blood. The authors concluded that, despite a number of similarities, the metals were absorbed by different mechanisms. The administration of cholecalciferol and of $1,25(OH)_2D_3$ to rachitic chicks increased the transfer of ^{203}Pb from the lumen of a ligated gut loop. The response was greatest in the duodenum and least in the ileum (Mykkänen and Wasserman, 1982).

XII. Myo-inositol

The *in vitro* transfer of myo-inositol into strips prepared from intestine removed from chickens fasted for 24 h was examined by Lerner and Smagula (1979). Myo-inositol was transported at low substrate concentrations by a saturable process (apparent K_m = 0·1 mM) and at high concentrations by diffusion. Phlorizin and actively transported sugars depressed the uptake, but the sugars have a low affinity for the transport system. The mediated myo-inositol transport was Na^+-sensitive and inhibited by a sulphydril group blocker. Large variations in the mediated transport were observed among individual intestines.

XIII. Choline

The uptake of choline into intestinal rings, prepared from 8- to 15-day-old chicks, was studied by Herzberg and Lerner (1973). Two processes were revealed, a mediated mechanism saturating at relatively low choline concentrations (apparent K_m = 110 μM) and a simple diffusion mechanism. Reducing the extracellular sodium concentration led to a doubling of the apparent K_m of the mediated component but no change in its J_{max}, suggesting that the carrier needs Na^+ for choline binding. The change, however, could also be caused by structural alterations in the enterocyte membrane induced by the low Na^+. The mediated transfer of choline was unaffected by amino acids or 3-O-methylglucose, but was completely inhibited by the choline analogue hemicholonium and by thiamine. Choline influx was unaffected by anaerobic conditions, ouabain, or oligomycin, indicating an independence from oxidative phosphorylation and Na^+/K^+ ATP-ase.

XIV. Vitamin B_{12}

Chickens possess two substances that bind vitamin B_{12}. One (mol. wt approx. 113 000) is in the plasma while the other is in the proventriculus (mol. wt approx. 96 000). Antibody elicited against the latter reacts against both (Sanneborn and Hansen, 1970), suggesting that the serum binder is from the proventriculus with an added "secretory" piece.

XV. Vitamin B_1 (Thiamin)

The uptake of radioactive B_1 (^{35}S-thiamin) was depressed in intestinal rings prepared from proximal jejunum of chickens (45 days old) fed on diets with added selenium (Lazarov *et al.*, 1980). Increasing the dosage of selenium (0·3 mg to 10 mg kg^{-1} food) increased the effect. The diets also depressed the alkaline phosphatase activity of the enterocytes which, according to the authors, is of functional importance for active thiamine transport.

Treating male chicks twice daily with lysine-vasopressin for 3 days increased the blood concentrations of ^{35}S-thiamine after its injection into the duodenal lumen (Lazarov, 1976). It was inferred that this indicated an enhanced absorption of the vitamin. Mucosal ATP-ase was also said to be increased and it was speculated that this may have been the cause of the enhancement. Obviously much more experimentation is necessary before such statements can be made.

XVI. Folic Acid and Folate

Eilam *et al.* (1981) investigated the uptake of folic acid in isolated (proximal) intestinal epithelial cells prepared from 2- to 6-week-old chicks. The cells accumulated folic acid (3 to 4 times medium level) by a saturable uptake mechanism (apparent $K_m = 3{\cdot}5 \times 10^{-5}$ M) which was sensitive to the extracellular Na^+ concentration; lowering the Na^+ reduced the uptake. The uptake of folic acid was strongly influenced by the medium pH, being greater at pH 5·8 than at 7·4, but accumulation was inhibited at acidic pH values with metabolic inhibitors. This result, contradicting previous inferences that energy was only needed to maintain an acid micro-environment for folic acid transfer, suggests that folic acid is accumulated by an active transfer mechanism (probably coupled to Na^+ movement). Because isolated cells were used it is not possible to conclude at which membrane (serosal/mucosal) the transport processes are based upon.

XVII. Absorption and Transfer in Germ-Free and Gnotobiotic Birds

Jayne-Williams and Fuller (1971) and Coates (1976) reviewed the influence of gut microflora on digestion and absorption in the chicken. Palmer and Rolls (1981) assessed the effects of microflora on the uptake and secretion of calcium by the enterocytes by a variety of *in vivo* and *in vitro* techniques. The conclusion was that the ability of the enterocyte to absorb calcium was unaffected by microbial presence or absence but in its absence the removal of calcium was reduced.

The influence of bacterial status on the absorption of methionine and the glucalogue 3-O-methylglucose was investigated *in vivo* in anaesthetized germ-free, gnotobiotic and conventional chicks, aged 2 to 3 weeks (Yokota and Coates, 1982). The results indicated that there was no difference in the jejunal uptake (actually luminal loss), from 20 mM of the glucalogue and 10 mM methionine per unit length of gut, but on a per gram basis the uptake of both solutes was less in conventional and gnotobiotic birds. It was concluded that micro-organisms did not impair the uptake of either solute. The results did not agree with earlier findings of the authors using intestine *in vitro* where they observed an increased serosal transfer of glucose and B complex vitamins (Ford and Coates, 1971).

Acknowledgements

Acknowledgements are given to the British Egg Marketing Board Scholarship and Research Fund and to the Agricultural Research Council, for financing some of the studies on amino acid and hexose absorption reported in this review.

References

Akester, A. R., Anderson, R. S., Hill, K. J. and Osbaldiston, G. W. (1967). *Br. Poult. Sci.* **8**, 209–212.

Bar, A. and Wasserman, R. H. (1974). *J. Nutr.* **104**, 1202–1207.

Bindslev, N. (1979). *J. Physiol., Lond.* **288**, 449–466.

Bindslev, N. (1981). *In* "Water Transport across Epithelia" (H. H. Ussing, N. Bindslev, N. A. Lassen and O. Sten-Knudsen, eds), pp. 468–484. Munksgaard, Copenhagen.

Boorman, K. N. (1976). *In* "Digestion in the Fowl" (K. N. Boorman and B. M. Freeman, eds), pp. 27–61. British Poultry Science Ltd., Edinburgh.

Burrill, P. H., Sattelmeyer, P. A. and Lerner, J. (1974). *Biochim. biophys. Acta* **373**, 265–276.

Burrill, P. H., Sattelmeyer, P. A. and Lerner, J. (1976). *Comp. Biochem. Physiol.* **53C**, 95–99.

Carew, L. B., Machemer, R. H., Sharp, R. W. and Foss, D. C. (1972). *Poult. Sci.* **51**, 738–742.

Carter-Su, C. and Kimmich, G. A. (1980). *Am. J. Physiol.* **237**, C73–C80.

Chosniak, I., Munck, B. G. and Skadhauge, E. (1977). *J. Physiol., Lond.* **271**, 489–504.

Christensen, O. and Bindslev, N. (1982). *J. Membrane Biol.* **65**, 19–30.
Coates, M. (1976). *In* "Digestion in the Fowl" (K. N. Boorman and B. M. Freeman, eds), pp. 179–191. British Poultry Science Ltd., Edinburgh.
Corradino, R. A. (1973). *Science, N.Y.* **179**, 402–405.
Corradino, R. A. (1974). *Endocrinology* **94**, 1607–1614.
Corradino, R. A. (1976). *Biochem. Pharmac.* **25**, 863–864.
Corradino, R. A. (1979). *Toxic. appl. Pharmac.* **48**, 257–261.
Corradino, R. A. and Wasserman, R. H. (1971). *Science, N.Y.* **172**, 731–733.
Cuthbert, A. W., Edwardson, J. M., Bindslev, N. and Skadhauge, E. (1982). *Pflügers Arch. ges. Physiol.* **392**, 347–351.
De Luca, H. F. (1979). "Vitamin D-Metabolism and Function." Springer-Verlag, New York.
Diez de los Rios, A., Baxendale, L. M. and Armstrong, W. McD. (1980). *Biochim. biophys. Acta* **603**, 207–210.
Eilam, Y., Ariel, M., Jablonska, M. and Grossowicz, N. (1981). *Am. J. Physiol.* **240**, G170–G175.
Fedde, M. R., Waibel, P. E. and Burger, R. E. (1960). *J. Nutr.* **70**, 447–452.
Ford, D. J. and Coates, M. E. (1971). *Proc. Nutr. Soc.* **30**, 10A.
Fox, J. and Heath, H. (1981). *Endocrinology* **108**, 1138–1141.
Freeman, C. P. (1976). *In* "Digestion in the Fowl" (K. N. Boorman and B. M. Freeman, eds), pp. 117–142. British Poultry Science Ltd., Edinburgh.
Gardner, M. L. G. and Atkins, G. L. (1982). *Clin. Sci.* **63**, 405–414.
Garrett, R. L. and Young, R. J. (1975). *J. Nutr.* **105**, 827–838.
Gauthier, A., Larbier, M. and Blum, J. C. (1979). *Annls Biol. anim. Biochim. Biophys.* **19**, 703–707.
Gous, R. M. (1977). *Br. J. Nutr.* **38**, 313–317.
Herzberg, G. R. and Lerner, J. (1973). *Biochim. biophys. Acta* **307**, 234–242.
Hill, K. J. (1971). *In* "Physiology and Biochemistry of the Domestic Fowl" (D. J. Bell and B. M. Freeman, eds), Vol. 1, pp. 25–49. Academic Press, London and New York.
Howe, C. L., Mooseker, M. S. and Graves, T. A. (1980). *J. Cell. Biol.* **85**, 916–923.
Hudson, D. A. and Levin, R. J. (1968). *J. Physiol., Lond.* **198**, 40P–41P.
Hudson, D. A., Levin, R. J. and Smyth, D. H. (1971). *In* "Physiology and Biochemistry of the Domestic Fowl" (D. J. Bell and B. M. Freeman, eds), Vol. 1, pp. 52–71. Academic Press, London and New York.
Hunter, B. and Chvapil, M. (1981). *Nutr. Rep. Int.* **24**, 867–874.
Hurwitz, S. (1976). *In* "Digestion in the Fowl" (K. N. Boorman and B. M. Freeman, eds), pp. 157–175. British Poultry Science Ltd., Edinburgh.
Hurwitz, S. and Bar, A. (1966). *Poult. Sci.* **45**, 345–352.
Hurwitz, S. and Bar, A. (1969). *J. Nutr.* **99**, 217–224.
Hurwitz, S. and Bar, A. (1972). *Am. J. Physiol.* **222**, 761–767.
Hurwitz, S., Bar, A. and Clarkson, T. W. (1970). *J. Nutr.* **100**, 1181–1188.
Hurwitz, S., Bar, A., Katz, M., Sklan, D. and Budowski, P. (1973). *J. Nutr.* **103**, 543–547.
Imondi, A. R. and Bird, F. H. (1966). *Poult. Sci.* **45**, 142–147.
Jayne-Williams, D. J. and Fuller, R. (1971). *In* "Physiology and Biochemistry of the Domestic Fowl" (D. J. Bell and B. M. Freeman, eds), Vol. 1, pp. 73–92. Academic Press, London and New York.

Kan, C. A. (1973). *Wld's Poult. Sci. J.* **31**, 46–56.
Kenny, A. D. (1982). "Intestinal Calcium Absorption and its Regulation." CRC Press Inc., Florida.
Kimmich, G. A. (1970). *Biochemistry* **9**, 3659–3668.
Kimmich, G. A. (1975). *In* "Methods in Membrane Biology" (E. D. Korn, ed.), Vol. 5, pp. 51–115. Plenum Press, New York.
Kimmich, G. A. (1981). *In* "Physiology of the Gastrointestinal Tract" (L. R. Johnson, ed.), pp. 1036–1061. Raven Press, New York.
Kimmich, G. A. and Carter-Su, C. (1978). *Am. J. Physiol.* **235**, C73–C81.
Kimmich, G. A. and Randles, J. (1975). *J. Membrane Biol.* **23**, 57–76.
Kimmich, G. A. and Randles, J. (1979). *Am. J. Physiol.* **237**, C56–C63.
Koike, T. I. and McFarland, L. Z. (1966). *Am. J. vet. Res.* **27**, 1130–1133.
Kushak, R., Zigure, D. and Kopman, E. (1973). *Latv. PSR Zinat. Akad. Vest.* **5**, 97–104.
Lasheras, B., Bolufer, J., Cenarruzabeitia, N., Lluch, M. and Larralde, J. (1980). *Revta esp. Fisiol.* **36**, 89–92.
Lawson, D. E. M. and Emtage, J. S. (1974). *Vitams Horm.* **32**, 277–298.
Lazarov, Y. (1976). *Anim. Sci., Sofia* **13**, 95–100.
Lazarov, Y., Stanchev, H. and Piperova, L. (1980). *Revta esp. Fisiol.* **36**, 377–382.
Lerner, J. (1971). *Tech. Bull. Life Sci. Agric. Exp. Stn, Univ. Maine* **50**.
Lerner, J. (1978). "A Review of Amino Acid Transport Processes in Animal Cells and Tissues." University Press, Orono, Maine.
Lerner, J. and Messier, D. L. (1980). *Comp. Biochem. Physiol.* **65A**, 363–365.
Lerner, J. and Smagula, R. M. (1979). *Comp. Biochem. Physiol.* **62A**, 939–945.
Lerner, J. and Steinke, D. L. (1977). *Comp. Biochem. Physiol.* **57A**, 11–16.
Lerner, J., Sattelmeyer, P. and Rush, R. (1975). *Comp. Biochem. Physiol.* **50A**, 113–120.
Lerner, J., Burrill, P. H., Sattelmeyer, P. A. and Janicki, C. F. (1976). *Comp. Biochem. Physiol.* **54A**, 109–111.
Levin, R. J. (1976). *In* "Digestion in the Fowl" (K. N. Boorman and B. M. Freeman, eds), pp. 63–116. British Poultry Science Ltd., Edinburgh.
Levin, R. J. (1979). *In* "Scientific Basis of Gastroenterology" (H. L. Duthie and K. G. Wormsley, eds), Chapter 11. Churchill Livingstone, Edinburgh.
Levin, R. J. (1982). *Scand. J. Gastroent.* **17** (Suppl. 74) 31–51.
Levin, R. J. (1983). *In* "Function and Dysfunction of the Small Intestine", (R. Batt and T. L. Lawrence, eds). Liverpool University Press, Liverpool.
Levin, R. J. and Mitchell, M. A. (1982). *In* "Mechanisms of Intestinal Adaptation" (J. W. L. Robinson, R. H. Dowling and E. O. Riecken, eds), pp. 103–110. MTP Press Ltd., Lancaster.
Levin, R. J., Mitchell, M. A. and Barber, D. C. (1983). *Comp. Physiol. Biochem.* **74A**, 961–966.
Lind, J., Munck, B. G., Olsen, O. and Skadhauge, E. (1980a). *J. Physiol., Lond.* **305**, 315–325.
Lind, J., Munck, B. G. and Olsen, O. (1980b). *J. Physiol., Lond.* **305**, 327–336.
McNab, J. M. (1973). *Wld's Poult. Sci. J.* **29**, 251–263.
Marti, M. T., Saiz, M. P., Mitjavila, M. T. and Planas, J. (1980). *Biol. Trace Element Res.* **2**, 255–267.
Matsumoto, T., Fontaine, O. and Rasmussen, H. (1980). *Biochim. biophys. Acta* **599**, 13–23.

Matthews, D. M. and Adibi, S. A. (1976). *Gastroenterology* **71**, 151–161.
Miller, D. S., Shehata, A. T. and Lerner, J. (1980). *J. Pharmac. exp. Ther.* **214**, 101–105.
Mitchell, M. A. and Levin, R. J. (1981). *Experientia* **37**, 265–266.
Mongin, P. and de Laage, X. (1977). *C. r. hebd. Séanc. Acad. Sci. Paris Ser. D.* **285**, 225–228.
Mooseker, M. S. (1976). *J. Cell. Biol.* **71**, 417–432.
Morley, M., Scanes, C. G. and Chadwick, A. (1980). *Comp. Biochem. Physiol.* **67A**, 695–697.
Morley, M., Scanes, C. G. and Chadwick, A. (1981). *Comp. Biochem. Physiol.* **68A**, 61–66.
Morrissey, R. L., Zolock, D. T., Bikle, D. D., Empson, R. N. and Bucci, T. J. (1978a). *Biochim. biophys. Acta* **538**, 23–33.
Morrissey, R. L., Zolock, D. T., Bucci, T. J. and Bikle, D. D. (1978b). *J. Histochem. Cytochem.* **26**, 628–634.
Munck, B. (1981). *In* "Physiology of the Gastrointestinal Tract" (L. R. Johnson, ed.), pp. 1097–1122. Raven Press, New York.
Murer, H. and Hildmann, B. (1981). *Am. J. Physiol.* **240**, G409–G416.
Mykkänen, H. M. and Wasserman, R. H. (1981). *J. Nutr.* **111**, 1757–1765.
Mykkänen, H. M. and Wasserman, R. H. (1982). *J. Nutr.* **112**, 520–527.
Nemere, I. and Norman, A. W. (1982). *Biochim. biophys. Acta* **694**, 307–327.
Norman, A. W. (1979). "Vitamin D—the Calcium Homeostatic Steroid Hormone." Academic Press, New York and London.
Palmer, M. F. and Rolls, B. A. (1981). *Br. J. Nutr.* **46**, 549–558.
Peterlik, M., Fuchs, R. and Cross, H. S. (1981). *In* "Calcium and Phosphate Transport across Biomembranes" (F. Bronner and M. Peterlik, eds), pp. 173–179. Academic Press, New York and London.
Porteus, J. W. (1979). *Environ. Health Pers.* **33**, 25–35.
Putkey, J. A., Spielvogel, A. M., Sauerheber, R. D., Dunlap, C. S. and Norman, A. W. (1982). *Biochim. biophys. Acta* **688**, 177–190.
Raheja, K. L., Tepperman, J. and Tepperman, H. M. (1977). *Comp. Biochem. Physiol.* **58A**, 245–248.
Rice, G. E. and Skadhauge, E. (1982a). *J. comp. Physiol.* **146**, 51–56.
Rice, G. E. and Skadhauge, E. (1982b). *J. comp. Physiol.* **147**, 65–69.
Riesenfeld, G., Sklan, D., Bar., A., Eisner, U. and Hurwitz, S. (1980). *J. Nutr.* **110**, 117–121.
Ruano, M. J., Larralde, J. and Lluch, M. (1974). *Revta esp. Fisiol.* **30**, 283–288.
Ruff, M. D. and Wyatt, R. D. (1976). *Toxic. appl. Pharmac.* **37**, 257–262.
Saiz, M. P., Marti, M. T., Mitjavila, M. T. and Planas, J. (1980). *Biol. Trace Element Res.* **2**, 269–280.
Sanneborn, D. W. and Hansen, H. J. (1970). *Science, N.Y.* **168**, 591–592.
Scharrer, E. (1972a). *Z. Tierphysiol. Tierernähr. Futtermittelk.* **29**, 334–342.
Scharrer, E. (1972b). *Z. Tierphysiol. Tierernähr. Futtermittelk.* **30**, 268–274.
Sepulveda, F. V., Burton, K. A. and Brown, P. D. (1982). *J. Cell. Physiol.* **111**, 303–308.
Shehata, A. T., Lerner, J. and Miller, D. S. (1981). *Am. J. Physiol.* **240**, G102–G108.
Skadhauge, E. (1973). *Dan. med. Bull.* **20** (Suppl. 1), 1–82.
Skadhauge, E. (1976). *In* "Digestion in the Fowl" (K. N. Boorman and B. M. Freeman, eds), pp. 143–156. British Poultry Science Ltd., Edinburgh.

Skadhauge, E. (1978). *In* "Comparative Physiology—Water, Ions and Fluid Mechanics" (K. Schmidt-Nielsen, L. Bolis and S. H. P. Maddrell, eds), pp. 195–205. Cambridge University Press, Cambridge.

Skadhauge, E. (1981a). *In* "Avian Endocrinology" (A. Epple and M. H. Stetson, eds), pp. 1–16. Academic Press, New York and London.

Skadhauge, E. (1981b). "Osmoregulation in Birds." Springer-Verlag, Berlin.

Sklan, D., Budowski, P., Ascarelli, I. and Hurwitz, S. (1973). *J. Nutr.* **103**, 1299–1305.

Sklan, D., Hurwitz, S., Budowski, P. and Ascarelli, I. (1975). *J. Nutr.* **105**, 57–63.

Spencer, R., Charman, M., Emtage, J. S. and Lawson, D. E. M. (1976a). *Eur. J. Biochem.* **71**, 399–409.

Spencer, R., Charman, M., Wilson, P. and Lawson, D. E. M. (1976b). *Nature, Lond.* **263**, 161–163.

Spencer, R., Charman, M., Wilson, P. W. and Lawson, D. E. M. (1978). *Biochem. J.* **170**, 93–101.

Tasaki, I. and Yokota, H. (1970). *Jap. J. Zootech.* **41**, 104–108.

Taylor, A. N. and Wasserman, R. H. (1965). *Nature, Lond.* **205**, 248–250.

Taylor, A. N. and Wasserman, R. H. (1970). *J. Histochem. Cytochem.* **18**, 107–115.

Thomas, D. H. (1982). *Comp. Biochem. Physiol.* **71A**, 527–535.

Thomas, D. H. and Skadhauge, E. (1979). *Pflügers Arch. ges Physiol.* **379**, 229–236.

Thomas, D. H. and Skadhauge, E. (1982). *In* "Electrolyte and Water Transport across Gastrointestinal Epithelia" (M. Case and A. Garner, eds), pp. 295–303. Raven Press, New York.

Thomas, D. H. and Jallageas, M., Munck, B. G. and Skadhauge, E. (1980). *Gen. comp. Endocr.* **40**, 44–51.

Thompson, E., Levin, R. J. and Jackson, M. J. (1970). *Biochim. biophys. Acta* **196**, 120–122.

Wasserman, R. H. Corradino, R. A., Fullmer, C. S. and Taylor, A. N. (1974). *Vitams Horm.* **32**, 299–324.

Wilson, P. W. and Lawson, D. E. M. (1980). *Pflügers Arch. ges Physiol.* **389**, 69–74.

Wiseman, G. (1968). *In* "Handbook of Physiology" (W. Heidel, ed.), Sect. 6, Vol. 3, pp. 1277–1307. American Physiological Society, Washington, D.C.

Wiseman, G. (1974). *In* "Biomembranes 4A, Intestinal Absorption" (D. H. Smyth, ed.), pp. 363–481. Plenum Press, London.

Yokota, H. and Coates, M. E. (1982). *Br. J. Nutr.* **47**, 349–356.

2 Metabolic Roles of the Vitamins

M. E. COATES

National Institute for Research in Dairying, University of Reading, England

I. Introduction

The classification of the vitamins into fat-soluble and water-soluble categories extends beyond their physical characteristics and is reflected in their metabolic properties. It is well established that vitamins B and C act mainly as

PHYSIOLOGY BIOCHEMISTRY DOMESTIC
FOWL, VOL. 5 ISBN 0-12-267105-8

co-factors in specific biochemical pathways, but the metabolic roles of the fat-soluble vitamins are much less clear. Present knowledge supports the idea that they may act as regulators of biological processes, and in fact the hormonal characteristics of vitamin D are now so well recognized that it is dealt with separately elsewhere in this volume (see Chapters 1 and 6).

II. Requirements

The basic dietary requirements of poultry for vitamins are still not firmly enough established to permit proper assessment of the effects of environmental and other factors that might modify them. Recommendations of adequacy have hitherto been based on gross physical characteristics such as growth and prevention of clinical signs of deficiency, but elucidation of the precise metabolic function of a vitamin makes it possible to use biochemical parameters such as activity of a specific enzyme as a measure of vitamin adequacy. Assessment of riboflavin status in chicks and pigs based on the activity of erythrocyte glutathione reductase has been recommended (Esch *et al.*, 1979). Such methods may be more sensitive, in that the biochemical lesion is likely to become apparent earlier than the clinical signs. For example, more vitamin B_6 was found to be required to maintain maximal activity of serum glutamic-oxalacetic transaminase than was needed to support chick growth (Sifri *et al.*, 1972).

In a critical review of published work concerning the interactions between disease and vitamin requirements of poultry, Wilgus (1980) concluded that dietary vitamin deficiencies can impair defence mechanisms and disease states can increase vitamin requirements. In certain circumstances the immune response is stimulated by high supplements of vitamin A (Tengerdy and Nockels, 1975) or vitamin E (Tengerdy and Nockels, 1983; Heinzerling *et al.*, 1974). In general, there is evidence for a positive interaction between vitamins A and K and parasitic diseases, and between vitamin C and certain viral and bacterial diseases. Environmental temperature also influences vitamin requirements, indirectly through food intake as well as through alterations in availability and utilization of vitamins. The margins of safety generally allowed in practical poultry diets are enough to compensate for many of the variations in requirement induced by environmental, disease and genetic factors.

III. Vitamin A

A. Systemic Role

The role of vitamin A in visual function is reasonably well-established, but this aspect involves quantitatively only a small part of the animal's total requirement of the vitamin. The effects of vitamin A deficiency are manifest in many tissues, and lesions in epithelial elements are among the first to become apparent. The biochemical mechanisms by which these are brought about are poorly understood, and subject to considerable controversy. In their review of recent research into the systemic mode of action of vitamin A Ganguly *et al.* (1980) drew attention to its importance in cell proliferation, as evidenced by studies in epithelia of the trachea, intestine, cornea, oestrogen-primed chick oviduct and regenerating liver cells. They suggest that vitamin A may have a common role in the normal proliferation and perhaps differentiation of cells in regenerating tissue.

Earlier work in rats and chicks suggested that vitamin A might be concerned in certain aspects of carbohydrate metabolism This has been supported by the finding that chicks on a low dietary intake of vitamin A had significantly raised concentrations of liver glycogen (Nockels and Phillips, 1971a,b) and a tendency for increased glycogen and ATP in white muscle. Glycogenolysis was not affected by the deficiency and red muscle showed no changes. It was later shown (Sundeen *et al.*, 1980) that a mild deficiency of vitamin A resulted in increased glycogen deposition and that this was related to isometric tension parameters of the muscle tissue. Shear value of the cooked muscle was increased by the deficiency, implying that vitamin A deprivation could have a deleterious effect on muscle tenderness.

B. Resistance to Infection

Further evidence has accumulated for a role of vitamin A in the immune response. Supplements of vitamins A or E protected chicks infected with a pathogenic strain of *Escherichia coli* by enhancing both humoral immunity and phagocytosis, but a combination of the two vitamins did not (Tengerdy and Nockels, 1975; Tengerdy and Brown, 1977). The mechanism of the apparent antagonism between vitamins A and E was not elucidated but a relationship with prostaglandin production was postulated.

C. Toxicity

High supplements of vitamin A in the diet of laying hens were reported to have adverse effects on egg production, egg size and hatchability (March *et al.*, 1972). Incubation time was prolonged when the dams were given 63 mg retinyl palmitate per kg diet. Injection of 0·37 mg retinol into eggs before incubation depressed hatchability and gave rise to abnormalities in the dead embryos and a high incidence of haemorrhages during the second and third weeks of incubation. Injection of retinyl palmitate, however, in considerably higher amounts had virtually no adverse effects.

IV. Vitamin E

A. Forms

The vitamin E content of a food is usually related to its content of α-tocopherol, but other tocopherols occur in the ingredients of poultry feeds, particularly cereal grains, and may contribute to the vitamin E intake. For instance, in bioassays with chicks, rats and hamsters γ-tocopherol had between 6 and 16% of the vitamin E activity of α-tocopherol, and in *in vitro* tests based on prevention of oxidative haemolysis it had 38% activity (Bieri and Farrell, 1976). The authors considered that the greater activity found by the *in vitro* test indicated a more rapid turnover of γ- than of α-tocopherol in the tissues.

B. Metabolic Roles

1. Vitamin E as an Antioxidant

The antioxidant properties of vitamin E have long been recognized, but the hypothesis that it acts as a non-enzymatic biological antioxidant is now held to be unlikely. Although many workers have established that vitamin E requirement increases with increasing unsaturation of the dietary fatty acids, there appears to be no simple linear relationship between the two. Vogtmann and Prabuki (1971) studied the deposition of vitamin E in hen's eggs and found a positive correlation with consumption of polyunsaturated fatty acids (PUFA) up to 4 g per egg produced, but as consumption exceeded this amount transfer of the vitamin to the egg decreased. Jager (1972) observed no relation between vitamin E requirement and dietary linoleic acid at low intakes of linoleic acid, but when linoleic acid exceeded one-fifth of the total energy intake, requirement for vitamin E was markedly increased. Results of experiments in several species of animal (quoted by Bieri and Farrell, 1976) indicate that the mechanism by which dietary PUFA increase vitamin E requirement involves both absorption and storage of the vitamin.

Electron microscope studies of jejunal epithelial cells in man and in ducklings have shown that vitamin E is involved in maintaining the integrity of cellular membranes (Molanaar *et al.*, 1972). The main effects of the deficiency appear to be reflected in the lipid rather than in the protein moiety of the membrane, as analysis of liver mitochondrial membranes of vitamin E-deprived ducklings showed a decrease in PUFA constituents, particularly arachidonic acid. The authors postulate several enzymic systems in which vitamin E might play a role to produce this result. Claims that the biological actions of α-tocopherol are related to its antioxidative properties are more strongly supported by evidence from *in vitro* than *in vivo* studies, which gives rise to the suggestion that it may have to be incorporated into biological membranes in order to function (Bieri and Farrell, 1976). Enzyme systems independent of vitamin E have been shown to be more important in controlling oxidative reactions.

The fact that vitamin E deficiency results in muscular dystrophy has led to the hypothesis that it may regulate the synthesis of specific proteins required for normal muscle function. In rabbits deprived of vitamin E the turnover rate of creatine phosphokinase was twice as great as in their normal controls. The nature of this enzyme in genetically dystrophic chicks and in chicks deprived of vitamin E was essentially similar (Olson, 1974). Increased *de novo* rate of synthesis of xanthine oxidase activity in vitamin E-deficient rabbits (Catigani *et al.*, 1974) also suggests a role for vitamin E in regulation of protein synthesis.

2. *Interrelationships with Selenium (Se)*

Many of the effects of vitamin E deficiency can be at least partially alleviated by supplements by selenites in the diet, and the interrelationship of the two substances has been the subject of much study (see review by Scott *et al.*, 1974). Detailed examinations of the pathology of vitamin E and Se deprivation are beginning to distinguish between the individual and interacting effects of each. In a recent study with broiler chicks deprived of Se and vitamin E the contents of cathepsin and protein, and the break strength, of the *Pectoralis major* muscle were measured and the effects of supplements of either nutrient, or both, were noted. Total catheptic activity and muscle protein increased with increasing supplements of vitamin E, but Se was ineffective. Muscle break strength was reduced by supplementation with either (Gill *et al.*, 1980). On a Se-deficient diet with the generally accepted adequate amount of vitamin E (15–20 mg kg^{-1}) atrophy and fibrosis of the pancreas occurred and many birds developed exeduative diathesis. Supplementation of the diet with 1 mg Se kg^{-1} restored the pancreas to its normal appearance and prevented the diathesis. Supplementation of the deficient diet with extra vitamin E prolonged the life of the birds and reduced the incidence and severity of the diathesis. It was concluded the Se deficiency alone is responsible for the pancreatic abnormality, but that this results in reduced efficiency of lipid digestion and therefore of absorption of vitamin E (Gries and Scott, 1972c). Noguchi *et al.* (1973) propose separate functions for Se and vitamin E in the prevention of exudative diathesis. Se participates in the activity of glutathione peroxidase (GSHP) (Rotruck *et al.*, 1973) and the concentration of GSHP in chick plasma is related to the Se content of the diet and the effectiveness of Se in preventing exudative diathesis. Plasma GHSP fell in Se deficient chicks irrespective of whether the diet contained vitamin E. The authors suggest that Se-dependent GHSP destroys lipid peroxides before they can attack the cell membrane, whereas vitamin E acts as an antioxidant at the site of their formation within the membrane itself.

V. Vitamin K

A. Metabolic Role

Vitamin K is exceptional among the fat-soluble vitamins in that a role as co-factor in a microsomal enzyme system has been ascribed to it. Recent knowledge concerning the action of vitamin K in mammalian systems has been reviewed by Suttie (1980). It has been shown in preparations of rat liver that vitamin K is required for the carboxylation of glutamyl residues of precursor proteins to γ-carboxyglutamyl residues in completed proteins. The discovery was based on the demonstration that prothrombin contained residues of γ-carboxyglutamic acid, an amino acid that had not previously been known. Since then, other tissue proteins containing this amino acid have been shown to be vitamin K-dependent, including a non-collagen protein in bone and a protein in the chorioallantoic membrane of the hen's egg (Suttie and Jackson, 1977). The presence of γ-carboxyglutamyl residues in prothrombin permits the interaction with Ca^{2+} and phospholipid on which the clotting mechanism depends. Although it has been assumed that the other vitamin K-dependent proteins may be involved in a similar type of reaction, no precise biochemical role has yet been elucidated for any of them.

VI. Vitamin B Complex

The metabolic defects resulting from deprivation of vitamins of the B complex are mostly very well known, so that only the important advances made in recent years are considered here.

A. Pathology

Although clinical signs of deficiency of the B vitamins are well documented, little attention has been paid so far to the accompanying morphological and histological changes. Detailed studies of the pathology of pyridoxin, thiamin, riboflavin, pantothenic acid and niacin deficiencies in chicks have been reported by Gries and Scott (1972a,b).

Birds deprived or given very low supplements of vitamin B_6 showed the expected nervous signs, but no pathological lesions were detected in the brain, spinal cord, peripheral nerves or other soft tissues. Chicks given somewhat higher, but still sub-optimal, doses of the vitamin did not develop nervous signs but showed a high incidence of perosis. The amount required to prevent signs of deficiency and to support normal growth was only 1·4 mg kg^{-1} of a diet containing 220 g kg^{-1} protein, but was increased five-fold when the diet contained 310 g protein kg^{-1}. This accords with the function of pyridoxin in transamination reactions. The type of dietary protein is also important, as shown by Kazemi and Kratzer (1980), who found the requirement of pyridoxin for normal growth of chicks was higher in a diet containing soya bean meal than in diets with safflower or cottonseed meal as the protein source.

Neurological lesions were similarly absent from birds deprived of thiamin, riboflavin, pantothenic acid or niacin, although the classic clinical signs of deficiency were observed in all instances (Gries and Scott, 1972b). All four deficiencies caused degeneration of the cells lining the crypts of Lieberkuhn and changes in the pancreatic acinar cells. Since all four vitamins are important co-factors in pathways of energy metabolism, it is reasonable to expect that the effects of deficiency are likely to be most severely felt in rapidly metabolizing cells, such as those in the pancreas or gut mucosa. Absence of neurological lesions implies that the clinical signs are preceded by the biochemical changes, which may result in the death of the birds before morphological abnormalities have time to develop.

B. Metabolic Roles

1. Thiamin

Some biochemical changes in the brain of chicks deprived of thaimin have been described (Nalini and Nayeemunnisa, 1976). Three regions of the brain—the cerebrum, cerebellum and medulla oblongata—were examined, and the effects of the deficiency varied with the region. Activity of pyruvate dehydrogenase decreased, and the magnitude of the decrease was greatest in the medulla and least in the cerebellum. Succinate dehydrogenase and glutamate dehydrogenase activities were augmented in all three regions by the deficiency, the former being most affected in the medulla and the latter in the cerebrum. The significance of the different responses of these oxidative enzymes in the different regions of the brain is not clear, but it is assumed that they result from disturbances in the tricarboxylic acid cycle.

2. Pantothenic Acid

The importance of pantothenic acid in the form of 4′-phosphopantetheine, the prosthetic group of co-enzyme A (CoA), is well known. Pantothenic acid is also a component of the acyl carrier proteins (ACP) of the fatty acid synthetase (FAS) complex which catalyses the *de novo* synthesis of long chain fatty acids from acetyl-CoA and malonyl-CoA. It also occurs in the prosthetic groups of citrate lyase and citromalate lyase. The isolation and properties of ACPs from avian, mammalian and yeast FAS, which differ in the structure of their protein components, have been described (Qureshi *et al.*, 1976).

FAS activity is low in the chick embryo but increases on hatching and even more markedly during the first few days of life (Joshi and Sidbury, 1975). By use of ^{125}I-labelled anti-synthetase the fraction of polysomes synthesizing FAS could be identified (Zehner *et al.*, 1977) and it was thereby established that the increased activity was due to increased synthesis of the enzyme at the level of translation.

Protein-bound forms of pantothenic acid exist in foodstuffs and may contribute to the bird's requirement for the vitamin. Microbiological methods of assay do not detect all the forms of pantothenic acid in poultry feeds that are available to the chick. It appears that the procedures used in the microbiological assay are not adequate in all instances to release the vitamin for use by the assay organism (Latymer and Coates, 1982).

An antagonism between high dietary supplements of copper sulphate and pantothenic acid metabolism in the chick has been observed. Evidence suggests that copper interferes with the synthesis of CoA, but not of FAS, from pantothenic acid (Latymer and Coates, 1981a).

A lower requirement for dietary pantothenic acid by germ-free compared with conventional chicks has been reported (Latymer and Coates, 1981b). This might be explained by the suggestion that the need to metabolize bacterial products would increase the host's metabolic burden, and hence its need for the vitamin co-factors such as CoA that are concerned in so many biochemical pathways.

3. Biotin

One of the most important advances in knowledge of the metabolic role of the B vitamins has been the elucidation of the part played by biotin enzymes in fatty liver and kidney syndrome (FLKS) of poultry. The topic has been extensively reviewed by Pearce and Balnave (1978) and only an outline is given here.

FLKS is a condition occurring in broiler chicks on high energy/low protein diets. Mortality is high, and on post mortem examination the livers and kidneys are found to be enlarged and fatty. Affected chicks are hypoglycaemic, and concentrations of free fatty acids and triglycerides are increased. Examination of various nutritional factors led to the demonstration that supplements of biotin, but not of any other vitamin, prevented the syndrome

(Whitehead *et al.*, 1976). Although the exact sequence of reactions leading to the syndrome of FLKS is not clear, there are biochemical similarities between biotin deficiency and FLKS. For instance, hepatic pyruvate carboxylase is one of the enyzmes most severely and rapidly affected by lack of its co-factor, biotin, with consequent reduction of gluconeogenesis (Arinze and Mistry, 1971). Gluconeogenesis is also reduced in FLKS, and death may occur as a result of lack of glucose for essential functions. Desaturation of fatty acids occurs in biotin deficiency, which is characterized by a rise in palmitoleic acid and concomitant fall in stearic acid (Balnave, 1971). The concentration of palmitoleic acid is also elevated in FLKS (Pearson *et al.*, 1976).

Occurrence of FLKS in the field may in part be due to the poor availability of biotin from some cereals (Frigg, 1976). The microbiological assay with *Lactobacillus plantarum* gives an accurate measure of the biotin content after suitable processing to release bound forms of the vitamin. Comparison of results with those by chick bioassay shows that, although the biotin in maize and milo is readily available to the bird, the biotin in wheat and barley is only poorly utilized.

VII. Ascorbic Acid

Although in normal circumstances the fowl is able to synthesize adequate amounts of ascorbic acid, there are many indications that under stress the bird is unable to produce enough for its metabolic needs. In particular, temperature stress has been implicated in increasing the bird's demand for ascorbic acid for growth, egg production and egg shell strength. In a review of the subject, Scott (1975) proposes that high environmental temperatures may increase the metabolic requirement for ascorbic acid, decrease the rate of its biosynthesis and affect endocrine systems controlling its retention and proper function. A relationship between vitamin C and the thyroid has been postulated (Abdel-Wahab *et al.*, 1975). Chicks subjected to a high environmental temperature were given supplements of 50 or 100 mg ascorbic acid per kg diet, which increased their thyroid activity as measured by uptake of ^{125}I. This result could be explained in terms of a reduction of thyroid activity due to the high temperature with consequent reduction in synthesis of ascorbic acid, but requires further study. The claim that very high supplements of vitamin C are protective against infection has led to investigation of its effect on immune response (McCorkle *et al.*, 1980). Cell mediated immunity and antibody response to sheep red blood cells, a T-cell dependent antigen, were not altered by a dietary supplement of 10 g ascorbic acid kg^{-1}. However, the antibody response to *Brucella abortus*, a T-cell independent antigen, was lowered in newly-hatched and raised in adult birds by the vitamin C supplement.

References

Abdel-Wahab, M. F., Abdo, M. S., Megahed, Y. M., Attia, M. El-S. and Farahat, A. A. (1975). *Zentbl. Vet Med.* **22**, 769–775.

Arinze, J. C. and Mistry, S. P. (1971). *Comp. Biochem. Physiol.* **38B**, 285–294.

Balnave, D. (1971). *Int. J. Biochem.* **6**, 17.

Bieri, J. and Farrell, P. M. (1976). *Vitams Horm.* **34**, 31–75.

Catignani, G. L., Chytil, F. and Darby, W. J. (1974). *Proc. natn. Acad. Sci.,USA* **71**, 1966–1973.

Esch, M. W., Corley, J. R., Bahr, J. M. and Easter R. A. (1979). *J. anim. Sci.* **49** (Suppl. 1) 90 (abs.).

Frigg, M. (1976). *Poult. Sci.* **55**, 2310–2318.

Ganguly, J., Rao, M. R. S., Murthy, S. K. and Sarada, K. (1980). *Vitams Horm.* **38**, 1–54.

Gill, T. A., Sundeen, G. B., Richards, J. F. and Bragg, D. B. (1980). *Poult. Sci.* **59**, 2088–2097.

Gries, C. L. and Scott, M. L. (1972a). *J. Nutr.* **102**, 1259–1268.

Gries, C. L. and Scott, M. L. (1972b). *J. Nutr.* **102**, 1269–1286.

Gries, C. L. and Scott, M. L. (1972c). *J. Nutr.* **102**, 1287–1296.

Heinzerling, R. H., Nockels, C. F., Quarles, C. L. and Tengerdy, R. P. (1974). *Proc. Soc. exp. Biol. Med.* **146**, 279–283.

Jager, F. C. (1972). *Ann. NY Acad. Sci.* **203**, 199–211.

Joshi, J. C. and Sidbury, J. B. (1975). *Devl. Biol.* **42**, 282–291.

Kazemi, R. and Kratzer, F. H. (1980). *Poult. Sci.* **59**, 95–99.

Latymer, E. A. and Coates, M. E. (1981a). *Br. J. Nutr.* **45**, 431–439.

Latymer, E. A. and Coates, M. E. (1981b). *Br. J. Nutr.* **45**, 441–449.

Latymer, E. A. and Coates, M. E. (1982). *Br. J. Nutr.* **47**, 131–137.

McCorkle, F., Taylor, R., Stinson, R., Day, E. J. and Glick, B. (1980). *Poult. Sci.* **59**, 1324–1327.

March, B. E., Coates, V. and Goudie, C. (1972). *Poult. Sci.* **51**, 891–896.

Molanaar, I., Vos, J. and Hommes, F. A. (1972). *Vitams Horm.* **30**, 45–82.

Nalini, U. P. and Nayeemunnisa (1976). *Experientia* **32**, 198–199.

Nockels, C. F. and Phillips, R. W. (1971a). *Poult. Sci.* **50**, 174–181.

Nockels, C. F. and Phillips, R. W. (1971b). *Poult. Sci.* **50**, 766–768.

Noguchi, T., Cantor, A. H. and Scott, M. L. (1973). *J. Nutr.* **103**, 1502–1511.

Olson, R. E. (1974). *Am. J. clin. Nutr.* **27**, 1117–1129.

Pearce, J. and Balnave, D. (1978). *Br. vet. J.* **134**, 598–609.

Pearson, J. A., Johnson, A. R., Hood, R. L. and Fogerty, A. C. (1976). *Aust. J. biol. Sci.* **29**, 419–428.

Qureshi, A. A., Lornitzo, F. A., Hsu, R. Y. and Porter, J. W. (1976). *Archs Biochem. Biophys.* **177**, 379–393.

Rotruck, J. T., Pope, A. L., Ganther, H. E., Swanson, A. B., Haferman, D. G. and Hoekstra, W. G. (1973). *Science, N.Y.* **179**, 588–590.

Scott, M. L. (1975). *Ann. N.Y. Acad. Sci.* **258**, 151–155.

Scott, M. L., Noguchi, T. and Combs, G. F. (1974). *Vitams Horm.* **32**, 429–444.

Sifri, M., Daghir, N. J. and Asmar, J. A. (1972). *Br. J. Nutr.* **28**, 173–182.

Sundeen, G., Richards, J. F. and Bragg, D. B. (1980). *Poult. Sci.* **59**, 2225–2236.

Suttie, J. W. (1980). *Fedn Proc. Fedn Am. Socs exp. Biol.* **39**, 2730–2735.

Suttie, J. M. and Jackson, C. M. (1977). *Physiol. Rev.* **57**, 1–70.

Tengerdy, R. P. and Brown, J. C. (1977). *Poult. Sci.* **56**, 957–963.
Tengerdy, R. P. and Nockels, C. F. (1973). *Poult. Sci.* **52**, 778–783.
Tengerdy, R. P. and Nockels, C. F. (1975). *Poult. Sci.* **54**, 1292–1296.
Vogtmann, H. and Prabucki, A. L. (1971). *Nutr. Met.* **13**, 274–291.
Whitehead, C. C., Blair, R., Bannister, D. W., Evans, A. J. and Morley Jones, R. (1976). *Res. vet. Sci.* **20**, 180–184.
Wilgus, H. S. (1980). *Poult. Sci.* **59**, 772–781.
Zehner, Z. E., Joshi, J. C. and Wakil, S. J. (1977). *J. biol. Chem.* **252**, 7015–7022.

3 The Pituitary Gland

C. G. SCANES,[1] A. STOCKELL HARTREE[2] and F. J. CUNNINGHAM[3]

[1]*Department of Animal Sciences, Rutgers—the State University, New Brunswick, USA*
[2]*ARC Institute of Animal Physiology, Animal Research Station, Cambridge, England*
[3]*Department of Physiology and Biochemistry, University of Reading, England*

PHYSIOLOGY BIOCHEMISTRY DOMESTIC
FOWL, VOL. 5 ISBN 0–12–267105–8

I. Introduction

The hypophysis or pituitary gland secretes hormones which are essential to normal metabolism or which co-ordinate other endocrine glands. The proximity of the pituitary gland to the hypothalamus is significant with regard to the regulation of the secretion of the pituitary hormones. A relatively small population of hypothalamic peptidergic neurones exert a key role in controlling anterior pituitary gland function. The activities of these peptidergic neurones may be modified by afferent neural stimuli conveying information about the external environment and by a variety of internal factors, including circulating hormone concentrations, peripheral nerve activity and endogenous rhythms. The hypothalamo-pituitary system integrates, processes and transduces information, resulting in an appropriate hormonal secretion by the pituitary gland. The axons of these hypothalamic neurones converge to a final common pathway at the median eminence. Here they discharge their specific products into a portal system of blood vessels which drain into the anterior pituitary gland, thereby completing the neurovascular link. Alternatively, the axons terminate in the neural lobe of the pituitary gland where the secretions are stored in the nerve terminals. An understanding of the complex neural interactions which govern the release of these peptides is only beginning to emerge.

II. Anatomy of the Avian Hypothalamo–Hypophysial Complex

The earlier anatomical literature relating to the avian hypothalamus has been described in detail (Ariens-Kappers *et al.*, 1936) and the monograph of Wingstrand (1951) remains the prime source of the details of the hypothalamo–hypophysial system in 69 species of birds.

A. Adenohypophysis

The adenohypophysis in birds consists of the pars distalis and the pars tuberalis. No structural pars intermedia exists (Wingstrand, 1951). The pars distalis forms the bulk of the adenohypophysis and is situated ventrally or rostroventrally to the neurohypophysis.

Two histologically different portions of the pars distalis were distinguished and referred to as the cephalic and caudal lobes (Rahn and Painter, 1941).

Since the publication of the original review (Stockell Hartree and Cunningham, 1971), much progress has been made in determining the ultrastructure (Mikami, 1969; Amin and Gilbert, 1970; Mikami *et al.*, 1973) and cytochemistry (see review by Tixier-Vidal and Follett, 1973) of the adenohypophyseal cells.

Six cell types are now recognized as a result of definition by three criteria: (*a*) comparison of alternate thin sections subjected to electron microscopy and thick sections to light microscopy; (*b*) changes in cell structure in different physiological states; and (*c*) the close resemblance between avian and mammalian pituitary cells.

Cells which contain glycoprotein-bearing granules (presumable gonadotrophs and thyrotrophs) stain predominantly with basic dyes and show a positive reaction with periodic acid-Schiff reagent (PAS), whereas those which contain simple protein-bearing granules stain predominantly with acidic dyes. Glycoprotein hormone (gonadotrophic and thyrotrophic) cells of the basophilic "PAS-positive" category appear to be distributed throughout both cephalic and caudal lobes. Prolactin and adrenocortrophin secretory cells are believed to be located in the cephalic lobe, whereas growth hormone-secreting cells are apparently confined to the caudal lobe.

The distribution of cell types within the pars distalis has also been examined by an immunocytochemical approach. In the domestic fowl, somatrophs are largely confined to the caudal lobe, while corticotrophs and lactotrophs are within the cephalic lobe (Tai and Chadwick, 1977; Jozsa *et al.*, 1979). This agrees well with light and electron microscopy studies. The location of the glycoprotein hormone-producing cells is less well established. In the domestic duck, cells which bound antisera against bovine β-TSH subunit were exclusively found in the cephalic lobe (Sharp *et al.*, 1979a). Studies in the domestic fowl in which the cephalic and caudal lobes were subjected to biological assay support the cephalic lobe being the principal location for the thyrotrophs (Radke and Chiasson, 1974). Follett *et al.*, (1978) have provided evidence by LH radioimmunoassay and LH radioreceptor assays that the caudal lobe of the pituitary gland is the major site for LH cells.

B. Neurohypophysis

The adenohypophysis and the neurohypophysis are separated by a connective tissue sheath. The neurohypophysis consists of a distinct neural lobe, and the median eminence and the infundibular stem, which are not directly separable. The neural lobe tissue consists of nerve fibres arising from the supraoptic, paraventricular and infundibular nuclei in the hypothalamus (Duncan, 1956)—see Fig. 1. The nerve endings contain granules of diameter 100 to 200 nm and are surrounded by processes of glial pituicytes. The infundibular stem can be considered to be a tubular project of the diencephalic wall which carried the neural lobe. In the fowl, the stem is morphologically distinct from the median eminence, which is the ventral or rostroventral wall of the diencephalon from the optic chiasma to the infundibular stem. The histological appearance of the median eminence and the infundibular stem are, however, closely related. The lumen of the neurohypophysis, referred to as the recessus infundibuli, extends throughout the infundibular stem and is continuous with the third ventricle. The recessus is wide and the entire organ appears as a thin walled wrinkled sac.

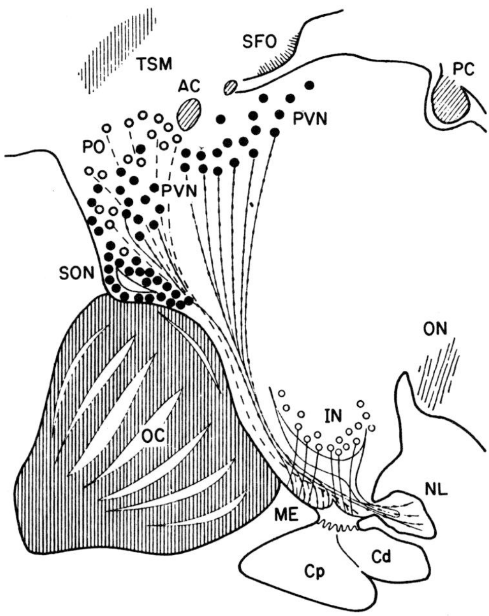

Fig. 1. The avian hypothalamo-pituitary system showing the neurosecretory pathways. (After Mikami, 1980.) Magnocellular supraoptic (SON) and paraventricular (PVN) nuclei (●) and parvocellular pre-optic (PO) and infundibular (IN) nuclei (○) send axons (······) into the neural lobe (NL) and the median eminence (ME). AC, anterior commissure; Cd, caudal lobe; Cp, cephalic lobe of the pars distalis; OC, optic chiasma; ON, oculomotor nerve; PC, posterior commissure; SFO, subfornical organ; TSM, septomesencephalic tract.

C. Hypothalamus

The hypothalamus, which forms a large portion of the ventral diencephalon, is a relatively small structure occupying about 3% of the total brain volume. It is separated dorsally from the thalamus by the hypothalamic sulcus, while its rostral and caudal limits lie just anterior to the optic chiasma and immediately posterior to the oculomotor nerve roots, respectively. Ventrally, it is bounded by the median eminence and infundibulum, and it is divided into two contralateral portions by the slit-like third ventricle.

The entire hypothalamus is extensively innervated by ascending and descending afferent fibres from other parts of the central nervous system. Some of these enter the lateral hypothalamus as distinct tracts (e.g. lateral forebrain bundles) before distributing terminals throughout the region, while many are diffuse in nature and therefore much less conspicuous. Massive and functionally important tracts, carrying most of the monoaminergic input to the hypothalamus, ascend from the brain stem (Fuxe and Ljunggren, 1965), but while similarly extensive projections from the forebrain and other adjacent structures are undoubtedly present in birds, they have only been described in detail for mammalian species. As in mammals, the medial periventricular zone of the hypothalamus contains relatively more neural perikarya than the lateral zones, which are dominated by the fibre tracts which run through them (Follett, 1973). While these perikarya generally form a diffuse array, some are sufficiently aggregated to be recognized anatomically as nuclei. However, the borders of these nuclei are ill-defined, showing only gradual transitions into relatively "cell-poor" zones. In view of the confusion in the earlier literature over the terminology used to describe different areas of the avian hypothalamus (see Follett, 1973), a simplified scheme has been proposed (Follett and Davies, 1975). In the anterior hypothalamus, the most prominent cell clusters include the pre-optic nucleus, supra-optic nucleus and the paraventricular nucleus, while those in the posterior or tuberal hypothalamus include the medial posterior hypothalamic nucleus and the infundibular nuclear complex (Fig. 1). All of these regions appear to be liberally innervated by fibres from adjacent nuclei and from more distant extrahypothalamic sites. Of these, only the monoaminergic fibre systems have been studied in birds (Fuxe and Ljunggren, 1965; Sharp and Follett, 1968).

Efferent projections from hypothalamic nuclei to the median eminence and neurohypophysis have been studied with varying degrees of thoroughness in at least 10 avian species (see reviews by Farner and Oksche, 1962; Dodd *et al.*, 1971; Kobayashi and Wada, 1973; Oksche and Farner, 1974). Before the recent advent of immunocytochemical methods, efforts to identify distinct neurosecretory cell-types in the hypothalamus involved selective staining and ultrastructural studies. Notably, Gomori's aldehyde fuschin and chrome alum haematoxylin stains enabled the identification of a group of axons originating from cell bodies in the paraventricular and supra-optic nuclei and projecting as a discrete supra-optico–hypophysial tract to the neurohypophysis. These so-called "Gomori-positive" magnocellular neurones are now known to manufacture the neurohypophysial hormones mesotocin and vasotocin, which are packaged into vesicles (100–200 nm diameter), transported by axoplasmic flow and stored in terminal depots in the neural lobe and to a lesser extent in the anterior division of the median eminence. Furthermore, this supra-optico–neurohypophysial system exists in essentially the same form in reptiles, birds and mammals (Kobayashi and Wada, 1973).

D. The Median Eminence and the Hypophysial Portal System

Anatomically, the avian median eminence, divisible into anterior and posterior portions, is an elongated structure which forms the floor of the third ventricle between the caudal margin of the optic chiasma and the infundibular stalk. Its organization is similar to that in mammals (Kobayashi and Wada, 1973); having both an external (comprised of palisade and reticular layers) and an internal zone (comprised of fibre, hypendymal and ependymal layers). Both ependymal and hypendymal cells exhibit cytoplasmic processes which extend towards the external zone, some terminating in close proximity to portal capillaries. While most "Gomori-positive" fibres of the supra-optic–hypophysial tract project caudally through the fibre layer towards the neurohypophysis, some descend to the outer palisade layers of the anterior division. "Gomori-negative" fibres, of diffuse origin, supply both the anterior and posterior divisions of the median eminence, with many terminals lying close to the capillaries of the primary portal plexus. Fluorescence histochemical studies have revealed that many of these fibres are monoaminergic (Sharp and Follett, 1968; Bjorklund *et al.*, 1968), while others are assumed to contain adenohypophysial regulatory peptides, or other neurotransmitters. Calas (1974) used a combination of immunocytochemical and autoradiographic techniques to study the relationship between neuronal elements containing noradrenaline, serotonin and luteinizing hormone-releasing hormone (LRHR) in the median eminence of the duck. Immunoreactive LHRH-containing fibres projected to the external zone of the anterior and posterior divisions, a finding confirmed by Bons *et al.* (1977, 1978a,b). However, while serotonin and noradrenaline-accumulating fibres were localized in the external and internal zones, respectively and appeared to make synaptic contact with various non-aminergic elements, including ependymal processes, it was not possible to demonstrate conclusively such contacts with neurones containing immunoreactive LHRH. Since the avian median eminence has been reported to possess very high cholinesterase activity and contains "Gomori-negative" fibres exhibiting small 30–50 nm diameter vesicles, tentatively ascribed to cholinergic neurones (see Kobayashi and Wada, 1973), it would appear that some of the tuberohypophysial fibres are cholinergic.

In birds, the ependymal cells of the median eminence and vascular organ of the terminal lamina extend small bulbous protrustions into the third ventricle. Kobayashi *et al.* (1972) have also shown that in the median eminence of quail, these modified ependymal cells ("tanycytes") are capable of absorbing peroxidase injected into the third ventricle and transporting it, via cytoplasmic processes, to the portal capillaries in the external zone. The observation that axons of LHRH (Bons, 1981) and monamine-containing cells (Sharp and Follett, 1968, 1970) in the anterior hypothalamus project to the vascular organ of the terminal lamina, therefore lend support to the proposal (Kobayashi *et al.*, 1972; Kobayashi and Wada, 1973) that the cerebrospinal fluid may prove an alternative route for the conveyance of neurohumoral factors to the hypophysial portal vessels. Indeed, the tentatively described synaptic contacts between monoaminergic terminals and tanycyte processes in the external zone of the duck median eminence (Calas, 1974) provide further support for this view, since they would constitute a nervous input to the tanycytes, whereby their secretory and absorptive activities could be regulated.

The blood supply and drainage of the avian hypothalamo–hypophysial system has been described (Green, 1951). Fig. 2 shows that the superior hypophysial arteries supply the primary capillary plexus on the median

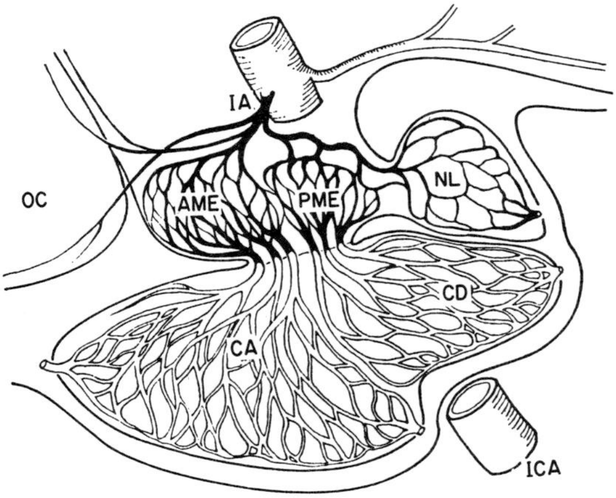

Fig. 2. The blood supply of the median eminence, pars distalis and neural lobe. (After Mikami, 1980.) AME, anterior division and PME, posterior divisions of median eminence; CA, cephalic and CD, caudal lobes of the pars distalis; IA, infundibular artery; ICA, internal carotid artery; OC, optic chiasma; NL, neural lobe.

eminence. The anterior and posterior divisions of the median eminence are drained respectively by distinct anterior and posterior primary portal plexuses. The anterior group of portal vessels is mainly distributed to the cephalic lobe of the adenohypophysis, while the posterior group is mainly distributed to the caudal lobe. Since the various adenohypophysial cell types are not equally distributed within the two lobes of the gland, it is possible that different releasing factors may be delivered to the two divisions of the median eminence.

E. Hypothalamic Peptidergic Neurones

Immunoreactive LHRH has been observed in the brain of the duck (Bons, 1981) and the chicken (deReviers and Dubois, 1974; Sterling and Sharp, 1982—see Fig. 3), with the majority of the LHRH-containing neurones in the anterior and posterior areas of the zona externa of the median eminence. McNeil *et al.* (1976) reported that in the domestic duck a population of

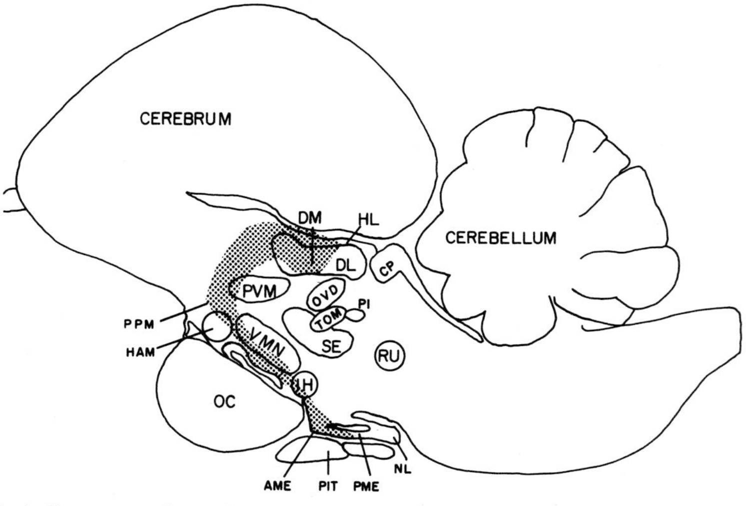

Fig. 3. A diagrammatic section of the brain of the domestic fowl showing the pituitary gland, hypothalamus and distribution of LHRH immunoreactive neurones (shaded). (Based on Sterling and Sharp, 1982.) AME, anterior median eminence; CP, choroid plexus; DL, nu. dorsolateralis; DM, nu. dorsomedialis; HAM, nu. hypothalamicus anterior medialis; HL, nu. habenularis lateralis; IH, nu. hypothalamic inferior; NL, neural lobe, OC, optic chiasma; OVD, nu. ovoidalis; PI, nu. paramedianus cortermedius; PIT, anterior pituitary; PME, posterior median eminence; PPM, nu. praeopticus paraventricularis magnocellularis, PVM, nu. paraventricularis magnocellularis; RU, nu. ruber; SE, stratum cellulare externum; TOM, Tr. occipitomesencephalicus; VMN, nu. ventromedialis.

LHRH-containing axons is also found in the arcuate nucleus. Bons *et al.* (1978a,b) found cell bodies and axons containing immunoreactive LHRH in the pre-optic nucleus of the domestic duck. These axons could be traced down the ventral hypothalamus into the external layer of the rostral and caudal median eminence in close proximity to the hypophysial portal system. Similar locations of LHRH cell bodies and axons have been found in fowl (Sterling and Sharp, 1982), see Fig. 3.

Somatostatin-immunoreactive neurones form a widely scattered system. In the domestic mallard and in Galliform species, these perikarya are found associated with the supra-optic and paraventricular nuclei and may extend as far as the lamina terminalis (Blahser *et al.*, 1978). In the rostral portion of the paraventricular nucleus, they are intermingled with vasotocin and mesotocin-immunoreactive cells. Some somatostatin axons project to the neurohaemal region of the median eminence, where they occupy a wide area. The somatostatin containing axons also show extensive extrahypothalamic projections. These ascending and descending pathways can be traced to different nuclear areas, where the neuropeptide could conceivably function as a neurotransmitter or "neuromodulator".

At the present time, TRH-containing neurones have not been localized in the avian brain. The localization of arginine vasotocin and mesotocin cell bodies and axons are considered in Section V.

III. Adenohypophysial Hormones

There is considerable evidence that polypeptide and protein hormones perform their biological functions by first interacting with a specific receptor in the target cell which in turn stimulates another reaction. Many receptors are known to be associated with the enzyme adenyl cyclase, which can mediate the action of hormones by production of cyclic AMP (see Wallis, 1975; Catt and Dufau, 1977; Dufau *et al.*, 1978). Avian pituitary hormones can be quantified using *in vivo* biological assay which often depends on a specified response in a target tissue in rodents. In addition, *in vitro* assays have been employed to determine the concentration of chicken hormones. These are often more sensitive, precise, convenient and economical than *in vivo* bioassays. *In vitro* systems are based on either the response of a target cell *in vitro* or on the ability of the hormone to inhibit binding or radio-labelled hormone to the receptor. The latter is a radioreceptor assay (RRA).

The adenohypophysial hormones are of two types: either glycoproteins, or proteins and polypeptides. Luteinizing hormone, follicle-stimulating hormone and thyroid-stimulating hormone are of the former class, while growth hormone, prolactin and adrenocorticotrophic hormone are of the latter.

A. Structure of Glycoprotein Hormones

The primary structure of several mammalian glycoprotein hormones has been studied in details and homologies have been demonstrated between the three hormones obtained from the same species. Each hormone is composed of two subunits, designated α and β, which alone possess negligible biological activity, but which can associate to form the active hormone. The α-subunits of LH, FSH and TSH from the same species have identical amino acid sequences while the β-subunits are the determinants of biological activity, with a different amino acid sequence for each hormone. There is substantial homology between β-subunits, about 40% of amino acid residues being found in identical positions in β-subunits derived from the same species (Pierce, 1971; Wallis, 1975; Pierce *et al.*, 1976; Stewart and Stewart, 1977). Each subunit contains carbohydrate attached at one or more positions in the peptide chain. There is evidence that the two subunits are synthesized separately in the mammalian pituitary gland.

The chicken pituitary glycoprotein hormones have not as yet been examined in such detail. However, there is evidence for similar structural relationships in lower vertebrate species. For instance, hybrid molecules prepared by combination of each subunit of turtle LH with a counterpart subunit from sheep LH were biologically active (Papkoff *et al.*, 1976) as were hybrids formed by combining each subunit of turkey LH with the appropriate sheep LH subunit (Burke *et al.*, 1979a,b). Further evidence for chemical similarities between mammalian and chicken LH and FSH is presented in the next section.

B. Luteinizing Hormone and Follicle-Stimulating Hormone

1. Chemistry

Since the separation by chromatographic fractionation of chicken LH and FSH (Stockell Hartree and Cunningham, 1969), these hormones have been, at least partially, purified in a number of laboratories. Two methods have been employed, both of which were initially developed for mammalian LH and FSH. In the first method, the glycoprotein hormones (LH, FSH and TSH) are extracted from adenohypophysial tissue in acid ethanolic ammonium acetate (yielding fraction GTN) and LH and FSH separated by ion-exchange chromatography on CM-Cellulose (Stockell Hartree and Cunningham, 1969; Scanes and Follett, 1972; Furuja and Ishii, 1974; Godden and Scanes, 1975; Sakai and Ishii, 1980).

The LH fraction (CM2) has been further purified (7-fold) by stepwise elution on DEAE-cellulose and Amberlite columns (Stockell Hartree and

Cunningham, 1969). The resulting preparation (IRC2) contained considerable TSH contamination in terms of an ovine standard (0·19 mg equivalent NIH-TSH-S6 per mg) (Scanes and Follett, 1972; Follett *et al.*, 1972). An alternative approach involved ion-exchange chromatography on DEAE-cellulose using a pH and salt gradient. This LH preparation (AEI) had a reduced TSH potency ($<$0·05 mg NIH-TSH-S6 per mg) (Scanes and Follett, 1972; Godden and Scanes, 1975), but had considerable LH potency with about 15% the activity of NIH-LH-S1 (ovine LH standard) by weight in both the rat ovarian ascorbic acid depletion assay (OAAD) (Scanes and Follett, 1972) and in a radioreceptor assay (RRA) for LH using rat gonadal tissue (Follett *et al.*, 1978). In avian assay systems, it is equipotent with NIH-LH-S1 in stimulating steroidogenesis *in vitro* by avian gonadal tissue (quail intestinal cell—Follett *et al.*, 1978; Jenkins *et al.*, 1978; chicken granulosa cells—Scanes and Fagioli, 1980) and uptake of ^{32}P-phosphate by chick testes *in vivo* (Scanes and Follett, 1972; Godden and Scanes, 1975). There is species specificity in the response of the assay systems used. The potency of chicken LH relative to ovine LH is much higher in stimulating avian gonadal tissues than in the widely used rodent assays.

An effective protocol for concentrating chicken FSH activity involves submitting the crude FSH fraction (CM1) to chromatography on calcium phosphate and DEAE-cellulose (e.g. Stockell Hartree and Cunningham, 1969; Godden and Scanes, 1975; Sakai and Ishii, 1980). The potency of this FSH preparation (CP1) was 67% that of the partially purified ovine standard (NIH-FSH-S1) in the Steelman-Pohley mouse ovarian hypertrophy assay (Stockell Hartree and Cunningham, 1969). Similar CP1 preparations were 4·7- and 1·9-fold more potent than the mammalian NIH-FSH-S1 standard in respectively an *in vitro* bioassay which employed mouse cells (Godden and Scanes, 1975) and in a RRA in which chickens testes were the source of receptors (Sakai and Ishii, 1980). Further purification of this FSH (CP1) preparation has been achieved by gel-filtration on Sephadex G100 (Stockell Hartree, unpublished; see also Follett *et al.*, 1972, 1978) with the resulting fraction (CP1 Seph) having a potency of 2·1 mg equivalents NIH-FSH-S1 per mg in the Steelman-Pohley assay. Subsequently, ion-exchange chromatography of fraction CP1 on DEAE-cellulose yielded a potent FSH (fraction DC3), which had a potency of 34 mg equivalents NIH-FSH-S1 per mg in an *in vitro* bioassay (Godden and Scanes, 1975). Sakai and Ishii (1980) have produced the most potent chicken FSH preparation (75 mg equivalents NIH-FSH-S1 per mg by RRA) by employing both this ion-exchange system and gel filtration chromatography. All these FSH preparations have low levels of contamination with LH (between 0·5 and 6% of the best LH preparation in both RRA and radioimmunoassays, RIA) (Follett *et al.*, 1972; Godden and Scanes, 1975; Sakai and Ishii, 1980). It may be noted that, compared with the ovine FSH standard (NIH-FSH-S1), the avian FSH preparations have similar activities to highly purified mammalian FSH preparations, in both *in vitro* bioassays and RRAs. However, in the *in vivo* Steelman-Pohley assay chicken FSH has a low activity. This may reflect its low carbohydrate content relative to other vertebrates (Follett *et al.*, 1978) and hence an increased metabolic clearance rate.

Chicken LH and FSH have also been purified by methods successfully employed for hormone purification in many lower vertebrate groups (Licht *et* al., 1977). This involved a series of extraction and salt precipitations, ion-exchange chromatography on sulfoethyl-Sephadex and DEAE-cellulose and gel filtration on Sephadex G100. The resulting LH preparation (W306B) was only 8% as active as NIH-LH-S1 in the *Xenopus in vitro* ovulation (LH) assay and respectively 8% as active as NIH-FSH-S1 in a chicken testis FSH RRA and 85% that of NIH-FSH-S1 in the *Anolis* lizard testis growth FSH assay. Their FSH preparation (W315C) had 2·1-fold and 4·3-fold the activity of NIH-FSH-S1 in the chicken FSH RRA and *Anolis* assays and had low LH contamination (activity in *Xenopus* assay <0·15% than of NIH-LH-S1) (Licht *et al.*, 1977; Burke *et al.*, 1979a).

It is difficult to compare preparations of LH and FSH from different laboratories due to the lack of standard assay procedures. To date 24 different systems have been used (including *in vivo* and *in vitro* bioassays, together with homologous and heterologous RRA and RIA systems). The use solely of radioligand assays (RRA and RIA) to follow the purification of LH and FSH can be criticized. For instance, the activity of a hormone in a RRA reflects the dissociation constant for its binding reaction to the receptor. This may not reflect the biological activity of the preparation, as activity depends on both the dissociation constant and the efficacy of its binding to the hormone receptor (efficacy being the ability of a hormone activated receptor to affect intracellular metabolism). Furthermore, the use of RIA to follow LH and FSH fractionation is fraught with problems, as it will detect the immunologically reactive, (including precursors, subunits and degraded products) as well as the biologically active, hormone.

Chicken LH and FSH are glycoproteins with similar properties to their mammalian homologues. The amino acid compositions of chicken LH and FSH are shown in Table 1. Irrespective of the laboratory where these hormones were isolated, chicken LH has more proline and less glutamate, asparate and histidine residues than FSH. Similarly, the carbohydrate constituents of chicken LH and FSH have been chemically determined, the total carbohydrate of LH being 13·7 g per 100 g glycoprotein (including 5·2 hexose, 7·1 hexosamine and 1·4 g $100g^{-1}$ sialic acid) and 7·1 for FSH (including 3·1 hexose, 3·2 hexosamine and 0·8 sialic acid) (Licht *et al.*, 1977). Additional evidence for the presence of sialic acid in chicken gonadotrophins comes from their decreased biological activity following neuraminidase treatment (Licht

Table 1
Amino acid composition of avian adenohypophyseal hormone

Amino acid	Chicken FSH (a)	Chicken FSH (b)	Chicken FSH (c)	Chicken LH (d)	Chicken LH (e)	Chicken GH (f)	Chicken GH (g)	Chicken PRL (h)
	Residues per 100 residues							
Lys	8·2	4·2	5·2	7·1	6·5	8·4	6·4	6·9
His	4·1	0·9	2·9	2·3	1·4	2·6	2·1	2·7
Arg	3·5	3·3	2·9	4·0	4·7	5·0	5·3	4·8
Asp	9·7	9·8	11·1	7·5	7·4	10·1	10·7	12·5
Thr	7·0	5·1	9·1	8·1	6·5	5·6	5·3	3·5
Ser	9·1	6·5	8·9	5·0	6·5	6·1	6·4	9·7
Glu	9·7	13·5	11·7	8·0	9·8	11·0	13·4	16·7
Pro	5·2	7·4	7·2	11·8	8·4	5·3	7·5	4·5
Gly	9·3	11·1	8·8	8·3	10·2	9·7	6·4	10·2
Ala	9·2	10·2	7·4	8·5	8·4	7·7	8·0	8·9
½ Cys	N.A.	6·5	1·7	7·0	7·4	N.A.	1·6	N.
Val	6·1	5·1	7·4	7·8	5·6	6·3	5·3	4·7
Met	1·1	1·4	1·1	2·5	1·9	0·7	2·1	N.A.
Ile	4·7	3·3	3·6	3·3	3·3	3·5	3·7	3·5
Leu	5·8	7·4	4·6	4·5	6·0	10·9	10·7	7·9
Tyr	3·1	2·3	2·2	3·6	1·4	2·1	1·6	1·8
Phe	3·1	2·3	4·3	3·8	3·7	4·9	4·8	2·5

N.A. Not available; (a) Godden and Scanes (1975); (b) Licht *et al.* (1977); (c) Sakai and Ishii (1980); (d) Godden and Scanes (1975); (e) Licht *et al.* (1977); (f) Harvey and Scanes (1977a–c); (g) Farner *et al.* (1974); (h) Scanes *et al.* (1975a,b).

and Papkoff, 1972; Scanes, 1972). Based on analogy with mammals and the turkey, chicken LH and FSH have molecular weights of about 28 300 daltons (Burke *et al.*, 1979a) and are composed of two distinct glycoprotein (an α and β) subunits (Burke *et al.*, 1979b).

2. Assay

All assay systems have disadvantages. Obviously a bioassay would be preferred, but this is usually precluded by the lack of sensitivity of the bioassay. However, the activities of LH and FSH in the plasma and pituitary gland have been followed through the ovulation cycle of the hen, respectively by the OAAD and Steelman-Pohley assays (Nelson *et al.*, 1965; Imai and Nalbandov, 1971). These studies required the assay of tissue or plasma combined from a number of hens at the same stage of the cycle. A further problem is that neither bioassay is specific for the estimation of circulating gonadotrophin concentration in birds. The OAAD assay detects arginine vasotocin as well as LH (Jackson and Nalbandov, 1969a), while the Steelman-Pohley assay appears to respond to both avian (turkey) LH and FSH (Burke *et al.*, 1979a). A somewhat more sensitive bioassay is the chick ^{32}P-phosphate testes incorporation assay (Breneman *et al.*, 1962; Follett and Farner, 1966). This has been used in some studies. For instance, an *in vitro* study demonstrated that gonadotrophin release from chicken pituitary glands is stimulated by chicken and quail hypothalamic extracts, but not by posterior pituitary hormones or neurotransmitters (Follett, 1970). The ^{32}P testis assay has the twin disadvantages of responding to both avian LH and FSH (Furr and Cunnigham, 1971; Scanes and Follett, 1972) and not being sensitive enough to determine gonadotrophins in small quantities of plasma.

The application of the technique of RIA to chicken LH and FSH has allowed the determination of these hormones in serial blood samples from an individual bird. The first RIA for a chicken pituitary hormone was developed by Follett *et al.* (1972). This is an homologous system using antisera raised against chicken LH and purified chicken LH as both tracer (following labelling with radioactive ^{125}I iodine) and standard. This assay is usually considered to be specific for measuring LH in plasma under normal physiological circumstances. It does not react with avian FSH and there is no evidence for any non-specific plasma effects. It is possible, however, that very high concentrations of TSH may affect the RIA, as plasma concentrations of immunoreactive LH are elevated in chickens treated with the potent goitrogen methimazole (Chiasson *et al.*, 1979). There are two other homologous avian LH RIAs: for turkey LH (Wentworth *et al.*, 1976) and chicken LH (Hattori and Wakabayshi, 1979). All these LH RIAs appear to have similar characteristics.

Radioimmunoassays have also been successfully developed for chicken FSH. Of these, two are homologous assays employing purified FSH as both tracer and standard and with antisera raised against chicken FSH (Scanes *et al.*, 1977a; Sakai and Ishii, 1980). The third assay is a heterologous system employing antisera to ovine FSH, radio-labelled rat FSH and rat FSH standard. This system has been validated with chicken gonadotrophin preparations and quail plasma (Croix *et al.*, 1974; Follett, 1976).

The RIAs for chicken LH and FSH have been extensively used in the study of the endocrinology of a number of avian species. For instance, in the male chicken, LH is released in an episodic manner (Wilson and Sharp, 1975a), and its secretion is increased by synthetic LH-releasing hormone (–RH) (Furr *et al.*, 1973a) and following castration (Follett *et al.*, 1972; Wilson and Sharp, 1975a) and depressed by testosterone, 5α-dihydrotestosterone and oestradiol (Balthazart and Henrick, 1978). In the domestic hen, plasma concentrations of LH are increased (approximately 2–2·5-fold) six to four hours prior to ovulation (Furr *et al.*, 1973b; Wilson and Sharp, 1973), by LHRH (e.g. Bonney *et al.*, 1974) and by progesterone positive feedback (e.g. Wilson and Sharp, 1975b). Circulating concentrations of LH vary over short periods due, in part, to the high disappearance rate from the circulation. In the chicken, LH has been reported to have a half life of 22 min on the basis of the decrease of injected ^{125}I-iodinated LH from the circulation (Scanes and Follett, 1973) and of 17 to 23 min on the decline in LH following an episodic release pulse (Wilson and Sharp, 1975a). Plasma FSH concentrations on the other hand are higher in male than female fowl and are further elevated by gonadectomy (Scanes *et al.*, 1977a). There are no major changes in plasma FSH concentrations during the ovulation cycle; a small increase is observed, however, 15 to 14 hours prior to ovulation (Scanes *et al.*, 1977a).

3. Physiology

The roles of LH and FSH in the fowl appear to be almost identical to those in mammals. Studies in the fowl and in the Japanese quail (*Coturnix coturnix japonica*) indicate that FSH acts to stimulate spermatogenesis and Sertoli cell function (fowl—Ishii and Yamamoto, 1976; quail—Brown *et al.*, 1975). In contrast, LH induces both the differentiation of the Leydig cells (fowl—Connell, 1972; quail—Brown *et al.*, 1975) and the testicular production of testosterone (fowl—Licht *et al.*, 1977; quail—Maung and Follett, 1977, 1978). Very high concentrations of FSH are reported to increase the *in vitro* production of testosterone from quail and chicken testes (Licht *et al.*, 1977; Maung and Follett, 1977). However, this may be due to the FSH preparations employed having a low, but significant, contamination with LH.

Gonadotrophins are essential for ovarian function. Considering first the production of progesterone, the major source of this is the granulosa layer of the three largest pre-ovulatory follicles (Shahabi *et al.*, 1975; Huang *et al.*, 1979). Progesterone synthesis is increased both *in vivo* and *in vitro* by mammalian LH (Shahabi *et al.*, 1975; Huang *et al.*, 1979; Scanes and Fagioli, 1980; Hammond *et al.*, 1980). Chicken LH fractions also strongly stimulate progesterone production; their potency in this being proportional to their LH content (Scanes and Fagioli, 1980). Avian and mammalian FSH preparations have some progesterone synthesis stimulating activity. However, much and possibly all, of this can be accounted for by the LH contamination in the FSH fractions (Huang *et al.*, 1979; Scanes and Fagioli, 1980; Hammond *et al.*, 1980). The relative roles of LH and FSH in the control of testosterone and oestrogen synthesis is less well established. Testosterone is produced by the major ovarian follicles, particularly the second and third largest follicles (Shahabi *et al.*, 1975; Huang *et al.*, 1979). Although both theca and granulosa cells can synthesize testosterone *de novo*, it is likely that testosterone is normally produced by the theca cell, using granulosa derived progesterone as the precursor (Huang *et al.*, 1979). LH elevates testosterone production *in vivo* (Shahabi *et al.*, 1975), *in vitro de novo* and *in vitro* from progesterone (Huang *et al.*, 1979). However, a role for FSH cannot be excluded as high concentrations of FSH increase testosterone production *in vitro* (Huang *et al.*, 1979). Oestrogens appear to be similarly produced by the second and third largest follicles (principally the theca cells). This can be stimulated to a limited extent by both LH and FSH (Huang *et al.*, 1979).

Follicular maturation does not occur in the absence of pituitary gonadotrophins. It has been suggested that FSH controls yolk deposition. This is supported by the observations that an impure chicken FSH preparation prevents the atrophy of the follicles which follow hypophysectomy (Mitchell, 1970) and that mammalian FSH increases follicular iodine uptake (quail—Robinson *et al.*, 1976; chicken—W. S. Newcomer, personal communication). Conversely, the ovulation of the mature follicle appears to be induced by LH. Evidence for this comes, for instance, from the high incidence of ovulation following LH but not FSH administration (Imai, 1973), the increased circulating concentration of LH four hours prior to ovulation (Furr *et al.*, 1973b) and the ability of antisera against chicken LH to inhibit ovulation (Sharp *et al.*, 1977; Landefeld and Kepa, 1979).

C. Thyrotrophin

1. Chemistry

Complete purification of chicken TSH and removal of LH contamination has not yet been achieved, and it is possible that similarities in the chemical structures of LH and TSH make difficult the final purification. Godden and Scanes (1975) reported on their separation of the two hormones by DEAE-cellulose chromatography at pH 9·5 in 5 mM glycine buffer, with elution of fractions by a pH and salt concentration gradient. Total gonadotrophic activity was estimated by the stimulation of testicular ^{32}P-phosphate incorporation in one-day-old chicks (Breneman *et al.*, 1962; Follett and Farner, 1966), and assay for TSH was by incorporation of ^{32}P-phosphorus by the chick thyroid (Greenspan *et al.*, 1956). Their most potent TSH fraction contained 328 μg mg^{-1} in terms of an ovine standard (NIH-TSH-S6), but it contained gonadotrophic activity that was 34% of their best LH preparation, suggesting appreciable LH contamination of their TSH fraction. Further attempts at separating the LH activity from TSH (A. Stockell Hartree and C. G. Scanes, unpublished) on DEAE-cellulose columns at pH 9·5 with varying concentrations of glycine buffer gave essentially similar results. An LH fraction with negligible TSH contamination was eluted by glycine concentrations up to 0·015 M, and at higher buffer concentration TSH activity was eluted along with significant LH activity. The LH:TSH ratio tended to be constant in the TSH fractions, so it is possible that chicken TSH possesses some intrinsic LH activity.

2. Assay

The absence of a pure chicken TSH has precluded the development of a homologous radioimmunoassay for the hormone. There is also no heterologous mammalian radioimmunoassay which has been validated for avian TSH. The most widely used bioassay for TSH depends on the uptake of ^{32}P-phosphate by the thyroid of one-day-old chicks (Lamberg, 1953). This system has been employed to monitor TSH activity during the purification of chicken LH (Scanes and Follett, 1972), and in the fractionation of TSH (see above). Radke and Chiasson (1974) used the assay to examine the distribution of TSH in the various portions of the chicken pars distalis. The cephalic lobe contained 60% more TSH than the middle portion and four times that in the caudal lobe. Similar studies in the Japanese quail indicate that most TSH activity is in the cephalic lobe in this species also (Radke and Chiasson, 1975). MacKenzie (1981) has developed an *in vivo* TSH bioassay in which the response measured is the plasma concentration of thyroxine following TSH administration. A significant release of T_4 is found with as little as 1 μg NIH-TSH-B4.

3. Physiology

As might be expected TSH acts in mammals and birds to increase thyroxine secretion from the thyroid gland. The plasma concentration of thyroxine is elevated in one-day-old chicks by preparations of bovine TSH and ostrich TSH with a maximal effect being observed after 5 h (MacKenzie, 1981). Similarly, mammalian TSH increases plasma thyroxine concentrations in chick embryos (Thommes and Hylka, 1978). Mammalian TSH stimulates the uptake of ^{131}I-iodide (as thyroxine) from the gland (Bates and Condliff, 1960). In addition mammalian TSH induces the *in vitro* release of cyclic AMP from thyroid lobes excised from one- and 13-day-old chickens (Tonoue and Kitoh, 1978). This may suggest that TSH exerts its effects with cyclic AMP as the secondary messenger.

D. Growth Hormone

1. Chemistry

Chicken GH has been isolated by methods developed for mammalian GH.

The purification of GH has involved its alkali extraction from pituitary glands, precipitation with ammonium sulphate (between 20 and 50% saturated) and both ion-exchange chromatography, on Amberlite and DEAE-cellulose with step wise elution, and gel-filtration on Sephadex G100 (Farmer *et al.*, 1974). Harvey and Scanes (1977a) prepared chicken GH by ion-exchange chromatography on DEAE-cellulose using a pH and salt gradient, following its alkali extraction and salt (ammonium sulphate) fractionation. Chicken GH resembles mammalian somatotrophin in terms of its amino acid composition (shown in Table 1), its molecular weight (22 000 to 23 000 as determined by gel-filtration or SDS polyacrylamide electrophoresis) and isoelectric point (pI 7·5) (Farmer *et al.*, 1974; Harvey and Scanes, 1977a; Burke and Papkoff, 1980).

2. *Assay*

Chicken GH is active in stimulating cartilage growth in hypophysectomized immature rats, in the tibia assay (Hazelwood and Hazelwood, 1961). It can also be estimated in a heterologous mammalian radioimmunoassay (Farmer *et al.*, 1974) or by densitometry following staining and analytical discontinuous polyacrylamide gel electrophoresis (Nicoll and Licht, 1971). A homologous radioimmunoassay capable of detecting GH in small volumes of chicken plasma (and also in pituitary tissue) has been developed (Harvey and Scanes, 1977a).

3. *Physiology*

Growth hormone exerts effects on both growth and on the short term control of metabolism. Growth of young chickens is markedly depressed following hypophysectomy (Nalbandov and Card, 1943) or after the administration of antisera raised against chicken GH (Scanes *et al.*, 1977b). The growth rate of chicks can also be increased by the administration of a trypsin treated preparation of bovine GH (Myers and Peterson, 1974), but not by bovine GH itself (Libby *et al.*, 1955). RNA metabolism in the chick liver is, however, enhanced by both bovine and chicken GH (Scanes *et al.*, 1977b). The plasma concentration of GH is high in young chickens during rapid post-hatching growth (Fig. 4) (Harvey *et al.*, 1979a).

Growth hormone increases muscle glycogen (Hazelwood and Lorenz, 1959). In addition, pituitary extracts or preparations of mammalian or chicken GH inhibit insulin-induced lipogenesis *in vitro* (Kompiang and Gibson, 1976; Harvey *et al.*, 1977). Avian GH-containing fractions also stimulate *in vitro* lipolysis (Langslow and Hales, 1969; Harvey *et al.*, 1977). It would seem, therefore, that GH mobilizes stored lipid and spares carbohydrate from use as a precursor for lipid synthesis.

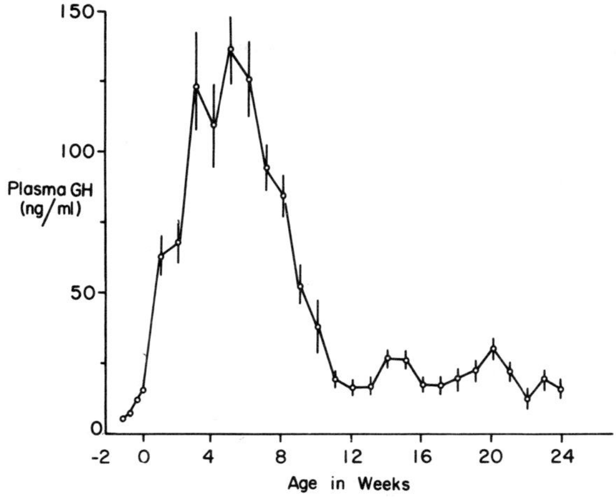

Fig. 4. Variation in plasma concentrations of GH through the growth and development of the male domestic fowl. Age is from the time of hatching. Data on plasma concentrations of GH is from Harvey *et al.*, 1979a (embryonic) and Scanes and Harvey, 1981c (post-hatching).

The clearance of GH from the circulation of the fowl follows a multi-exponential curve, characterized by the first half-life of 2·0 min, second half-life of 12·3 min and third half-life of 194 min; the metabolic clearance rate is 1·5 ml min^{-1} kg^{-1} (Harvey and Scanes, 1977b).

E. Prolactin

1. Chemistry

Chicken prolactin has been purified by methods developed for mammalian prolactin (Scanes *et al.*, 1975b), as has turkey prolactin (Burke and Papkoff, 1980). Both these fractionations have involved the alkali extraction of prolactin and its subsequent purification by ion-exchange chromatography on DEAE-cellulose and gel filtration on Sephadex G100. Chicken prolactin resembles prolactin from other species in both amino acid composition (shown in Table 1) and pI (5·6) (Scanes *et al.*, 1975b). Its molecular weight is probably 22 000–26 000, a similar value being reported for the turkey hormone (Burke and Papkoff, 1980).

2. Assay

Prolactin stimulates the crop sac gland of the pigeon. This response is employed in the biological assay of prolactin (e.g. Nicoll, 1967), for instance, in its purification (Scanes *et al.*1975b; Burke and Papkoff, 1980). In addition, pituitary prolactin can be estimated (e.g. Hall *et al.*, 1975) by densitometry, following its staining and separation by analytical discontinuous polyacrylamide gel electrophoresis (Nicoll *et al.*, 1969; Nicoll and Nichols, 1971). The concentration of prolactin in both plasma and media from incubation of chicken pituitary tissue can be estimated by homologous radioimmunoassay (Scanes *et al.*, 1976a), and there is also a heterologous mammalian system (McNeilly *et al.*, 1978) which detects avian prolactin.

3. Physiology

Prolactin has been proposed to have a number of roles in the fowl, including the regulation of reproduction, the adrenal cortex, osmoregulation, growth and skin metabolism. Prolactin does not appear to affect gonadal functioning in the male chicken (Shani *et al.*, 1973), but it inhibits reproduction in the hen. Broodiness can be induced by prolactin (Riddle *et al.*, 1935); broody chickens have increased concentrations of prolactin in the pituitary gland (Burrows and Byerly, 1936; Saeki and Tan be, 1953) and in the plasma (Chadwick, 1979; Sharp *et al.*, 1979a). Prolactin suppresses the induction of ovulation by exogenous LH in the chicken (Tanaka *et al.*, 1971). Moreover, in another Galliform, the turkey, prolactin depresses the effects of LH and FSH on ovarian steroidogenesis (Camper and Burke, 1977). It may also be noted that during the ovulation cycle, the plasma concentrations of prolactin are reduced at the time of the pre-ovulatory surges of LH secretion and ovarian steroidogenesis (Scanes *et al.*, 1977c). These reports are consistent with prolactin inhibiting gonadal functioning in the hen.

Prolactin reduces the metabolism of corticosterone by chicken (R. V. Carcia, S. Malamed and C. G. Scanes, unpublished) and rat adrenal tissue (Ogle and Kitay, 1979), presumably by inhibiting 5α-reductase. The evidence for the involvement of prolactin in the control of growth and osmoregulation/salt balance in the chicken rests either on analogy with other avian and lower vertebrate species, or on correlations between high circulating prolactin concentrations and various physiological states. For instance, the plasma concentration of prolactin in chickens is elevated by salt loading (Scanes *et al.*, 1976a) and following water deprivation (Harvey *et al.*, 1979a). Moreover, the plasma concentration of prolactin is high during the early rapid phase of growth in the chicken (Harvey *et al.*, 1979a; Scanes *et al.*, 1980).

Prolactin also affects chicken skin and in particular the uropygeal glands which are analogous to the sebaceous glands of mammals. Prolactin administration increases the rate of mitosis and decreases the wax content of chicken uropygeal glands (Chakraborty *et al.*, 1979).

F. Adrenocorticotrophin and Biosynthetically Related Hormones

1. Chemistry

For some years structural similarities have been apparent between certain pituitary polypeptide hormones, which include *α*- and *β*-melanocyte stimulating hormones (*α*-MSH, *β*-MSH), ACTH, *β*- and *γ*-lipotrophin (*β*-LPH, *γ*-LPH), *β*-endorphin and enkephalin. It seemed likely that the smaller peptides were produced by specific enzymatic cleavage of the larger ones (Lowry and Scott, 1975; Chrétien and Seidah, 1981). The demonstration by Eipper *et al.* (1976) that mouse tumour cells produce a high molecular weight glycoprotein form of ACTH led to the concept of a common precursor molecule for these related polypeptide hormones. The techniques of DNA cloning and nucleotide sequence analysis have been used to determine the complete amino acid sequence of the bovine precursor (Nakanishi *et al.*, 1979), which has been referred to as pro-opiocortin or pro-opiomelanocortin (Chang *et al.*, 1980). The results suggest a precursor protein consisting of around 260 amino acid residues, with the carboxyl-terminal sequence of 134 residues containing the polypeptide hormones listed above. The precursor is processed to different end products in the anterior and intermediate lobes of the pituitary by enzymatic cleavage between pairs of basic amino acids (Fig. 5). In mammals, it has been reported that the anterior pituitary lobe produces preferentially ACTH and *β*-LPH, while the intermediate lobe producers mainly *α*-MSH and *β*-endorphin (Lowry and Scott, 1975; Chrétien and Seidah, 1981).

The relationships between these hormones have not yet been studied in the domestic fowl. There is a preliminary report on the amino acid composition of chicken ACTH (Lowry and Scott, 1975), but it contains no information on the

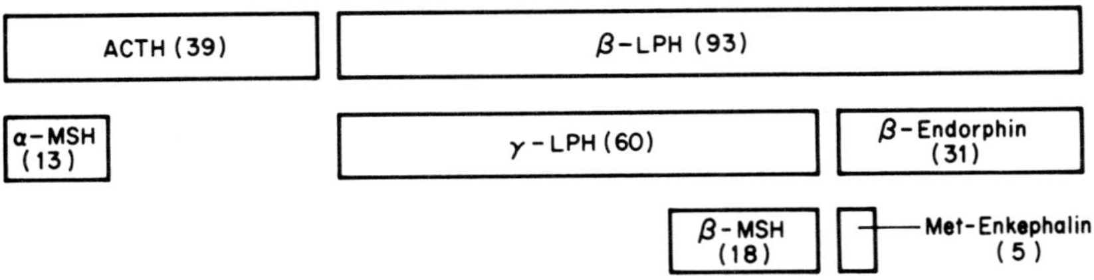

Fig. 5. Schematic representation of the related peptide hormones derived from bovine pro-opiomelanocortin. The length of the peptide chain is proportional to the horizontal length of each rectangle, and the figures in parentheses are the number of amino acid residues in each hormone. The position of each rectangle indicates the portion of the parent molecule from which it is derived . (Adapted from Nakanishi *et al.*, 1979.) ACTH, adrenocorticotrophin; LPH, lipotrophin; MSH, melanocyte stimulating hormone.

purification procedure or on the biological properties of this hormone. More information is available on ACTH from turkey and also from ostrich pituitaries. The two species of ACTH were purified by procedures similar to those used for the mammalian hormone, which include successively—acid/acetone extraction, fractionation with NaCl, ion-exchange chromatography on CM-cellulose, and gel filtration (Naudé and Oelofsen, 1977; Chang *et al.*, 1980). The purified ostrich hormone had a potency of 77 IU mg^{-1} when compared to a standard preparation of pig ACTH (Naudé and Oelofsen, 1977), in an *in vitro* assay based on stimulation of corticoid production by isolated rat adrenals (Saffran and Schally, 1955). The purified turkey ACTH was 82% as potent as sheep ACTH (Chang *et al.*, 1980), in an assay based on steroidogenesis in rat adrenal cells (Rao *et al.*, 1978).

The amino acid sequence of ostrich ACTH was determined by Li and Chung (1978) and that of turkey ACTH by Chang *et al.* (1980). Like mammalian and dogfish ACTH, avian ACTH contains 39 amino acids (Table 2); residues 1–24 (the sequence required for full biological activity) are similar in all species, except for a few conservative substitutions. In the remainder of the molecule there are a number of differences when the avian sequences are compared with each other or with ACTH from other vertebrates (Table 2). It is noteworthy that the amino acid composition of chicken ACTH (Lowry and Scott, 1975) is virtually identical to that of turkey ACTH (Chang *et al.*, 1980).

Although β-LPH and γ-LPH are known to have lipid mobilizing properties, the physiological significance of this activity in mammalian and avian species is uncertain. Attention has been focused mainly on their functions as precursors to the smaller peptide hormones shown in Fig. 5. The endorphin and enkephalin peptides have potent opiate or morphine-like effects in mammals and will specifically bind to opiate receptors in mammalian brain tissue (Chrétien and Seidah, 1981). The amino acid sequence required for opiate activity in these peptides is Tyr-Gly-Gly-Phe-X, where X is methionine (Met-enkephalin) or leucine (Leu-enkephalin). Turkey β-LPH was purified and characterized by Chang *et al.* (1980). Its lipolytic activity was only 5% as high as sheep β-LPH when assayed *in vitro* using isolated rabbit fat cells. Hydrolysis of turkey β-LPH with trypsin resulted in the appearance of opiate activity when tested with a guinea pig ileum preparation. β-endorphin itself was not detected in any of the turkey pituitary fractions, presumably because the pituitaries had been frozen immediately after decapitation, thus preventing enzymic activity which might produce β-endorphin from β-LPH. From amino acid analysis and preliminary sequence data, turkey β-LPH was of the same molecular size as ovine β-LPH and included a β-endorphin-like sequence. Turkey β-LPH was inactive in an ovine β-LPH radioimmunoassay, but it showed a low degree of cross-section in an immunoassay for human β-endorphin (Chang *et al.*, 1980).

Table 2

Amino acid sequences of ACTH

	5 10 15 20
Turkey ACTH	H-Ser-Tyr-Ser-Met-Glu-His-Phe-Arg-Trp-Gly-Lys-Pro-Val-Gly-Arg-Arg-Lys-Arg-Pro-Ile-Lys-Val-Tyr-Pro-
Ostrich ACTH	————————————————Lys-Arg——— Val————
Porcine ACTH	———————————————Lys-Lys-Arg——— Val————
Ovine ACTH	———————————————Lys-Lys-Arg——— Val————
Dogfish ACTH	——————————————Met———Lys-Arg————————

	25 30 35 39
Turkey ACTH	-Asn-Gly-Ser-Val-Asx-Glx-Glx-Gln-Ala-Ser-Tyr-Pro-Val-Glu-Phe-OH
Ostrich ACTH	——— Val-Gln-Glu-Glu-Thr-Ser-Glu-Gly-Phe——Leu————
Porcine ACTH	——— Ala-Glu-Asp-Glu-Leu-Ala-Glu-Ala-Phe——Leu————
Ovine ACTH	——— Ala-Glu-Asp-Glu-Ser-Ala-Gln-Ala-Phe——Leu————
Dogfish ACTH	—— Ser-Phe-Glu-Asp-Glu-Ser-Val-Glu-Asn-Met-Gly-Pro——Leu-OH

The sequence of the turkey hormone is shown in full. The solid lines indicate regions of each sequence that are identical to turkey ACTH. Amino acid residues that are different are shown on the figure. References for the sequence data are as follows: turkey ACTH, Chang *et al.* (1980); ostrich ACTH. Li and Chung (1978); porcine ACTH, Riniker *et al.* (1972); ovine ACTH, Jöhl *et al.* (1974); dogfish ACTH, Lowry *et al.* (1974).

A side-fraction with potent opiate activity, obtained during purification of ostrich ACTH, was further studied by Naudé *et al.* (1980). Preparative paper electrophoresis of the fraction yielded a purified peptide with opiate activity, similar to that of porcine β-endorphin when tested on a guinea pig ileum, as evidenced by a dose-related inhibition of the twitch response which was specifically antagonized by naloxone (Naudé *et al.*, 1980). The ostrich β-endorphin was nearly three times more active than camel β-endorphin in a receptor binding assays using rat brain membrane preparations (Naudé *et al.*, 1981). The amino acid sequence of the ostrich hormone shows substantial homology with mammalian β-endorphins. Like them, it contains 31 amino acids with the pentapeptide sequence of Met-enkephalin at the amino terminus of the peptide chain; ostrich β-endorphin is different mainly in the sequence from residues 9 to 12 inclusive (Naudé *et al.*, 1981).

Acetylation of the N-terminal amino group of β-endorphin results in loss of opiate activity in mammals (Smyth *et al.*, 1979), and this inactive form predominates in the intermediate lobe of the pig pituitary. The active form of β-endorphin is produced together with ACTH in the pig anterior lobe, suggesting that the mechanisms for processing the common precursor molecule differ in various regions of the gland (Smyth and Zakarian, 1980). In mammals, enkephalins are also derived from another precursor protein found in a variety of tissues (Udenfriend, 1981). The demonstration of β-LPH and ACTH together in the turkey adenohypophysis and the presence of ACTH and β-endorphin together in the ostrich adenohypophysis suggest that in avian species there are similarities to the mammalian biosynthetic pathway shown in Fig. 5.

Two different forms of melanocyte-stimulating hormone (MSH), which causes darkening of the skin particularly in amphibia and fish, are derived from ACTH and from γ-LPH (Fig. 5). This activity is normally found in the intermediate lobe of species that possess this structure, but in the avian pituitary this structure is absent. Kleinholz and Rahn (1940) and Betz *et al.* (1976) reported that MSH activity is concentrated in the cephalic portion of the chicken anterior pituitary gland. The partial purification from duck anterior lobes of biologically active fractions with molecular size similar to mammalian ACTH, α-MSH and β-MSH has been reported (Estivariz *et al.*, 1980), and it was concluded that α-MSH is the major source of the activity in this species. Further studies, with antibody labelling techniques, demonstrated that α-MSH and ACTH co-exist in the same cells, which are found mainly in the cephalic lobe of the duck pituitary (Iturriza *et al.*, 1980). Whether or not these cells secrete both hormones is uncertain, but these studies suggest that a particular cell population within the avian adenohypophysis fulfils the function of the absent intermediate lobe. In those species where it has been determined, the sequence of α-MSH is that of the N-terminal 13 amino acids of

ACTH (see Fig. 5). It is homologous with β-MSH, which has 18 amino acids, and there are four amino acid differences when α-MSH is compared with the homologous portion of β-MSH (Chrétien and Seidah, 1981).

2. Assay

Despite the isolation of ACTH from the chicken (Lowry and Scott, 1975), ostrich (Naudé and Oelofsen, 1977) and turkey (Chang *et al.*, 1980), there are no reports of the development of homologous radioimmunoassays of avian ACTH. Furthermore, heterologous mammalian systems have not been validated or applied to the measurement of ACTH in chicken plasma. Biological activity has been followed during the purification of avian ACTH by the ability to stimulate corticosterone secretion *in vitro* from the rat adrenal gland or isolated adrenal cells (Naudé and Oelofsen, 1977; Chang *et al.*, 1980).

3. Physiology

Adrenocorticotrophin, as its names applies, stimulates the adrenal cortex. Purified mammalian ACTH and also crude chicken pituitary extracts stimulate the secretion *in vitro* of corticosterone and aldosterone from chicken adrenal tissue (de Roos and de Roos, 1964). The *in vivo* effects of porcine ACTH in the immature chicken are, a transitory increase in the plasma concentrations of corticosterone (and cortisol), some depression in growth after repeated injection, decreased adrenal cholesterol, and involution of lymphoid tissue (Freeman *et al.*, 1979; Davison *et al.*, 1979; Kalliecharan, 1981). Genetic differences in the magnitude of adrenal response to ACTH have been observed in chickens (Edens and Siegel, 1975) and in turkeys (Brown and Nestor, 1973). There is little information on the role of MSH, lipotrophin or the opioid peptides in the fowl or other avian species.

IV. Control of Adenohypophysial Function

The functional activity of the vertebrate pituitary gland is primarily controlled by the central nervous system. A variety of external and internal environmental stimuli converges on the hypothalamus and thus influences the adenohypophysis. The release of specific neurohumoral substances from nerve endings in the median eminence into a portal vascular system provides the link between the brain and peripheral endocrine organs. Accordingly, hypophysiotrophic hormones are synthesized by peptidergic neurones in the hypothalamus and are transported by axoplasmic flow to nerve endings in the median eminence, where they are released from nerve terminals which are in close contact with the endothelia of the primary capillary plexus. The neurohormones are then distributed to the anterior pituitary gland via the portal blood flow (Harris, 1955). Four of these hypothalamic hypophysiotrophic factors or hormones, thyrotrophin releasing hormone (TRH), LHRH, growth release inhibiting hormone (somatostatin) and corticotrophin releasing factor (CRF), have been isolated from mammalian hypothalamic tissue.

In 1969, thyrotrophin releasing factor of both ovine and porcine origin was reported to be a tripeptide with the following structure (Burgus *et al.*, 1969):

(Pyro)-Glutamyl-Histidyl-Proline-amide

Shortly afterwards the tripeptide was synthesized and absolute chemical identity with the natural preparation established (Boler *et al.*, 1969). Later, a single gonadotrophin releasing factor (LHRH) was isolated from porcine (Schally *et al.*, 1971) and ovine (Burgus *et al.*, 1972) hypothalamic tissue. LHRH was found to be a decapeptide with identical structure in both species:

(Pyro)-Glu-His-Trp-Ser-Try-Gly-Leu-Arg-Pro-Gly-NH_2

The decapeptide was subsequently synthesized (Matsuo *et al.*, 1971) and shown to possess LH and follicle-stimulating hormone (FSH) releasing activity (Schally *et al.*, 1971). The third factor to be isolated from hypothalamic tissue was growth hormone release-inhibiting factor (somatostatin) which was identified as a cyclic tetradecapeptide (Brazeau *et al.*, 1973). Corticotrophin releasing factor has been isolated and characterized as a polypeptide with 41 amino acid residues (Vale *et al.*, 1981).

A. Gonadotrophins

1. Effects of Hypothalamic Lesions

The involvement of a neural mechanism in the control of gonadotrophin secretion in birds was first indicated by the ability of phenobarbital sodium and dibenamine (an adrenergic blocker) to suppress ovulation in the hen (Fraps, 1953; Tienhoven *et al.*, 1954). The role of the direct vascular connection with the hypothalamus was demonstrated by the regression of the ovary and comb following transection of the hypophysial portal vessels (Shirley and Nalbandov, 1956).

Lesioning of the hypothalamus of the domestic fowl has indicated some of the nuclei and pathways controlling LH-releasing hormone (LHRH) secretion, and hence gonadotrophin release. In domestic fowl, Ralph (1959) and Ralph and Fraps (1959a) found that electrolytic lesions in the medial pre-optic region and ventral portion of the paraventricular nucleus consistently resulted in an immediate cessation and prolonged interruption of ovulation. Posterior hypothalamic regions are also involved in the regulation of gonadal function. In male domestic fowl, lesions located in the ventral infundibular region induced testicular regression (Ravona *et al.*, 1973).

Davies and Follett (1975a,b,c, 1980) have used lesioning, deafferentation and electrical stimulation techniques to localize hypothalamic regions involved in photo-induced gonadal growth, gonadal maintenance and ovulation in Japanese quail. In males lesions which destroyed either the pre-optic region or the posterior-dorsal part of the infundibular nuclear complex prevented gonadal growth, while electrical stimulation of the same two regions was followed by rapid release of LH from the adenohypophysis. These sites appear to contain LHRH neurones in ducks and chickens (Bons, 1981; Sterling and Sharp, 1982) (Fig. 3). The posterior projections from the pre-optic area have been studied by deafferentation using a rotating microknife. Deafferentation immediately posterior to the pre-optic region blocked testicular growth, but extensive cuts designed to sever most of its connections with the forebrain were without effect. Several types of cuts in the mid-hypothalamic region designed to sever direct contacts between the pre-optic region and the posterior division of the infundibular nuclear complex also failed to prevent gonadal growth. These findings suggest that projections from the pre-optic region which are functionally important for gonadal growth must fan out immediately posterior to the region and enter the tuberal hypothalamus in a diffuse manner. Similar studies have been made on the tuberal hypothalamus. Complete surgical deafferentation of the tuberal (posterior) hypothalamus prevented testicular growth. This effect was reproduced by partial cuts which only deafferentated the anterior and anterio-lateral borders of the tuberal hypothalamus.

In sexually mature female quail, lesions of the pre-optic region and infundibular nuclear complex, or deafferentation of the tuberal hypothalamus blocked ovulation and resulted in marked regression of the ovary and oviduct. However, although lesions confined to the supra-optic region also blocked ovulation, the ovary and oviduct did not undergo regression, with the result that a polyfollicular syndrome ensued. This suggests that damage to the supra-optic region can block the surge of LH required for ovulation without interfering with the tonic release of LH/FSH required to maintain the ovary and stimulate follicular maturation.

Essentially, Davies and Follett's results in Japanese quail are consistent with and complement many of the earlier conclusions drawn from lesioning experiments (see Stockell Hartree and Cunningham, 1971). It is clear that at least two discrete hypothalamic centres are involved in gonadal growth and maintenance, the pre-optic region and infundibular nuclear complex, particularly its posterio-dorsal division. When surgically isolated from the rest of the brain, the tuberal hypothalamus cannot autonomously maintain the gonads. It also seems likely that the supra-optic region, while not directly involved in the mechanism controlling tonic gonadotrophin secretion and gonadal maintenance, does actively participate in the initiation of the LH surge required for ovulation.

2. *Factors Affecting Gonadotrophin Secretion*

Plasma concentrations of LH in chickens have been observed to increase following synthetic LHRH (see Section IV.A.3) and α-adrenergic agonists (Buonomo and Scanes, 1983), and to be depressed by handling stress (Wilson and Sharp, 1975a; Buonomo and Scanes, 1983), starvation for one or two days (Scanes *et al.*, 1976c), feeding a protein-deficient diet (Buonomo *et al.*, 1982) and pharmacological inhibition of noradrenaline/adrenaline synthesis or action (α-receptors) (Buonomo *et al.*, 1981; Buonomo and Scanes, 1982; Knight *et al.*, 1982). There are also changes in the plasma concentration of LH during growth and puberty (Sharp *et al.*, 1977). This probably reflects maturation of both the hypothalamus and of the pituitary, together with changes in feedback from gonadal steriods. The effects of gonadal steroids on gonadotrophin secretion are considered below. It appears that most of these factors act at the level of the central nervous system to influence the release of LHRH from the median eminence, and hence LH secretion. It is likely that not only the amount of LH released will be affected but also the episodic pattern of LH secretion (Wilson and Sharp, 1975a) may be modified. Furthermore, LHRH release itself is probably, directly or indirectly, stimulated by adrenergic neurones.

3. *Avian LHRH*

In vitro studies using cockerel anterior pituitary tissue established that extracts of chicken hypothalamic, but not of cerebral cortex, tissue contained an LH-releasing factor (Tanaka *et al.*, 1969). In a similar series of studies Jackson and Nalbandov (1969a) observed that extracts of chicken hypothalamic tissue induced the release of LH (as measured by the OAAD bioassay) from rat anterior pituitary tissue. Using a different assay system for gonadotrophins, namely the method which depends on the uptake of ^{32}P from the testis of one-day-old chicks, Follett (1970) observed that extracts of chicken hypothalamic tissue provoked the release of gonadotrophin from cockerel pituitary tissue *in vitro*. This assay method, unlike the OAAD assay (Jackson and Nalbandov, 1969b), does not respond to arginine vasotocin, but has the disadvantage that it measures the combined effects of LH and FSH. Jackson (1971a,b) purified chicken LH-releasing activity by chromatography on

Sephadex G25 and CM-Sephadex. Comparison of the chromatographic behaviour of avian LH-releasing activity and that from rat hypothalami indicated that chicken and rat LHRH are similar but have distinct chemical differences. On the other hand, the chromatographic results of Jeffcoate *et al.* (1974) pointed to a chemical similarity between mammalian LHRH and avian LH-releasing activities.

King and Millar (1982) isolated and characterized chicken LHRH as having the following structure:

$$(\text{Pyro})\text{-Gly-His-Try-Ser-Tyr-Gly-Leu-GlN-Pro-Gly-NH}_2$$

Thus avian LHRH differs from mammalian LHRH by a single amino acid residue substitution (at position 8—GlN for Arg).

Effect of synthetic mammalian LHRH. Synthetic LHRH induced premature ovulation in laying hens (Tienhoven and Schally, 1972; Reeves *et al.*, 1973; Etches and Cunningham, 1976) and promoted a rapid release of LH in both male and female birds (Furr *et al.*, 1973a; Bonney *et al.*, 1974; Wilson and Sharp, 1975a). Similarly, enzymatically-dispersed chicken anterior pituitary cells release LH in response to LHRH, under static incubation conditions (Bicknell and Follett, 1975; Bonney and Cunngingham, 1977a,b).

Mechanism of LHRH. The mechanism of action of LHRH at the level of the avian gonadotrope is not fully established. A role for adenosine 3,5-monophosphate (cyclic AMP) is supported by the ability of dibutyryl cyclic AMP to stimulate, both basal and LHRH stimulated, LH release from chicken pituitary cells *in vitro* (Bonney and Cunningham, 1977a). Similarly, *in vitro* LH secretion was shown to be enhanced by increasing the cellular concentration of cyclic AMP, by agents which inhibit phosphodiesterase (Bonney and Cunningham, 1977a). There is also evidence for a role for calcium ions in the action of LHRH on LH secretion. Not only is the presence of calcium required for LHRH to stimulate LH release *in vitro* (Bonney and Cunningham, 1977b), but also LH release is provoked by calcium ionophores (Luck and Scanes, 1980). In addition, depolarizing concentrations of potassium have been shown to increase LH release (Bonney and Cunningham, 1977b).

4. Feedback Regulation of Gonadotrophin Secretion

Feedback mechanisms play a fundamental role in the regulation of pituitary function and are particularly important in relation to the control of reproduction. In the context of the hypothalamus–pituitary–gonadal axis, three levels of feedback control have been established. Hypothalamic LHRH may influence its own secretion by an "ultrashort-loop" feedback. Secondly, pituitary gonadotrophins may modify the secretion of LHRH from the median eminence by acting on the hypothalamus via a "short-loop' feedback. The third, and most thoroughly investigated, component is the so-called "long-loop" feedback system, whereby circulating steroid hormones of gonadal origin interact with the hypothalamo–pituitary complex and exert both positive and negative feedback influences on gonadotrophin secretion (see Everett, 1964). The negative feedback action of gonadal steriods is primarily responsible for regulating basal gonadotrophin concentrations, whilst positive feedback mechanisms are responsible for triggering the pre-ovulatory discharges of gonadotrophin in the female. Although the crucial role of gonadal feedback has now been established beyond doubt, the degree to which "short" and "ultra-short" feedback loops are involved in normal physiological situations has yet to be investigated; indeed their existence in avian species has yet to be demonstrated.

Negative feedback action of gonodal steroids. The concept of a reciprocal relationship between gonadal steroids and pituitary gonadotrophins is long established. Removal of the gonads in chickens relieves the hypothalamo–pituitary complex of a major restraining influence. This is then reflected by an increase in the circulating concentration of plasma LH (Wilson and Sharp, 1976; Wilson, 1978). Conversely, the post-castration increase in plasma gonadotrophin content can be suppressed by treatment with gonadal steroids.

Endogenous plasma concentrations of LH were observed to be depressed by the administration of testosterone, 5α-dihydrotestosterone (DHT) and oestradiol (Balthazart and Hendrick, 1978). In castrated Japanese quail, Davies *et al.* (1980) found that plasma LH concentrations were depressed by testosterone, DHT, 5α-andostane-3α-17β-diol, androstenedione, 5α-androstane-3,17-dione, 5α-androstan-3β-ol-17-one, 5α-androstan-3α-ol-17-one and oestradiol. 5β-Dihydrotestosterone, 5β-androstane, 3α,17β-diol, 5α-androstane-3β,17β-diol, 5β-androstane-3,17-dione, androst-5-ene-3β,17β-diol and androst-5-en-3β-ol-17-one were ineffective.

Whether the hypothalamus or the pituitary gland represents the major target for negative gonadal feedback is controversial. Compelling evidence for a central site of action comes from studies involving implantation of steroids into the hypothalamus or pituitary gland. These implants tend only to be effective in suppressing gondotrophic function when placed in the hypothalamus. Testosterone has been implanted in the hypothalamus of male avian species, including ducks (Kordon and Gogan, 1964) and quail (Stetson, 1972a; Wada, 1972). Mediobasal hypothalamic implants were consistently found to inhibit photo-induced testicular growth, whereas implants in other regions were much less effective. In female quail, oestradiol-17β implants into the hypothalamus (pre-optic/supra-optic, median eminence and ventral region of the infundibular nuclear complex) and the anterior pituitary gland inhibited ovulation (Stetson, 1972b).

Positive feedback effects of gonadal steroids on gonadotrophin secretion. In mammals, the facilitatory role of gonadal steroids on gonadotrophin secretion is well established with oestrogen having a stimulatory effect on LH release. In the female fowl, the predominant positive feedback effect is due to progesterone. Progesterone can readily induce ovulation (Fraps and Dury, 1943) and the LH surge (Etches and Cunningham, 1975, 1976; Wilson and Sharp, 1975b) (see also Fig. 6) when injected at an appropriate stage of the ovulatory cycle. In addition, the administration of antisera to either progesterone or testosterone, but not oestradiol, can block ovulation in laying hens (Furr and Smith, 1975). However, testosterone only induces ovulation in a proportion of cases, while oestrogen does not induce ovulation (Fraps, 1955; Etches, 1975). Fraser and Sharp (1978) showed that the injection of an antiserum to LHRH blocked the progesterone-induced increase of LH in laying hens. This was clear evidence that the positive feedback action of progesterone in the hen requires LHRH to be available.

It has been shown in the hen that between 8 and 4 h before ovulation plasma concentration of LH (Furr *et al.*, 1973b), progesterone (Peterson and Common, 1971; Furr *et al.*, 1973b) (see Fig. 6), oestrogens (Peterson and Common, 1972; Senior and Cunningham, 1974) and testosterone (Etches and Cunningham, 1977) are higher than at any other time during the ovulation cycle (see Fig. 6). Any direct casual relationships between these increased levels of gonadal steroids and the pre-ovulatory LH surge have, therefore, been difficult to establish. Wilson and Sharp (1976) clarified this situation somewhat by

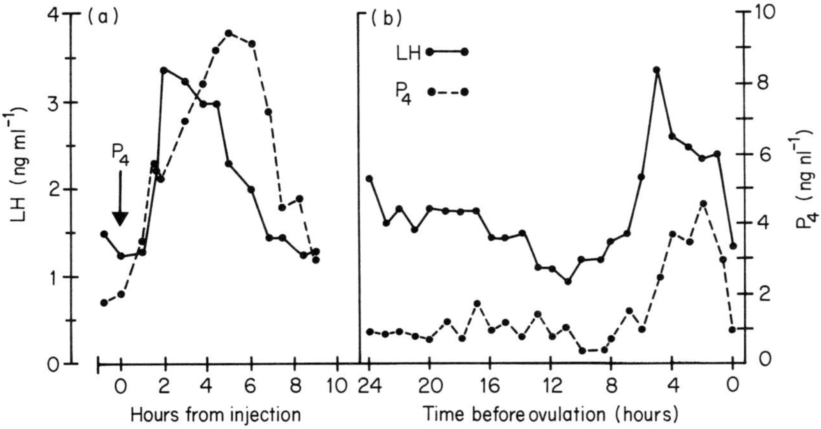

Fig. 6. (A) Effect of progesterone administration on the plasma concentration of LH in the domestic hen. (Re-drawn from Etches and Cunningham, 1975.) (B) Plasma concentrations of LH and progesterone through the ovulation cycle of the domestic hen. (Re-drawn form Furr *et al.*, 1973b.)

examining the effects of exogenous steroids on LH secretion in ovariectomized hens. Single injections of progesterone, oestrogen, or testosterone alone had no effect on LH secretion. However, after priming the birds for one week with oestrogen and progesterone, a single injection of progesterone, but not oestrogen or testosterone, promoted an increase in plasma LH. It would appear, therefore, that in the hen the release of LH is facilitated by increasing concentrations of progesterone, but only when the hypothalamo–pituitary complex has been exposed to both oestrogen and progesterone.

The pre-optic region has been implicated as a major site for the positive gonadal feedback responsible for triggering cyclic gonadotrophin release (an area containing LHRH neurones in the domestic fowl—Sterling and Sharp, 1982). In the hen, injection of progesterone directly into the pre-optic region induced premature ovulation (Ralph and Fraps, 1960) and lesions of the same region blocked the ability of a systemic injection of progesterone to induce premature ovulation (Ralph and Fraps, 1959b). The absence of a direct involvement of the pituitary gland was shown by Rothchild and Fraps (1949) and Ralph and Fraps (1960), who were able to induce premature ovulation by intra-pituitary injection of progesterone.

Whilst it is clear that gonadal steroids exert a stimulatory influence on the neural mechanism governing the cyclic discharge of LHRH, there is also compelling evidence in several species, including the rat (Aiyer and Fink, 1974), sheep (Reeves *et al.*, 1971a,b) and chicken (Bonney and Cunningham, 1977a), that gonadal steroids, particularly oestrogen, can directly enhance the responsiveness of the pituitary to LHRH. In the chicken, Bonney and Cunningham (1977a) found that pre-treatment with oestradiol, but not with progesterone or testosterone, enhanced the pituitary responsiveness to synthetic LHRH under both *in vivo* and *in vitro* experimental conditions. Therefore, it seems reasonable to speculate that, during the ovulatory cycle of the hen, progesterone triggers LH release via a neural mechanism involving the pre-optic region (Ralph and Fraps, 1959b, 1960), while oestradiol facilitates its release at the level of the anterior pituitary gland.

Gonadal steroid receptors in hypothalamus and pituitary gland. The presence and topographical distribution of gonadal steroid retention sites in the brain and pituitary gland of a variety of vertebrates have been examined by means of autoradiography (Morrell *et al.*, 1975; Martinez-Vargas *et al.*, 1976; Barfield *et al.*, 1978). It has emerged that marked similarities exist between different vertebrate classes with respect to the neuro-anatomical distribution of receptors binding gonadal steroids. In mammals and birds of either sex the lateral septal, pre-optic, medial anterior and medial basal hypothalamic regions consistently show an accumulation of testosterone and oestradiol, while more variable sites of uptake were found in the limbic system and in other parts of the hypothalamus and mesencephalon. Furthermore, in several mammals, a marked uptake of oestradiol and testosterone by adenohypophysial basophils has also been reported. While progesterone-concentrating structures have been less amenable to autoradiographic localization and receptor characterization studies, the existence of cytoplasmic progesterone receptors in the hypothalamus and adenohypophysis of the hen has recently been demonstrated (Kawashima *et al.*, 1979). Moreover, the concentration of progesterone-binding sites was greater in laying than in non-laying hens, and showed two peaks during the ovulatory cycle at 18 and 8 h before ovulation.

B. Thyrotrophin

Thyrotophin secretion in the fowl is under stimulatory hypothalamic control. This is supported by studies on the effect of electrolytic lesions in the hypothalamus (particularly within the anterior hypothalamus) on thyroid histology (Egge and Chiasson, 1963; Kanematsu and Mikami, 1970). Moreover acid extracts of chicken hypothalami stimulate the release of TSH from hen pituitaries *in vitro*, as does the synthetic mammalian thyrotrophin-releasing hormone (TRH), L-pyroglutamyl-L-histidyl-L-proline amide (Scanes, 1974). *In vivo*, synthetic TRH increases the circulating concentrations of thyroxine (T_4) and triiodothyronine (T_3) (Klandorf *et al.*, 1978). Evidence that pyroglutamyl-histidyl-proline amide is the avian TRH comes from the presence of immunoreactive (IR-) mammalian TRH in the chicken hypothalamus (Jackson and Reichlin, 1974) and the presence of receptors to ovine TRH in chicken pituitary tissue (Thompson *et al.*, 1981).

A substantial component of TSH secretion appears to be independent of the hypothalamus, as the surgical transection of the portal blood vessel does not affect thyroid histology (Ma and Nalbandov, 1963).

Further progress on the control of TSH awaits the development of assay systems capable of detecting the hormone in small quantities of plasma. Although estimates of circulating concentrations of T_4 and T_3 may indicate changes in TSH, these could be due to metabolic effects particularly deiodination of T_4 and T_3.

C. Growth Hormone

The secretion of GH from the chicken pituitary is under dual stimulating and inhibitory control by the hypothalamus, as is the case in mammals. Extracts of the chicken hypothalamus, but not other areas of the brain, stimulate *in vitro* GH release from chicken pituitary glands, as determined both by densitometry after polyacrylamide gel electrophoresis of the incubation media

(Hall and Chadwick, 1976a) and by radioimmunoassay (Harvey *et al.*, 1979b). Synthetic mammalian TRH increases GH secretion *in vitro* (Hall *et al.*, 1975; Harvey *et al.*, 1978a) and *in vivo* in young chickens (Harvey *et al.*, 1978a). Evidence for an avian hypothalamic somatostatin (GHRIH) comes in part from studies using synthetic mammalian GHRIH and from the distribution of immunoreactive GHRIH in the pigeon brain and gastrointestinal tract (Vale *et al.*, 1976). GHRIH suppresses the *in vitro* increases in GH secretion found in the presence of either chicken hypothalamic extract (Hall and Chadwick, 1975; Harvey *et al.*, 1979c) or synthetic TRH (Hall and Chadwick, 1976b; Harvey *et al.*, 1978b). In addition, GHRIH reduces the increase in circulating GH concentrations following TRH administration (Harvey *et al.*, 1978a).

The neurotransmitter serotonin exerts an inhibitory effect on GH secretion in the young chicken, presumably acting at the hypothalamic level (Rabii *et al.*, 1981). Plasma concentrations of GH are increased by inhibiting serotonin synthesis (by parachlorophenylanaline) or by serotonergic antagonists and they are depressed by serotonin antagonists and precursors (Rabii *et al.*, 1981). There is evidence that catecholamines both stimulate and inhibit GH secretion. Administration of adrenaline to young cockerels is marked by a decreased plasma concentration of GH, the adrenaline acting via β-adrenergic receptors (Harvey and Scanes, 1978). In contrast, the catecholamine depletor, reserpine, and an inhibitor of noradrenaline synthesis, diethyldithiocarbamate, both decrease the circulating concentrations of GH in young chickens (Harvey *et al.*, 1978a; Scanes *et al.*, 1982).

The circulating concentration of GH in young domestic fowl is reduced by a number of stimuli which might be classed as stressful. These include insulin, glucagon (Harvey *et al.*, 1978c), adrenaline (Harvey and Scanes, 1978), prostaglandin E_1 and E_2 (Scanes *et al.*, 1978; Scanes and Harvey, 1981a) and anaesthetics, including ether (Harvey and Scanes, 1977c). Plasma GH concentration increases in chicks subjected to one day of starvation (Harvey *et al.*, 1978c) or to a chronic restriction in food intake (Engster *et al.*, 1979) or protein–energy deficiencies (Scanes *et al.*, 1981). Plasma GH concentrations are also increased in young hypothyroid chickens, irrespective of whether the hypothyroidism is due to auto-immune thyroiditis (Scanes *et al.*, 1976b) or to goitrogen administration (Chiasson *et al.*, 1979).

D. Prolactin

Prolactin release is under predominantly stimulatory hypothalamic control in birds. This differs from the inhibitory control in mammals. Extracts of chicken hypothalami, but not other areas of the brain, increase the concentrations of immunoreactive (IR-)-prolactin in the plasma of chickens and in media following *in vitro* incubation of chicken hemi-pituitary glands (Harvey *et al.*, 1979b). Chicken hypothalamic extract has also been demonstrated to stimulate *in vitro* prolactin secretion from chicken pituitary glands, as determined by bioassay (Hall *et al.*, 1975) and by densitometry following polyacrylamide gel electrophoresis (Hall *et al.*, 1975; Hall and Chadwick, 1976a), and from dispersed adenohypophysial cells, as determined by radioimmunoassay (Harvey *et al.*, 1979c).

The identity of the avian prolactin releasing factor (PRF) is unknown. Synthetic mammalian TRH increases prolactin release from chicken pituitary glands (Hall *et al.*, 1975; Harvey *et al.*, 1978). However, TRH does not appear to be the avian PRF, as its concentration in the hypothalamus (Jackson and Reichlin, 1974) is too low to account for the ability of hypothalamic extract to stimulate prolactin release (Harvey *et al.* 1979b).

The role of neurotransmitters, either in the direct control of prolactin secretion or acting via the hypothalamus has not been fully established. Serotonin stimulates prolactin release *in vivo* (Rabii *et al.*, 1981; Scanes *et al.*, 1982) and *in vitro* from coincubations of anterior pituitary glands and hypothalamic fragments (Harvey *et al.*, 1982). *In vivo* prolactin release is also increased by serotonin agonists and precursors (Rabii *et al.*, 1981). Catecholamines may inhibit prolactin secretion, as reserpine increases the circulating concentration of prolactin in the fowl (Harvey *et al.*, 1978b).

The circulating concentration of IR-prolactin is increased by a number of stimuli, including glucagon (Harvey *et al.*, 1978c), prostaglandin E_2 (Scanes *et al.*, 1978), thyroid insufficiency due to auto-immune thyroiditis (Scanes *et al.*, 1976b) or goitrogen administration (Chiasson *et al.*, 1979), salt loading (Scanes *et al.*, 1976a) and withholding drinking water (Harvey *et al.*, 1979a). The plasma IR-prolactin concentration is decreased by short periods (12 to 48 h) of starvation (Harvey *et al.*, 1978c).

E. Adrenocorticotrophic Hormone

Despite the fact that CRF was the first hypothalamic releasing factor to be proposed (Saffran and Schally, 1955b) following the demonstration that the addition of hypothalamic extract to pituitary tissue cultures caused a discharge of ACTH into the medium, the structure of this putative releasing factor has only recently been elucidated (Vale *et al.*, 1981). In addition, vasopressin is known to provoke the release of ACTH from the pituitary gland. Evidence for the existence of widespread CRF activity in the duck (*Anas platyrhynchos*) was obtained by Stainer and Holmes (1969), who found that extracts of hypothalamus, cerebrum and spinal cord provoked the release of ACTH in a duck pituitary incubation system. The significance of these findings is dubious since there is a likelihood of non-specificity of the response. Although there is no information on CRF in the domestic fowl, it is likely that the effects of synthetic mammalian CRF in birds will be characterized in the near future.

V. Neurohypophysial Hormones

A. Vasotocin and Mesotocin

All vertebrates possess at least one neurohypophysial polypeptide hormone which is analogous to, or identical with, the following structure of oxytocin:

$$\overline{\text{CyS}\text{-Tyr-Ile-Gln-Asn-}\text{CyS}}\text{-Pro-Leu-Gly}(\text{NH}_2)$$

1 2 3 4 5 6 7 8 9

In mammals, the chief neurohypophysial hormones are oxytocin and vasopressin (with Phe at position 3 and Arg or Lys at position 8). In avian species, vasotocin (8-arginine oxytocin) predominates, but mesotocin (8-isoleucine oxytocin) is also present (see Sawyer, 1977).

Biological methods of assay for these hormones have been reviewed by Sawyer (1966). "Oxytocic" activity can be assayed by its stimulation of the contraction of the mammalian uterus (Munsick *et al.*, 1960). Vasopressin elicits antidiuretic and vasoconstrictor responses. In lower vertebrates, including the domestic fowl, the hybrid molecule vasotocin can produce both "oxytocic" and "vasodepressor" responses. These include oviduct stimulation, water retention and vasoconstriction. Because these hormones have similarities in chemical structure as well as in biological activities, bioassays for a particular hormone have not normally been very specific. Somewhat better specificity, as well as improved sensitivity, has been claimed for radioimmunoassays. Rosenbloom and Fisher (1974) have described a radioimmunoassay for vasotocin which employs a rabbit antiserum raised against lysine vasopressin conjugated to bovine thyroglobulin. Although the antiserum reacts equally well with arginine vasopressin and vasotocin, it can be used for assay of the latter hormone in avian and other lower vertebrate species where vasopressin is absent. This radioimmunoassay has been employed by Koike *et al.* (1977) to study the effect of water deprivation on plasma vasotocin concentrations in conscious chickens. Dehydration for 96 h caused weight loss and increased plasma osmolality and plasma vasotocin. The maximum concentration of the hormone ($3{\cdot}9\ \mu U\ ml^{-1}$) observed after 74 h of dehydration was about six times greater than under normal hydration states. In order to study the effect of a rise in plasma osmolality on vasotocin concentrations in the absence of reductions in vascular volume, Koike *et al.*

(1979) infused hyperosmotic saline and observed a five-fold increase in plasma vasotocin. They concluded that an increase in plasma osmolality and/or sodium concentration stimulates secretion of vasotocin in chickens. Raffel *et al.* (1976) found that a strain of White Leghorn chickens with hereditary diabetes insipidus responded to injections of vasotocin, and they suggested that the genetic defect affects the quantity of vasotocin produced. Rzasa *et al.* (1974) reported that injection of vasotocin (0·1 μg kg^{-1} body weight) into normal cockerels led to increases in blood volume and plasma Na^+ concentration while plasma K^+ decreased.

The abrupt decrease in vasotocin content of the hen neurohypophysis (Tanaka and Nakajo, 1962) with a corresponding increase in blood vasotocin (Sturkie and Lin, 1966) shortly before oviposition, provided evidence for a role for the hormone in oviposition in the domestic fowl. The physiological function of fowl mesotocin is not known. The hormone is known to have "oxytocic" activity (Sawyer, 1977) and has been isolated from the neurohypophysis of the chicken, goose and turkey (Acher *et al.*, 1970). There is no convincing evidence for the occurrence of oxytocin in birds, and most of the oxytocic activity in the fowl is attributed to vasotocin. High affinity binding sites or receptors have been observed in various mammalian target tissues for oxytocin (summarized by Soloff *et al.*, 1977) and for vasopressin (Hechter *et al.*, 1978). There is evidence that cyclic AMP serves as an intracellular mediator for the actions of mammalian neurohypophysial hormones (see Dousa, 1977; Hechter *et al.*, 1978). It seems likely that a similar mechanism exists in the fowl, although this has not yet been investigated.

In mammals, specific carrier proteins, the neurophysins, are found associated with vasopressin and oxytocin (see Burford and Pickering, 1973; North and Mitchell, 1981). There is evidence that each hormone is synthesized together with its specific neurophysin as a larger precursor protein and that the separate hormone and neurophysin molecules are produced by proteolytic cleavage (Russell *et al.*, 1980). Carrier proteins for lower vertebrate neurohypophysial hormones have not as yet been investigated.

B. Control of Neurohypophysial Hormone Secretion

Immunohistochemical procedures have been used to localize neurohypophysial peptides. Vasotocin and mesotocin are found in separate neurones of the avian hypothalamus (Goosens *et al.*, 1977), in accordance with the one neurone/one neurohormone concept. Neurones containing vasotocin predominate in the rostral portion of the supra-optic nucleus, whereas mesotocin-containing neurones are most numerous in the lateral division of the supra-optic nucleus and particularly in the paraventricular nucleus.

The neurohypophysial hormones are secreted particularly in response to the changing needs of the internal environment. For instance, the osmoregulatory functions of the mammalian neurohypophysis are well known and it is satisfying that a similar role has been identified in the fowl. Wingstrand (1951) first showed that the time of appearance of antidiuretic activity during embryonic life is largely coincident with the appearance of chrome-haematoxylin stainable material in the neural lobe median eminence and supra-optic nucleus.

Legait and Legait (1955) and Legait (1959) demonstrated that osmoregulatory activity resulted in changes in the hypothalamo-hypophysial system of hens. These were comparable with changes found in other vertebrates. For example, dehydration was associated with a marked decrease in the amount of neurosecretory material which could be detected both within the neurones which form the supra-optic hypophysial tract and the neural lobe itself. Conversely, lesions of the hypothalamus lead to polydipsia and diuresis in chickens (Koike and Lepkovsky, 1967). Release of neurohypophysial hormones can also result from stimulation of specific areas of the hypothalamus. Opel (1964) reported that electrical stimulation of the pre-optic area of the hypothalamus induced premature oviposition of the terminal egg of the two-egg sequence. Opel (1966) later established that the induced oviposition was associated with a release of vasotocin but not of oxytocin. The immediate stimulus leading to the apparent release of the neurohypophysial hormone at the time of oviposition has not been identified. Distention and contraction of the oviduct failed to stimulate release as did premature oviposition induced by acetylcholine or sodium pentobarbitone. The question thus remains as to what causes the release of vasotocin at the time of oviposition.

References

Acher, R., Chauvet, J. and Chauvet, M. T. (1970). *Eur. J. Biochem.* **17**, 509–513.

Aiyer, M. S. and Fink, G. (1974). *J. Endocr.* **62**, 553–572.

Amin, S. O. and Gilbert, A. B. (1970). *Br. Poult. Sci.* **11**, 451–458.

Ariens-Kappers, C. V., Huber, C. G. and Crosby, E. C. (1936). "The Comparative Anatomy of the Nervous System of Vertebrates, Including Man." MacMillan, New York.

Balthazart, J. and Hendrick, J. C. (1978). *J. Endocr.* **77**, 149–150.

Barfield, R. J., Ronay, G. and Pfaff, D. W. (1978). *Neuroendocrinology* **26**, 297–311.

Bates, R. W. and Condliffe, P. G. (1960). *Recent Prog. Horm. Res.* **16**, 309–352.

Betz, T. W., Enemar, A. and Röhss, M. (1976). *Can. J. Zool.* **54**, 1554–1558.

Bicknell, R. J. and Follett, B. K. (1975). *Gen. comp. Endocr.* **26**, 141–152.

Bjorklund, A., Falck, B. and Ljunggren, L. (1968). *Z. Zellforsch. mikrosk. Anat.* **89**, 193–200.

Blahser, S., Fellman, D. and Bugnon, C. (1978). *Cell. Tiss. Res.* **195**, 183–187.

Boler, J., Engmann, F., Folkers, K. Bowers, C. Y. and Schally, A. V. (1969). *Biochem. biophys. Res. Comm.* **37**, 705–710.
Bonney, R. C. and Cunningham, F. J. (1977a). *Mol. Cell. Endocr.* **7**, 233–244.
Bonney, R. C. and Cunningham, F. J. (1977b). *Mol. Cell. Endocr.* **7**, 245–251.
Bonney, R. C., Cunningham, F. C. and Furr, B. J. A. (1974). *J. Endocr.* **63**, 539–547.
Bons, B. (1981). *In* "Recent Advances of Avian Endocrinology" (G. Pethes, P. Peczely and R. Rudas, eds), pp. 15–23. Pergamon Press, London.
Bons, N., Kerdelhue, B. and Assenmacher, I. (1978b). *C. r. hebd. Séanc. Acad. Sci., Paris* **285**, 1327–1330.
Bons, N., Kerdelhue, B. and Assenmacher, I. (1978a). *Cell. Tiss. Res.* **188**, 99–106.
Bons, N., Kerdelhue, B. and Assenmacher, I. (1978b). *C. r. hebd. Séanc. Acad. Sci., Paris* **287**, 145–148.
Brazeau, P., Vale, W., Burgus, R., Ling, N., Butcher, M., Rivier, J. and Guillemîn, R. (1973). *Science, N.Y.* **179**, 77–79.
Breneman, W. R., Zeller, F. J. and Creek, R. O. (1962). *Endocrinology* **71**, 790–798.
Brown, K. I. and Nestor, K. E. (1973). *Poult. Sci.* **52**, 1948–1954.
Brown, N. L., Bayle, J. D., Scanes, C. G. and Follett, B. K. (1975). *Cell Tiss. Res.* **156**, 499–520.
Buonomo, F. C. and Scanes, C. G. (1983). *Gen. comp. Endocr.* **49**, 358–363.
Buonomo, F. C., Rabii, J. and Scanes, C. G. (1981). *Gen. comp. Endocr.* **45**, 162–166.
Buonomo, F. C., Griminger, P. and Scanes, C. G. (1982). *Poult. Sci.* **61**, 800–803.
Burford, G. D. and Pickering, B. T. (1973). *Biochem. J.* **136**, 1047–1052.
Burgus, R., Dunn, T., Desiderio, D. and Guillemin, R. (1969). *C. r. hebd. Séanc. Acad. Sci. Paris,* **269**, 1870–1875.
Burgus, R., Butcher, M., Amoss, M., Ling, N., Monohan, M. Rivier, J., Fellows, R. Blackwell, R., Vale, W. and Guillemin, R. (1972). *Proc. natn. Acad. Sci., U.S.A.* **69**, 278–282.
Burke, W. H. and Papkoff, H. (1980). *Gen. comp. Endocr.* **40**, 297–307.
Burke, W. H., Licht, P., Papkoff, H. and Gallo, A. B. (1979a). *Gen. comp. Endocr.* **37**, 508–520.
Burke, W. H., Papkoff, H., Licht, P. and Gallo, A. B. (1979b). *Gen. comp. Endocr.* **37**, 501–507.
Burrows, W. H. and Byerly, T. C. (1936). *Proc. Soc. exp. Biol. Med.* **34**, 841–844.
Calas, A. (1974). *Thèse, Académie de Montpellier.*
Camper, P. M. and Burke, W. H. (1977). *Gen. comp. Endocr.* **32**, 72–77.
Catt, K. J. and Dufau, M. L. (1977). *A. Rev. Physiol.* **39**, 529–557.
Chadwick, A. (1979). *Gen. comp. Endocr.* **39**, 270–271.
Chakraborty, S., Maiti, B. R. and Bhattacharjya, S. P. (1979). *Gen. comp. Endocr.* **38**, 461–465.
Chang, A. C. Y., Cochet, M. and Cohen, S. N. (1980). *Proc. natn. Acad. Sci., U.S.A.* **77**, 4890–4894.
Chang, N. C., Chung, D. and Li, C. H. (1980). *Int. J. Peptide Protein Res.* **15**, 261–270.
Chiasson, R. B., Sharp, P. J., Klandorf, H., Scanes, C. G. and Harvey, S. (1979). *Poult. Sci.* **58**, 1575–1583.
Chrétien, M. and Seidah, N. G. (1981). *Mol. Cell. Biochem.* **34**, 101–127.
Connell, C. J. (1972). *Z. Zellforsch. mikrosk. Anat.* **128**, 139–151.
Croix, D., Hendrick, J. C., Balthazart, J. and Franchimont, P. (1974). *C. r. Séanc. Soc. Biol.* **168**, 136–140.

Davies, D. T. and Follett, B. K. (1975a). *Proc. R. Soc.* **B191**, 285–301.
Davies, D. T. and Follett, B. K. (1975b). *Proc. R. Soc.* **B191**, 303–315.
Davies, D. T. and Follett, B. K. (1975c). *J. Endocr.* **67**, 431–438.
Davies, D. T. and Follett, B. K. (1980). *Gen. comp. Endocr.* **40**, 220–225.
Davies, D. T., Massa, R. and James, R. (1980). *J. Endocr.* **84**, 211–222.
Davison, T. F., Scanes, C. G., Flack, I. H. and Harvey, S. (1979). *Br. Poult. Sci.* **20**, 575–585.
DeReviers, M. and Dubois, M. P. (1974). *Horm. Met. Res.* **6**, 494.
DeRoos, R. and de Roos, C. C. (1964). *Gen. comp. Endocr.* **4**, 602–607.
Dodd, J. M., Follett, B. K. and Sharp, P. J. (1970). *Adv. Physiol. Biochem.* **4**, 114–220.
Dousa, T. P. (1977). *Fedn. Proc. Fedn. Am. Socs. exp. Biol.* **36**, 1867–1871.
Dufau, M. L., Hayshi, K., Sala, G., Baukal, A. and Catt, K. J. (1978). *Proc. natn. Acad. Sci., U.S.A.* **75**, 4769–4773.
Duncan, D. (1956). *Anat. Rec.* **125**, 457–471.
Edens, F. W. and Siegel, H. S. (1975). *Gen. comp. Endocr.* **25**, 64–73.
Egge, A. S. and Chiasson, R. B. (1963). *Gen. comp. Endocr.* **3**, 346–361.
Eipper, B. A., Mains, R. E. and Guenzi, D. (1976). *J. biol. Chem.* **251**, 4121–4126.
Engster, H. M., Carew, L. B., Harvey, S. and Scanes, C. G. (1979). *J. Nutr.*, **109**, 330–338.
Estivariz, F. E., Levitin, H. P. and Iturriza, F. C. (1980). *Gen. comp. Endocr.* **40**, 123–127.
Etches, R. J. (1975). Ph.D. thesis, University of Reading.
Etches, R. J. and Cunningham, F. J. (1975). *J. Endocr.* **64**, 47P–48P.
Etches, R. J. and Cunningham, F. J. (1976). *J. Endocr.* **71**, 51–58.
Etches, R. J. and Cunningham, F. J. (1977). *Acta endocr. Copenh.* **84**, 357–366.
Everett, J. W. (1964). *In* "Major Problems in Neuroendocrinology" (E. Bajasz and G. Jasmin, eds), pp. 346–366. Karger, Basel.
Farmer, S. W., Papkoff, H. and Hayashida, T. (1974). *Endocrinology* **95**, 1560–1565.
Farner, D. S. and Oksche, A. (1962). *Gen. comp. Endocr.* **2**, 113–147.
Follett, B. K. (1970). *Gen. comp. Endocr.* **15**, 165–179.
Follett, B. K. (1973). *In* "Breeding Biology of Birds" (D. S. Farner, ed.), pp. 209–243. National Academy of Sciences, Washington, D.C.
Follett, B. K. (1976). *J. Endocr.* **69**, 117–126.
Follett, B. K. and Davies, D. T. (1975). *Symp. Zool. Soc., Lond.* **35**, 199–225.
Follett, B. K. and Farner, D. S. (1966). *Gen. comp. Endocr.* **7**, 125–131.
Follett, B. K., Scanes, C. G. and Cunningham, F. J. (1972). *J. Endocr.* **21**, 329–334.
Follett, B. K., Davis, D. T., Gibson, R., Hodges, K. J., Jenkins, N., Maung, S. L., Redshaw, M. R. and Sumpter, J. P. (1978). *Pavo 16*, 34–55.
Fraps, R. M. (1953). *Poult. Sci.* **32**, 899.
Fraps, R. M. (1955). *Mem. Soc. Endocr.* **4**, 205–219.
Fraps, R. M. and Dury, A. (1943). *Proc. Soc. exp. Biol. Med.* **52**, 346–349.
Fraser, H. M. and Sharp, P. J. (1978). *J. Endocr.* **76**, 181–182.
Freeman, B. M., Manning, A. C. C. and Flack, I. H. (1979). *Br. Poult. Sci.* **20**, 391–399.
Furr, B. J. A. and Cunningham, F. J. (1971). *Br. Poult. Sci.* **11**, 7–13.
Furr, B. J. A. and Smith, G. K. (1975). *J. Endocr.* **66**, 303–304.
Furr, B. J. A., Onuoro, G. I., Bonney, R. C. and Cunningham, F. J. (1973a). *J. Endocr.* **59**, 495–502.

Furr, B. J. A., Bonney, R. C., England, R. J. and Cunningham, F. J. (1973b). *J. Endocr.* **57**, 159–169.
Furuja, T. and Ishii, S. (1974). *Endocr. jap.* **21**, 329–334.
Fuxe, K. and Ljunggren, J. (1965). *J. comp. Neurol.* **125**, 355–382.
Godden, P. M. M. and Scanes, C. G. (1975). *Gen. comp. Endocr.* **27**, 538–542.
Goosens, N., Blasher, S. Okshe, A., Vandesande, F and Dierick, K. (1977). *Cell. Tiss. Res.* **184**, 1–13.
Green, J. D. (1951). *Am. J. Anat.* **88**, 225–311.
Greenspan, F. S., Kriss, J. P., Moses, L. E. and Lew, W. (1956). *Endocrinology* **58**, 767–776.
Hall, T. R. and Chadwick, A. (1975). *IRCS Med. Sci.* **3**, 631.
Hall, T. R. and Chadwick, A. (1976a). *Gen. comp. Endocr.* **37**, 333–342.
Hall, T. R. and Chadwick, A. (1976b). *J. Endocr.* **68**, 163–164.
Hall, T. R., Chadwick, A., Bolton, N. J. and Scanes, C. G. (1975). *Gen. comp. Endocr.* **25**, 298–306.
Hammond, R. W., Todd, T. and Hertelendy, F. (1980). *Gen. comp. Endocr.* **41**, 467–476.
Harris, G. W. (1955). "Neural Control of the Pituitary Gland" Arnold, London.
Harvey, S. and Scanes, C. G. (1977a). *J. Endocr.* **73**, 321–329.
Harvey, S. and Scanes, C. G. (1977b). *Horm. Met. Res.* **9**, 340–341.
Harvey, S. and Scanes, C. G. (1977c). *Experientia* **33**, 1242–1243.
Harvey, S. and Scanes, C. G. (1978). *Experientia* **34**, 1096–1097.
Harvey, S., Scanes, C. G. and Howe, T. (1977). *Gen. comp. Endocr.* **33**, 322–328.
Harvey, S. Scanes, C. G., Chadwick, A. and Bolton, N. J. (1978a). *Neuroendocrinology* **26**, 249–260.
Harvey, S., Scanes, C. G., Chadwick, A. and Bolton, N. J. (1978b). *J. Endocr.* **79**, 153–154.
Harvey, S., Scanes, C. G., Chadwick, A. and Bolton, N. J. (1978c). *J. Endocr.* **76**, 501–506.
Harvey, S., Scanes, C. G., Chadwick, A. and Bolton, N. J. (1979a). *Br. Poult. Sci.* **20**, 9–17.
Harvey, S., Scanes, C. G., Chadwick, A., Border, G. and Bolton, N. J. (1979b). *J. Endocr.* **82**, 193–197.
Harvey, S., Scanes, C. G., Chadwick, A. and Bolton, N. J. (1979c). *Experientia* **35**, 694–695.
Harvey, S., Chadwick, A., Border, G., Scanes, C. G. and Phillips, J. G. (1982). *In* "Aspects of Avian Endocrinology" (C. G. Scanes, M. A. Ottinger, A. D. Kenney, J. Balthazart, J. Cronshaw, and I. Chester Jones, eds), pp. 41–64. Texas Technical Press, Lubbock, Texas.
Hattori, M. and Wakabayashi, K. (1979). *Gen. comp. Endocr.* **39**, 215–221.
Hazelwood, R. L. and Lorenz, F. W. (1959). *Am. J. Physiol.* **197**, 47–51.
Hazelwood, R. L. and Hazelwood, B. S. (1961). *Proc. Soc. exp. Biol. Med.* **108**, 10–12.
Hechter, O., Terada, S., Nakahara, T., Flouret, G. and Bergman, R. N. (1978). *J. biol. Chem.* **253**, 3219–3229.
Huang, E. S. R., Kao, K. J. and Nalbandov, A. V. (1979). *Biol. Reprod.* **20**, 454–461.
Imai, K. (1973). *J. Reprod. Fert.* **33**, 91–98.
Imai, K. and Nalbandov, A. V. (1971). *Endocrinology* **88**, 1218–1223.
Ishii, S. and Yamamoto, K. (1976). *Gen. comp. Endocr.* **29**, 506–510.

Iturriza, F. C., Estivariz, F. E. and Levitin, H. P. (1980). *Gen. comp. Endocr.* **42**, 110–115.
Jackson, G. L. (1971a). *Endocrinology* **89**, 1454–1459.
Jackson, G. L. (1971b). *Endocrinology* **89**, 1460–1463.
Jackson, G. L. and Nalbandov, A. V. (1969a). *Endocrinology* **84**, 1218–1223.
Jackson, G. L. and Nalbandov, A. V. (1969b). *Endocrinology* **84**, 1262–1265.
Jackson, I. M. D. and Reichlin, S. (1974). *Endocrinology* **95**, 854–862.
Jeffcoate, S. L., Sharp, P. J., Fraser, H. M., Hall, D. T. and Gunn, A. (1974). *J. Endocr.* **62**, 85–91.
Jenkins, N., Sumpter, J. P. and Follett, B. K. (1978). *Gen. comp. Endocr.* **35**, 309–321.
Jöhl, A., Riniker, B. and Schlenkel-Hulliger, L. (1974). *FEBS Letts*, **45**, 172–174.
Jozsa, R., Scanes, C. G., Vigh, S. and Mess, B. (1979). *Gen. comp. Endocr.* **39**, 158–163.
Kalliecharan, R. (1981). *Gen. comp. Endocr.* **44**, 249–251.
Kanematsu, S. and Mikami, S. (1970). *Gen. comp. Endocr.* **14**, 25–34.
Kawashima, M. Kamiyoshi, M., and Tanaka, K. (1979). *Biol. Reprod.* **20**, 581–585.
King, J. A. and Millar, R. P. (1982). Program of the 64th Annual Meeting of the Endocrine Society.
Klandorf, H., Sharp, P. J. and Sterling, R. (1978). *Gen. comp. Endocr.* **34**, 377–379.
Kleinholz, L. H. and Rahn, H. (1940). *Anat. Rec.* **76**, 157.
Knight, P. G., Wilson, S. C., Glandwell, R. T. and Cunningham, F. J. (1982). *J. Endocr.* **94**, 295–304.
Kobayashi, H. and M. Wada. (1973). *In* "Avian Biology" (D. S. Farner and J. R. King, eds), Vol. III, pp. 287–348. Academic Press, New York and London.
Kobayashi, H., Wada, M., Ueumura, H. and Ueck, M. (1972). *Z. Zellforsch. mikrosk. Anat.* **127**, 545–551.
Koike, T. and Lepkovsky, S. (1967). *Gen. comp. Endocr.* **8**, 397–402.
Koike, T. I., Pryor, L. R., Neldon, H. L. and Venable, R. S. (1977). *Gen. comp. Endocr.* **33**, 359–364.
Koike, T. I., Pryor, L. R. and Neldon, H. L. (1979). *Gen. comp. Endocr.* **37**, 451–458.
Kompiang, I. K. and Gibson, W. R. (1976). *Horm. Met. Res.* **8**, 340–345.
Kordon, C. and Gogan, F. (1964). *C. r. Séanc. Soc. Biol.* **158**, 1759–1798.
Lamberg, B. A. (1953). *Acta med. scand. Suppl.* **279**, 1–79.
Landefeld, T. D. and Kepa, J. (1979). *Biochem. biophys. Res. Commun.* **90**, 1111–1118.
Langslow, D. R. and C. N. Hales, (1969). *J. Endocr.* **43**, 285–294.
Legait, E. and Legait, H. (1955). *C. r. Ass. Anat.* **84**, 188–199.
Legait, H. (1959). *Thèse, Louvain, Nancy.*
Li, C. H. and Chung, D. (1978). *Biochem. biophys. res. Commun.* **81**, 900–905.
Libby, D. A., Meites, J. and Schaible, J. (1955). *Poult. Sci.* **34**, 1329–1331.
Licht, P. and Papkoff, H. (1972). *Gen. comp. Endocr.* **19**, 102–114.
Licht, P., Papkoff, H., Farmer, S. W., Muller, C. H. Tsui, H. W. and Crews, D. (1977). *Recent Prog. Horm. Res.* **33**, 169–243.
Lowry, P. J. and Scott, A. P. (1975). *Gen. comp. Endocr.* **26**, 16–23.
Lowry, P. J., Bennett, H. P. J., McMartin, C. and Scott, A. P. (1974). *Biochem. J.* **141**, 427–437.
Luck, M. R. and Scanes, C. G. (1980). *Gen. comp. Endocr.* **41**, 260–265.
MacKenzie, D. (1981). *Poult. Sci.* **60**, 2136–2143.
McNeill, T. H., Kozlowski, G. P., Abel, J. H. and Zimmerman, E. A. (1976). *Endocrinology* **99**, 1323–1332.

McNeilly, A. S., Etches, R. J. and Frieson, H. G. (1978). *Acta endocr. Copenh.* **89**, 60–69.
Ma, R. C. S. and Nalbandov, A. V. (1963). *In* "Advances in Neuroendocrinology" (A. V. Nalbandov, ed.), pp. 306–311. University of Illinois Press, Urbana.
Martinez-Vargas, M. C., Stumpf, W. E. and Sar, M. (1976). *J. comp. Neurol.* **167**, 83–104.
Matsuo, H., Baba, Y., Nair, R. N. G., Arimura, A. and Schally, A. V. (1971). *Biochem. biophys. Res. Comm.* **43**, 1334–1339.
Maung, Z. W. and Follett, B. K. (1977). *Gen. comp. Endocr.* **33**, 242–253.
Maung, S. L. and Follett, B. K. (1978). *Gen. comp. Endocr.* **36**, 79–89.
Mikami, S. (1969). *Gunma Symp. Endocr.* **6**, 151–170.
Mikami, S. (1980). *In* "Biological Rhythms in Birds: Neural and Endocrine Aspects" (Y. Tanuabe, K. Tanaka and T. Ookawa, eds). pp. 17–32. Springer-Verlag, Berlin.
Mikami, S., Hashikawa, T. and Farner, D. S. (1973). *Z. Zellforsch. mikrosk. Anat.* **138**, 299–314.
Mitchell, M. E. (1970). *J. Reprod. Fert.* **22**, 233–241.
Morrell, J. I., Kelley, D. B. and Pfaff, D. W. (1975). *J. comp. Neurol.* **164**, 63–78.
Munsick, R. A., Sawyer, W. H. and van Dyke, H. B. (1960). *Endocrinology* **66**, 860–871.
Myers, W. R. and Fleck, A. (1974). *Poult. Sci.* **53**, 508–514.
Myers, W. R. and Peterson, R. A. (1974). *Poult. Sci.* **53**, 508–514.
Nakanishi, S., Inoue, A., Kita, T., Nakamura, M., Chang, A. C. Y., Cohen, S. N. and Numa, S. (1979). *Nature. Lond.* **278**, 423–427.
Nalbandov, A. V. and Card, L. E. (1943). *J. exp. Zool.* **94**, 387–415.
Naudé, R. J. and Oelofsen, W. (1977). *Biochem. J.* **165**, 519–523.
Naudé, R. J., Oelofsen, W. and Maske, R. (1980). *Biochem. J.* **187**, 245–248.
Naudé, R. J., Chung, D., Li, C. H. and Oelofsen, W. (1981). *Biochem. biophys. res. Commun.* **98**, 108–114.
Nelson, D. M., Norton, H. W. and Nalbandov, A. V. (1965). *Endocrinology* **77**, 889–896.
Nicoll, C. S. (1967). *Endocrinology* **80**, 641–655.
Nicoll, C. S. and Licht, P. (1971). *Gen. comp. Endocr.* **17**, 490–507.
Nicoll, C. S. and Nichols, C. W. (1971). *Gen. comp. Endocr.* **17**, 300–310.
Nicoll, C. S., Parsons, J. A., Fiorindo, R. P. and Nicholls, C. W. (1969). *J. Endocr.* **45**, 183–196.
North, W. G. and Mitchell, T. I. (1981). *FEBS Lett.* **126**, 41–44.
Ogle, T. F. and Kitay, J. I. (1979). *Endocrinology* **104**, 40–44.
Oksche, A. and Farner, D. S. (1974). *Ergebn. Anat. EntwGesch.* **48/4**, 1–136.
Opel, H. (1964). *Endocrinology* **74**, 193–200.
Opel, H. (1966). *Anat. Rec.* **154**, 396.
Papkoff, H., Farmer, S. W. and Licht, P. (1976). *Endocrinology* **98**, 767–777.
Peterson, A. J. and Common, R. H. (1971). *Can. J. Zool.* **49**, 599–604.
Petersen, A. J. and Common, R. H. (1972). *Can. J. Zool.* **50**, 395–404.
Pierce, J. G. (1971). *Endocrinology* **89**, 1331–1344.
Pierce, J. G., Faith, M. R., Giudice, L. C. and Reeve, J. R. (1976). *In* "Polypeptide Hormones: Molecular and Cellular Aspects" (R. Porter and D W. Fitzsimons, eds), pp. 225–250. Elsevier/Excerpta Medica/North-Holland, Amsterdam.
Rabii, J., Buonomo, F. C. and Scanes C G. (1981). *J. Endocr.* **90**, 355–358.
Radke, W. J. and Chiasson, R. B. (1974). *J. Endocr.* **60**, 187–188.
Radke, W. J. and Chiasson, R. B. (1975). *Gen. comp. Endocr.* **26**, 274–276.

Raffel, L. J., Buss, E. G. and Clagett, C. O. (1976). *Poult. Sci.* **55**, 1834–1840.
Rahn, H. and Painter, B. T. (1941). *Anat. Rec.* **79**, 297–311.
Ralph, C. L. (1959). *Anat. Rec.* **134**, 411–431.
Ralph, C. L. and Fraps, R. M. (1959a). *Endocrinology* **65**, 819–824.
Ralph, C. L. and Fraps, R. M. (1959b). *Am. J. Physiol.* **197**, 1279–1283.
Ralph, C. L. and Fraps, R. M. (1960). *Endocrinology* **66**, 269–272.
Rao, A. J., Long, J. A. and Ramachandran, J. (1978). *Endocrinology* **102**, 371–378.
Ravona, H., Snapir, N. and Perek, M. (1973). *Gen. comp. Endocr.* **20**, 112–124.
Reeves, R. R., Arimura, A. and Schally, A. V. (1971a). *J. Anim. Sci.* **32**, 123–126.
Reeves, J. J., Arimura, A. and Schally, A. V. (1971b). *Biol. Reprod.* **4**, 88–92.
Reeves, J. J., Harrison, P. C. and Casey, J. M. (1973). *Poult. Sci.* **52**, 1883–1886.
Riddle, O., Bates, R. W. and Lahr, E. L. (1935). *Am. J. Physiol.* **111**, 352–360.
Riniker, B., Sieber, P., Rittel, W. and Zuber, H. (1972). *Nature, New Biol.* **235**, 114–115.
Robinson, G. A. Wasnidge, D. C., Floto, F. and Downie, S. E. (1976). *Poult. Sci.* **55**, 1665–1671.
Rosenbloom, A. A. and Fisher, D. A. (1974). *Endocrinology* **95**, 1726–1732.
Rothchild, I. and Fraps, R. M. (1949). *Endocrinology* **44**, 141–149.
Russell, J. T., Brownstein, M. J. and Gainer, H. (1980). *Endocrinology* **107**, 1880–1891.
Rzasa, J., Niezgoda, J. and Kahl, S. (1974). *Br. Poult. Sci.* **15**, 261–265.
Saeki, Y. and Tanabe, Y. (1954). *Poult. Sci.* **34**, 909–919.
Saffran, M. and Schally, A. V. (1955a). *Endocrinology* **56**, 523–532.
Saffran, M. and Schally, A. V. (1955b). *Can. J. Bioch. Physiol.* **33**, 408–415.
Sakai, H. and Ishii, S. (1980). *Gen. comp. Endocr.* **42**, 1–8.
Sawyer, W. H. (1966). *In* "The Pituitary Gland" (G. W. Harris and B. T. Donovan, eds), Vol. 3, pp. 307–329. Butterworths, London.
Sawyer, W. H. (1977). *Fedn Proc. Fedn Am. Socs. exp. Biol.* **36**, 1842–1847.
Scanes, C. G. (1972). Ph.D. thesis, University of Wales.
Scanes, C. G. (1974). *Neuroendocrinology* **15**, 1–9.
Scanes, C. G. and Fagioli, J. H. (1980). *Gen. comp. Endocr.* **41**, 1–17.
Scanes, C. G. and Follett, B. K. (1972). *Br. Poult. Sci.* **13**, 603–610.
Scanes, C. G. and Follett, B. K. (1973). *J. Endocr.* **58**, 125–126.
Scanes, C. G. and Harvey, S. (1981a). *Horm. Met. Res.* **12**, 641–642.
Scanes, C. G. and Harvey, S. (1981b). *Life Sci.* **28**, 2895–2902.
Scanes, C. G. and Harvey, S. (1984). *Experientia* (in press).
Scanes, C. G., Telfer, S. B., Hackett, A. F., Nightingale, R. and Sharifuddin, B. A. K. (1975a). *Br. Poult. Sci.* **16**, 405–408.
Scanes, C. G., Bolton, N. J. and Chadwick, A. (1975). *Gen. comp. Endocr.* **27**, 371–379.
Scanes, C. G., Chadwick, A. and Bolton, N. J. (1976a). *Gen. comp. Endocr.* **30**, 12–20.
Scanes, C. F., Gales, L., Harvey, S., Chadwick, A. and Newcomer, W. S. (1976b). *Gen. comp. Endocr.* **30**, 419–423.
Scanes, C. G., Harvey, S. and Chadwick, A. (1976c). *IRCS Med. Sci.* **4**, 371.
Scanes, C. G., Godden, P. M. M. and Sharp, P. J. (1977a). *J. Endocr.* **73**, 473–481.
Scanes, C. G., Harvey, S. and Chadwick, A. (1977b). *In* "Growth and Poultry Meat Production" (K. N. Boorman and B. J. Wilson, eds), pp. 79–85. British Poultry Science Ltd, Edinburgh.
Scanes, C. G., Sharp, P. J. and Chadwick, A. (1977c). *J. Endocr.* **72**, 401–402.
Scanes, C. G., Harvey, S., Bolton, N. J. and Chadwick, N. J (1978). *IRCS Med. Sci.* **6**, 58.

Scanes, C. G., van Middelkoop, J. H., Sharp, P. J. and Harvey, S. (1980). *Poult. Sci.* **59**, 159–163.
Scanes, C. G., Buonomo, F. C. and Griminger, P. (1981). *Proc. Soc. exp. Biol. Med.* **168**, 334–337.
Scanes, C. G., Rabii, J. and Buonomo, F. C. (1982). *In* "Aspects of Avian Endocrinology" (C. G. Scanes, M. A. Ottinger, A. Kenny, J. Cronshaw, I. Chester-Jones and J. Balthazart, eds) pp. 13–31. Texas Tech University Press.
Schally, A. V., Arimura, A., Kastin, A. J., Matsuo, H., Baba, Y., Redding, T. W., Nair, R. M. G., Debeljuk, L. and White W. F. (1971). *Science, N.Y.* **173**, 1036–1038.
Senior, B. E. and Cunningham, F. J. (1974). *J. Endocr.* **60**, 201–202.
Shahabi, N. A., Bahr, J. M. and Nalbandov, A. V. (1975). *Endocrinology* **96**, 969–972.
Shani, J., Furr, B. J. A. and Forsyth, I. A. (1973). *J. Reprod. Fert.* **34**, 167–170.
Sharp, P. J. and Follett, B. K. (1968). *Z. Zellforsch. mikrosk. Anat.* **90**, 245–262.
Sharp, P. J. and Follett, B. K. (1970). *In* "Aspects of Neuroendocrinology" (W. Bargman and B. Scharrer, eds), pp. 95–103. Springer Verlag, Berlin.
Sharp, P. J., Culbert, J. and Wells, J. W. (1977). *J. Endocr.* **74**, 467–476.
Sharp, P. J., Scanes, C. G. and Gilbert, A. B. (1978). *Gen. comp. Endocr.* **34**, 296–299.
Sharp, P. J., Chaisson, R. B., El Tounsy, M. M., Klandorf, H. and Radke, W. J. (1979a). *Cell Tiss. Res.* **198**, 53–63.
Sharp, P. J., Scanes, C. G., Williams, J. B., Harvey, S. and Chadwick, A. (1979b). *J. Endocr.* **80**, 51–57.
Shellabarger, C. J. (1954). *J. appl. Physiol.* **6**, 721–723.
Shirley, H. V. and Nalbandov, A. V. (1956). *Endocrinology* **58**, 477–483.
Smyth, D. G. and Zakarian, S. (1980). *Nature, Lond.* **288**, 613–615.
Smyth, D. G., Massey, D. E., Zakarian, S. and Finnie, M. D. A. (1979). *Nature, Lond.* **279**, 252–254.
Soloff, M. S., Schroeder, B. T., Chakraborty, J. and Pearlmutter, A. F. (1977). *Fedn Proc. Fedn Am. Socs. exp. Biol.* **36**, 1861–1866.
Stainer, I. M. and Holmes, W. N. (1969). *Gen. comp. Endocr.* **12**, 350–359.
Sterling, R. J. and Sharp, P. J. (1982). *Cell. Tiss. Res.* **222**, 283–298.
Stetson, M. H. (1972a). *Gen. comp. Endocr.* **19**, 37–47.
Stetson, M. H. (1972b). *J. Reprod. Fert.* **31**, 205–213.
Stewart, M. and Stewart, F. (1977). *J. mol. Biol.* **116**, 175–179.
Stockell Hartree, A. and Cunningham, F. J. (1969). *J. Endocr.* **43**, 609–616.
Stockell Hartree, A. and Cunningham F. J. (1971). *In* "Physiology and Biochemistry of the Domestic Fowl" (D. J. Bell and B. M. Freeman, eds), pp. 426–457. Academic Press, London and New York.
Sturkie, P. D. and Lin, Y. C. (1966). *J. Endocr.* **35**, 325–326.
Tai, S. W. and Chadwick, A. (1977). *Proc. Leeds phil. lit. Soc.* **10**, 209–220.
Tanaka, K. and Nakajo, S. (1962). *Endocrinology* **70**, 453–458.
Tanaka, K., Kamiyoshi, M. and Tagami, M. (1969). *Poult. Sci.* **48**, 1985–1987.
Tanaka, K., Kamiyoshi, M. and Tanabe, Y. (1971). *Poult. Sci.* **50**, 63–66.
Thommes, R. C. and Hylka, V. W. (1978). *Gen. comp. Endocr.* **34**, 193–200.
Thompson, D. F., Taylor, R. L. and Burt, D. R. (1981). *Gen. comp. Endocr.* **44**, 77–81.
Tienhoven, A. van and Schally, A. V. (1972). *Gen. comp. Endocr.* **19**, 594–595.
Tienhoven, A. van, Nalbandov, A. V. and Norton, H. W. (1954). *Endocrinology* **54**, 605–611.

Tixier-Vidal, A. and Follett, B. K. (1973). *In* "Avian Biology" (D. S. Farner and J. R. King, eds), Vol. 3, pp. 110–182. Academic Press, New York and London.
Tonoue, T. and Kitoh, J. (1978). *Endocr. jap.* **25**, 105–109.
Undenfriend, S. (1981). *Biochem. Soc. Trans.* **9**, 23P.
Vale, W., Leng, N., Rivier, J., Villareal, J., Rivier, C., Douglas, C. and Brown, M. (1976). *Metabolism* **25** (Suppl.), 1491–1494.
Vale, W., Spiess, J., Rivier, C. and Rivier, J. (1981). *Science N.Y.* **213**, 1394–1397.
Wada, M. (1972). *Z. Zellforsch. mikrosk. Anat.* **124**, 507–519.
Wallis, M. (1975). *Biol. Rev.* **50**, 35–98.
Wentworth, B. S., Burke, W. H. and Birrenkoff, G. P. (1976). *Gen. comp. Endocr.* **29**, 119–127.
Wilson, S. C. (1978). *Gen. comp. Endocr.* **35**, 481–490.
Wilson, S. C. and Sharp, P. J. (1973). *J. Reprod. Fert.* **35**, 561–564.
Wilson, S. C. and Sharp, P. J. (1975a). *J. Endocr.* **64**, 77–86.
Wilson, S. C. and Sharp, P. J. (1975b). *J. Endocr.* **67**, 59–70.
Wilson, S. C. and Sharp, P. J. (1976). *J. Endocr.* **71**, 87–98.
Wingstrand, K. G. (1951). "The Structure and Development of the Avian Pituitary", Gleerup, Lund.

4 The Thyroid Glands

I. R. FALCONER

School of Biological Sciences, University of New England, Armidale, Australia

I. Introduction

The major developments in avian thyroid research during the seventies and early eighties have been in the fields related to the impact of the environment on the bird. In particular, variations in thyroid function during the diurnal rhythm, during changes in ambient temperature and during stressful stimuli have received attention. The complex issue of the relationship of the thyroid to food intake has also been scrutinized.

PHYSIOLOGY BIOCHEMISTRY DOMESTIC FOWL, VOL. 5 ISBN 0–12–267105–8

II. Basic Thyroid Physiology

A. Ultrastructure

The ultrastructure of the thyroid of the domestic fowl is very similar to that of mammals (French and Hodges, 1977). This is to be expected, since thyroid function developed in the earliest vertebrates, and so occurs in all the vertebrates (Barrington, 1979).

B. Thyrotrophin-releasing Hormone

In 1970, a hormone originating in the hypothalamus was found, which controlled the pituitary secretion of thyroid stimulating hormone (TSH) in the mammal (Burgus *et al.*, 1970). Subsequently, it was shown that this hormone, named thyrotrophin-releasing hormone, will also cause the release of TSH from the avian pituitary (Scanes, 1974). Administration of 100 ng of thyrotrophin-releasing hormone to laying hens increased circulating thyroxine (T_4) and triiodothyronine (T_3) concentrations, both reaching a peak about one hour after injection, although only the T_3 increase was statistically significant (Klandorf *et al.*, 1978b). It is reasonable to conclude that in the bird the control of TSH release and subsequent thyroid activation is essentially the same as in mammals.

The TSH molecule contains two subunits, one (α) which is in common with the α-subunit of the gonadotrophins and the other (β) which provides the hormone specificity. This β-subunit has an immunological resemblance in both the mammals and birds. Studies in the domestic drake have established that the TSH-containing cells are mostly found in the rostral (beak) lobe of the anterior pituitary (Sharp *et al.*, 1979).

C. Thyroid Hormones and their Transport

One major difference between birds and mammals in thyroid function is in the serum transport of T_4 and T_3. Mammals possess a thyroid-hormone binding α_2-globulin which has a high affinity and capacity for T_4 in particular. It is not present in birds. As a consequence, mammalian blood contains 80–100 ng ml^{-1} of T_4, compared with 10–15 ng ml^{-1} in hens (Klandorf *et al.*, 1978b), and more than 99·5% of circulating mammalian T_4 is protein-bound. Studies of protein-binding of T_4 and T_3 in avian blood have shown 70–75% of protein-bound T_4 to be in the albumin, with about 10% in α-globulin and the remainder largely in pre-albumin (Davison *et al.*, 1978). The proportion of circulating T_4 bound to proteins in avian blood is lower than in mammals due to lower binding affinities of the plasma proteins, leading to a shorter half-life in birds (138 min—Davison, 1978) than in goats (20 to 30 h—Abdullah and Falconer, 1977). Triiodothyronine is the quantitatively minor form of thyroid hormone in circulation in birds or mammals, with a concentration of about 1 ng ml^{-1} in hen plasma (Klandorf *et al.*, 1978b). It is, however, highly important in the physiological response to thyroid stimulation (see Section IV).

III. Thyroid Function and Growth

The function of the thyroid during hatching has been studied by Davison (1976), who showed a marked peak in T_4 concentration (30 ng ml^{-1}) in the 1-day-old chick and a decline thereafter. The ratio of T_4 to T_3 at this time was 4:1, which is a higher proportion of T_3 than is seen in adult hens (about 10:1). Significant increases in metabolic rate and in the concentrations of T_4 and T_3 in the plasma have been observed during pipping and hatching in the turkey. After emergence from the shell the plasma concentrations of both hormones decreased, but the ratio of T_4 to T_3 showed an elevation of T_3 in the hatched as compared to unhatched chick (Christensen *et al.*, 1982). Between 3 and 9 weeks of age cockerels showed no significant changes in circulating T_4, which averaged 20 ng ml^{-1}. Plasma T_3 showed a reduction over this period from 3 ng ml^{-1} to about 1·5 ng ml^{-1} at 9 weeks (Chiasson *et al.*, 1979).

Suppression of thyroid secretion by feeding methimazole (1%) in the diet decreased the concentration of T_4 and T_3 in the plasma, and significantly reduced growth of broiler cockerels (Chaisson *et al.*, 1979). Injection of propylthiouracil to growing cockerels reduced body weight, muscle weight and bone length, effects that were reversed by the administration of thyroxine (King and King, 1973). Thyroidectomy, as would be expected, also significantly reduced growth (Davison *et al.*, 1980). Related studies in the sheep showed a curvilinear relationship between growth rate and thyroid function in animals fed *ad libitum*. At the hypothyroidic end of the range of thyroid activities growth was limited, presumably due to the reduction of metabolic rate in hypothyroidism. At the hyperthyroidic end of the range a decrease in growth also occurred (Draper *et al.*, 1968). It is likely that over a fairly wide range of thyroid activities growth rate is independent of the thyroid, and influenced primarily by food intake and composition. However, under conditions of hypo- or hyperthyroidism of genetic or nutritional origin, growth retardation may occur.

Malnutrition has a depressing effect on the thyroid secretion in domestic animals and birds, which is assumed to be exerted at the level of the secretion of TSH (Abdullah and Falconer, 1977; Penn and Huston, 1968; Poczopko *et al.*,

1977). Withdrawal of food initially leads to a decrease in the concentration of T_3 in the blood, probably reflecting higher rates of utilization of this hormone (May, 1978). A 4-h delay in the regular daily feeding of quail resulted in decreased plasma T_4 and T_3 concentrations, without changing the plasma TSH. The authors concluded that the altered thyroid hormone concentrations were not a consequence of changes in pituitary secretion and hence imply altered metabolism of the hormones (Almeida and Thomas, 1981). Wide variations in dietary iodide can be tolerated by growing chickens; Newcomer (1978) added 0 to 100 $\mu g I^-$ per g to a semi-synthetic diet and observed normal growth in all groups, though thyroid gland activity changed markedly to compensate for the lack of availability of iodide in the groups fed on the diets containing least iodide.

IV. Thyroid Function and the Environment

A. Photoperiod and Diurnal Variation

Krebietke (1975a,b,c) examined diurnal changes in thyroid activity in 4- or 5-week-old cockerels exposed to a normal light period from 05.00 to 20.00 h. A maximum uptake of ^{131}I was observed at 03.00 h, when maxima of thyroid colloid content and circulating protein-bound ^{131}I were also present. A minimum of protein-bound ^{131}I was observed at 12.00 h, rising to a second peak at 21.00 h. More detailed investigations, in which plasma T_4 and T_3 were measured independently in chickens on a very similar regime (14 h light, 10 h dark), showed clear sinusoidal variations in both T_3 and T_4 concentration, which were effectively opposite to each other. The T_4 concentration peak occurred at 04.00 h (11·5 ng ml^{-1}), coincident with the minimum T_3 concentration of 1·5 ng ml^{-1}. Measurements of heart rate also showed a marked sinusoidal pattern resembling that of T_3 concentration, indicating T_3 is the metabolically active hormone in the fowl (Klandorf *et al.*, 1978a). Further work (Klandorf *et al.*, 1981), in which hens were held at 20°C or 32°C and subjected to 14 h light—10 h dark, showed that the higher temperature depressed heat production and plasma T_3 concentration, but not T_4 concentration. Fasting also depressed heat production and plasma T_3 concentration. They concluded that plasma T_3 concentration was directly related to metabolic rate in the hen. A possible interpretation of the authors' data is that thyroid secretion and iodide uptake increase during the dark period to a maximum just before dawn. Progressive deiodination of T_4 and T_3 occurs in peripheral tissues during the light period, corresponding to increased heart rate and resulting in peak concentration of T_3 about 12.00 h. Thereafter, the decreased T_4 concentration reduces the production of T_3 until the secretion of T_4 rises again during the dark period.

It is of interest that cockerels held under constant darkness for 32 days had greater T_3 concentrations than birds held under a 14-h light: 10-h dark regime (Osol *et al.*, 1980), and that surgical removal of the pineal had no effect on T_4 and T_3 concentrations.

B. Influence of Cold and Hot Environments

In a study of the response of the quail to cold (−1 to −6°C) and warmth (34 to 35°C) ambient temperatures over a period of 48 h, Bobek *et al.* (1980) found that blood flow through the thyroid increased sharply within two hours of cold exposure, returning to almost the initial rate by 48 h. Thyroxine concentration decreased from 14 ng ml^{-1} to 10 ng ml^{-1} initially, and then increased to 18 ng ml^{-1} by 12 h. Triiodothyronine concentration increased three-fold in the first two hours, then decreased to a steady concentration about twice the initial value. Oxygen consumption was approximately doubled during the second 24 h of cold exposure.

The data are consistent with a rapid increase in metabolism of T_4 to T_3 immediately on cold exposure. This is supported by the decreased half life of T_4, and increased plasma inorganic iodide observed in chicks exposed to cold (7·2°C) by May *et al.* (1974). Less severe cold exposure was also shown to increase T_3 concentration in chicks, during a progressive decline in temperature from 26·5°C to 17·5°C. In these experiments, T_4 concentration was only seen to increase after the temperature was reduced to 12·5°C (Kuhn and Nouwen, 1978). An intravenous injection of 25 ng of thyrotrophin-releasing hormone was shown to increase both T_3 and T_4 in a manner similar to acute exposure of chicks to 10°C. Persistent cold stress induced 80% defeathering of hens, resulting in increased heat production, thyroid mass and plasma T_4 concentration (Pietras, 1981).

The cold response is thus comparable to that seen in mammals, in which a rapid activation of the thyroid occurs through TSH release from the pituitary (Williams *et al.*, 1977) stimulating the increased secretion of thyroid hormones, and compensating increase in hormone synthesis. This was also recorded in chickens, by measurement of the conversion of inorganic to organic iodine during cold exposure (Jastrzebski and Barowicz, 1975).

The increased conversion of T_4 to T_3 and raised oxygen consumption are components of the metabolic adaptation to cold. The essential nature of this role of the thyroid was demonstrated by Davison *et al.* (1980), who showed that thyroidectomized 4- to 5-week-old chicks could not maintain body temperature at an ambient temperature of 12°C, and even at 30°C had depressed heat production and body temperature.

Exposure of quail to 34°C–35°C decreased thyroid blood flow and plasma T_4

concentrations. Triiodothyronine concentration fluctuated over a narrow range with no clear trend, although oxygen consumption was clearly reduced by 48 h of exposure to warm temperature (Bobek *et al.*, 1980). Moss and Balnave (1978) measured plasma thyroxine and thyroid weight in chicks kept at 22°C (normal) and 30°C for 28 days. They observed a progressive increase in T_4 from 8·0 ng mg^{-1} to 17·5 ng mg^{-1} in birds at 30°C compared to 8·0 ng mg^{-1} to 8·6 ng mg^{-1} in birds at 22°C. This was associated with a 30% reduction in thyroid weight to 36 mg kg^{-1} body weight at the higher temperature

Since thyroid weight is likely to reflect TSH stimulation of the gland over this period, it is probable that the thyroid secretion rate had actually decreased at the higher temperature, possibly due to feedback from the raised circulating T_4. The increased concentration of T_4 could be due to decreased peripheral metabolism to T_3, as a result of the elevated temperature or the reduced food intake. These experiments point to the deceptive nature of measurements of circulating hormone concentrations, which may change reciprocally to the actual rate of hormone secretion and gland activity. When food intake changes in an experiment, as occurred in the experiments of Moss and Balnave (1978), the enterohepatic circulation of thyroxine also changes, leading to increased conservation of T_4 at a reduced food intake (Abdullah and Falconer, 1977).

Other experimenters have observed similar effects, indicating a suppression of thyroid activity at elevated temperatures (Chiasson and Combest, 1979; Cogburn and Harrison, 1980).

V. Seasonal Changes in Thyroid Function

While the commercial poultry producer endeavours to standardize the environment as far as possible, it is of interest to observe the natural seasonal fluctuations of thyroid activity in a feral population of birds. In Ruffed grouse (*Bonasa umbellus*), both T_4 and T_3 concentrations in the plasma were least during the cold winter months and increased sharply at the onset of gonadal development in early spring. The peak concentrations occurred at about the time of egg laying and incubation, and T_3 in particular showed a fall during the brooding-moulting period in mid- to late-summer (Garbutt *et al.*, 1979). The apparent difference between these data, and those for chicks and hens exposed to cold, may reflect the slow physiological adaptation to cold in a natural environment, in which hormone utilization may rise considerably, together with increased secretion, while plasma concentrations actually fall.

VI. Thyroid Responses to Non-specific Stressors

With increasing refinements in techniques for measuring endocrine function, many investigators have become concerned that simply handling their experimental animals or birds causes changes to the indices of function that are being measured. That the thyroid gland is highly susceptible to a variety of non-injurious stressors, such as mild fright (Falconer and Hetzel, 1964) and restraint (Falconer, 1976), has been known for some years. In the fowl, several investigations have shown effects of handling on plasma thyroid hormone concentrations (Klandorf *et al.*, 1978b; Bobek *et al.*, 1980); they indicate an inhibition of secretion due to repeated bleeding or to a new environment. Similarly, the effect of immobilizing hens was a fall in plasma T_3 from 3–4 ng ml^{-1} to 0·5–2·0 ng ml^{-1}, within 3 to 5 h, and an increase in plasma corticosterone. Even the stress of crowding hens in battery cages significantly reduced plasma T_3 concentration and affected behaviour during the first week, but after two weeks both T_3 and behaviour patterns had returned to normal (Wodzicka-Tomaszewska *et al.*, 1980).

In these changes, the fowl shows a thyroid inhibition in response to stress similar to that seen in the laboratory rabbit (Brown-Grant *et al.*, 1954) and quite different to that in the sheep, in which an initial activation of the gland has been observed (Falconer and Hetzel, 1964). Where dietary changes also occur as a result of stress, experimental results can be further affected by changes in iodide supply and in hydration of the bird.

References

Abdullah, R. and Falconer, I. R. (1977). *Aust. J. biol. Sci.* **30**, 207–215.

Almeida, D. F. X. and Thomas, D. H. (1981). *Gen. comp. Endocr.* **44**, 508–513.

Barrington, E. J. W. (1979). "Hormones and Evolution". Academic Press, New York and London.

Bobek, S., Neizgoda, J., Pietras, M., Kacinska, M. and Ewy, Z. (1980). *Gen. comp. Endocr.* **40**, 201–210.

Brown-Grant, K., Harris, G. W. and Reichlin, S. (1954). *J. Physiol., Lond.* **126**, 29–40.

Burgus, R., Dunn, T. F., Desiderio, D., Ward, D. M., Vale, W. and Guillemin, R. (1970). *Nature, Lond.* **226**, 321–325.

Chiasson, R. V., Sharp, P. J., Klandorf, H., Scanes, C. G. and Harvey, S. (1978). *Poult. Sci.* **58**, 1575–1583.

Chiasson, R. B. and Combest, W. L. (1979). *Life Sci.* **25**, 1551–1556.

Christensen, V. L., Biellier, H. V. and Forward, J. F. (1982). *Poult. Sci.* **61**, 367–374.

Cogburn, L. A. and Harrison, P. C. (1980). *Poult. Sci.* **59**, 1132–1141.

Davison, T. F. (1976). *Gen. comp. Endocr.* **29**, 21–27.

Davison, T. F. (1978). *Gen. comp. Endocr.* **36**, 380–387.

Davison, T. F., Flack, I. H. and Butler, E. J. (1978). *Res. vet. Sci.* **25**, 280–283.

Davison, T. F., Misson, B. H. and Freeman, B. M. (1980). *J. therm. Biol.* **5**, 197–202.

Draper, S. A., Falconer, I. R. and Lamming, G. E. (1968). *J. Physiol., Lond.* **197**, 659–665.

Falconer, I. R. (1976). *Aust. J. biol. Sci.* **29**, 117–123.

Falconer, I. R. and Hetzel, B. S. (1964). *Endocrinology* **75**, 42–48.
French, E. I. and Hodges, R. D. (1977). *Cell Tiss. Res.* **178**, 397–410.
Garbutt, A., Leatherland, J. F. and Middleton, A. L. A. (1979). *Can. J. Zool.* **57**, 2022–2027.
Jastrzebski, M. and Barowicz, T. (1975). *Pol. Arch. Wet.* **18**, 87–95.
King, D. B. and King, C. R. (1973). *Gen. comp. Endocr.* **21**, 517–529.
Klandorf, H. P., Sharp, J. and Duncan, I. J. H. (1978a). *Gen. comp. Endocr.* **36**, 238–243.
Klandorf, J., Sharp, P. J. and Sterling, R. (1978b). *Gen. comp. Endocr.* **34**, 377–379.
Klandorf, H., Sharp, P. J. and Macleod, M. G. (1981). *Gen. comp. Endocr.* **45**, 513–520.
Krebietke, P. (1975a). *Endocrinology* **65**, 34–41.
Krebietke, P. (1975b). *Endocrinology* **65**, 42–52.
Krebietke, P. (1975c). *Endocrinology* **65**, 53–59.
Kuhn, E. R. and Nouwen, E. J. (1978). *Gen. comp. Endocr.* **34**, 336–342.
May, J. D. (1978). *Gen. comp. Endocr.* **34**, 323–327.
May, J. D., Kubena, L. F. and Deaton, J. W. (1974). *Poult. Sci.* **53**, 687–691.
Moss, B. and Balnave, D. (1978). *Comp. Biochem. Physiol.* **60B**, 157–161.
Newcomer, W. S. (1978). *Am. J. Physiol.* **234**, E168–E176.
Osol, J. G., Foss, D. C. and Carew, L. B., Jr. (1980). *Poult. Sci.* **59**, 647–653.
Penn, R. P. and Huston, T. M. (1968). *Poult. Sci.* **47**, 1432–1437.
Pietras, M. (1981). *Acta physiol., pol.* **32**, 455–460.
Poczopko, P., Keller, J., Piekarzewska, A. and Witkowska, H. (1977). *Bull. Acad pol.* 423–427.
Scanes, C. G. (1974). *Neuroendocrinology* **15**, 1–9.
Sharp, P. J., Chiasson, R. B., El Tounsey, M. M., Klandorf, H. and Radke, W. J. (1979). *Cell Tiss. Res.* **198**, 53–63.
Singh, Ajit, Reineke, E. P. and Ringer, R. K. (1968). *Poult. Sci.* **47**, 212–219.
Williams, D. D., Marques, P., Illner, P., Steiner, R. A., Green, W. L., Davis, S. O., Kendall, J. W., Johnson, D. G. and Gale, C. C. (1977). *In* "Drugs, Biogenic Amines and Body Temperature" (K. E. Cooper, P. Lomas and E. Schoenbaum, eds) pp. 62–65. Karger, Basal.
Wodzicka-Tomaszewska, M., Cumming, R. B. and Stelmasiak, T. (1980). *S. Pacific Poult. Sci. Conv.*, 171–176.

5 The Endocrine Pancreas: Control of Secretions and Actions of the Hormones

G. CRAMB[1] and D. R. LANGSLOW[2]

[1]*Department of Physiology and Pharmacology, University of St Andrews, Scotland*
[2]*Chief Scientist's Team, Nature Conservancy Council, Huntingdon, England*

PHYSIOLOGY BIOCHEMISTRY DOMESTIC FOWL, VOL. 5 ISBN 0–12–267105–8

I. Introduction

Early experiments involving pancreatectomy in the bird indicated that the avian dependence on pancreatic hormone action was qualitatively different from that in the mammal. The post-operative hypoglycaemia found after total pancreatectomy in the bird resulted in questions being asked about the role of the pancreatic hormones, particularly insulin, in the control of carbohydrate metabolism. Only in the past few years, with the development of new techniques *in vitro*, has information become available concerning the direct control of pancreatic hormone secretion, as well as the molecular mechanisms of hormone action in tissues isolated from birds. The main aim of this chapter is to review these experiments although reference has been made to the earlier observations *in vivo* where relevant. This review is predominantly concerned with experiments carried out using the domestic fowl. However, it was often necessary, for comparative purposes, to refer to experiments carried out on other birds, such as the duck and goose, as well as to the well documented results from mammalian systems.

II. Structure of the Endocrine Pancreas

Both phylogenetic and ontogenetic studies indicate that the vertebrate endocrine pancreas has evolved from the gastro-intestinal tract (Falkmer and Patent, 1972; Pictet and Rutter, 1972; Falkmer and Ostberg, 1977; Bonner-Weir and Weir, 1979). The avian pancreas, situated in the duodenal loop, comprises three morphologically distinct lobes; splenic, dorsal and ventral. In some species, including the chicken, an additional lobe, confusingly named the "third lobe", is found between the dorsal and ventral lobes (Oakberg, 1949; Mikami and Ono, 1962).

Histologically, the endocrine parenchyma is composed of several types of granulated cells, which are distributed in defined heterogeneous clusters, interspersed between a labyrinth of vascular capillaries. Due to this physical arrangement of cells and capillaries, these regions were designated the Islets (or Islands) of Langerhans, after the anatomy was first described by Paul Langerhans in 1869.

In birds, the islets of Langerhans are larger and more numerous in the splenic and third lobes than in the dorsal or vental lobes of the pancreas. The cellular composition and distribution is markedly different from other vertebrates, with minimal variations between species. In all birds so far studied, the cell composition of the islet depends on its position within the lobes. Due to these regional differences, islets have been grouped into three types. This classification is unduly complicated by the same Greek symbols being used for both the islet and individual cell types. This, however, has been circumvented by a second classification system for the cells. The dark, or α, islets comprise predominantly A(α_2)- and D(α_1)-cells; the light, or β, islets comprise mainly B(β)-cells, with smaller numbers of D(α_1) cells and the occasional A(α_2)-cell; and the mixed islets contain significant numbers of all three cell types.

In the chicken, dark islets are almost exclusively restricted to the splenic and third lobes, whereas the light islets are distributed evenly throughout the gland (Oakberg, 1949; Mikami and Ono, 1962). Several other species also show a preponderance of dark islets in the splenic lobe, although dark islets are also found in the other lobes (Guha and Gosh, 1978). Immunochemical studies indicate that the larger light islets of the third and splenic lobes have a cell ratio of 80B:10A:10D, whereas the smaller light islets of the dorsal and ventral lobes have a cell ratio of 75B:25D (Bonner-Weir and Weir, 1979).

The A-cells contain small, uniformly sized granules containing glucagon. The D-cells also have a characteristic granular composition and contain somatostatin. Compared with mammals, the avian pancreas contains a relatively large number of these cell types (Guha and Gosh, 1978). The B-cells contain insulin and are easily distinguished under the electron microscope by the crystalline zinc–insulin cores within the granules. Other cell types are also present in the endocrine parenchyma but their functions and composition have not been so well investigated. The PP, or F, cells are found singly or in small groups around the islets of the dorsal and ventral lobes, particularly in the duodenal area (Larsson *et al.*, 1974; Aluments *et al.*, 1978), with few, if any, elsewhere (Bonner-Weir and Weir, 1979). Their granulated appearance is very similar to that of the D-cell (Rawdon and Andrew, 1979; Andrew and Rawdon, 1980). Large numbers of PP-cells are also found in close contact with the acinar cells of the exocrine pancreas (Aluments *et al.*, 1978). The PP-cells contain avian pancreatic polypeptide (APP), which has been extracted and purified (Kimmel *et al.*, 1968). PP-cells are also present in mammalian pancreata (Larsson *et al.*, 1976) as well as in those of cartilagenous and bony fishes (van Noorden and Patent, 1978; Klein and van Noorden, 1980). A few agranular cells are also distributed throughout the gland, but their function is unknown (Boquist and Falkmer, 1970).

The topological arrangement of islet cells within the endocrine pancreas may be of importance in both intercellular (via the extracellular space—paracrine system) and intracellular (via ion channels between cells—gap junctions) communication necessary for the regulation of hormone secretion (see Section IV). The blood flow through the capillary network may also play a role in intra-pancreatic regulation (via endocrine mechanisms) of hormone secretion. The islet cells of various mammals show a non-random distribution within the pancreas. Generally A-cells (glucagon-secretory) and D-cells (somatostatin-secretory) are dispersed towards the periphery of the islet tissue, whereas B-cells (insulin-secretory) are found centrally (Unger *et al.*, 1978). The peripheral location and close proximity of A- and D-cells may be important in the regulation of hormone release. In the chicken, the capillaries of the small islets of the dorsal and ventral lobes (mainly light islets) continue through the capillary bed to the exocrine tissue (Bonner-Weir and Weir, 1979). Hormones secreted in this region probably influence exocrine function. PP-cells are almost exclusively situated in the dorsal and ventral lobes. In general, glucagon, somatostatin and pancreatic polypeptide inhibit and insulin stimulates exocrine secretions (Henderson *et al.*, 1981; Lonovics *et al.*, 1981). Hormones secreted by the large islets of the splenic and third lobes, which are not in contact with the exocrine system, enter the portal bloodstream.

Investigation of the chicken pancreas has shown that it is highly innervated, with four types of synaptic terminals. Although fewer nerve terminals are located in the endocrine tissue than in the exocrine tissue, the nerve axons come into close contact with islet cell membranes and the D-cells are highly innervated (Watanabe and Yasuda, 1977).

III. Hormone Composition, Biosynthesis and Structure

A. Insulin

1. Composition

The chemical properties of insulin have been reviewed (Humbel *et al.*, 1972). Bovine insulin, MW 5734, has two polypeptide chains of 21 and 30 amino acids, linked by disulphide bridges (Ryle *et al.*, 1955). Except for the guinea pig hormone, there are only slight variations in amino acid sequence between different mammalian insulins (Humbel *et al.*, 1972). The amino acid sequence of chicken insulin varies in six positions from that of the bovine hormone (Smith, 1966), and is reported as more potent than the mammalian hormones (Humbel *et al.*, 1972; Simon *et al.*, 1977b; McCumbee and Hazelwood, 1978), especially when administered to chickens (Hazelwood *et al.*, 1968). Turkey insulin has the same primary sequence (Weitzel *et al.*, 1972), but the duck hormone shows three positional variations (Markusson and Sundby, 1973).

2. Biosynthesis

The mechanism of insulin biosynthesis has been elucidated from experiments using both mammalian and fish islet tissue. Despite the large evolutionary gap, the processes are almost identical, indicating that a similar mechanism is likely in birds. Insulin biosynthesis has been extensively reviewed (Steiner, 1977; Tager *et al.*, 1980). A large single chain precursor (preproinsulin), MW 11 500, is synthesised in the rough endoplasmic reticulum of the B-cell. Messenger RNA precursors for preproinsulin have been isolated from rat (Lomedico *et al.*, 1979; Chan *et al.*, 1979; Cordell *et al.*, 1979), human (Bell *et al.*, 1979, 1980), angler fish (Shields, 1981) and chicken (Perler *et al.*, 1980), and the coded amino acid sequences show large regions of homology. Rapid post-translational modification of preproinsulin results in the removal of the hydrophobic *N*-terminal of 24 amino acids, yielding proinsulin (MW 8700). This hydrophobic region of the amino acid chain is thought to be a "leader sequence" which is essential for translocation of the peptide into the cisternum of the rough endoplasmic reticulum (Steiner *et al.*, 1980; Tager *et al.*, 1980). The resulting proinsulin chain adopts a characteristic low energy three dimensional conformation which allows the correct disulphide bond formation. An energy-dependent transfer step takes the packaged proinsulin from the endoplasmic reticulum to the Golgi apparatus. Hydrolytic enzymes then specifically cleave at pairs of basic amino acids in the precursor chain, resulting in the formation of biologically active insulin and the C-peptide remnant. Concomitantly, immature granules or progranules are formed from the Golgi apparatus and these gradually mature as insulin is formed. As the C-peptide is released, zinc ions are sequestered forming organo-metallic complexes eventually leading to crystallization of the zinc–insulin within the granule. The crystalline rhombohedral unit cells contain two zinc ions chelated by the B10 histidines from six insulin molecules.

3. Content

The concentration of insulin in the chicken pancreas is only 10 to 30 ng mg^{-1} wet weight tissue compared with 100 to 150 ng mg^{-1} wet weight in the mammalian pancreas (Kimmel *et al.*, 1968; Langslow *et al.*, 1973; Weir *et al.*, 1976). A regional variation in concentration exists, with over five times the mean concentration found in the splenic lobe (Weir *et al.*, 1976).

B. Glucagon

1. Composition

Bromer (1972a,b) has reviewed the structure and chemistry of glucagon. Glucagons isolated from various mammalian species consist of a single polypeptide chain of 29 amino acids, which are identical in sequence (MW 3485; Bromer *et al.*, 1971; Thompson *et al.*, 1972). Chicken and turkey glucagons have the same amino acid sequence as the mammalian hormone except that serine replaces asparagine at position 28 (Markusson *et al.*, 1972; Pollock and Kimmel, 1975; Hazelwood, 1976). In addition, duck glucagon also differs at position 16, where threonine replaces serine (Sundby *et al.*, 1972; Hazelwood, 1976). It is not clear whether this difference in the amino acid sequence alters biological potency; chicken glucagon has been reported to have increased activity *in vivo* (Hazelwood *et al.*, 1973) and decreased activity *in vitro* (McCumbee and Hazelwood, 1978).

2. *Biosynthesis*

Glucagon is initially synthesised as a larger molecular weight precursor within the pancreatic A-cell. The reported size of the precursor protein is variable, with two peptides of MW 11 400 and 9000 reported for angler fish (Noe and Bauer, 1971, 1975) and MW 18 000 for the precursor isolated from the rat (Tager *et al.*, 1980) and guinea pig (Hellerstrom *et al.*, 1972). A MW 69 000 form of glucagon has also been reported in extracts of pigeon islets (Tung, 1973) with intermediate breakdown products of MW 6000 and 9000 (Tung, 1974). The MW 9000 component has an amino acid composition similar to, but not identical with, proglucagon isolated from the angler fish (Tung *et al.*, 1976). The mechanism by which the precursor peptide is processed to form glucagon is unknown, although using rat islets, pulse-chase studies have indicated an initial increase in the molecular weight of the precursor from 18 000 to 19 000 followed by a four-step enzymatic cleavage (again at pairs of basic amino acids) resulting in the active hormone (Tager *et al.*, 1980).

3. *Content*

Reports on the glucagon content of the avian pancreas are inconsistent. Early studies indicated up to 10 times more immunoassayable glucagon in chicken or duck pancreas than the mammalian gland (Vuylsteke and De Duve, 1953; Samols *et al.*, 1969; Falkmer and Marques, 1972; Hazelwood, 1973). More recent studies by Weir *et al.* (1976) report concentrations in the chicken pancreas of 8 ng mg^{-1} wet weight which is similar to that found in mammals. Pollock and Kimmel (1975) report recoveries of glucagon around 1 ng mg^{-1} during extraction procedures, but no corrections were made for handling losses. Like insulin, a distributional difference is found, with 75 times the mean concentration found in the large islets of the splenic lobe, and almost no immunoassayable material present in either the dorsal or ventral lobes (Weir *et al.*, 1976).

C. Somatostatin

1. Composition

The amino acid sequence of the cyclic tetra-decapeptide (MW 1638) isolated from pigeon pancreas is identical to that isolated from the ovine (Brazeau *et al.*, 1973; Burgus *et al.*, 1973) and porcine (Schally *et al.*, 1976) hypothalamus. Although mammalian pancreatic somatostatin has not been sequenced, biological and immunological studies indicate that the structure is conserved both throughout the different secretory glands and also throughout all vertebrates. Larger forms of somatostatin (prosomatostatins), 25 and 28 amino acids and still retaining biological activity have also been isolated (Esch *et al.*, 1980; Meyers *et al.*, 1980; Schally *et al.*, 1980).

2. Biosynthesis

As with insulin and glucagon, a large precursor protein is synthesized, followed by post-translational cleavage to form the active peptide within the secretory granule. Using pulse chase experiments in rat islets, a large protein of MW 12 500 has been detected (Tager *et al.*, 1980) and a tryptic digest yields various peptide fragments, some of which are identical with that found after tryptic digest of somatostatin. Fletcher *et al.* (1980) also reported high molecular weight peptides with somatostatin-like immunoreactivity associated with the microsomes and secretory granules of angler fish islets. A membrane-bound thiol protease, specific for arginine residues, was also detected in the extract and may be the specific processing enzyme. High molecular weight proteins with somatostatin-like immunoreactivity ("big-somatostatin") are also found in the blood (Patel *et al.*, 1980). Messenger RNA precursors, coding for high molecular weight proteins having somatostatin immunoreactivity, have been isolated from angler fish (Lundt *et al.*, 1980; Goodman *et al.*, 1980; Shields, 1981).

High molecular weight preprosomatostatins, with reported molecular weights ranging from 14 000 to 18 000, are processed to the lower molecular weight prosomatostatin when incubated with microsomal membranes. A large somatostatin-like peptide of molecular weight 11 000 to 12 500 has been detected in pigeon pancreas (Spiess *et al.*, 1979), but no information is yet available into its biosynthesis or post-translational modification. Large molecular weight forms of somatostatin have been reported in hypothalamus, pancreatic islets, stomach and cerebral cortex (Patel and Reichlin, 1978), as well as in the median eminence and neurohypophysis (Zingg and Patel, 1979) of the rat. How these prosomatostatins are then processed to yield the active tetradecapeptide is unknown.

3. Content

The avian pancreas contains a large number of D-cells (Orci *et al.*, 1975) and, as a result, the somatostatin content of the chicken pancreas is over 20-fold higher than that found in the rat, with concentrations of 3·8 ng mg^{-1} wet weight (Weir *et al.*, 1976). Regional variations in concentration exist, with over five times this concentration found in the islets of the splenic lobe (Weir *et al.*, 1976). A large amount of somatostatin has also been reported to be present in the pigeon pancreas (Vale *et al.*, 1976).

D. Avian Pancreatic Polypeptide (APP)

1. Composition

This hormone was first extracted as a contaminating protein during the isolation of chicken insulin (Kimmel *et al.*, 1968). The peptide comprises a single polypeptide chain (MW 4258) of 36 amino acids (Kimmel *et al.*, 1971, 1975). Although the peptide bears no homology with insulin, a slight amino acid sequential homology does exist with glucagon (Kimmel *et al.*, 1975; Pollock and Kimmel ,1975).

2. Biosynthesis

No information is available on the mechanism of synthesis of this hormone. However, details of post-translational cleavage of a large precursor molecule isolated from the canine pancreas have been reported (Schwartz and Tager, 1981).

3. Content

The APP content of the chicken pancreas ranges from 40 to 80 ng mg^{-1} wet weight (Kimmel *et al.*, 1971, 1975; Langslow *et al.*, 1973). Similar values are found for goose, duck and guinea-fowl (Langslow *et al.*, 1973). Similar peptides have also been isolated from bovine (BPP), porcine (PPP), ovine (OPP) and human (HPP) pancreas (Lin and Chance, 1974). Unlike somatostatin, the structure of which is totally conserved, the amino acid sequence of the mammalian hormones, although themselves similar, are very different from APP, with only 16 of the 36 amino acids in the sequence being conserved (Kimmel *et al.*, 1975). This is reflected in the poor cross-reactivity between antisera raised against APP and BPP (Langslow *et al.*, 1973).

IV. Hormone Secretion

The concentrations of the pancreatic hormones in the peripheral blood of chickens range up to 2 nM for insulin, 0·4 nM for glucagon and 3 nM for APP (Cramb, 1980). The concentration limits are found at the extremes of metabolic demand for these hormones. Concentrations in the portal blood will be substantially higher and, therefore, the liver will respond to higher concentrations than the peripheral tissues (e.g. muscle and adipose tissue. No information on avian blood somatostatin concentrations is available. However, secretions from the isolated chicken pancreas–duodenum preparations range from 0·06 to 0·48 nM (Honey and Weir, 1979). Somatostatin-like immunoreactivity in the rat ranges from 0·06 to 0·36 nM in the portal blood, with around 10% of these concentrations found in the peripheral circulation. Nearly 50% of the immunoreactivity in the portal blood and over 90% in the peripheral blood is attributable to a larger molecular weight form of somatostatin (Patel *et al.*, 1980).

A. Mechanism of Hormone Release

The release of the pancreatic hormones from islet cells results from a movement of the storage granules within the cells to the plasma membrane followed by the discharge of their contents into the extracellular space or directly into a blood capillary. The study of the molecular mechanisms of hormone secretion has been confined mainly to insulin, although the other pancreatic hormones are probably released by a similar mechanism. Experimental evidence suggests that the microtubular and microfilament structures associated with the plasma membrane and surrounding cytosol of the B-cell serve as a cytoskeleton, guiding the secretory granules along defined routes to the exocytotic sites on the plasma membrane (Somers *et al.*, 1979; Malaisse and Orci, 1979; Kanazawa *et al.*, 1980). Once in contact with the plasmalemma, membrane fusion occurs followed by the release of the packaged hormones by exocytosis. Evidence suggests that the rupture of the plasma membrane at the site of granule fusion follows increased anion uptake into the granule, causing osmotic lysis (Orci and Malaisse, 1980). Hormones and metabolites (e.g. glucose) regulate the rate of insulin release by stimulating intracellular concentrations of cyclic adenosine monophosphate (cAMP) and calcium. The mechanisms involved and the roles of cAMP and calcium in microtubular assembly and granule movement have been reviewed (Malaisse *et al.*, 1971; Sharp *et al.*, 1975; Sharp, 1979; Hedeskov, 1980). A vitamin D-dependent calcium binding protein has also been found in the B-cell (Roth *et al.*, 1982) and it may have a regulatory role in insulin biosynthesis or secretion or both.

B. Control of Hormone Release

Control mechanisms for the regulation and co-ordination of pancreatic hormone secretion may be grouped into three categories: peripheral metabolic control, intra-pancreatic regulation and nervous control.

1. Peripheral Metabolic Control

Fluctuations in the blood concentrations of metabolites, particularly glucose and amino acids, can alter the rate of hormone secretion. Studies on insulin secretion in the chicken, using the isolated perfused pancreas or pancreas–duodenum preparations, indicate a relative insensitivity to circulating glucose concentrations. Compared with the rapid and large increases in insulin secretion in response to glucose in mammals (Malaisse *et al.*, 1967), concentrations of perfusate glucose of 30 to 40 mM (some two to three times the normal physiological concentration) are required to induce a modest stimulation (King and Hazelwood, 1976; Naber and Hazelwood, 1977; Honey *et al.*, 1980b; Colca and Hazelwood, 1981). Even with prolonged glucose perfusion, increased insulin secretion is only of a transient nature, and diminishing responses are found to repeated glucose challenges (King and Hazelwood, 1976; Naber and Hazelwood, 1977) which again contrasts with the situation in mammals.

Similar findings were reported *in vivo* in both chickens (Langslow *et al.*, 1970; Simon and Rosselin, 1978) and ducks (Samols *et al.*, 1969). Perfusion of arginine in the presence of physiological glucose concentrations improves the rate of insulin release four-fold (Honey *et al.*, 1980b). Perfusion of microfragments of chicken pancreas with lysine, phenylalanine or arginine induces a prolonged response, whereas leucine or isoleucine only transitionally stimulate insulin secretion (Colca and Hazelwood, 1982). Since the regulation of insulin release is qualitatively similar in birds and mammals (King and Hazelwood, 1976; Simon and Rosselin, 1978), the low insulinogenic potential of the avian pancreas may be due to, either a diminished sensitivity to circulating glucose or to a decreased number of mature insulin-containing granules within the cell available for secretion. Since both amino acids and acetylcholine (see IVB3) can induce large responses, the former is more likely.

Perfusion of the chicken pancreas with low glucose concentrations (3 mM–four times lower than normal physiological concentrations) results in glucagon concentrations of up to 1 ng mg^{-1} (0·29 nM) in the perfusate. Increasing the perfusate glucose concentrations from 3 to 40 mM causes a rapid and prolonged decrease in these glucagon concentrations, by as much as 40-fold. Under the same conditions, the somatostatin output increases four-fold from around 0·15 ng ml^{-1} to 0·6 ng ml^{-1}. In contrast, the perfusion of arginine

(10 nM) in the presence of physiological glucose concentrations results in increases in both glucagon and somatostatin secretion. Although somatostatin secretion gradually decreases, glucagon secretion is sustained throughout the time of arginine perfusion, but then rapidly decreases to basal values following withdrawal of the amino acid (Honey *et al.*, 1980b).

Increasing the glucose concentration in the isolated perfused pancreas does not affect APP secretion (Colca and Hazelwood, 1981). Although the amino acids, leucine, isoleucine, phenylalanine and valine produce sustained APP release from chicken pancreas *in vitro*, no changes in blood APP concentration are found after intravenous injection of these amino acids (Colca and Hazelwood, 1982). Glucose and arginine both fail to induce PP secretion in the isolated perfused canine pancreas (Gingerich *et al.*, 1978); however, glucose ingestion in man increases circulating HPP concentrations (Marco *et al.*, 1977).

2. *Intra-pancreatic Regulation*

The pancreatic hormones can regulate the secretion of each other. This type of regulation is a rapid control mechanism, either attenuating (by negative feedback mechanisms) or accentuating (by positive feedback mechanisms) hormone secretion. Although there is as yet no direct evidence, three types of cell–cell communication between islet cells have been proposed.

(a) The paracrine system—communication between different cell types via hormone secretion into the extracellular space. The cellular composition and distribution within the islets would be of great importance in such regulation.

(b) The endocrine system—communication via hormones secreted directly into the bloodstream and carried through the capillary channels to sites of action on other endocrine cells. The route taken by the capillaries throughout the gland would be important.

(c) Gap junctions—cells in physical contact with each other, including cells of the same type, could be in constant communication via gap junctions (ion channels between the two cells). The extent of different cell contact within the islets would be important. Homo- and heterocellular coupling via such junctions has been implicated in the rat pancreas (Meda *et al.*, 1982). Such intracellular communication may be responsible for the regulation of basal insulin release (Halban *et al.*, 1982).

In the presence of high glucose concentrations, perfusion of glucagon in the isolated chicken pancreas causes a marked improvement in the duration and extent of insulin release (King and Hazelwood, 1976; Naber and Hazelwood, 1977). Injections of glucagon, but not APP, results in a bimodal stimulation of insulin release *in vivo* (Hazelwood and Langslow, 1978). Somatostatin is known to inhibit pancreatic insulin release in mammals (Koerker *et al.*, 1974;

Sakuri *et al.*, 1974; Guillerman and Gerich, 1976; Johnson *et al.*, 1975), ducks (Strosser *et al.*, 1980) and chickens (Honey *et al.*, 1980a).

Insulin suppresses the high rates of glucagon secretion when the pancreas is perfused with sub-physiological concentrations of glucose (Honey and Weir, 1979; Honey *et al.*, 1980a) although the effects on glucagon secretion are less pronounced than with high concentrations of glucose alone (Honey *et al.*, 1980b). Despite this finding, insulin injections result, *in vivo*, in a bimodal increase in circulating glucagon (Hazelwood and Langslow, 1978). However, this bimodal increase in blood glucagon is paralleled by a decrease in blood glucose, as a direct result of the insulin injection. Inhibition of glucagon release by an injection of insulin has been reported in the starved goose (Sitbon and Mialhe, 1978). However, with injections of large amounts of insulin, the resulting hypoglycaemia stimulates glucagon release, thus masking the direct inhibitory effect of insulin. The major controlling factor regulating glucagon secretion is blood glucose, although intra-pancreatic control by insulin does have an attenuating effect. Although APP injection failed to alter blood glucose concentrations (Hazelwood *et al.*, 1973), the hormone significantly lowered circulating glucagon concentrations. Glucagon injection also decreased the circulating APP concentration *in vivo* (Hazelwood and Langslow, 1978). No effect on the analogous mammalian polypeptide has been found in the isolated perfused canine pancreas (Weir *et al.*, 1979). Since APP does not affect insulin release (Hazelwood and Langslow, 1978), a direct negative feedback mechanism may exist between PP- and A-cells in the chicken pancreas.

Very little is known of any intra-pancreatic control mechanisms existing between APP and somatostatin in the bird. However, somatostatin secretion is stimulated by both insulin, at low glucose concentrations (Honey and Weir, 1979; Honey *et al.*, 1980a), and glucagon (Honey *et al.*, 1980a). Somatostatin is reported to stimulate glucagon release and inhibit insulin release in the duck (Strosser *et al.*, 1980), but to inhibit both glucagon and insulin secretion in the chicken (Honey *et al.*, 1980a) and mammalian pancreas (Koerker *et al.*, 1974; Johnson *et al.*, 1975; Guillerman and Gerich, 1976; Weir *et al.*, 1979). Infusion of somatostatin antiserum in the isolated perfused chicken pancreas results in significant stimulation of both insulin and glucagon secretion (Honey *et al.*, 1981) indicating that somatostatin continually inhibits hormone release from A- and B-cells. A high affinity receptor site for somatostatin has been detected on hamster B-cells (Reibi *et al.*, 1982). Stimulation of insulin and glucagon secretion from chick pancreas as a result of the phosphodiesterase inhibitor theophylline is not antagonised by somatostatin (Foltzer *et al.*, 1982). The action of somatostatin on pancreatic A- and B-cells is, therefore, possibly a result of an inhibitory action on receptor stimulated cyclic AMP production. A larger form of somatostatin consisting of 28 amino acids (SS-28) is reported to be longer acting and more selective than the tetradecapeptide (SS-14) at inhibiting insulin secretion (Tannenbaum *et al.*, 1982), and may constitute the major bioactive form of the peptide involved in intrapancreatic regulation *in vivo*. Somatostatin injection inhibits PP secretion in man (Marco *et al.*, 1977), but there are no reports of similar actions in the bird. More information is needed before any conclusions can be reached on the intrapancreatic control exerted by somatostatin, although a major difference is apparent in its effects on duck pancreas compared with that found in chicken and mammals.

3. Control by the Nervous System

The autonomic nervous system is known to be involved in regulating the endocrine pancreas (Woods and Porte, 1974; Steffens, 1981; Bereiter *et al.*, 1981). Secretion can be regulated by electrical stimulation of vagal and splanchnic nerves and by both the sympathetic and parasympathetic neurotransmitters. Acetylcholine, the parasympathetic neurotransmitter, stimulates insulin and glucagon secretion in mammals (Iverson, 1973; Samols *et al.*, 1978, 1981). The effect of neurotransmitters on mammalian somatostatin release is uncertain, with both inhibition (Samols *et al.*, 1978, 1981) and stimulation (Hermansen *et al.*, 1979) being reported. In experiments using the isolated chicken pancreas–duodenum, Honey and Weir (1980) have shown that acetylcholine, when given in conjunction with physiological or high glucose concentrations, stimulated insulin release nearly ten times more than the glucose alone. Moreover, this response was lost when the glucose concentration fell below physiological concentrations.

The parasympathetic nervous system may be an important physiological regulator of insulin secretion in the chicken (Honey and Weir, 1980). Since chickens tend to eat regularly through the light period (Hill, 1971), storing the excess ingested food in the crop, a constant rate of digestion can be maintained. The consequence is that chickens may never be faced with the large nutrient loads found in most mammals after meals. Therefore, low insulin demands would be necessary over long periods to regulate blood glucose concentrations. A lower pancreatic insulin reserve and/or rate of secretion would meet metabolic requirements. Birds of prey generally have spasmodic eating patterns and, therefore, will be challenged with high nutrient loads. This may be the reason for the Great Horned Owl, *Bubo virginianus*, having at least four times the pancreatic insulin content of the chicken (Langslow *et al.*, 1973) and, unlike most granivorous birds, it becomes hyperglycaemic after total pancreatectomy (Nelson *et al.*, 1942). Of the few reported pancreatectomies carried out on carnivorous birds, all workers have observed signs of diabetes mellitus with marked glucosuria and hyperglycaemia (see review by Sitbon *et al.*, 1980), a condition which is not normally induced in birds after pancreatectomy (Langslow and Hales, 1971).

Acetylcholine also stimulates glucagon secretion at physiological or high glucose concentrations, but at low glucose concentrations glucagon secretion is already maximally stimulated (Honey and Weir, 1980). Somatostatin secretion can be stimulated up to three-fold by acetylcholine independent of the perfusate glucose concentrations (Honey and Weir, 1980). Acetylcholine may be an important regulator of somatostatin secretion in the bird, since the D-cells of the pancreas are highly innervated (Watanabe and Yasuda, 1977). Cholinergic control of APP secretion has not yet been investigated in the chicken, but both vagal and cholinergic stimulations of polypeptide secretion have been reported in pig and man (Schwartz *et al.*, 1978).

The catecholamines, including noradrenaline (the sympathetic neurotransmitter) have long been known to affect the functions of the mammalian endocrine pancreas (Woods and Porte, 1974; Steffens, 1981). Both α- and β-adrenergic receptors are present in the mammalian pancreas. Although there is general agreement concerning adrenergic effects on insulin secretion, the actions of the catecholamines on the release of the other hormones remains unsettled. β-Agonists have been shown to stimulate the release of somatostatin, glucagon and insulin in dogs (Samols *et al.*, 1978; Samols and Weir, 1979) and pancreatic polypeptide (Feurle *et al.*, 1980) and insulin (Robertson and Porte, 1973) secretion in man. In the isolated canine pancreas, α-adrenergic agonists also stimulate the release of glucagon but depress the release of both somatostatin and insulin (Samols *et al.*, 1978; Samols and Weir, 1979; Samols *et al.*, 1981). Few data are available regarding the action of catecholamines on the avian pancreas. As far as we are aware, the only reports on catecholamine action have been carried out *in vivo* with ducks. As with mammals, α-adrenergic agonists were found to stimulate glucagon and inhibit the release of insulin, but β-adrenergic antagonists had the opposite effect, with decreased glucagon and enhanced insulin secretion (Tyler and Kajinuma, 1972). Since injection of β-agonists also resulted in the increase of plasma glucose concentrations, the decrease in blood glucagon may have been a response to the hyperglycaemia. Injection of adrenaline (having both α- and β-effects) into ducks had no effect on plasma insulin concentration, but increases both plasma glucagon and plasma glucose concentrations (Samols *et al.*, 1972). Clearly, further information is needed before any conclusions can be made as to the role of the catecholamines on the avian pancreas.

V. Hormone Action

A. Actions *In Vivo*

It is now generally accepted that glucagon is more effective than insulin in birds, which exhibit a marked insulin insensitivity. This may partly explain the relatively high blood glucose concentrations of 12–15 mM which are two to three times greater than mammals. Total pancreatectomy in birds results in only a transient hyperglycaemia or prolonged hypoglycaemia, in contrast to the intensive and prolonged hyperglycaemia found in mammals. Although insulin is essential for the normal regulation of avian carbohydrate metabolism (Langslow and Freeman, 1972), its effects on metabolic processes are not so widespread nor as sensitive as found in mammals. Birds exhibit a high resistance to insulin, surviving up to 1000 times the dose per kilogram body weight which induces hypoglycaemic convulsions in rabbits (Chen *et al.*, 1945). Starvation markedly increases the blood concentrations of glucagon and to a lesser extent insulin (Simon and Rosselin, 1978). The increased insulin concentrations are probably the result of the high circulating glucagon concentrations. As the glucose tolerance of starved birds is impaired (Simon and Rosselin, 1978), starvation must reduce the capacity for further insulin secretion or decrease the insulin sensitivity of the responsive tissues. Apart from a slight hypoglycaemic action, insulin stimulated plasma free fatty acid concentrations and increased plasma uric acid concentrations, suggesting enhanced amino acid catabolism. The former effect is probably the result of the increased glucagon concentrations, induced by the hypoglycaemic action of insulin *in vivo* (Hazelwood and Langslow, 1978).

Little is known about the metabolic actions of APP and somatostatin. Injection of physiological doses of APP (1 to 25 μg kg^{-1} body weight) into chickens stimulated gastric secretion, with increased proventricular fluid volume, release of pepsin, free acid and total protein (Hazelwood *et al.*, 1973; Turner and Hazelwood, 1974). At higher doses (50 to 100 μg kg^{-1} body weight) APP also induced hepatic glycogenolysis and plasma hypoglycerolaemia, but did not effect blood glucose (Hazelwood *et al.*, 1973). In mammals, pancreatic polypeptide may be involved in the regulation of the rhythm of the migrating myoelectric complex of the gastrointestinal tract (Bueno *et al.*, 1982).

No actions *in vivo* of somatostatin in birds have been reported; effects on mammals have been reviewed by Schusdziarra (1980). Actions include a further decrease in blood glucose concentrations after starvation in both man (Gerich *et al.*, 1975) and dog (Altszuler *et al.*, 1976). The site and molecular mechanism of action are yet to be determined.

B. Mechanism of Hormone Action

The site of insulin and glucagon action on target tissues is well known. Both hormones bind to specific receptor sites on the plasma membrane of target cells. The insulin receptor isolated from rat adipose tissue is a glycoprotein of molecular weight about 300 000 (Cuatrecasas, 1971). Similarities in physical and kinetic characteristics of the insulin receptor isolated from several sources, including fat and liver cell membranes (Cuatrecasas, 1972a,b), lymphocytes (Gavin *et al.*, 1973) and avian erythrocytes (Ginsberg *et al.*, 1976; 1977), indicates that all target issues contain a very similar if not identical protein (Kahn, 1975). Insulin receptors have been found in tissues which are not considered major target sites for the hormone, such as human granulocytes (Fussganger *et al.*, 1976), lymphocytes (Gavin *et al.*, 1972; van Obberghen *et al.*, 1976) and blood monocytes (Schwartz *et al.*, 1975), as well as various placental tissues Posner, 1974; Cuatrecasas and Hollenberg, 1976), mouse mammary glands (O'Keefe and Cuatrecasas, 1974), avian erythrocytes (Ginsberg, *et al.*, 1976) and thymocytes from the rat (Goldfine *et al.*, 1972), mouse (Soll *et al.*, 1976) and chicken (Simon, 1979). The reason for the existence of these high affinity binding sites is unclear.

The mechanism of transfer of the signal to the cell cytosol following the binding of insulin to its receptor has not been resolved: for a review of the possible mechanisms of insulin action in the control of metabolism see Larner *et al.* (1982). Evidence suggests that insulin-receptor internalization by absorptive pinocytosis (Silverstein *et al.*, 1977) is necessary for the mediation of hormone action on intracellular processes (Steiner, 1977; Terries *et al.*, 1979). Autoradiographic analysis has shown a time and temperature dependent incorporation of ^{125}I-insulin, or degraded insulin fragments, into the intracellular environment (Goldfine *et al.*, 1978; Gordon *et al.*, 1978; Bergeron *et al.*, 1979) which may explain the reports of specific ^{125}I-insulin binding to sites in the cisternum of the Golgi apparatus (Posner *et al.*, 1978; Bergeron *et al.*, 1978). The actions of insulin on membrane transport processes are, however, probably mediated at the level of the plasma membrane, and hence may not require prior internalization of the hormone.

The signal transfer mechanism induced by glucagon binding to its specific receptor is well characterized. Binding to the receptor site on the external surface of the cell leads to an activation of adenylate cyclase situated on the inner half of the membrane lipid bilayer (Houslay and Palmer, 1978; Houslay *et al.*, 1980; Ross and Gilman, 1980). Glucagon binding and activation of adenylate cyclase is also regulated by guanine nucleotide-sensitive proteins which associate with the receptor and adenylate cyclase moieties (Rodell, 1980). In various mammalian tissues the elevated intracellular cAMP concentrations induce dissociation and activation of cAMP-dependent protein kinase(s), resulting in the phosphorylation of certain enzymes or functional proteins within the cell. Cyclic AMP binding proteins are present at relatively high concentrations in the chicken liver (Kwast-Welfeld and Kaniuga, 1979) and protein kinase activity is probably associated with one or a number of these proteins. Phosphorylation results in alteration of the activities of key regulatory enzymes, leading to changes in metabolic flux. The earliest report of a reversible phosphorylation of an enzyme leading to altered activity was for glycogen phosphorylase (Fischer and Krebs, 1955). Since then over 20 other enzymes have been found to be regulated by phosphorylation–dephosphorylation mechanisms carried out by specific protein kinases and phosphoprotein phosphates. Their regulation and action have been reviewed (Nimmo and Cohen, 1977; Krebs and Beavo, 1979; Cohen, 1980). Not only cAMP but cGMP and calcium-dependent protein kinases have been found. The calcium sensitivity of protein kinase is induced via a specific calcium binding protein, calmodulin (Cheung, 1980a,b; Means and Dedman, 1980). Any fluctuations in basal intracellular concentrations of cAMP, cGMP or free calcium may activate a particular protein kinase causing enzyme phosphorylation and thus alter basal metabolism.

C. Sites of Hormone Action

1. Liver

(a) Insulin. Simon *et al.* (1977a) have reported fewer insulin receptor sites per cell and per unit surface area of plasma membrane in chicken hepatocytes than in rat hepatocytes. Half maximum binding constants of 1·3 nM and 3·2 nM were found from isolated chicken hepatocytes and chicken plasma membranes respectively. These values are similar to those found by the same group of workers (Freychet *et al.*, 1974) when using rat hepatocytes and rat liver membranes. However, when analysing the hormone binding data in terms of both high- and low-affinity binding sites, much lower values are found, with a dissociation constant (K_d) of 0·3 nM (Cramb, 1980; Cramb *et al.*, 1982a). Such an analysis separates the high affinity binding component from the low affinity non-physiological binding components found during experimentation. It, therefore, reflects a value much closer to the true physiological affinity of the hormone receptor complex. Similar analysis of insulin binding data for rat hepatocytes or liver membranes also resulted in higher affinity values with the K_d ranging from 0·4 nM to 0·5 nM (Kahn, 1976; Gammeltoft *et al.*, 1978). Although different methods of analysis are used, the receptor affinity of the chicken liver insulin receptor is about the same as that in rat liver whether the data are treated as arising from single or multicomponent sites. Reported binding capacities are also dependent on the method of data analysis. Results analysed with respect to two classes of binding site yield capacities of 15 × 10^3 sites per cell (Gammeltoft *et al.*, 1978) or 4 × 10^{10} sites per mg membrane protein (Kahn, 1976) for rat liver and 2 × 10^3 sites per cell (Cramb, 1980; Cramb *et al.*, 1982a) for chicken liver. Analysis in terms of a single class of receptor sites results in higher capacities, with rat liver having 80 to 90 × 10^3 sites per cell or 160 × 10^{10} sites per mg membrane protein (Freychet *et al.*,

1974; Freychet, 1976) and chicken liver with $4{\cdot}6 \times 10^3$ sites per cell or 30×10^{10} sites per mg membrane protein (Simon *et al.*, 1977a). Since the average diameters of rat and chicken hepatocytes are 24 μm and 12 μm respectively (Capuzzi *et al.*, 1974; Dickson and Langslow, 1978), there is a two to five fold decrease in receptor density on the surface of the chicken hepatocyte depending on the mathematical treatment of the binding data.

Therefore, the chicken liver insulin receptor has approximately the same binding affinity as that of rat liver, but the receptor number per unit surface area of plasma membrane is decreased at least two fold. Since mammalian insulins were used in these binding studies, and chicken insulin has been reported to be twice as potent as mammalian insulins (Simon *et al.*, 1977b; McCumbee and Hazelwood, 1978), this apparent decrease in receptor number could well be counteracted by the increased binding affinity of chicken insulin.

Insulin circulates in the peripheral blood in the range 10^{-10} to 10^{-9}M and higher concentrations are obviously present in the portal blood. Since the true affinity of the chicken liver insulin receptor *in vivo* may be higher due to partial degradation of the receptor on cell isolation coupled with the higher affinity of chicken insulin then, even at the lowest physiological concentrations of the hormone, a large proportion of the insulin receptors will be occupied.

Insulin, like many other hormones, including glucagon, plays an important role in the regulation of its own receptor density on target cells. A prolonged increase in the concentration of the circulating hormone results in a reduction in the number of insulin receptors on the target cell surface; a phenomenon known as "down regulation" of receptor number (see review by Van Obberghen and Roth, 1981). Reduction in receptor number results from the binding and uptake of both hormone and receptor into the cells, followed by intralysosomal degradation. In chicken liver, however, the intracellular degradation of insulin exceeds that of its receptor by over 200-fold, indicating that after internalization of the hormone-receptor complex the receptor is recycled unchanged back into the plasma membrane (Krupp and Lane, 1982). This may explain why a substantial number of receptors still exist on the hepatocyte despite the high levels of receptor occupancy indicated in the chicken liver *in vivo*.

Despite the existence of high affinity receptor sites, insulin (porcine or chicken) is without a short-term intracellular action in hepatocytes isolated from 4- to 8-week-old birds. Negative responses have been found for effects on cAMP or cGMP concentrations, glycogenolysis, glycogen synthesis, gluconeogenesis or lipogenesis, either in the presence or absence of sub-saturating glucagon concentrations (Anderson and Langslow, 1975; Dickson *et al.*, 1978; Cramb, 1980; Cramb *et al.*, 1982b). Although Capuzzi *et al.* (1974) reported a small stimulation in the rate of lipogenesis by insulin, this could not be repeated (Cramb *et al.*, 1982b). The lack of effect of insulin in the chicken liver is in sharp contrast to the immediate and pronounced effects found in rat liver preparations (Exton and Park, 1972; Garrison and Haynes, 1973; Pilkis *et al.*, 1974; Westwood and Siddle, 1979; Beynen *et al.*, 1979, 1980). As a high affinity receptor exists in the chicken liver, the effector mechanism is either absent or non-functional, resulting in a lack of insulin action in the short term control of carbohydrate and lipid metabolism in the chicken.

Although insulin was devoid of an action in the adult chicken liver, cultures of liver slices isolated from 20-day-old chick embryos were insulin sensitive, with the hormone inducing a four-fold increase in stearoyl CoA desaturase activity (Joshi and Aranda, 1979a) and a five-fold increase in fatty acid synthetase activity (Joshi and Aranda, 1979b). Increases in the activities of both enzymes were attributable to enhanced protein synthesis. It must, therefore, be concluded that either the insulin effector system becomes non-functional around hatching, or the effector mechanism in chicken liver is specifically lost or damaged during hepatocyte isolation procedures. Alternatively, the receptor sites present on the chicken hepatocyte may exist only for the long term control of metabolism by means of protein biosynthesis, having no short term effects on carbohydrate and lipid metabolism. Although no conclusive evidence exists, the last possibility seems the most likely.

(b) Glucagon. Concentrations of glucagon in the peripheral blood of starved chickens can reach 0·4 nM. The hormone binds specifically to a high affinity receptor present in the isolated chicken hepatocyte, with a dissociation constant of 9·4 nM. There are about 13 000 sites per cell (Cramb, 1980; Cramb *et al.*, 1982a). Even assuming a 10-fold increase in the glucagon concentration in the portal blood, only a small population of the total receptor number would be occupied at the highest possible physiological concentration of the hormone, especially since chicken glucagon seems to be less active than porcine glucagon (McCumbee and Hazelwood, 1978).

Glucagon stimulates adenylate cyclase in the chicken hepatocyte, but the control of cAMP production and extracellular release is dependent on the method of cell isolation (Langslow and Siddle, 1979; Cramb *et al.*, 1982b). Cyclic nucleotide concentrations of under 1 pmol per 10^6 cells (resulting in theoretical intracellular concentrations of 5 to 10 μM) can be stimulated, after 10 min, to a maximum of 60-fold with glucagon, but only 20-fold with adrenaline (Cramb, 1980; Cramb *et al.*, 1982b). These effects were not additive. Depending on the cell isolation technique, intracellular cAMP is either rapidly increased and then abruptly attenuated, with concomitant release to the external medium (Cramb *et al.*, 1982b), or produced slowly over a prolonged period, and does not leak from the cell (Langslow and Siddle, 1979). Induction of this second messenger shows half maximum stimulation at 13 nM, which compares favourably with the value found for the dissociation constant of hormone binding. A parallel relationship exists between hormone binding and induction of cAMP accumulation, and since the maximum effects of cAMP production by glucagon cannot be enhanced by adrenaline (Cramb, 1980; Cramb *et al.*, 1982b) the high affinity glucagon receptor adenylate cyclase ratio is near unity, as in rat hepatocytes (Bataille *et al.*, 1974; Soman and Felig, 1978; Sonne *et al.*, 1978).

Relatively small increases in intracellular cAMP are responsible for the initiation of the metabolic effect. Using cell preparations of similar sensitivity, half maximum effects of glucagon were found at 0·9 nM, 0·4 nM and 1·0 nM respectively for the stimulation of glycogenolysis, gluconeogenesis and the inhibition of lipogenesis (Cramb, 1980; Cramb *et al.*, 1982b). Glycogenolysis was stimulated up to 300%, gluconeogenesis stimulated by 30% and lipogenesis from acetate inhibited by 90%. Inhibition of lipogenesis by glucagon was suggested to act by inhibition of acetyl CoA carboxylase as a result of increased cAMP synthesis (Allred and Roehrig, 1972; Capuzzi *et al.*, 1974; Beynen *et al.*, 1979; Clarke *et al.*, 1979). A bimodal effect of cAMP on lipogenesis in chicken liver slices has been reported (Bhat *et al.*, 1978a) with stimulation at low concentrations (10^{-6} to 10^{-8}M) and inhibition at higher concentrations (10^{-3}M). The significance of the effect at low cAMP concentrations is unknown, particularly since the concentrations reported are over five-fold lower than basal concentrations of the nucleotide in the isolated cells (Cramb *et al.*, 1982b). It is possible that most or all of the intracellular cAMP is bound by one of the many cAMP binding proteins found in chicken liver (Kwast-Welfeld and Kaniuga, 1979) which may not be associated with protein kinase activity. The fall in lipogenesis corresponds with the maximum decrease (90%) in intracellular citrate concentration found in glucagon-treated chicken hepatocytes (Watkins and Lane, 1976; Watkins *et al.*, 1977; Clarke *et al.*, 1979). The decrease in intracellular citrate (an allosteric activator of acetyl CoA carboxylase–Meredith and Lane, 1978) is caused by an inhibition of glycolysis, possibly at the level of phosphofructokinase and/or pyruvate kinase (Harris *et al.*, 1978; Clarke *et al.*, 1979; Fister *et al.*, 1982). This action lowers the concentrations of intracellular substrates for the tricarboxylic acid cycle. Besides this allosteric inactivation, Beynen *et al.* (1979) also report on direct effects of glucagon on acetyl CoA carboxylase. Cyclic AMP inhibition of lipogenesis from malonate in chicken liver slices has also been reported (Bhat *et al.*, 1978b), indicating that an additional control step exists beyond the level of acetyl CoA carboxylase. Cyclic AMP also induces a differential inhibition in the synthesis of various phospholipids in chicken liver (Bhat *et al.*, 1979), with 60% inhibition in the synthesis *de novo* of the major phospholipid components, phosphatidylcholine and phosphatidylethanolamine. Cyclic AMP also stimulates lipolytic breakdown of the triglyceride-rich vesicles found in chicken hepatocytes, resulting in ketogenesis with the release of substantial amounts of acetoacetate and β-hydroxybutyrate (Mooney and Lane, 1981). Like the inhibition of lipogenesis, inhibition of glycolytic flux by increased cyclic AMP may also be responsible for the stimulation of lipolysis within the hepatocyte (Mooney and Lane, 1982).

Inhibition of lipogenesis and stimulation of glycogenolysis have parallel dose–response curves, with metabolic effects saturating when only 10% of the total receptor sites are occupied (1300 sites per cell) and 10% of the total possible cAMP produced (3 to 4 pmol per 10^6 cells—a theoretical intracellular concentration of around 50 μM). Although similar concentrations of glucagon are necessary for minimum stimulations of both glycogenolysis and gluconeogenesis, the latter effect saturates at half the concentration required to saturate the former (Cramb, 1980).

(c) APP. No high affinity receptor for APP is present in the isolated chicken hepatocyte (Cramb, 1980; Cramb *et al.*, 1982a) which is in conformity with the lack of effect of this hormone on liver metabolism, even at high concentrations (McCumbee and Hazelwood, 1977; Cramb *et al.*, 1982b). The increasing rate of hepatic glycogenolysis found *in vivo* after APP injection (Hazelwood *et al.*, 1973) must arise as an indirect effect of the hormone, possibly by stimulating glucagon secretion (Hazelwood and Langslow, 1978); the reason for the lack of a simultaneous increase in blood glucose concentration is unresolved.

(d) Somatostatin. No metabolic actions of somatostatin have yet been reported for the chicken liver. Actions of somatostatin in mammalian liver remain controversial. Although some believe that somatostatin antagonizes glucagon-stimulated cAMP production (Oliver and Wagle, 1975; Oliver *et al.*, 1976), other disagree (Sacks *et al.*, 1977; Canivet *et al.*, 1979). Since high somatostatin concentrations are necessary for a response, it is doubtful that this hormone plays any direct role in the regulation of glucose metabolism in the liver.

2. *Adipose Tissue*

(a) Insulin. In mammals insulin is powerfully lipogenic (Glieman *et al.*, 1975) and anti-lipolytic (Hales *et al.*, 1978), antagonizing the actions of the catecholamines. Insulin administration to chicken *in vivo* increases blood free fatty acid concentrations (Langslow *et al.*, 1970), possibly as a result of enhanced glucagon secretion (see section IVB2). Although there are no reports of insulin binding to chicken adipose tissue plasma membranes, numerous reports are available for similar mammalian preparations (Cuatrecasas, 1971; Kono and Barham, 1971; Glieman and Sonne, 1978; Kahn and Baird, 1978). Insulin at physiological concentrations induced significant increases in glucose uptake,

oxidation and incorporation into triglycerides in chicken adipocytes (Gomez-Capilla and Langslow, 1977), but failed to antagonize the lipolytic actions of glucagon or adrenaline in chicken adipose tissue (Goodridge, 1968; Langslow and Hales, 1969; Langslow, 1971). McCumbee and Hazelwood (1978) found no effects of insulin on glucose utilization or on basal or glucagon-stimulated lipolysis in chicken adipocytes, even at concentrations three orders of magnitude higher than required for action in rat adipocytes. The metabolic actions of insulin are secondary to those of glucagon, but more evidence is required before the true metabolic balance exerted by these two hormones on lipid metabolism in adipose tissue can be determined.

(b) Glucagon. Glucagon is the main lipolytic hormone in birds and contrasts with the greater lipolytic action of the catecholamines in mammals (Langslow and Hales, 1971). Both hormones act by stimulating adipocyte adenylate cyclase and result in the gradual and prolonged elevation of intracellular cAMP (Langslow, 1972; Boyd *et al.*, 1975; Hales *et al.*, 1978; Langslow *et al.*, 1979). The sensitivity of chicken adipose tissue to glucagon increases 10-fold during hatching and is possibly associated with the increased capacity for cAMP accumulation within the adipocyte and/or an increase in lipase sensitivity to cAMP accumulation (Langslow *et al.*, 1979). Since phosphodiesterase activity is unaltered, the increased capacity for synthesizing cAMP is probably due to enhanced adenylate cyclase activity. Glucagon concentrations of 4 nM induce half maximum stimulation of cAMP production in both chick and chick embryo adipocytes (Langslow *et al.*, 1979), whereas stimulation of lipolysis was half maximal at 0·1 nM and 1·0 nM respectively (Langslow, 1972). As in chicken hepatocytes, only a small increase in the total possible cAMP production is necessary to induce the maximum metabolic effect. An increase in the number of receptor sites linked to adenylate cyclase in the plasma membrane would increase the sensitivity of the adipocyte to low concentrations of glucagon by increasing cAMP production at any hormone concentration. It is not known whether there is an increase in the number of glucagon receptors or adenylate cyclase molecules per unit surface area, over the hatching period.

(c) APP. Despite being devoid of actions in the chicken hepatocyte, APP binds to isolated chicken adipocytes with both high affinity (K_d – 5·6 nM) low capacity (40×10^3 sites per cell) and low affinity (K_d – 0·83 μM) high capacity (2×10^6 sites per cell) sites being reported (McCumbee and Hazelwood, 1977). The binding data have been analysed in terms of two classes of binding site, and it is most likely that only the high affinity site is of any physiological significance. This receptor is probably responsible for the transmission of the antagonistic effects of APP on glucagon -stimulated cAMP production and

enhanced rates of lipolysis (McCumbee and Hazelwood, 1977). This antilipolytic action *in vivo* may help explain the decreased plasma glycerol concentrations found *in vivo* after APP injection (Hazelwood *et al.*, 1973).

(d) Somatostatin. No direct actions of somatostatin on avian or mammalian adipose tissue have been reported.

VI. Summary and Conclusions

With the introduction of new perfusion techniques, considerable progress has been made over the past ten years regarding the secretion and action of insulin, glucagon and APP in the chicken. Somatostatin has only recently been discovered in both mammalian and avian hypothalamus and pancreas and thus little information is available about the control of its secretion or its metabolic function.

The heterogeneous distribution of islets throughout the chicken pancreas is now well documented. Similar heterogeneous clusters of different islets are also found in mammals. The complex arrangement of cells within the endocrine gland may well be an important factor in the intrapancreatic control of hormone secretion by direct communication between cells. Although there is now much information concerning the external factors which regulate pancreatic hormone release, possible control mechanisms exerted within the pancreas itself await the development of more sophisticated experimental techniques, possibly involving homogeneous populations of isolated islet cells.

Although blood glucose concentrations are under the direct control of hormones secreted by the avian pancreas, there are major differences in the mechanism of this control compared with the mammalian system. It is apparent that in the chicken, and many other species of granivorous birds, insulin plays only a minor role in the control of carbohydrate and lipid metabolism. The avian pancreas responds very poorly to insulinogenic signals, such as high glucose concentrations, carried by the bloodstream. However, insulin release by the chicken pancreas is highly sensitive to the neurotransmitter acetylcholine, indicating that the parasympathetic nervous system may play an important part in controlling insulin release in the bird. The mild hypoglycaemic action of insulin in the bird is in contrast to its immediate and assertive effects on blood glucose concentrations in mammals. When avian blood glucose concentrations are reduced to any extent, the resulting increased rates of pancreatic glucagon secretion quickly compensate for the mild hypoglycaemic effect of insulin. This rather poor response may be partly attributed to the lack of an effect *in vitro* of insulin in liver and, perhaps adipose tissue.

Despite the presence of high affinity insulin receptors on the liver cell membrane, no metabolic actions of insulin have been found, suggesting the absence of an intracellular effector system for this hormone. Since the dissociation constant for the receptor–hormone interaction is lower than the portal blood insulin concentrations, the receptor sites are probably always occupied *in vivo*. Hence, an alternative explanation would be that the liver could be maximally activated by this hormone at all times, with the regulation of carbohydrate and lipid metabolism depending solely on the antagonistic actions of glucagon. Isolation of the hepatocytes for the experiments *in vitro* may remove the insulin from its specific receptor on the cell surface but the effector system may remain maximally activated. Long term culturing of these cell suspensions would be necessary to test this hypothesis.

Since it is unlikely that insulin injection *in vivo* would result in enhanced glucose uptake in liver, the hypoglycaemic effect of this hormone is probably due to actions on the other main target tissue, muscle. Further experiments are needed to examine this possibility. Glucagon therefore appears the more potent of the two hormones *in vivo* and *in vitro*, with immediate and pronounced effects found in the liver and adipose tissue. Evolution of the digestive system of granivorous birds has resulted in an almost continuous slow digestion of the food reserves in the crop. Since the bird is never faced with large nutrient loads as found in mammals, there is no immediate requirement for a rapid release of insulin to act on target tissues as in mammalian liver and adipose tissue.

Experiments with isolated cells indicate that APP has no direct action on the chicken liver. However, a high affinity receptor is present in adipose tissue which may be responsible for the transmission of the antagonistic effect of APP on glucagon-stimulated lipolysis. This antilipolytic effect of the hormone is also found *in vivo*. Whether this is the only effect of APP on adipose tissue or on other tissues in the bird awaits further experimentation. The stimulation of proventricular secretion appears to be a major action of APP in the chicken. However, other receptor sites for the hormone have been found in the pancreas, duodenum, ileum, spleen and bone marrow (Kimmel and Pollock, 1981).

Work on somatostatin has only just begun. No conclusive evidence has yet been presented of any actions of somatostatin in liver or adipose tissue, in birds or mammals. From those experiments already carried out, it is unlikely that somatostatin plays any direct role in the control of carbohydrate and lipid metabolism in avian liver or adipose tissue, although the hormone may be important in the intra-pancreatic control of hormone secretion.

Acknowledgements

The authors would like to thank the British Egg Marketing Board, the

Medical Research Council and the University of Edinburgh for research grants.

References

Allred, J. B. and Roehrig, K. L. (1972). *Biochem. Biophys. Res. Commun.* **46**, 1135–1139.
Altszuler, N., Gottlieb, B. and Hampshire, J. (1976). *Diabetes* **25**, 116–121.
Aluments, J., Hakanson, R. and Sundler, F. (1978). *Cell Tiss. Res.* **194**, 377–386.
Anderson, C. E. and Langslow, D. R. (1975). *Biochem. Soc. Trans.* **3**, 1037–1039.
Andrew, A. and Rawdon, B. B. (1980). *Histochemistry* **65**, 261–267.
Bataille, D., Freychet, P. and Rosselin, G. E. (1974). *Endocrinology* **95**, 713–721.
Bell, G. I., Swain, W. F., Pictet, R., Cordell, B., Goodman, H. M. and Rutter, W. J. (1979). *Nature, Lond.* **282**, 525–527.
Bell, G. I., Pictet, R., Rutter, W. J., Cordell, B., Tischer, E. and Goodman, H. M. (1980. *Nature, Lond.* **284**, 26–32.
Bereiter, D. A., Rohner-Jeanrenaud, F., Berthoud, H. R. and Jeanrenaud, B. (1981). *Diabetologia Suppl.* **20**, 417–425.
Bergeron, J. J. M., Posner, B. I., Josefsberg, Z. and Sikstrom, R. (1978). *J. biol. Chem.* **253**, 4058–4066.
Bergeron, J. J. M., Sikstrom, R., Hand, A. R. and Posner, B. I. (1979). *J. Cell. Biol.* **80**, 427–443.
Beynen, A. C., Vaartjes, W. J. and Geelen, M. J. H. (1979). *Diabetes* **28**, 828–835.
Beynen, A. C., Vaartjes, W. J. and Geelen, M. J. H. (1980). *Horm. Metab. Res.* **12**, 425–430.
Bhat, N. R., Madhava Rao, A. and Murthy, S. K. (1978a). *Indian J. Biochem. Biophys.* **15**, 39–42.
Bhat, N. R., Madhava Rao, A. and Murthy, S. K. (1978b). *Indian J. Biochem. Biophys.* **15**, 487–488.
Bhat, N. R., Madhava Rao, A., Kulkarni, G. R. and Murthy, S. K. (1979). *Indian J. Biochem. Biophys.* **16**, 288–293.
Bonner-Weir, S. and Weir, G. C. (1979). *Gen. comp. Endocr.* **38**, 28–37.
Boquist, L. and Falkmer, S. (1970). *In* "The Structure and Metabolism of the Pancreatic Islets" (S. Falkmer, B. Hellman and I. B. Taljedal, eds), pp. 25–35. Pergamon Press, New York.
Boyd, T. A., Wieser, P. B. and Fain, J. N. (1975). *Gen. comp. Endocr.* **26**, 243–247.
Brazeau, R., Vale, W. Burgus, R., Ling, N., Butcher, M., Rivier, J. and Guillemin, R. (1973). *Science, N.Y.* **179**, 77–79.
Bromer, W. W. (1972a). *In* "Handbook of Physiology—Section 7, Endocrinology" (R. O. Greep and E. B. Astwood, eds), Vol. 1, pp. 133–138. Waverly Press, Baltimore.
Bromer, W. W. (1972b). *In* "Glucagon; Molecular Physiology, Clinical and Therapeutic Implications" (P. J. Lefebvre and R. H. Unger, eds), pp. 27–30. Pergamon Press, New York.
Bromer, W. W., Boucher, M. E. and Koffenberger, J. E. (1971). *J. biol. Chem.* **246**, 2822–2827.
Bueno, L., Fioramonti, J., Rayner, V. and Puckenburch, Y. (1982). *Gastroenterology* **82**, 1395–1402.
Burgus, R., Ling, N., Butcher, M. and Guilleman, R. (1973). *Proc. natn. Acad. Sci., USA* **70**, 684–688.

Capuzzi, D. M., Rothman, V. and Margolis, S. (1974). *J. biol Chem.* **249**, 1286–1294.

Canivet, B., LeCam, A. and Freychet, P. (1979). *Diabete Metab.* **5**, 17–19.

Chan, S. J., Noyes, B. E. Agarwal, K. L. and Steiner, D. F. (1979). *Proc. natn. Acad. Sci., USA* **76**, 5036–5040.

Chen, K. K., Anderson, R. C. and Maze, N. (1945). *J. Pharmac. exp. Ther.* **84**, 74–77.

Cheung, W. Y. (1980a). *Science, N.Y.* **207**, 19–27.

Cheung, W. Y. (ed.), (1980b). "Calcium and Cell Function—Vol. 1, Calmodulin." Academic Press, New York and London.

Clarke, S. D., Watkins, P. A. and Lane, M. D. (1979). *J. Lipid Res.* **20**, 974–985.

Cohen, P. (ed.), "Molecular Aspects of Cellular Regulation" Vol. 1. Elsevier, North Holland.

Colca, J. R. and Hazelwood, R. L. (1981). *Gen comp. Endocr.* **45**, 482–490.

Colca, J. R. and Hazelwood, R. L. (1982). *Gen. comp. Endocr.* **47**, 104–110.

Cordell, B., Bell, G. I., Tischer, E., DeNoto, F. M., Ullrich, A., Pictet, R., Rutter, W. J. and Goodman, H. M. (1979). *Cell* **18**, 533–543.

Cramb, G. (1980). *Ph.D. thesis, University of Edinburgh.*

Cramb, G., Langslow, D. R. and Phillips, J. H. (1982a). *Gen. comp. Endocr.* **46**, 297–309.

Cramb, G., Langslow, D. R. and Phillips, J. H. (1982b). *Gen. comp. Endocr.* **46**, 310–321.

Cuatrecasas, P. (1971). *J. biol. Chem.* **246**, 6532-6542.

Cuatrecasas, P. (1972a). *Diabetes* **21**, 396–402.

Cuatrecasas, P. (1972b). *Proc. natn. Acad. Sci. USA* **69**, 318–322.

Cuatrecasas, P. and Hollenberg, M. D. (1976). *Adv. Protein Chem.* **30**, 251–451.

Dickson, A. J. and Langslow, D. R. (1978). *Mol. Cell. Biochem.* **22**, 162–181.

Dickson, A. J., Anderson, C. E. and Langslow, D. R. (1978). *Mol. Cell. Biochem.* **19**, 81–92.

Esch, F., Ohlen, B., Ling, N., Benoit, R., Brazeau, P. and Guillemin, P. (1980). *Proc. natn. Acad. Sci. USA* **77**, 6171–6174.

Exton, J. H. and Park, C. R. (1972). *In* "Handbook of Physiology—Section 7, Endocrinology" (R. O. Greep and E. B. Astwood, eds), Vol. 1, pp. 437–455. Waverley Press, Baltimore.

Falkmer, S. and Marques, M. (1972). *In* "Glucagon; Molecular Physiology, Clinical and Therapeutic Implications" (P. J. Lefebvre and R. H. Unger, eds) pp. 343–361. Pergamon Press, New York.

Falkmer, S. and Ostberg, Y. (1977). *In* "The Diabetic Pancreas" (B. Volk and K. F. Wellman, eds) pp. 15–60. Plenum Press, New York.

Falkmer, S. and Patent, G. J. (1972). *In* "Handbook of Physiology—Section 7, Endocrinology" (R. O. Greep and E. B. Astwood, eds), Vol. 1, pp. 1–23. Waverly Press, Baltimore.

Feurle, G. E., Wirth, A., Diehm, C. Lorenzen, M. and Schlier, F. G. (1980). *Eur. J. clin. Invest.* **10**, 249–251.

Fister, P., Eigenbrodt, E. and Schomer, W. (1982). *Mol. Cell. Endocr.* **26**, 19–30.

Fletcher, D. J., Noe, B. D., Bauer, G. E. and Quigley, J. P. (1980). *Diabetes* **29**, 593–599.

Foltzer, C., Haffen, K., Kedinger, M. and Mialhe,, P. (1982). *Gen. comp. Endocr.* **47**, 213–220.

Fischer, E. H. and Krebs, E. G. (1955). *J. biol. Chem.* **216**, 121–132.

Freychet, P. (1976). *In* "Methods in Receptor Research, Part II" (M. Blecher, ed.), pp. 385–428. Dekker, New York.

Freychet, P., Rosselin, G., Rancon, F., Fouchereau, M. and Broer, Y. (1974). *Horm. Metab. Res.* **5** (Suppl.), 72–78.

Fussganger, R. D., Kahn, C. R., Roth, J. and DeMeyts, P. (1976). *J. biol. Chem.* **251**, 2761–2769.

Gammeltoft, S., Kristensen, L. O. and Sestoft, L. (1978). *J. biol. Chem.* **253**, 8406–8413.

Garrison, J. C. and Haynes, R. C. (1973). *J. biol. Chem.* **248**, 5333–5343.

Gavin, J. R., III, Roth, J., Jen, P. and Freychet, P. (1972). *Proc. natn. Acad. Sci. USA* **69**, 747–751.

Gavin, J. R., III, Gorden, P., Roth, J., Archer, J. A. and Buell, D. N. (1973). *J. biol. Chem.* **248**, 2202–2207.

Gerich, J. E., Lorenzi, M., Hane, J., Gustafson, G., Guillerman, R. and Forsham, P. H. (1975). *Metabolism* **24**, 175–182.

Gingerich, R. L., Lacy, P. E., Chance, R. E. and Johnson, M. G. (1978). *Diabetes* **27**, 96–101.

Ginsberg, B. H., Kahn, C. R. and Roth, J. (1976). *Biochim. biophys. Acta* **443**, 227–246.

Ginsberg, B. H., Kahn, C. R. and Roth, J. (1977). *Endocrinology* **100**, 82–90.

Glieman, J. and Sonne, O. (1978). *J. biol. Chem.* **253**, 7857–7863.

Glieman, J., Gammeltoft, S. and Vinten, J. (1975). *J. biol. Chem.* **250**, 3368–3374.

Goldfine, I. D., Gardner, J. D. and Neville, D. M., Jnr. (1972). *J. biol. Chem.* **247**, 6919–6926.

Goldfine, I. D., Jones, A. L., Hradek, G. T., Wong, K. Y. and Monney, J. S. (1978). *Science, N.Y.* **202**, 760–763.

Gomez-Capilla, J. A. and Langslow, D. R. (1977). *Int. J. Biochem.* **8**, 417–420.

Goodman, R. H., Lund, P. K., Jacobs, J. W. and Habener, J. F. (1980). *J. biol. Chem.* **225**, 6549–6552.

Goodridge, A. G. (1968). *Am. J. Physiol.* **214**, 897–901.

Gorden, P., Carpentier, J. L., Freychet, P., LeCam, A. and Orci, L. (1978). *Science, N.Y.* **200**, 782–785.

Guha, B. and Gosh, A. (1978). *Gen. comp. Endocr.* **34**, 38–44.

Guillerman, R. and Gerich, J. E. (1976). *A. Rev. Med.* **27**, 379–388.

Halban, P. A., Wollheim, C. B., Blondel, B., Meda, P., Niesor, E. M. and Mintz, D. M. (1982). *Endocrinology* **111**, 86–94.

Hales, C. N., Luzio, J. P. and Siddle, K. (1978). *Biochem. Soc. Symp.* **43**, 97–135.

Harris, R. A., Mapes, J. P., Ochs, R. S., Crabb, D. W. and Stropes, L. (1978). *Adv. exp. Med. Biol.* **111**, 17–42.

Hazelwood, R. L. (1973). *Am. Zool.* **13**, 699–709.

Hazelwood, R. L. (1976). *In* "Avian Physiology" (P. D. Sturkie, ed.), pp. 210–232. Springer-Verlag, New York.

Hazelwood, R. L. and Langslow, D. R. (1978). *J. Endocr.* **76**, 449–459.

Hazelwood, R. L., Kimmel, J. R. and Pollock, H. G. (1968). *Endocrinology* **83**, 1331–1336.

Hazelwood, R. L., Turner, S. D., Kimmel, J. R. and Pollock, H. G. (1973). *Gen. comp. Endocr.* **21**, 485–497.

Hedeskov, C. J. (1980). *Physiol. Rev.* **60**, 442–509.

Hellerstrom, C., Howell, S. L., Edwards, J. C. and Anderson, A. (1972). *FEBS Lett.* **27**, 97–101.

Henderson, J. R., Daniel, P. M. and Fraser, P. A. (1981). *Gut* **22**, 158–167.

Hermansen, K., Christensen, S. E. and Orskov, H. (1979). *Diabetologia* **16**, 261–266.

Hill, K. J. (1971). *In* "Physiology and Biochemistry of the Domestic Fowl" (D. J. Bell and B. M. Freeman, eds), Vol. 1, pp. 25–49. Academic Press, London and New York.
Honey, R. N. and Weir, G. C. (1979). *Life Sci.* **24**, 1747–1750.
Honey, R. N. and Weir, G. C. (1980). *Endocrinology* **107**, 1065–1068.
Honey, R. N., Fallon, M. B. and Weir, G. C. (1980a). *Metabolism* **29**, 1242–1246.
Honey, R. N., Schwarz, J. A., Mathe, C. J. and Weir, G. C. (1980b). *Am. J. Physiol.* **238**, E150–156.
Honey, R. N., Arimura, A. and Weir, G. C. (1981). *Endocrinology* **109**, 1971–1974.
Houslay, M. D. and Palmer, R. W. (1978). *Biochem. J.* **174** 909–919.
Houslay, M. D., Dipple, I. and Elliot, K. R. F. (1980). *Biochem. J.* **186**, 649–658.
Humbel, R. E., Bosshard, M. R. and Zahn, H. (1972). *In* "Handbook of Physiology—Section 7, Endocrinology" (R. O. Greep and E. B. Astwood, eds) Vol. 1, pp. 111–132. Waverly Press, Baltimore.
Iverson, J. (1973). *Diabetes* **22**, 381–387.
Johnson, D. G., Ensinick, J. W., Koerker, D., Palmer, J. and Goodner, C. J. (1975). *Endocrinology* **96**, 370–374.
Joshi, V. C. and Aranda, L. P. (1979a). *J. biol. Chem.* **254**, 11779–11782.
Joshi, V. C. and Aranda, L. P. (1979b). *J. biol. Chem.* **254**, 11783–11786.
Kahn, C. R. (1975). *In* "Membrane Receptors for Polypeptide Hormones" (E. D. Korn, ed.), pp. 81–146. Plenum Press, New York.
Kahn, C. R. (1976). *J. Cell. Biol.* **70**, 261–286.
Kahn, C. R. and Baird, K. (1978). *J. biol. Chem.* **253**, 4900–4906.
Kanazawa, Y., Kawazu, S., Ikeuch, M. and Kosaka, K. (1980). *Diabetes* **29**, 953–959.
Kimmel, J. R. and Pollock, H. G. (1981). *Endocrinology* **109**, 1693–1699.
Kimmel, J. R., Pollock, H. G. and Hazelwood, R. L. (1968). *Endocrinology* **83**, 1323–1330.
Kimmel, J. R., Pollock, H. G. and Hazelwood, R. L. (1971). *Fedn. Proc. Fedn. Am. Socs. exp. Biol.* **30**, 1318.
Kimmel, J. R., Hayden, L. J. and Pollock, H. G. (1975). *J. biol. Chem.* **250**, 9369–9376.
King, D. L. and Hazelwood, R. L. (1976). *Am. J. Physiol.* **231**, 1830–1839.
Klein, C. and van Noorden, S. (1980). *Cell. Tiss. Res.* **205**, 187–198.
Koerker, D. J., Ruch, W., Chideckel, E., Palmer, J., Goodner, C. J., Ensinck, J. and Gale, C. C. (1974). *Science, N.Y.* **184**, 482–484.
Kono, T. and Barham, F. W. (1971). *J. biol. Chem.* **246**, 6210–6216.
Krebs, E. G. and Beavo, J. A. (1979). *A. Rev. Biochem.* **44**, 923–959.
Krupp, M. N. and Lane, M. D. (1982). *J. biol. Chem.* **257**, 1372–1377.
Kwast-Weldfeld, J. and Kaniuga, Z. (1979). *Int. J. Biochem.* **10**, 403–410.
Langslow, D. R. (1971). *Biochim. biophys. Acta.* **239**, 33–37.
Langslow, D. R. (1972). *Comp. Biochem. Physiol.* **43B**, 689–701.
Langslow, D. R. and Hales, C. N. (1969). *J. Endocr.* **43**, 285–294.
Langslow, D. R. and Hales, C. N. (1971). *In* "Physiology and Biochemistry of the Domestic Fowl" (D. J. Bell and B. M. Freeman, eds), Vol. 1, pp. 521–547. Academic Press, London and New York.
Langslow, D. R. and Freeman, B. M. (1972). *Diabetologia* **8**, 206–210.
Langslow, D. R. and Siddle, K. (1979). *Gen. comp. Endocr.* **39**, 521–526.
Langslow, D. R., Butler, E. J., Hales, C. N. and Pearson, A. W. (1970). *J. Endocr.* **46**, 243–260.

Langslow, D. R., Kimmel, J. R. and Pollock, H. G. (1973). *Endocrinology* **93**, 558–565.
Langslow, D. R., Cramb, G. and Siddle, K. (1979). *Gen. comp. Endocr.* **39**, 527–533.
Larner, J., Cheng, K., Schwartz, C., Kikuchi, K., Tamuras, A., Creacy, S., Dubler, R., Galaskp, G., Pullin, C. and Katz, M. (1982). *Recent Progr. Horm. Res.* **38**, 511–556.
Larsson, L-I., Sundler, F., Hakanson, R., Pollock, H. G. and Kimmel, J. R. (1974). *Histochemistry* **42**, 377–382.
Larsson, L-I., Sundler, F. and Hakanson, R. (1976). *Diabetologia* **12**, 211–226.
Lin, T. M. and Chance, R. E. (1974). *Gastroenterology* **67**, 730–755.
Lomedico, P., Rosenthal, N., Efstratiadis, A., Gilbert, W., Kolodner, R. and Tizard, R. (1979). *Cell* **18**, 545–558.
Lonovics, J., Guzman, S., Devitt, P. G., Mejtmancik, K. E., Suddith, R. L. Rayford, P. L. and Thompson, J. C. (1981). *Endocrinology* **108**, 1925–1930.
Lundt, P. K., Goodman, R. H., Jacobs, J. W. and Habener, J. F. (1980). *Diabetes* **29**, 583–586.
McCumbee, W. D. and Hazelwood, R. L. (1977). *Gen. comp. Endocr.* **33**, 518–525.
McCumbee, W. D. and Hazelwood, R. L. (1978). *Gen. comp. Endocr.* **34**, 421–427.
Malaisse, W. J. and Orci, L. (1979). *Meth. Archiv. exp. Path.* **9**, 112–136.
Malaisse, W. J., Malaisse-Lagae, F. and Wright, P. H. (1967). *Endocrinology* **80**, 99–108.
Malaisse, W. J., Malaisse-Lagae, F., Walker, M. O. and Lacy, P. E. (1971). *Diabetes* **20**, 257–265.
Marco, J., Hedo, J. H. and Villanueva, M. L. (1977). *Life Sci.* **21**, 789–792.
Markusson, J. and Sundby, F. (1973). *Eur. J. Biochem.* **34**, 401–408.
Markusson, J., Frandsen, E., Heding, L. G. and Sundby, F. (1972). *Horm. Metab. Res.* **4**, 360–363.
Means, A. R. and Dedman, J. R. (1980). *Nature, Lond.* **285**, 73–77.
Meda, P., Kohen, E., Kohen, C. and Orci, L. (1982). *C.r. Séanc. Acad. Sci. Ser. III* **293**, 607–610.
Meredith, M. J. and Lane, M. D. (1978). *J. biol. Chem.* **253**, 3381–3383.
Meyers, C. A., Murphy, W. A., Redding, T. W., Coy, D. H. and Schally, A. V. (1980). *Proc. natn. Acad. Sci. USA* **77**, 6171–6174.
Mikami, S-I. and Ono, K. (1962). *Endocrinology* **71**, 464–473.
Mooney, R. A. and Lane, M. D. (1981). *J. biol. Chem.* **256**, 11724–11733.
Mooney, R. A. and Lane, M. D. (1982). *Eur. J. Biochem.* **121**, 281–288.
Naber, S. P. and Hazelwood, R. L. (1977). *Gen. comp. Endocr.* **32**, 495–504.
Nelson, N., Elgart, S. and Mirsky, I. A. (1942). *Endocrinology* **31**, 119–123.
Nimmo, H. G. and Cohen, P. (1977). *Adv. Cyclic. Nuc. Res.* **8**, 145–266.
Noe, B. D. and Bauer, G. E. (1971). *Endocrinology* **89**, 642–651.
Noe, B. D. and Bauer, G. E. (1975). *Endocrinology* **97**, 868–877.
Oakberg, E. F. (1949). *Am. J. Anat.* **84**, 279–310.
O'Keefe, E. and Cuatrecasas, P. (1974). *Biochim. biophys. Acta* **343**, 64–77.
Oliver, J. R. and Wagle, S. R. (1975). *Biochem. biophys. Res. Commun.* **62**, 772–777.
Oliver, J. R., Long, K., Wagle, S. R. and Allen, D. O. (1976). *Proc. Soc. exp. Biol. Med.* **153**, 367–369.
Orci, L. and Malaisse, W. (1980). *Diabetes* **29**, 943–944.
Orci, L., Baetens, D., Dubois, M. P. and Rufener, C. (1975). *Horm. Metab. Res.* **7**, 400–402.
Patel, Y. C. and Reichlin, S. (1978). *Endocrinology* **102**, 523–530.

Patel, Y. C., Wheatley, T., Fitz-Patrick, D. and Brock, G. (1980). *Endocrinology* **107**, 306–313.
Perler, F., Efstradiadis, A., Lomedico, P., Gilbert, W. Kolodner, R. and Dodgson, J. (1980). *Cell* **20**, 555–566.
Pictet, R. and Rutter, W. J. (1972). *In* "Handbook of Physiology—Section 7, Endocrinology" (R. O. Greep and E. B. Astwood eds), Vol. 1, pp. 25–66. Waverly Press, Baltimore.
Pilkis, S. J., Claus, T. H., Johnson, R. A. and Park, C. R. (1974). *Biochim. biophys. Acta* **343**, 250–267.
Pollock, H. G. and Kimmel, J. R. (1975). *J. biol. Chem.* **250**, 9377–9380.
Posner, B. I. (1974). *Diabetes* **23**, 209–217.
Posner, B. I., Josefsberg, Z. and Bergeron, J. J. M. (1978). *J. biol. Chem.* **253**, 4067–4073.
Rawdon, B. B. and Andrew, A. (1979). *Histochemistry* **59**, 181–197.
Reubi, J-C., Rivier, J ., Perrin, M., Brown, M. and Vale, W. (1982). *Endocrinology* **110**, 1049–1051.
Robertson, R. P. and Porte, D. (1973). *Diabetes* **22**, 1–8.
Rodbell, M. (1980). *Nature, Lond.* **284**, 17–22.
Ross, E. M. and Gilman, A. G. (1980). *A. Rev. Biochem.* **49**, 533–564.
Roth, J., Bonner-Weir, S., Norman, A. W. and Orci, L. (1982). *Endocrinology* **110**, 2216–2218.
Ryle, A. P., Sanger, F., Smith, L. F. and Kitai, R. (1955). *Biochem. J.* **60**, 541–556.
Sacks, H., Waligora, K., Matthew, J. and Pimstone, B. (1977). *Endocrinology* **101**, 1751–1759.
Sakuri, H., Dobbs, R. and Unger, R. H. (1974). *J. clin. Invest.* **54**, 1395–1402.
Samols, E. and Weir, G. C. (1979). *J. clin. Invest.* **63**, 230–238.
Samols, E., Tyler, J. M., Marks, V. and Mialhe, P. (1969). "Proceedings of the 3rd International Conference on Endocrinology, Mexico", pp. 206–219. Excerpta Medica, Amsterdam.
Samols, E., Taylor, J. M. and Marks, V. (1972). *In* "Glucagon: Molecular Physiology, Clinical and Therapeutic Implications" (P. J. Lefebvre and R. H. Unger, eds) pp. 151–173. Pergamon Press, New York.
Samols, E., Weir, G. C., Ramseur, R., Day, J. A. and Patel, Y. C. (1978). *Metabolism* **27** (Suppl. 1), 1219–1221.
Samols, E., Stagner, J. I. and Weir, G. C. (1981). *Diabetologia* **20** (Suppl.), 388–392.
Schally, A. V., Dupont, A., Arimura, A., Redding, T. W., Nishi, N., Linthicum, G. L. and Schlesinger, D. H. (1976). *Biochemistry* **15**, 509–514.
Schally, A. V., Huang, N. Y., Chang, R. C., Arimura, A. and Redding, T. W. (1980). *Proc. natn. Acad. Sci., USA* **77**, 4489–4493.
Schusdziarra, V. (1980). *Horm. Metab. Res.* **12**, 563–577.
Schwartz, R. H., Bianco, A. R. and Handwerger, B. S. (1975). *Proc. natn. Acad. Sci. USA* **72**, 474–478.
Schwartz, R. H., Holst, J. J., Fahrenkrug, J., Jensen, S. L., Nielson, O. V., Rehfeld, J. F., DeMuckadell, O. B. and Stadil, F. (1978). *J. clin. Invest.* **61**, 781–789.
Schwartz, T. W. and Tager, H. S. (1981). *Nature, Lond.* **294**, 589–591.
Sharp, G. W. G. (1979). *Diabetologia* **16**, 287–296.
Sharp, G. W. G., Wollheim, C., Muller, W. A., Gutzeit, A., Trueheart, P. A., Blonden, B., Orci, L. and Renold, A. E. (1975). *Fedn. Proc. Fedn. Am. Socs. exp. Biol.* **34**, 1537–1548.

Shields, D. (1981). *Biochem. biophys. Res. Commun.* **98**, 242–249.
Shushevich, S. I., Khustochka, L. N., Khalmuradov, A. G. and Fomenko, A. I. (1981). *Ukr. biochem. Zh.* **53**, 101–105.
Silverstein, S. C., Steinman, R. M. and Cohn, Z. A. (1977). *A. Rev. Biochem.* **46**, 669–722.
Simon, J. (1979). *Biochim. biophys. Acta* **585**, 563–574.
Simon, J. and Rosselin, G. (1978). *Horm. Metab. Res.* **10**, 93–98.
Simon, J., Freychet, P. and Rosselin, G. (1977a). *Diabetologia* **13**, 219–228.
Simon, J., Freychet, P., Rosselin, G. and DeMeyts, P. (1977b). *Endocrinology* **100**, 115–121.
Sitbon, G. and Mialhe, P. (1978). *Horm. Metab. Res.* **10**, 473–477.
Sitbon, G., Laurent, F., Mialhe, A., Krug, E., Karmann, H., Gross, R., Strosser, M. T., Cohen, L., Jean-Marie, P., Foltzer, C. and Mialhe, P. (1980). *Horm. Metab. Res.* **12**, 1–9.
Smith, L. F. (1966). *Am. J. Med.* **40**, 662–666.
Soll, A. H., Goldfine, I. D., Roth, J., Kahn, C. R. and Neville, D. M. (1974). *J. biol. Chem.* **249**, 4127–4131.
Soman, V. and Felig, P. (1978). *Nature, Lond.* **272**, 829–832.
Somers, G., Blondel, B., Orci, L. and Malaisse, W. J. (1979). *Endocrinology* **104**, 255–264.
Sonne, O., Berg, T. and Christoffersen, T. (1978). *J. biol. Chem.* **253**, 3203–3210.
Spiess, J., Rivier, J. E., Rodkey, J. A. Bennett, C. D. and Vale, W. (1979). *Proc. natn. Acad. Sci. USA* **76**, 2974–2978.
Steffens, A. B. (1981). *Diabetologia* **20** (Suppl.), 411–416.
Steiner, D. F. (1977). *Diabetes* **26**, 322–340.
Steiner, D. F., Quinn, P. S., Chan, S. J., Marsh, J. and Tager, H. S. (1980). *Ann. N.Y. Acad. Sci.* **343**, 1–16.
Strosser, M. T., Cohen, L., Harvey, S. and Mialhe, P. (1980). *Diabetologia* **18**, 319–322.
Sundby, F., Frandsen, E. K., Thomson, J., Kristiansen, K. and Brunfeldt, K. (1972). *FEBS. Letts* **26**, 289–293.
Tager, H. S., Patzelt, C., Assoian, R. K., Chan, S. H., Duguid, J. R. and Steiner, D. F. (1980). *Ann. N.Y. Acad. Sci.* **343**, 133–147.
Tannenbaum, G. S., Ling, N. and Brazeau, P. (1982). *Endocrinology* **111**, 101–107.
Terris, S., Hofmann, C. and Steiner, D. F. (1979). *Can. J. Biochem.* **57**, 459–468.
Thompsen, J., Kristiansen, K., Brunfeldt, K. and Sundby, F. (1972). *FEBS. Letts.* **21**, 315–319.
Tung, A. K. (1973). *Horm. Metab. Res.* **5**, 416–424.
Tung, A. K. (1974). *Can. J. Biochem.* **52**, 1081–1086.
Tung, A. K., Rosenzweig, S. A. and Foa, P. P. (1976). *Proc. Soc. exp. Biol. Med.* **153**, 344–349.
Turner, S. D. and Hazelwood, R. L. (1974). *Comp. Biochem. Physiol.* **47A**, 303–313.
Tyler, J. M. and Kajinuma, H. (1972). *Diabetes* **21**, 332 (abs.).
Unger, R. H., Dobbs, R. E., Orci, L. (1978). *A. Rev. Physiol.* **40**, 307–343.
Vale, W., Ling, N., Rivier, J., Villarreal, J., Rivier, C., Douglas, C. and Brown, M. (1976). *Metabolism* **25** (Suppl.), 1491–1494.
Van Noorden, S. and Patent, G. J. (1978). *Cell. Tiss. Res.* **188**, 521–525.
Van Obberghen, E. and Roth, J. (1981). *In* "Receptor Regulation" (R. J. Lefkowitz, ed.), pp. 7–40. Chapman and Hall, London.
Van Obberghen, E., DeMeyts, P. and Roth, J. (1976). *J. biol. Chem.* **251**, 6844–6851.

Vuylsteke, C. A. and DeDuve, C. (1953). *Arch. int. Physiol.* **61**, 273–274.
Watanabe, T. and Yasuda, M. (1977). *Cell Tiss. Res.* **180**, 453–465.
Watkins, P. A. and Lane, M. D. (1976). *Fedn. Proc. Fedn. Am. Socs. exp. Biol.* **45**, 1428 (abs.).
Watkins, P. A., Tarlow, D. M. and Lane, M. D. (1977). *Proc. natn. Acad. Sci. USA* **74**, 1497–1501.
Weir, G. C., Goltsos, P. C., Steinberg, E. P. and Patel, Y. C. (1976). *Diabetologia* **12**, 129–132.
Weir, G. C., Samols, E., Loo, S., Patel, Y. C. and Gabbay, K. H. (1979). *Diabetes* **28**, 35–40.
Weitzel, G., Renner, R. Kemmler, W. and Rager, K. (1972). *Hoppe-Seylers, Z. physiol. Chem.* **353**, 980–986.
Westwood, S. A. and Siddle, K. (1979). *Biochem. Soc. Trans.* **7**, 1032–1033.
Woods, S. C. and Porte, B. D. Jnr. (1974). *Physiol. Rev.* **54**, 596–619.
Zingg, H. H. and Patel, Y. C. (1979). *Biochem. biophys. Res. Commun.* **90**, 466–472.

6 Calcium Metabolism and its Regulation

T. G. TAYLOR[1] and C. G. DACKE[2]

[1]*School of Biochemical and Physiological Sciences, University of Southampton, Southampton, England*
[2]*Physiology Department, Marischal College, University of Aberdeen, Aberdeen, Scotland*

PHYSIOLOGY BIOCHEMISTRY DOMESTIC
FOWL, VOL. 5 ISBN 0–12–267105–8

I. Introduction

As in mammals, calcium metabolism in birds is under the control of three major hormones, parathyroid hormone (PTH), calcitonin (CT) and 1,25-dihydroxycholecalciferol ($1,25(OH)_2D_3$), the active metabolite of vitamin D_3, but prostaglandins, reproductive steroids and some other hormones also exert a significant influence. Furthermore, the amounts of calcium and vitamin D in the diet have profound effects on the metabolism of the mineral. Since the mid-seventies, the central role of $1,25(OH)_2D_3$ in the control of calcium metabolism has come to be recognized. Advances in knowledge of the metabolism and mechanism of action of vitamin D during this period have been truly spectacular, and most of the basic research has been carried out using birds.

In this chapter, the basic physiology of the major calcium-regulating hormones will first be discussed and in the subsequent sections the way in which these hormones function together to achieve calcium homoeostasis in periods of physiological stress will be considered.

II. Parathyroid Hormone

Advances in knowledge of parathyroid physiology and biochemistry in avian species have been handicapped by the absence of a sensitive method for assaying PTH in physiological fluids. Bioassays for PTH have been reported using chicks (Lewis and Taylor, 1972; Parsons *et al.*, 1973) or Japanese quail (Dacke and Kenny, 1973), but these methods are not sufficiently sensitive for measuring the concentration of hormone in small samples of blood. The measurement of changes in the rate of secretion of PTH in relation to diet and in different physiological states must await the development of a radioimmunological, or of an equally sensitive, assay. Meanwhile, the main experimental tools available for studying parathyroid function in birds are parathyroidectomy and the use of PTH injections.

A. Chemistry and Biosynthesis

Information on the biosynthesis and secretion of PTH relates primarily to mammals, but the work of MacGregor *et al.* (1973) on chicken PTH suggests that similar mechanisms may operate in birds; these mechanisms have been reviewed by Habener (1981) and will be summarized here.

PTH is a polypeptide containing 84 amino acids that is synthesized from a precursor molecule, pro-PTH, by removal of an NH_2-terminal sequence of six amino acids in the Golgi apparatus of the secretory cell. Pro-PTH is itself derived from a precursor polypeptide with 115 residues, known as pre-pro-PTH, by the removal of 25 amino acids from the NH_2-terminal end of the molecule during its translation in the rough endoplasmic reticulum. Further breakdown of PTH occurs both before and after release from the cells of the parathyroid gland giving rise to a large number of fragments of different sizes, many of which react in immunoassay systems even though they may have no biological activity. This phenomenon complicates the interpretation of results obtained by immunoassays. The NH_2-terminal 1–34 peptide possesses near-maximal activity and up to seven amino acids can be removed from the carboxyl terminus without serious loss of activity. Removal of even one amino acid from the NH_2-terminal results in a marked decrease in activity.

B. Physiological Action

The concentration of ionic calcium in the extracellular fluid is the most powerful regulator of PTH secretion but a number of other factors, including magnesium, catecholamines and prostaglandins, act as modulators of hormone secretion. Cyclic AMP appears to be a secondary messenger in the control of PTH secretion by calcium, and intracellular concentrations of cyclic AMP increase in parallel with increases in the rate of PTH secretion under the influence both of hypocalcaemia and secretagogues, such as adrenaline, dopamine and prostaglandin E_2. Furthermore, agents that suppress PTH release, for example, α-adrenergic agonists and prostaglandin $F_{2\alpha}$, decrease intracellular concentrations of cyclic AMP (see Habener, 1981, for review).

The primary targets for PTH in birds, as in mammals, are kidney and bone, and the physiological action of the hormone on these tissues appears to be similar. In laying birds fed on a high-calcium diet (50 gCa kg^{-1}), which probably inhibited the endogenous secretion of PTH, Mueller *et al.* (1973) demonstrated transient hypocalcaemic and hypophosphataemic responses to PTH, 2·5 and 5 min after a single injection of the hormone. The plasma values had returned to the base-line value by 7·5 min and the normal hypercalcaemic and hyperphosphataemic phase peaked at 30 min. Boelkins *et al.* (1976) showed that changes in the blood flow to the leg bones following PTH injection paralleled the changes in calcium and phosphorus concentrations. Three minutes after the injection, blood flow to the leg bones was reduced by 16 to 18% relative to pre-injection values, while at 30 min blood flow increased by 15 to 50%, depending on the type of PTH preparation used.

A major role for PTH is the regulation of the metabolism of vitamin D and this aspect is discussed in Section IV.

III. Calcitonin

The publication by Cutler *et al.* (1974) of a sensitive radioimmunoassay for chicken calcitonin (CT) using synthetic salmon CT for raising the antibody should have provided a great stimulus to CT research in birds, but workers have been disappointingly slow to exploit this technique. Nevertheless, there have been some important developments in this field.

A. Embryological Origins

Within five years of its discovery, the embryonic source of calcitonin (CT) was identified as the ultimobranchial bodies which, in birds, remain more or less discrete (Copp *et al.*, 1967). However, like PTH-secreting cells, it seems that the ultimate source of CT-secreting (C) cells lies in the neuro-ectoderm of the neural crest. Thus, C-cells, in common with other peptide-secreting cells of neuro-ectodermal origin, are able to take up and decarboxylate amine precursors, the so-called APUD (amine precursor uptake and decarboxylation) phenomenon (Pearse, 1976). In the same review, Pearse gives details of the comparative morphology and cytochemistry of vertebrate ultimobranchial bodies.

Until recently, the first phylogenic appearance of CT was thought to be in the lower orders of vertebrates (Dacke, 1979), but it is now apparent that immunoreactive CT is also present in the central nervous systems of several protochordates (Fritsch *et al.*, 1979; Girgis *et al.*, 1980). In birds, it seems to be located predominantly in the hypothalamus and mid-brain (Galan *et al.*, 1981). The latter authors have accordingly ascribed a possible neuromodulator function to CT, though whether it is produced locally or is simply bound to specific receptors in these areas of the CNS is not yet clear. Hoyt *et al.* (1972) assayed chicken thyroid, parathyroid and ultimobranchial glands for CT using a rat bioassay technique and observed that the potency of the parathyroids/g fresh tissue was about the same as in the ultimobranchial glands; CT was not detected in the thyroid, but it was present in the cervical nerves. The localization of CT in the pigeon was slightly different.

B. Chemistry

Amino acid sequences for CTs from several sources have been elucidated. The basic molecule is consistently a chain of 32 amino acids (MW 3000) with a seven membered ring at the N-terminus. Unlike PTH, all 32 amino acids are necessary for the expression of biological activity (Potts and Aurbach, 1976).

Major differences exist between the amino acid composition of CT from different species and even within species different forms of the hormone may exist. Surprisingly, the amino acid sequence for chicken and other avian CTs is not completely elaborated, although the amino acid composition is known to be quite similar to that of the eel or salmon hormones. Moreover, in radioimmunoassay, the chicken and salmon hormones give completely parallel curves, indicating a high degree of immunological homogeneity (Cutler *et al.*, 1974). Immunological and structural studies tend to group avian and teleost CTs together as advanced types, while of the mammalian CTs, the major human molecule appears to be relatively primitive.

Small amounts of a human CT-like hormone in the ultimobranchial and thyroid glands of the fowl have recently been detected at concentrations of 1% and 3·75% respectively of the avian type of CT present in these glands (Perez Cano *et al.*, 1982).

C. Changes with Age in Circulating CT

Dacke *et al.* (1976) studied the changes with age that occur in the concentration of CT in the plasma of Japanese quail. There was a three-fold increase in the concentration of CT at 6 weeks of age in both sexes, shortly before sexual maturity. When the females came into lay, the concentration of CT decreased and a slight decrease was also observed in the cock birds once they were sexually mature (Fig. 1). Castration of mature cocks at 8 weeks of age resulted in a marked lowering of plasma CT levels, but castration at 4 weeks of age had little effect. The authors suggested that the increase in androgenic activity at the time of sexual maturity may play an important part in the CT surge observed at 6 weeks of age. Boelkins and Kenny (1973) had earlier shown that

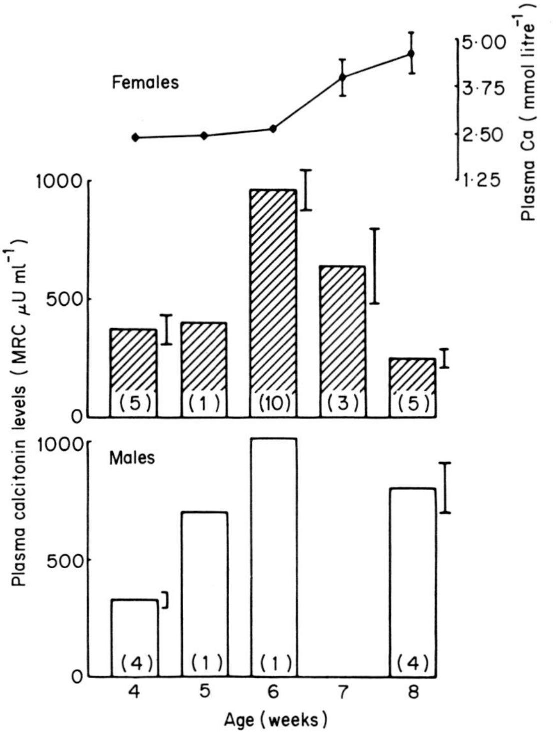

Fig. 1. Changes in plasma calcitonin concentrations in Japanese quail in relation to sexual maturity . (From Dacke *et al.*, 1976.) Note that the maximum (6-week) values occur before sexual maturity is reached in both sexes. The numbers in parentheses denote the number of samples.

adult male quail have greater concentrations of CT in their plasma than adult females, in spite of the fact that the plasma concentration of Ca^{2+} is greater in females.

Baimbridge and Taylor (1981) studied the effects of different amounts of dietary calcium on plasma CT concentrations in chicks from 6 to 10 weeks of age. The amount of CT in the control birds given 11 g calcium per kg diet varied from 1·05 to 1·64 ng ml^{-1}. This concentration rose to a maximum of 2·5 ng ml^{-1} at the highest rate of inclusion of dietary calcium (60 g kg^{-1}). The concentrations in the plasma of both CT and total calcium increased progressively as the amount of calcium in the diet increased and the plasma inorganic phosphorus concentration showed a progressive decline. There were no consistent differences between the sexes in any of these variables. These results confirm that CT secretion in chicks is stimulated by hypercalcaemia, but indicate that CT is unable to restore the plasma calcium to normal when the chicks are fed with diets rich in calcium.

D. Control of CT Secretion

Short loop negative feedback control of CT secretion by the plasma Ca^{2+} concentration seems less important, particularly in avian and other sub-mammalian species, than it is for PTH secretion. Much of the information concerning the mechanisms of CT secretion in birds has been summarized by Care and Bates (1972) and by Dacke (1979). While it is clear that secretion of this hormone from the avian ultimobranchial body is stimulated by hypercalcaemia, it is also apparent that the gland, at least in geese, is less responsive to this stimulus than the mammalian thyroid (Fig. 2). The resting rate of CT

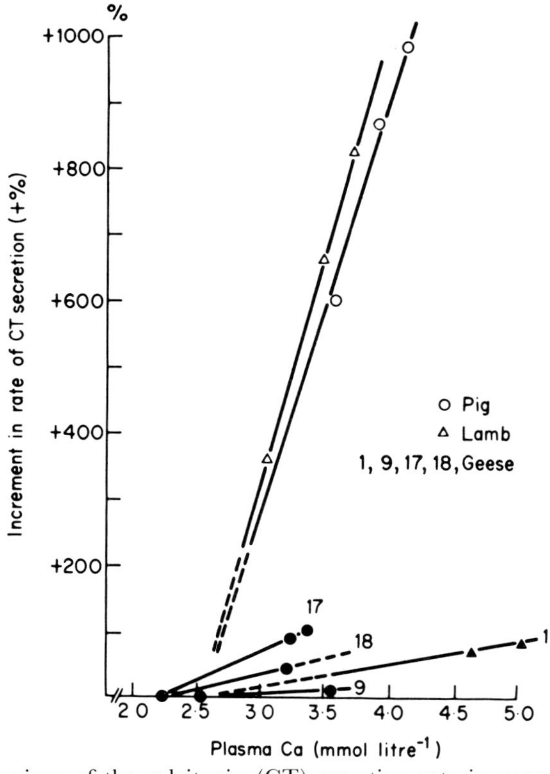

Fig. 2. Comparison of the calcitonin (CT) secretion rate in goose, pig and lamb. Doubling the plasma calcium concentration caused a much greater increase in CT secretion from porcine and ovine thyroids than from anserine ultimobranchial glands. (From Care and Bates, 1972.)

secretion in the goose (2 MRC mU min^{-1} kg^{-1}) is, however, about twenty five times higher on a body weight basis than that reported for pigs and sheep (Bates *et al.*, 1969).

Ziegler *et al.* (1970) found that cyclic AMP can stimulate CT release in birds. Only β-adrenergic compounds such as isoproterenol have been found to activate adenylate cyclase in avian C-cells, but this may be significant when the complex innervation (compared with mammals) of avian ultimobranchial bodies is considered (Hodges, 1970). Care and Bates (1972) demonstrated that vagal stimulation results in as much as a three-fold increase in the rate of CT secretion in birds, indicating an important neural element in the control of secretion. CT secretion has also been studied *in vitro* in cultures of chicken ultimobranchial bodies (Feinblatt and Raisz, 1972; Nieto *et al.*, 1975), and it is stimulated both by an increase Ca^{2+} concentration and by dibutyryl cyclic AMP (2×10^{-3} mol $litre^{-1}$).

In mammals, the rate of CT secretion is very sensitive to secretagogue hormones of gastrointestinal origin, such as glucagon (Care *et al.*, 1969), pancreozymin-cholecystokinin (Care *et al.*, 1971) and gastrin (Cooper *et al.*, 1971), all of which are released in response to food ingestion. This aspect of CT secretion has not been studied in birds.

E. Ultimobranchial Extirpation

Copp *et al.* (1970) demonstrated that ultimobranchialectomy in young turkeys seriously reduced their ability to maintain plasma Ca^{2+} concentrations during infusions of calcium (Fig. 3).

F. Calcitonin Injection

Plasma calcium concentrations of normocalcaemic birds are remarkably refractory to CT injection (Dacke, 1979). Two reasons may be suggested to explain the failure of most workers (e.g. Gonnerman *et al.*, 1972) to observe a hypocalcaemic action for CT in normal birds: the first is that only total calcium was measured rather than ionic calcium; the second possible explanation is that, due to the speed with which PTH acts in birds (Candlish and Taylor, 1970), the hypocalcaemia initially induced by CT was rapidly overcome, too rapidly for it to be detected. Luck *et al.* (1980) reported that salmon CT (40 MRC U per bird) reduced the plasma Ca^{2+} concentration in laying hens by about 18% (but not total Ca), when injected 15 to 16 h after ovulation, and Baimbridge and Taylor (1980) observed a significant hypocalcaemia in

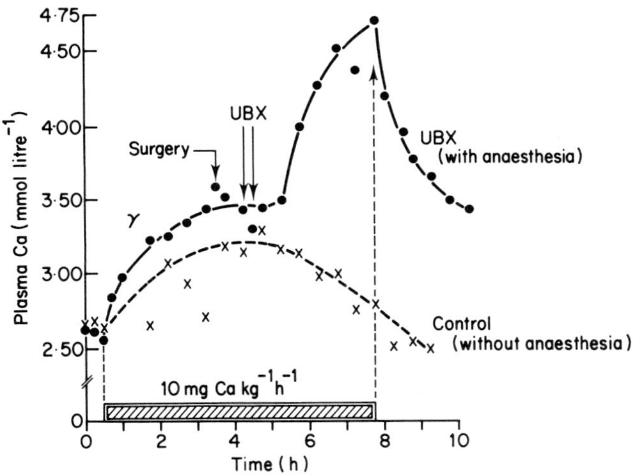

Fig. 3. The effect on plasma total calcium of bilateral ultimobranchialectomy (UBX) in a young turkey during the course of a calcium infusion at the rate of 10 mg Ca kg^{-1} h^{-1} (solid line). In the control bird (broken line), the concentration of plasma calcium reached a peak about 4 h after the start of the infusion and then fell, presumably under the influence of calcitonin. When UBX was carried out half way through the infusion, the plasma calcium concentration increased markedly and remained well above normal 2 h after the calcium infusion had ceased. (From Copp *et al.*, 1970.)

chick embryos in which endogenous release of CT was stimulated by isoprenaline.

G. General Conclusions

Since the first review in this series was published (Simkiss and Dacke, 1971), our understanding of the function of CT in birds has greatly increased. Although CT does not induce a lowering of the plasma calcium concentration in normocalcaemic birds, there is now little doubt that the hormone plays an important role in calcium homoeostasis in birds and Baimbridge and Taylor (1981) have emphasized that one of the true physiological roles of CT in birds, as in mammals, is to *combat hypercalcaemia* rather than to *induce hypocalcaemia*. The other major role of CT in mammals is the protection of the skeleton from excessive resorption in times of calcium stress, for example, in pregnancy and lactation (Taylor *et al.*, 1975). The possibility that CT may play an analagous role in egg-laying birds is considered in Section VII. Other putative functions for this hormone in vertebrates include those of osmoregulation and phosphate regulation (Dacke, 1979).

IV. Vitamin D

A. Introduction

It has been shown that vitamin D is metabolized to active compounds which endocrinologists now recognize as hormonal in character, and avian studies, particularly with chickens and Japanese quail, have provided the main source of information on the metabolism and physiological actions of the vitamin. For detailed reviews see Lawson (1978), De Luca (1979a) and Dacke (1979) (comparative aspects).

B. Chemistry

Vitamin D_3 (cholecalciferol) and its metabolites are fat-soluble compounds classed as secosteroids. Conversion of the steroid precursor 7-dehydrocholesterol to D_3 under the influence of ultra violet (u.v.) light over the range of wave length 256–313 nm is well known in mammals, and is thought to occur also in birds, when the preen gland oil containing 7-dehydrocholesterol, is spread over the feathers and irradiated by U.V. light before oral ingestion of the vitamin (Sebrell and Harris, 1954). The photolysis reaction converts 7-dehydrocholesterol to previtamin D_3 which is in chemical equilibrium both with D_3 and with its precursor molecule (Fig. 4). The conversion of previtamin D_3 to D_3 is a slow process and in mammals equilibrium is not reached for about 36 h (Holick *et al.*, 1977). The next step is a hydroxylation at the 25 position yielding 25-hydroxycholecalciferol ($25(OH)D_3$). This reaction occurs mainly in microsomal fractions of liver cells, but Tucker *et al.* (1973) have presented evidence that some hydroxylation occurs also in the kidney and intestines of chicks.

C. Metabolism in the Liver

There is no general agreement as to the mechanisms by which production of $25(OH)D_3$ by the liver is regulated, or indeed as to whether it is regulated at all (Holick and Clark, 1978). Bhattacharyya and De Luca (1974), however, showed that, whereas a small dose of D_3 administered to rachitic chicks did not alter the activity of the 25-hydroxylase, a large dose decreased its activity to 17% of that observed in control D_3-deficient birds after 24 h. Later, *in vitro* work with D_3-replete Japanese quail (Nicholson *et al.*, 1979) showed that the activity of the 25-hydroxylase in the liver of immature and adult male birds was very low and that D_3 was mainly converted into unknown compounds,

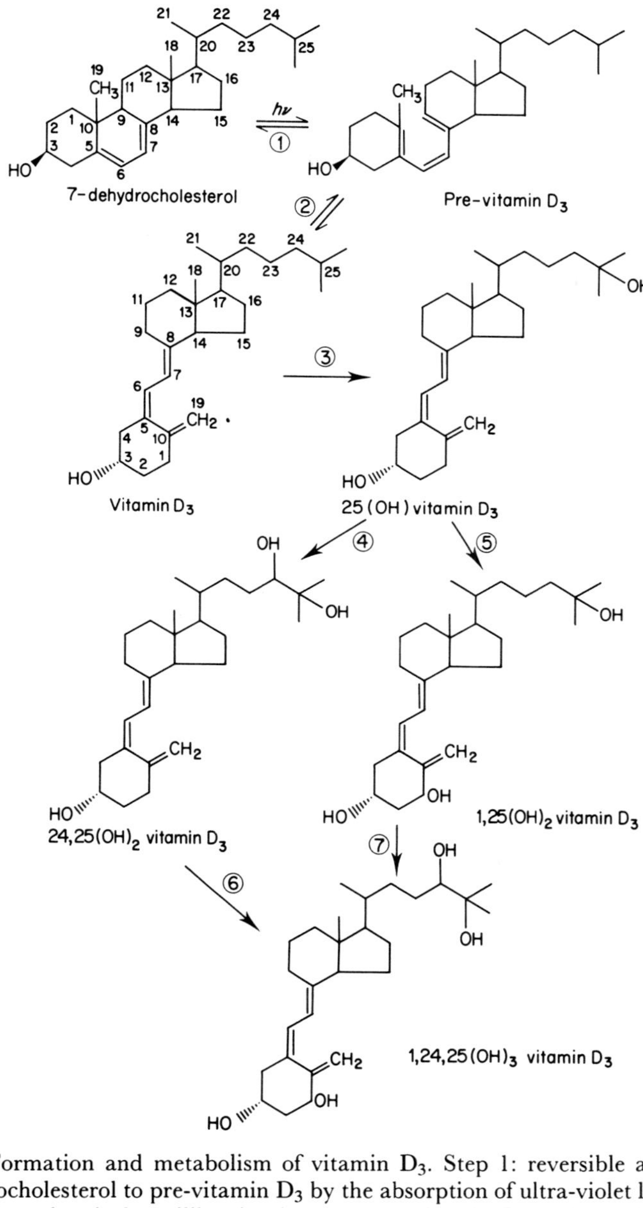

Fig. 4. Formation and metabolism of vitamin D_3. Step 1: reversible activation of 7-dehydrocholesterol to pre-vitamin D_3 by the absorption of ultra-violet light energy. Step 2: slow chemical equilibration between pre-vitamin D_3 and the vitamin itself. Step 3: hydroxylation of vitamin D_3 in the 25 position by liver microsomes. Step 4: under normo- and hyper-calcaemic conditions kidney mitochondria hydroxylate $25(OH)D_3$ to $24,25(OH)_2D_3$. Step 5: under hypocalcaemic conditions kidney mitochondria hydroxylate $25(OH)D_3$ to $1,25(OH)_2D_3$ the "active metabolite" of vitamin D_3. Steps 6 and 7: the dihydroxy metabolites may be further hydroxylated in the kidney to give $1,24,25(OH)_3D_3$.

some of which were water-soluble, probably representing degradation products. The 25-hydroxylase was, however, found to be active in laying birds and in oestrogen-treated quail of both sexes. Oestrogen not only stimulated the 25-hydroxylation of D_3, but also protected both D_3 and $25(OH)D_3$ from degradation by the enzymic pathways active in immature and adult male birds, thus ensuring a more efficient conversion of D_3 to $25(OH)D_3$ in laying than in non-laying birds.

D. Metabolism in the Kidney

The second and more important step in the activation of D_3 takes places in the kidney (Fraser and Kodicek, 1970) to convert $25(OH)D_3$ to 1α,25-dihydroxy D_3 ($1,25(OH)_2D_3$). The enzyme responsible for this conversion is localized exclusively in the mitochondria of cells of the kidney cortex (Midgett *et al.*, 1973), and production of what is now regarded as the key calcium-regulating hormone under its influence is regulated by a number of ionic and hormonal mechanisms. When demands of the body for calcium are low as, for example, in normo- and hyper-calcaemic conditions, production of $1,25(OH)_2D_3$ by the kidney is also low. Under these conditions, the major hydroxylation product of $25(OH)D_3$ is $24,25(OH)_2D_3$ (Boyle *et al.*, 1973). There is a reciprocal relation between the 1- and the 24-hydroxylases in the kidney: conditions that stimulate the 1-hydroxylase, e.g. a deficiency of vitamin D, suppress the 24-hydroxylase and *vice-versa* (Omdahl *et al.*, 1972; Henry *et al.*, 1974). The physiological significance of $24,25(OH_2)D_3$ and of a number of other metabolites of D_3 that have been identified in recent years, including $25,26(OH)_2D_3$ and $1,24,25(OH)_3D_3$, is not known for certain (De Luca, 1979b, 1980), but there is evidence that $24,25(OH)_2D_3$ inhibits the secretion of PTH in mammals (Bates *et al.*, 1975; Canterbury *et al.*, 1978). The formation of D_3 from its precursors and the main steps by which it is metabolized to its hydroxylated forms are shown in Fig. 4.

E. Control of $1,25(OH)_2D_3$ Synthesis

It is now accepted that virtually all the actions originally attributed to D_3 are in fact brought about by $1,25(OH)_2D_3$, and a great deal of research has, therefore, been concentrated on the mechanisms that regulate the production of this metabolite, requirements for which are closely linked to the requirements of the birds for calcium. In hypocalcaemic conditions, induced by a dietary deficiency either of calcium or of vitamin D, production of

$1,25(OH)_2D_3$ is greatly increased. Norman *et al.* (1980) reported a diurnal fluctuation in activity of $25(OH)D_3$-1-hydroxylase in chicks fed on a calcium-deficient diet. When these birds were maintained on 18 h light 6 h dark cycles, a peak of $1,25(OH)_2D_3$ synthesis occurred at the end of each light period. This rhythm persisted to some extent under conditions of continuous light. It was at one time thought that a low concentration of Ca^{2+} stimulated the 1-hydroxylase directly, as occurs *in vitro* in preparations of kidney tissue. The weight of evidence now supports the view that the control of enzyme activity of Ca^{2+} is exercised indirectly by way of PTH. In studies on the development of vitamin D deficiency in chicks from hatching to 27 d of age, Fraser and Kodicek (1973) showed that the activity of the 1-hydroxylase in the kidney was substantially raised after 6 and 9 days on the deficient diet, whereas the fall in the concentration of blood calcium did not occur before day 12 and in some chicks it remained normal until day 18. The role of the parathyroid glands in mediating the activity of the enzyme was confirmed in experiments involving parathyroidectomy and ultimobranchialectomy and the injection of PTH. Garabedian *et al* (1972) had earlier demonstrated the role of PTH in modulating the renal hydroxylation step in experiments with thyro-parathyroidectomized rats. There is some disagreement about the time-course of the stimulatory action of PTH on the 1-hydroxylase: whereas Sedrani *et al.* (1981) observed a significant increase in the activity of the enzyme in Japanese quail 2 h after injection of 100 USP units bovine parathyroid extract (PTE) per kg and a peak response after 3 h, Baksi and Kenny (1979) did not detect an effect on either the 1- or the 24-hydroxylase until 12 h after the PTE (30 USP units kg^{-1}) was administered to their quail. Sedrani *et al.* (1981) observed a significant reduction in the activity of the 24-hydroxylase after only 1 h, a reduction that lasted for 5 h.

Before a direct physiological role can with certainty be assigned to a particular hormone, an appropriate action on its target tissue must be demonstrated both *in vivo* and *in vitro*. *In vivo* studies alone cannot distinguish between direct and indirect effects mediated by the hormone. This criterion has been fulfilled for PTH in that the hormone has been shown to stimulate the production of $1,25(OH)_2D_3$ *in vitro* in preparations of isolated kidney tubules (Rasmussen *et al.*, 1972), in primary cultures of chick kidney cells (Trechsel *et al.*, 1979) and in chick kidney slices (Rost *et al.*, 1981). In the latter study, evidence was obtained for the involvement of cyclic AMP in stimulating the 1-hydroxylase.

A number of other hormones has been implicated in regulating the production of $1,25(OH)_2D_3$, namely, prolactin, growth hormone, insulin, glucocorticoids, CT, reproductive steroids and $1,25(OH)_2D_3$ itself and the evidence for a significant trophic influence for these hormones is greater for some than for others.

Spanos *et al.* (1976a,b) were the first to report that prolactin may be involved in controlling the hydroxylation of 25(OH)D_3. They observed that injection of 70 μg ovine prolactin doubled the activity of the kidney 1-hydroxylase in 1-day-old chicks after 1 h and that this enhancement had disappeared 3 h after the injection. In addition, they demonstrated that plasma concentrations of 1,25$(OH)_2D_3$ were increased 1 h after the last injection of prolactin in 3-week-old D_3-deficient and D_3-supplemented chicks that had been injected with ovine prolactin (100 μg day^{-1}) for 5 days. Bikle *et al.* (1980) studied the effect of turkey and ovine prolactin on the production of 1,25$(OH)_2D_3$ *in vitro* by isolated renal tubules and by kidney slices and observed that 8 ng turkey prolactin ml^{-1} stimulated 1,25$(OH)_2D_3$ production in both preparations: with tissue slices the response was immediate (within 20 min), but a 3-h pre-incubation period in the presence of the hormone was necessary before the response occurred with the tubules. Ovine prolactin produced similar responses, but higher concentrations of the hormone were required. Spanos *et al.* (1981), using primary chick kidney cells grown in culture media containing 1,25$(OH)_2D_3$ to suppress the activity of the 1-hydroxylase, obtained a significant stimulation of the enzyme with as little as 1 ng ovine prolactin ml^{-1}. This response reached a maximum with 100 ng hormone ml^{-1} and the activity of the 24-hydroxylase was unaffected. A time-course study revealed that prolactin stimulated the 1-hydroxylase within 30 min, the response reaching a maximum between 1–2 h and disappearing by 4 h.

In vitamin D-deficient birds, the activity of the 25(OH)D_3-1-hydroxylase in the kidney is very high, whereas that of the 24-hydroxylase is low and administration of D_3 or 1,25$(OH)_2D_3$ *in vivo* results in a decrease in 1-hydroxylase and an increase in 24-hydroxylase activity. These changes are brought about both by the direct action of 1,25$(OH)_2D_3$ on the kidney and indirectly by suppressing PTH secretion. Spanos *et al.* (1978b) and Trechsel *et al.* (1979), among others, have demonstrated a direct action of 1,25$(OH)_2D_3$ in chick kidney cells growing in culture to suppress the 1-hydroxylase and activate the 24-hydroxylase, and 1,25$(OH)_2D_3$ has been shown to exert feedback inhibition on PTH production both *in vivo* (Chertow *et al.*, 1975) and *in vitro* (Dietal *et al.*, 1979). A similar feedback inhibition on prolactin production by the pituitary has also been demonstrated in experiments on rat pituitary cells grown in culture (Murdoch and Rosenfeld, 1981).

Hypophysectomy depresses the production of 1,25$(OH)_2D_3$ in rats and replacement therapy with growth hormone largely overcomes this depression (Spencer and Tobiassen, 1977; Spanos *et al.*, 1978a). It is doubtful, however, whether growth hormone exerts a direct action on 1,25$(OH)_2D_3$ production. Bikle *et al.* (1980) could not obtain any response to bovine growth hormone in their *in vitro* preparations of chick kidneys and Spanos *et al.* (1981) observed only a slight stimulation of the 1-hydroxylase in chick kidney cell cultures with high concentrations of human growth hormone, which may have been due to the prolactin-like activity of the hormone. Impure (50%) chick growth hormone increased the activity of the 1-hydroxylase in these cultures, but pituitary hormones other than growth hormone may have been responsible for this effect.

Schneider *et al.* (1977a,b) observed that streptozotocin-induced diabetes resulted in a significant reduction in the circulating concentration of $1,25(OH)_2D_3$ in rats that can be restored by injecting insulin, but similar studies have not been carried out in birds. Henry (1981) reported that insulin was required for PTH to stimulate the production of $1,25(OH)_2D_3$ by cultures of chick kidney cells. There is no suggestion, however, that the role of insulin in vitamin D metabolism is other than permissive.

It is well established that corticosteroids have an inhibitory effect on intestinal calcium transport (Luckert *et al.*, 1973; Kimberg *et al.*, 1981) and it is difficult to reconcile this with reports that these hormones activate the 1-hydroxylase. Thus, Spanos and MacIntyre (1977) reported a 20-fold increase in the activity of this enzyme, coupled with an almost complete inhibition of the 24-hydroxylase in chicks after a single injection of cortisone. They also showed that corticosterone, the major adrenal steroid in birds, stimulated the 1-hydroxylase within 5 h. Evidence for a direct action of glucorticoids on the kidney enzymes is lacking.

Galante *et al.* (1972) reported that injection of CT into intact rats stimulated $1,25(OH)_2D_3$ production and this observation was confirmed by Lorence *et al.* (1977). The latter workers showed that the CT action was abolished after thyroparathyroidectomy and they suggested that this effect is mediated via the parathyroids, i.e. that the hypocalcaemia induced by CT elicits the secretion of PTH which in turn activates the 1-hydroxylase. There is no reason to believe that CT has any direct influence on the metabolism of vitamin D in birds.

Reproductive steroids have most profound effects on the production of $1,25(OH)_2D_3$ in the kidneys of birds and these effects will be discussed in Section VII.

F. Mode of Action of $1,25(OH)_2D_3$

A young bird that is seriously deficient in vitamin D develops rickets; in this condition the plasma concentrations of both calcium and inorganic phosphorus are so reduced that the growing bones fail to calcify. The main role of the active metabolite of vitamin D is to elevate the plasma concentrations of these minerals to levels that will support normal mineralization of the skeleton. This is achieved mainly by increasing the absorption of calcium and phosphate from the intestines by stimulating the active transport of these ions across the intestinal epithelial cells (see Bikle *et al.* (1981) for a review). In addition, $1,25(OH)_2D_3$ working in conjunction with PTH mobilizes calcium and phosphorus from the skeleton when the concentration of Ca^{2+} in the plasma decreases. $1,25(OH)_2D_3$ may also stimulate the reabsorption of calcium from the kidney tubules, although this is still a matter for controversy.

Since 1965, when it was shown that actinomycin D, an inhibitor of protein synthesis, blocks the physiological actions of vitamin D in rats (Zull *et al.*, 1965) and in chicks (Norman, 1965), major advances have been made in elucidating the mode of action of $1,25(OH)_2D_3$ in stimulating calcium transport in the intestines. The first vitamin D-dependent protein to be identified was the cytoplasmic calcium-binding protein, CaBP (Wasserman and Taylor, 1966). It was subsequently shown that in many, but by no means all, physiological situations there was a strong correlation between the rate of calcium transport and the concentration of CaBP in the intestinal tissue. The role of CaBP in calcium transport was a matter for intense discussion and experimentation for many years after its discovery: how is it possible for a cytoplasmic protein to control the rate at which calcium is transported from the intestinal lumen into the epithelial cells? The probable answer is that CaBP is not in fact concerned in transporting calcium across the cell membrane. A more likely role for this protein is in buffering the Ca^{2+} that enter the cell, so that the concentration of these ions in the cytoplasm is kept within physiological limits in spite of large changes in calcium flux across the intestinal cells. In a key experiment, that clearly demonstrated a dissociation between CaBP and calcium transport, Spencer *et al.* (1976) injected $1,25(OH)_2D_3$ intracardially into rachitic chicks and showed that $1,25(OH)_2D_3$-stimulated calcium transport could be demonstrated 1 h after the injection: 3 h later, transport was proceeding at more than 50% of the maximum rate, at a time when CaBP could not be detected in the tissue. The highest concentration of CaBP was reached after 24–28 h, by which time calcium transport had returned to its basal level (Fig. 5).

Vitamin D-dependent membrane-bound proteins, which are thought to be integral components of the calcium transport mechanism, were later identified in rat (Kowarski and Schachter, 1975, 1980) and chick (Wilson and Lawson, 1977, 1981) intestines. In the rat, these membrane proteins consist of a complex of three components: a calcium-dependent ATPase, a *p*-nitrophenylphosphatase (alkaline phosphatase) and a calcium-binding protein of high affinity. The vitamin D-dependent proteins in the brush borders of chick intestines appear to be different from the ones described in the rat: one of these proteins is actin (Wilson and Lawson, 1978) and another, one with a molecular weight of 84 000, is rapidly phosphorylated by ATP under the stimulus of $1,25(OH)_2D_3$ (Wilson and Lawson, 1981). Whereas $1,25(OH)_2D_3$ stimulates the synthesis of CaBP by initiating DNA transcription of its mRNA

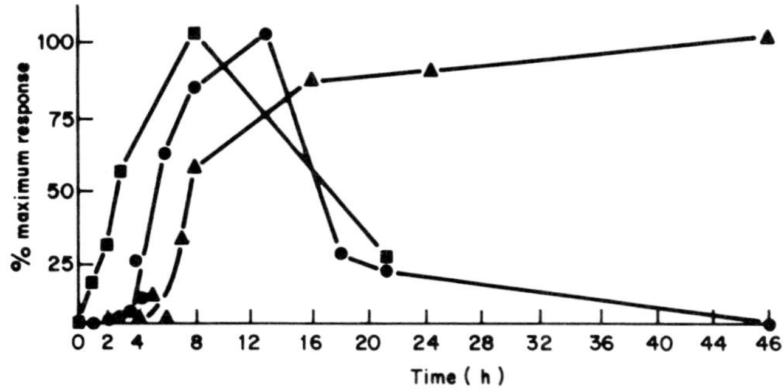

Fig. 5. Time-course study of the effects of a single intracardial injection of 125 ng $1,25(OH)_2D_3$ on intestinal functions in rachitic chicks: ■, Calcium transport *in vitro*; ●, CaBP mRNA activity; ▲, CaBP concentration in intestinal cytosol. (From Spencer *et al.*, 1976.)

(Spencer *et al.*, 1976), the classical mechanism by which steroid hormones exert their action, the stimulation of intestinal calcium transport, would appear to be mediated by a direct action of the hormone on the brush border membrane, possibly by phosphorylating a calcium-dependent ATPase, a component of the calcium pump.

General aspects of vitamin D_3 interactions with bone have been reviewed by Stern (1980). While D_3, through its major metabolite $1,25(OH)_2D_3$, permits normal calcification in bone, its major direct effect on the skeleton is, paradoxically, to bring about bone resorption. Under normal conditions *in vivo*, PTH and $1,25(OH)_2D_3$ work together to facilitate the transfer of calcium from the fluid bathing the bone crystals to the extracellular fluid compartment to maintain normal plasma calcium levels (Talmage, 1970). However, $1,25(OH)_2D_3$ exerts a calcium-mobilizing action both *in vitro* on bone growing in organ culture (Reynolds *et al.*, 1973) and *in vivo* (Wong *et al.*, 1972). It seems probable that $1,25(OH)_2D_3$ can act on bone independently of PTH, provided that its concentration is sufficiently high (Reynolds *et al.*, 1976). Whether or not this action of $1,25(OH)_2D_3$ independent of PTH occurs normally *in vivo* is uncertain: Hughes *et al.* (1976) have demonstrated normal serum concentrations of $1,25(OH)_2D_3$ in patients intoxicated with vitamin D, and $25(OH)D_3$, which induces bone resorption at high concentrations (Reynolds *et al.*, 1973), is probably responsible for the hypercalcaemia observed in this condition.

Little is known of the precise mechanism by which the metabolite induces bone resorption, but it is clear that it is direct, since radio-labelled $1,25(OH)_2D_3$ is concentrated into bone cell nuclei of rachitic chicks (Weber *et al.*, 1971). It is also apparent that inhibitors of DNA-directed RNA synthesis, such as actinomycin D, block D_3-induced bone resorption (Norman and Henry, 1974), while Kream *et al.* (1977) demonstrated the presence of a specific receptor protein for $1,25(OH)_2D_3$ in bones of both rats and chicks.

Unlike PTH and CT, D_3 metabolites do not appear to influence cyclic AMP in bone (Stern, 1980), and the alternative metabolite $24,25(OH)_2D_3$ is not active in bone resorption in either chicks or rats (Henry *et al.*, 1976).

G. Transport of Vitamin D and its Metabolites

Cholecalciferol and $25(OH)D_3$ are transported in association with plasma albumin and, in some species of bird, with α- and β-globulins as well (Hay and Watson, 1976). These plasma transport proteins do not bind pre-vitamin D_3. Edelstein *et al.* (1973) reported that chick plasma contains two vitamin D-binding proteins (DBP), one mainly responsible for transporting $25(OH)D_3$ and the other for D_3 itself, and Lawson *et al.* (1976) identified three such proteins. Later work (Bouillon *et al.*, 1980) largely resolved this disagreement by showing that, whereas chick serum contains two 4S and one 6S forms of DBP, carefully prepared plasma, avoiding haemolysis, contains only 4S forms. The 6S form is a 1 : 1 molar complex of DBP with G-actin and the two 4S forms appear to differ in the number of neuraminic acid residues present. The DBP probably has a single binding site for all vitamin D compounds and its affinity for $25(OH)D_3$ and $24,25(OH)_2D_3$ are similar: $25(OH)D_3$ and $1,25(OH)_2D_3$ have a 3- and 10-fold lower affinity respectively. No evidence was found that any one form of DBP had a higher affinity for D_3 than any other. The concentration of DBP was more than twice as high in the plasma of laying hens than in immature birds or adult cocks.

It has been known for many years that egg yolk is a rich source of vitamin D and Fraser and Emtage (1976) have shown that, of the total vitamin D present, 90% is in the form of D_3 itself and 5% as $25(OH)D_3$. Unless there is a specific mechanism for regulating the transport of the two forms of vitamin D across the vitelline membrane, it is to be expected that the proportion in which these compounds occur in eggs reflects the proportion in which they are present in plasma. The amounts of D_3 circulating in the blood of laying hens have not been determined, but they would be expected to vary according to the amounts present in the diet. Abe *et al.* (1979) have reported, however, that the plasma concentrations of $25(OH)D_3$, $1,25(OH)_2D_3$ and $24,25(OH)_2D_3$ in laying hens with an egg in the shell gland are, respectively, $14{\cdot}0 \pm 2{\cdot}0$ ng ml^{-1}, $0{\cdot}14 \pm 0{\cdot}02$ ng ml^{-1} and $0{\cdot}63 \pm 0{\cdot}18$ ng ml^{-1} (mean $\pm$ SE). Thus, one might expect to find 100 times as much $25(OH)D_3$ as $1,25(OH)_2D_3$ in egg yolk.

H. Ergocalciferol (Vitamin D_2)

The anti-rachitic potency of D_2 is much less than that of D_3 for chicks, although both forms of D are equipotent in most mammals. Estimates of the relative potency of D_2 vary greatly according to the precise response criteria used. The minimum estimate of the $D_3 : D_2$ potency ratio is about 10 : 1 (Chen and Bosmann, 1964), but earlier workers (*e.g.* McChesney, 1943) observed potency ratios of 35–40. The precise way in which birds discriminate against D_2 is not known, but it has been shown by Imrie *et al.* (1967) using D_2 and D_3 labelled with different radioactive isotopes that, although the initial rate of uptake of label by the target tissues is equally as good for D_2 as for D_3, metabolites of D_2 are excreted in the bile far more rapidly than those of D_3, suggesting that the low antirachitic potency of D_2 is the result of rapid metabolism and excretion. A major biliary metabolite of D_2 has been shown to be 25(OH)D_2-β-D-25-glucuronic acid (Le Van, 1980).

I. Summary of Calcium Homoeostasis

PTH, CT and 1,25$(OH)_2D_3$ work together to control the concentration of Ca^{2+} in the plasma, more particularly in the extra-cellular fluid, within narrow limits. The way in which these hormones interact in the control of hypo- and hypercalcaemia are shown, respectively, in Figs 6 and 7.

J. Calcium–Phosphorus Interactions

The metabolism of these two minerals is so closely interrelated that it is not possible to consider either one in isolation. For many years it was thought that vitamin D influenced phosphorus metabolism indirectly by way of its effect on calcium metabolism, but it is now known that phosphorus has a direct action on D_3 metabolism independent of calcium and that 1,25$(OH)_2D_3$ stimulates intestinal absorption of phosphorus (Chen *et al.*, 1974). When chicks are fed on a diet deficient in phosphorus (>3 g/P kg^{-1}), the rate of calcium absorption from the small intestine increases and this is accompanied by an increased accumulation of 1,25$(OH)_2D_3$ in the intestinal mucosa (Edelstein *et al.*, 1975; Friedlander *et al.*, 1977) and by an increase in the activity of the renal 25(OH)D_3-1-hydroxylase (Baxter and De Luca, 1976; Somerville *et al.*, 1978). The latter authors compared the effects of dietary calcium and phosphorus deficiency on the metabolism of 25(OH)D_3 in the chick and observed that *in vitro* renal production of 1,25$(OH)_2D_3$ increased eightfold in the calcium-deficient and threefold in the phosphorus-deficient chicks compared with controls. The *in vivo* accumulation of 1,25$(OH)_2D_3$ in the gut mucosa, the

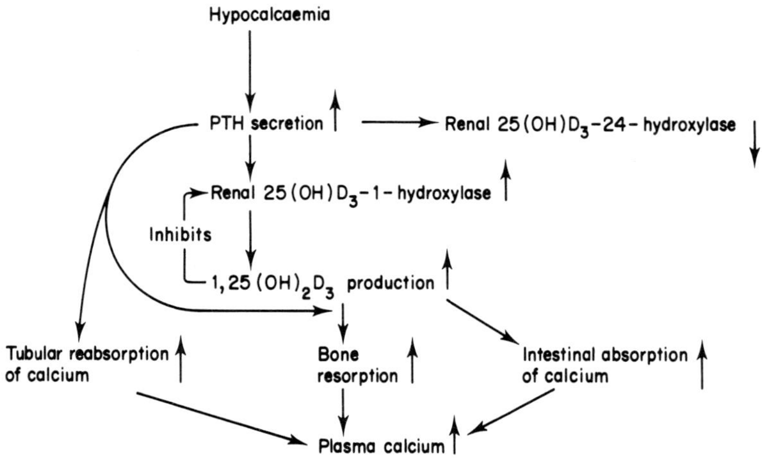

Fig. 6. The control of hypocalcaemia. Of the three sources of additional calcium for restoring the concentration of plasma calcium, bone resorption is controlled by PTH and 1,25(OH)$_2$D$_3$ working together and intestinal absorption by 1,25(OH)$_2$D$_3$ alone. Whether PTH works alone or in concert with 1,25(OH)$_2$D$_3$ in stimulating tubular reabsorption of calcium has not been conclusively resolved. The quantitative significance of these three sources depends on the magnitude of the original hypocalcaemia, and a mild hypocalcaemia (provoking a low level of PTH secretion) may be controlled without involving the bone.

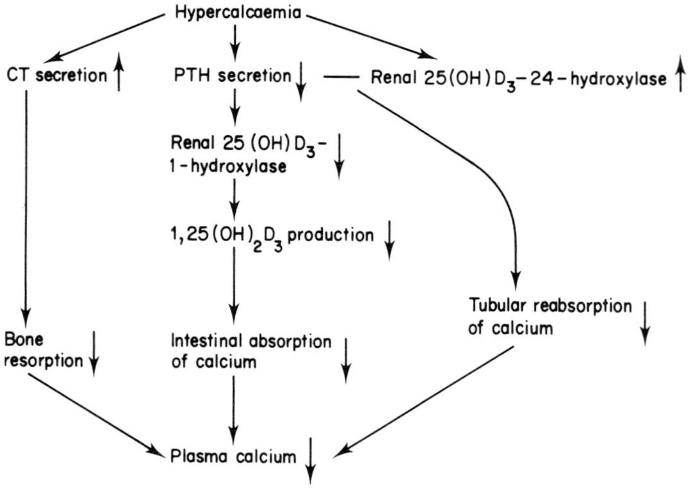

Fig. 7. The control of hypercalcaemia. The plasma calcium is restored by increasing the urinary excretion, by decreasing intestinal absorption and by bone mineralization removing calcium from the blood at the normal rate. (CT inhibits bone resorption, thus depressing the rate at which calcium is released, but the rate of bone formation is unchanged.)

CaBP activity and the rate of calcium absorption from the duodenum increased by a similar extent in both experimental groups, but the accumulation of $1,25(OH)_2D_3$ in bone increased threefold in the low-calcium chicks and showed no change in the low-phosphorus birds. These results are consistent with the view that the adaptation to a low-phosphorus diet depends primarily on the ability of the intestinal mucosa to accumulate $1,25(OH)_2D_3$ rather than on an increased renal production of the metabolite. The results of these experiments confirm the work of Bar and Wasserman (1973), Bar *et al.* (1975) and Ribovich and De Luca (1975), which showed that bypassing the 1-hydroxylation control step in the kidney by feeding dihydrotachysterol, $1\alpha(OH)D_3$ or $1,25(OH)_2D_3$, respectively, abolished the adaptive response to a low-calcium but not to a low-phosphorus diet, expressed as an increased ability of the intestine to absorb calcium and, presumably, to absorb phosphate, though this response was not studied.

Whereas a low-calcium diet stimulates PTH secretion, a low-phosphorus diet results in an increase in the concentration of ionized calcium in the plasma, which depresses PTH secretion. The effects of this depression are to conserve phosphorus (by reducing the PTH inhibition of tubular reabsorption of phosphate) and to permit the urinary excretion of the additional calcium absorbed from the gut during the low-phosphorus regimen. In addition, the mammalian kidney possesses a mechanism independent of PTH and vitamin D, whereby tubular reabsorption of phosphate is markedly increased under conditions of hypophosphataemia (Steele and De Luca, 1976), but it is not known whether this mechanism operates in birds.

V. Prostaglandins

It has been recognized for more than a decade that prostaglandins (PGs) influence calcium and bone metabolism in mammals. A number of PGs are osteolytic in bones growing in organ culture, PGE_2 being the most potent (Klein and Raisz, 1970; Dietrich *et al.*, 1975), and there is circumstantial evidence that the hypercalcaemia, independent of the parathyroids which is a common feature of certain neoplastic diseases, may be mediated by PGs. Thus, treatment of tumour-bearing hypercalcaemic mice, rabbits or humans with indomethacin, a potent inhibitor of PG biosynthesis, was generally found to lower the plasma concentration of calcium (Tashjian *et al.*, 1972; Voelkel *et al.*, 1975; Seyberth *et al.*, 1975). In young rats, infusion of PGE_2 for 4 h produces modest hypercalcaemic responses under some circumstances (Franklin and Tashjian, 1975), and a stable analogue, 16-16 dimethyl PGE_2, causes resorption of a chronic ^{45}Ca label from bone, but not hypercalcaemia (Vanderwiel and Talmage, 1979).

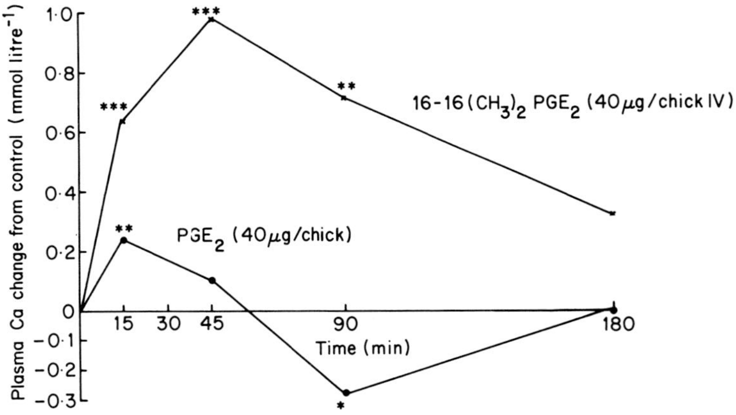

Fig. 8. Hypercalcaemic response duration curves for native PGE_2 and 16-16 dimethyl PGE_2 in chicks, shown as mean changes from controls. Significance compared with controls: $*P < 0{\cdot}02$, $**P < 0{\cdot}01$, $***P < 0{\cdot}001$. (From Dacke and Willins, in press.)

Early data from chickens and quail indicated that plasma calcium concentrations in these species might be refractory to injected or infused PGEs (Dacke and Kenny, 1982), but more recent work (Dacke and Willins, in press), clearly indicates that intravenous injection of 16-16 dimethyl PGE_2 into young (10-day-old) chickens causes a profound hypercalcaemic response. In comparison, the response to native PGE_2 is much smaller and of shorter duration (Fig. 8). Ongoing experiments, using either acute or chronic (6-day) ^{45}Ca labelling, suggest that these responses are due partly to a decrease in the efflux of calcium from the extracellular pool and partly to an increased bone resorption (G. C. Kirby and C. G. Dacke, unpublished). Qualitatively they are similar to responses obtained with PTH in immature birds (Kenny and Dacke, 1974). Histological studies of foetal rat bones growing in organ culture suggest that bone resorption under the influence of PGE_2, $1,25(OH)_2D_3$ and PTH is mediated by the same mechanism, i.e. by increasing activity of pre-existing osteoclasts (Holtrop and Raisz, 1979).

VI. Chick Embryos

About 80% of the calcium present in the chick at hatching is derived from the egg shell (see Simkiss, 1967). The process of shell resorption begins at day 10 or 11 of incubation. Calcium is accumulated rapidly by the embryo for bone formation between day 13 or 14 of incubation and hatching (Johnston and Comar, 1955). The mechanism by which the calcite of the shell is dissolved is not known, but it may involve the secretion of an acid, possibly hydrochloric

(Crooks and Simkiss, 1974). During normal development, the 15-d embryo accumulates calcium at a rate of about 7·3 μmole h^{-1} (Crooks and Simkiss, 1974) by a process of active transport across the chorio-allantoic membrane. This transport process occurs at a rate of 116 nmole cm^{-2} h^{-1} in 15-day embryos (Crooks and Simkiss, 1975). $1,25(OH)_2D_3$ may be involved in its regulation, since Narbaitz *et al.* (1980) observed that tritiated $1,25(OH)_2D_3$ was concentrated in nuclei of the chorionic epithelium with a distribution that suggested that they were those of calcium-absorbing cells.

Narbaitz (1979), however, had earlier produced data using shell-less chick embryos cultured *in vitro* which indicated that both $1,25(OH)_2D_3$ and PTH still retained strong hypercalcaemic activity, despite the fact that this type of preparation lacks the chorio-allantoic membrane. These results indicate that both hormones can raise plasma calcium concentrations via target organs other than the chorio-allantoic membrane.

In spite of this rapid flux of calcium through the embryo, the concentrations of plasma calcium show remarkably small changes during incubation. On days 14 and 15 of incubation the mean value is 2·42 mmol $litre^{-1}$: from day 16 the concentration rises slowly, reaching a plateau of 2·61 mmol $litre^{-1}$ which is maintained from days 18–20. At hatching the concentration decreases to 2·55 mmol $litre^{-1}$ and one day later it is 2·52 mmol $litre^{-1}$ (Baimbridge and Taylor, 1980). These changes are shown in Fig. 9.

The relative constancy of plasma calcium concentrations during embryonic development suggests that endocrine mechanisms are involved in their regulation. Observations on the ultrastructure of the parathyroid glands (Narbaitz, 1972) indicate that they are active after the 10th day of incubation and chick embryos show a hypercalcaemic response to PTH at day 15 (Narbaitz, 1975) and even at day 11 (Narbaitz, 1979). Embryos parathyroidectomized at day 18 develop a significant hypocalcaemia 7 h after the operation (Clark and Mok, 1981). The results of all these experiments strongly suggest that PTH is actively involved in maintaining the plasma concentration of calcium in embryos during the latter half of incubation.

It has been known for many years that egg production is low in hens deficient in vitamin D and that the eggs they produce hatch poorly. Sunde *et al.* (1978) fed laying hens on diets supplemented with D_3, $25(OH)D_3$ or $1,25(OH)_2D_3$ and observed that D_3 and $25(OH)D_3$ supported egg production and hatchability equally well. Whereas egg production and shell thickness were normal in hens given $1,25(OH)_2D_3$, the hatchability of the eggs declined to the level observed in eggs from vitamin D-deficient hens. The major abnormality in the embryos that failed to hatch was a fore-shortening of the upper mandible. The results of this experiment suggest that $1,25(OH)_2D_3$ is not transported into the developing ovarian follicle in significant amounts. They are consistent with the observations of Fraser and Emtage (1976) noted

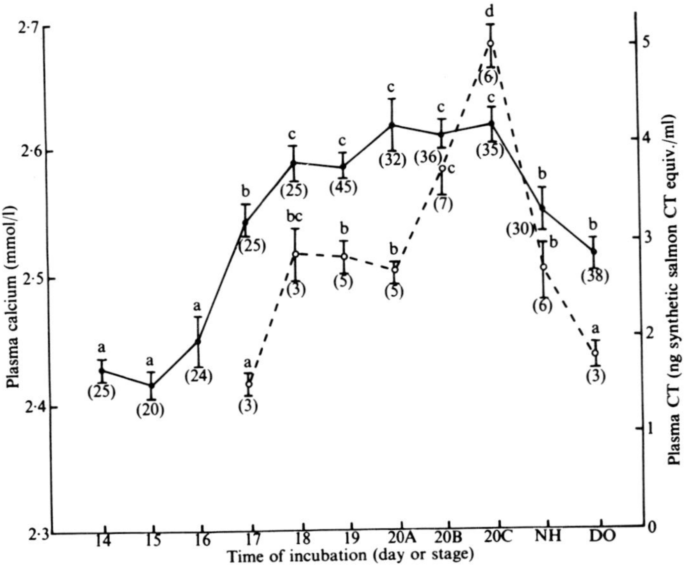

Fig. 9. Changes in the concentration of total Ca (●) and calcitonin (CT) (○) in the plasma of chick embryos during incubation. Number of samples in parentheses. Means with different letters differ significantly from one another. CT was undetectable before day 17 and after day 22 (2-day-old chicks). 20A, Shell (Chorio-allantoic) respiration; 20B, lung respiration; 20C, shell pipped; NH newly hatched at 21 days; DO, 1-day-old chick. (From Baimbridge and Taylor, 1980.)

above that most of the vitamin D in egg yolk is present as D_3 together with a small amount of 25(OH)D_3.

Relatively little work has been reported on the metabolism of vitamin D in embryos, but Taylor and Wasserman (1972) were able to detect CaBP in the kidney tissue of chick embryos from day 10 of incubation, which suggests that 1,25$(OH)_2D_3$ was being produced at this stage of development, athough direct evidence for the 25- and 1-hydroxylation steps has only been reported for 18-day embryos (Moriuchi and De Luca, 1974). However, intestinal CaBP does not appear until day 21, the day of hatching (Corradino *et al.*, 1969), in spite of the fact that the 1,25$(OH)_2D_3$ cytosolic receptor can be detected in intestinal tissue at day 17 (Oku *et al.*, 1975) and that CaBP can be induced by 1,25$(OH)_2D_3$ in embryos injected *in ovo* at day 18 (Corradino and Wasserman, 1974) and in embryonic duodenum grown in organ culture (Corradino, 1973). These observations, taken together, suggest that the failure of the chick embryo intestine to produce CaBP until hatching is due, not to a lack of synthetic capability, but to an inadequate amount of circulating 1,25$(OH)_2D_3$ reaching the target cells.

Studies on the ultimobranchial bodies of chick embryos suggest that these glands are active during the latter half of incubation (Narbaitz, 1972), but CT cannot be detected in the circulation until day 17, the earliest stage of incubation at which the mean plasma calcium concentration exceeded 2·5 mmol litre^{-1} (Cutler *et al.*, 1974; Baimbridge and Taylor, 1980). The concentration of CT rises progressively from day 17, reaching a peak value at the "pipping" stage, falling rapidly thereafter until it is no longer detectable in 2-day-old chicks. These changes are shown in Fig. 9, together with the corresponding changes in the concentration of plasma calcium.

In other experiments, Baimbridge and Taylor (1980) showed that, when embryos were injected with calcium, CT secretion was stimulated but the level induced was substantially less than the peak observed at "pipping" although an extreme degree of hypercalcaemia developed. When CT was temporally removed from the circulation by injecting anti-CT plasma, a mild but statistically significant hypercalcaemia was observed and in another study exogenous CT significantly decreased an artificially-induced hypercalcaemia. These results are consistent with the view that CT is secreted in response to hypercalcaemia and that its role is to restrict the hypercalcaemia resulting from the large and rapid transfer of calcium from the eggshell to the developing embryo and to its yolk sac.

There is evidence that the secretion of CT is also stimulated by a β-adrenergic mechanism, since the β-antagonist, propranolol, decreases and the β-agonist, isoprenaline, increases the concentration of circulating CT (Baimbridge and Taylor, 1980). Taylor *et al.* (1975) suggested that the release of catecholamines in response to increasing hypoxia or increasing respiratory acidosis may provide the stimulus for the high rate of CT secretion during the period immediately prior to "pipping". Experimental support for this hypothesis is, however, lacking.

In summary, it would appear that the control of calcium metabolism in the embryo is not fundamentally different from that in hatched birds. The same three hormones are involved, and any difference in their relative importance is mainly due to the fact that the major source of calcium is the eggshell rather than the diet. However, much remains to be learned about the mechanisms of fine control that are responsible for regulating the circulating level of calcium and the supply of calcium for bone mineralization.

VII. Laying Hens

Calcium metabolism in laying birds is dominated by the demands of the uterus for shell formation. The intense metabolism of calcium associated with the formation of the shell is supported by the high capacity of the intestines to absorb calcium and by the phenomenal ability of the skeleton to mobilize its mineral reserves whenever the rate of calcium absorption from the gut is less than the rate at which it is deposited on the calcifying shell (see reviews by Taylor, 1970a; Simkiss, 1975; Dacke, 1979). Under normal conditions, i.e. when a high-calcium diet is being fed, it is the medullary bone that is resorbed whenever supplies of calcium from the gut are insufficient to provide for the demands of the shell gland; this occurs mainly in the early hours of the morning when most of the calcium from the previous day's food has been absorbed (Tyler, 1954). Medullary bone is formed under the combined influence of oestrogen and androgen (Common *et al.*, 1948), and it is probably mobilized by an increase in the secretion of PTH (Taylor and Belanger, 1969), stimulated by the fall in the plasma concentration of ionic calcium during shell formation (Luck and Scanes, 1979).

Although the broad features of calcium metabolism in relation to shell formation summarized above are generally accepted, the precise details of the hormonal mechanisms by which the supplies of calcium from the gut and from the skeleton are regulated in relation to the requirements for shell formation are not fully understood. The greatest uncertainties relate to the mechanisms by which the production of $1,25(OH)_2D_3$ is regulated.

A. $1,25(OH)_2D_3$ Production and its Endocrine Control

The circulating concentration of $1,25(OH)_2D_3$ is significantly higher in laying hens than in immature or in non-laying adult hens: the concentration in immature pullets is 30–50 pg ml^{-1} and in laying birds 120–300 pg ml^{-1} (Spanos *et al.*, 1976a, Abe *et al.*, 1979). Both Castillo *et al.* (1979) and Abe *et al.* (1979) have reported circadian rhythms in circulating $1,25(OH)_2D_3$ during the egg cycle, but there is disagreement as to the form this rhythm takes. The former authors observed maximum concentrations of about 200 pg ml^{-1} from 4–10 h after ovulation, after which the concentration fell to about 100 pg ml^{-1} and remained at this level until 2 h after oviposition, while Abe *et al.* (1979) observed a peak value of 300 pg ml^{-1} 14–16 h after ovulation (in the middle of the night). It is not possible to reconcile these two reports, but one would expect circulating concentrations of $1,25(OH)_2D_3$ to be highest when the demands for calcium for shell formation are at a maximum, i.e. during the period 10–24 h after ovulation, rather than the earlier period reported by Castillo *et al.* (1979).

The activity of the renal $25(OH)D_3$-1-hydroxylase increases greatly with the onset of reproductive activity in chickens (Montecuccoli *et al.*, 1977; Castillo *et al.*, 1979) and in Japanese quail (Montecuccoli *et al.*, 1977; Sedrani, 1979): the latter author observed an activity approximately six-fold higher in

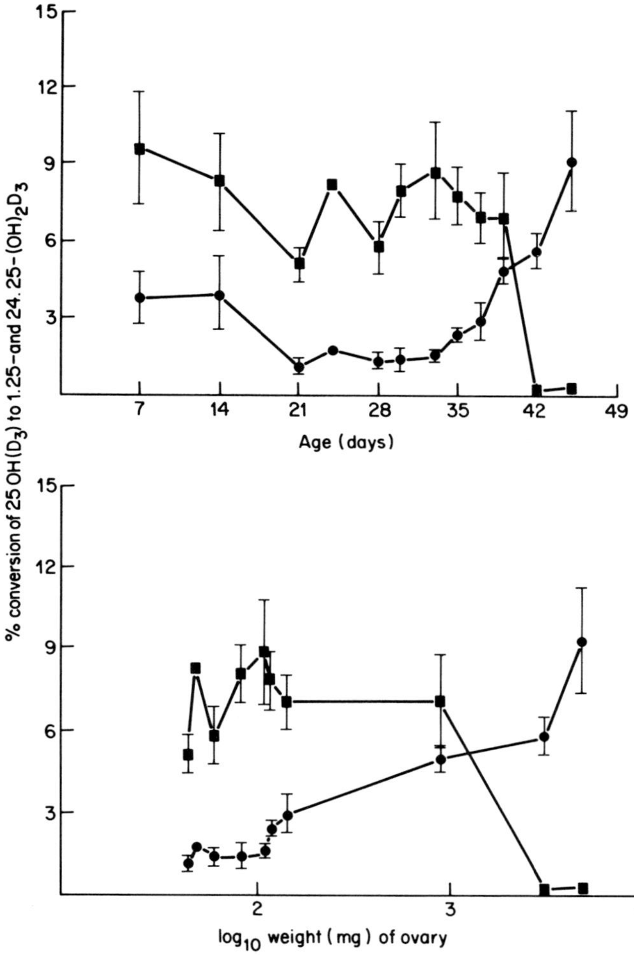

Fig. 10. Changes with age (top) and with ovarian development (bottom) in the activity of the $25(OH)D_3$ 1- and 24-hydroxylases in the kidneys of Japanese quail measured *in vitro* in terms of the % conversion of substrate. $1,25(OH)_2D_3$, ●; $24,25(OH)_2D_3$, ■. (From Sedrani, 1979.)

laying compared with pre-laying (21- to 33-day-old) birds (Fig. 10). Similar observations have been made by Turner *et al.* (1979). The ability of renal tissue from female birds that are temporarily out of lay to synthesize $1,25(OH)_2D_3$ *in vitro* is very much less than in birds that are in lay (Castillo *et al.*, 1977). Under all these conditions the reciprocal relationship between the production of 1,25- and $24,25(OH)_2D_3$ is maintained.

The activity of the 1-hydroxylase shows a circadian rhythm during the egg cycle. Abe *et al.* (1979) observed peak activity at the same time as the peak of circulating $1{,}25(OH)_2D_3$, namely, at 14–16 h after ovulation, whereas Castillo *et al.* (1979) reported maximum activity during the period 0–2 h after ovulation; the activity at this time was approximately twice as great as it was during the rest of the egg cycle. Resolution of these conflicting results must await further work. Abe *et al.* (1979) also reported cyclic changes in circulating $25(OH)D_3$ with a peak at the time of ovulation and minimum values 5–7 h later, shortly after the egg had entered the shell gland. Concentrations of $24{,}25(OH)_2D_3$ remained constant throughout the egg cycle.

The hormonal control of vitamin D metabolism in the laying bird has been the subject of intensive research, and interest has centred on the reproductive steroids, PTH and prolactin. Any comprehensive scheme that seeks to relate the control of $1{,}25(OH)_2D_3$ production to the physiology of reproduction in the pullet must take account of the fact that considerable increases in the rates at which calcium is absorbed from the intestinal tract and stored in the skeleton occur during the 14 days or so before the first egg is laid (Hurwitz, 1964). The actual amount of calcium stored during the pre-laying period is somewhat variable but it is usually within the range 2 to 6 g with a mean of 4 g, representing an increase in the dry fat-free skeletal weight of nearly 20 g (Taylor and Moore, 1954, 1958). Before the rapid phase of calcium storage begins medium-hybrid pullets have a mean skeletal weight of about 80 g, so that the skeleton increases in weight by about 25% during the pre-laying period and it must be assumed that medullary bone accounts for most of this increase. The primary role of $1{,}25(OH)_2D_3$ during the pre-laying period is to make available the increased amounts of calcium required for the mineralization of the medullary bone by increasing calcium absorption from the gut and there is no reason to suppose that it is required for the bone-forming process itself.

There is general agreement that oestrogen administered *in vivo* increases the activity of the $25(OH)D_3$-1-hydroxylase in avian kidney and inhibits the 24-hydroxylase (Tanaka *et al.*, 1976, 1978; Baksi and Kenny, 1977, 1978a; Sedrani *et al.*, 1981). One possible explanation for this effect is that oestrogen increases the production of enzyme protein by stimulating the transcription of the specific mRNA which directs its biosynthesis, i.e. according to the classical mechanism whereby steroid hormones exert their action. In all these experiments esters of 17β-oestradiol were used and the enzyme activities were measured 24 h or more after the first hormone injection. Baksi and Kenny (1978b), however, observed a significant increase in the activity of the 1-hydroxylase and a significant decrease in the 24-hydroxylase after only 4 h in Japanese quail injected with a high dose of oestradiol benzoate. P. J. Williams and T. G. Taylor (unpublished) have demonstrated a significant increase in the 1-hydroxylase after only 3 h using the free steroid. The speed with which the hormone can act suggests, therefore, that it may not operate by way of the protein biosynthetic machinery of the cell and it seems more likely that its action is indirect. The regulatory effects of oestrogen on renal $25(OH)D_3$ hydroxylases is eliminated in birds raised on low-calcium diets (Baksi and Kenny, 1978a). Spanos *et al.* (1978b) were unable to demonstrate an effect of oestrogen on the 1-hydroxylase in chick kidney cells grown in culture, and Spanos *et al.* (1976a,b) suggested that oestrogens may activate the enzyme by stimulating the release of prolactin.

Oestrogen has been shown to increase the circulating level of prolactin in non-laying turkey hens three-fold within 30 min after the injection, but not in laying turkeys (McNeilly *et al.*, 1978). The plasma concentration of prolactin was approximately ten times higher in the laying than in the non-laying turkeys, and it is possible that the maximum level of pituitary response to oestrogen had already been reached by the laying birds before the injections were given.

There is some disagreement as to the role of testosterone in regulating the activity of the 1-hydroxylase. Whereas Baksi and Kenny (1978a) and Sedrani *et al.* (1981) observed that injections of testosterone inhibit the *in vitro* production of $1,25(OH)_2D_3$ and stimulate the production of $24,25(OH)_2D_3$, Tanaka *et al.* (1976, 1978) reported that either testosterone or progesterone are necessary for oestrogen to activate the renal 1-hydroxylase. Tanaka *et al.* (1978) observed a maximum stimulation of this enzyme with a combination of oestrogen, androgen and progesterone, precisely that combination of reproductive steroids whose concentrations are elevated during the reproductive period. Both Tanaka *et al.* (1976) and Sedrani *et al.* (1981) found a marked synergism between PTH and the oestrogen–androgen combination in activating the 1-hydroxylase.

In the experiments summarized above, the dosage levels and the ratios between the different steroids varied considerably. Some workers used chickens, others quail, some worked with immature birds, others with castrates, so that the endogenous production of reproductive steroids may have influenced the outcome of some of the experiments. Further work is clearly needed to define more exactly the precise combination of those steroids responsible for the increased activity of $25(OH)D_3$-1-hydroxylase in laying compared with immature birds, but there seems little doubt that they are together responsible for controlling the basal rate of $1,25(OH)_2D_3$ production and, therefore, the basal rate of calcium absorption during the laying period.

The absorption of calcium from the gut of laying hens is much greater when shell formation is in progress than when the shell gland is inactive (Taylor and Kirkley, 1967; Hurwitz *et al.*, 1973; Bar *et al.*, 1976) and possible mechanisms whereby this differential rate of absorption is achieved must now be considered. The $1,25(OH)_2D_3$-dependent CaBP is unlikely to be involved in what essentially is a short-term control of calcium absorption (Bar and Hurwitz, 1975), and the role of $1,25(OH)_2D_3$ itself is uncertain in spite of the variations in the circulating levels of hormone during the egg cycle that have been reported (Castillo *et al.*, 1979; Abe *et al.*, 1979). In hens and Japanese quail that are laying regularly, the activity of the 1-hydroxylase is similar in birds in which shell calcification is and is not proceeding (Montecuccoli *et al.*, 1977). Furthermore, the difference in calcium absorption in relation to shell formation is maintained when the renal 1-hydroxylation control mechanism is by-passed by feeding 1α-$(OH)D_3$ as the sole source of vitamin D (Bar *et al.*, 1976). It is possible that the increased rate of calcium absorption during shell formation is dependent on the increased calcium concentration gradient across the gut. Luck and Scanes (1979) reported a decrease in Ca^{2+} ion concentration from a mean of 1·60 mmol $litre^{-1}$ when shell calcification was not occurring to a minimum value of 1·14 mmol $litre^{-1}$ during shell formation, a decrease of more than 25% (Fig. 11).

During a one-day pause between successive clutches there is no significant decrease in the activity of the $25(OH)D_3$-1-hydroxylase in Japanese quail (Montecuccoli *et al.*, 1977; Sedrani and Taylor, 1977), but in laying hens there is a significant reduction in enzyme activity 20 h after the last oviposition when the yolk of the first egg of the next clutch is in the magnum (Montecuccoli *et al.*,

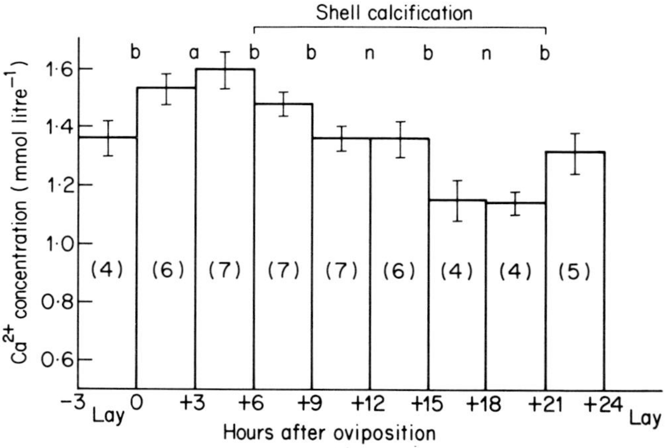

Fig. 11. Mean concentrations (±SE) of ionized calcium in the plasma of hens during a laying cycle in the middle of an egg sequence. Observations are grouped in 3-h periods relative to the time of oviposition of the earlier egg. The significance of difference between adjacent groups (from analysis of variance) are indicated as follows: a, $p < 0{\cdot}05$; b, $P < 0{\cdot}001$; n, non-significant. The significant rise in Ca^{2+} concentration during the 3-h period immediately prior to oviposition is consistent with a slowing of the rate of shell formation at this time. (From Luck and Scanes, 1979.)

1977). When ovulation is inhibited in Japanese quail by administration of the drug methallibure, there is a progressive decline in renal 1-hydroxylase activity with increasing length of drug treatment (Sedrani *et al.*, 1981), and Montecuccoli *et al.* (1977) have reported that the activity of the enzyme decreases by more than 50% in hens treated with nicarbazin to arrest ovulation.

When Japanese quail are given a diet containing 3 g sulphanilamide kg^{-1} diet they lay normally, but shell thickness is reduced by 20 to 30%. In these birds the activity of the renal 1-hydroxylase is significantly reduced, but it is restored almost to normal 3 h after an injection of parathyroid extract (Sedrani *et al.*, 1981). Since the treated birds continued to lay normally, these authors assumed that all the hormones involved in follicle growth and development and in ovulation (gonadotrophins, oestrogen, androgen, progesterone and prolactin) were secreted normally, but that, because of the impairment of shell calcification, PTH secretion was likely to have been reduced. They concluded that

(i) the reproductive steroids are mainly responsible for the increase in renal 1-hydroxylase activity in laying compared with non-laying birds and, therefore, for the large increase in calcium absorption that occurs in female birds with the onset of reproductive activity, and
(ii) PTH is responsible for the short-term increase in the activity of the enzyme during shell formation reported by Abe *et al.* (1979).

Bar *et al.* (1978) had earlier arrived at somewhat similar conclusions, although they placed less emphasis on the role of oestrogen than most other workers. They showed that the plasma concentration of oestradiol was similar in laying and in mature, pre-laying pullets, whereas the amount of CaBP, an index of $1,25(OH)_2D_3$ production, was far greater in the laying than in the pre-laying birds. In hens in which egg production had been arrested by nicarbazin, the circulating concentration of oestradiol was similar to that in control birds, but the kidney 1-hydroxylase activity had fallen to less than a quarter of that observed in the controls and the intestinal CaBP was reduced to one tenth. In both Japanese quail and pullets, the kidney 1-hydroxylase was significantly more active in laying than in mature, pre-laying birds and the concentration of $1,25(OH)_2D_3$ in the intestines was more than three times as great in laying as in pre-laying quail. These observations were confirmed and extended by Bar and Norman (1981) in experiments in which quail were injected with tritium-labelled $25(OH)D_3$. The concentrations of labelled $1,25(OH)_2D_3$ were much higher in the plasma, intestinal mucosa and shell gland of laying than in pre-laying birds. The authors concluded that the massive transport of calcium by the shell gland may be vitamin D dependent, and that changes in gonadal activity during maturation have only minor effects on the metabolism of $25(OH)D_3$ by the kidney.

It is clear that much more research is required to elucidate the complex interactions between the numerous hormones that influence the amount of $1,25(OH)_2D_3$ produced by the kidneys of laying birds in response to varying calcium requirements.

B. Bone Metabolism

The role of the skeleton in the provision of calcium for egg shell calcification in the domestic fowl was discussed at some length in Volume 2, but a short summary of the conclusions reached in that chapter will be given here as a background against which recent work can be discussed.

Interest centres on the mechanisms whereby the formation and destruction of medullary bone are regulated in relation to calcium requirements. It is now thought that both processes occur simultaneously and continuously at adjacent sites on the spicules of medullary bone, and that it is the relative rate at which they proceed during the egg cycle that changes in relation to the demands for calcium for shell formation. The earlier ideas that periods of medullary bone destruction (during shell formation) alternate with periods of bone formation (between the calcification of successive eggs) in response to changes in plasma oestrogen concentration cannot be sustained in the light of newer knowledge of changes in the circulating concentrations of reproductive steroid during the egg cycle (see Chapter 10), particularly since peaks of oestrogen and androgen, which are together responsible for the induction of medullary bone, are known to occur at the height of shell formation. The available evidence, largely circumstantial but relatively strong nevertheless, suggests the resorption of medullary bone is induced by an increase in the circulating concentration of PTH, secretion of which is stimulated by the fall in Ca^{2+} concentration that occurs during shell formation.

Simkiss (1967, 1975) finds difficulty in accepting that control of medullary bone resorption during the egg cycle is exercised by PTH largely because, in his view, it does not provide a satisfactory explanation for the observations of Taylor and Moore (1954) that, in hens laying on a calcium-deficient diet, the amount of medullary bone present remains virtually the same in birds that have laid two, four or six eggs on the deficient diet as in the controls, whereas the cortical bone shows a pregressively increasing loss of weight according to the number of eggs laid. Taylor (1970a) sought to explain this paradox in terms of

(i) differences in the sensitivity of cortical and medullary bone to PTH and
(ii) differences in the circulating concentrations of PTH on high- and low-calcium diets.

But an additional point requires to be made, namely, that medullary bone formation was proceeding normally in the calcium-deficient birds, which all had active ovaries and, presumably, normal circulating levels of oestrogen and androgen. In other words, medullary bone was maintained at the expense of cortical bone, although the extent to which the new medullary tissue was calcified decreased as the calcium deficiency became more severe and its Ca : P ratio also decreased (Taylor and Moore, 1954). In two of the calcium-deficient birds the ash percentage of the medullary bone fell from a control value greater than 40% to 17%.

During a calcium deficiency, erosion of cortical bone occurs at the endosteal surface and the thickness of the cortex is thereby reduced. There is no mechanism by which bone tissue can be restored at this site, but Luck (1978) observed that when hens were fed on a low-calcium diet (0·3 g calcium kg^{-1}) for 9 weeks, having ceased egg production within a week or so of the introduction of the experimental diet, a relatively thick layer of loosely packed columns of sub-periosteal bone developed, presumably serving a mechanical function. The medullary bone persisted but it remained poorly calcified (Fig. 12).

The greater sensitivity of medullary bone to PTH, measured in terms of collagenolytic response, was demonstrated by Bannister and Candlish (1973), in an experiment in which laying hens were injected with parathyroid extract. Five minutes after the injection the response in the medullary bone was far greater than in the cortical bone. It is worthy of note that a significantly higher titre of collagenolytic activity (to a synthetic peptide) was observed in both fractions of bone during shell calcification than when the oviduct was quiescent, suggesting that some mobilization of calcium from cortical bone occurs at this time.

The suggestion that medullary bone formation takes place continuously at particular sites on the surfaces of the medullary bone trabeculae is supported by the results of an experiment in which laying hens fed on a normal high-calcium diet were injected with a tetracycline drug immediately after oviposition and killed 24 h or so later after the next egg of the sequence was laid (Jean Kirkley and T. G. Taylor, unpublished). Ground sections of undecalcified bone from the femurs were examined in a fluorescent miscroscope (Fig. 13) and the tetracycline-labelled medullary bone laid down during the 24 h period following the injection showed up as bright yellow fluorescent areas. Adjacent areas on the bone surfaces showed only background fluorescence: these were areas which were either inactive or which were undergoing resorption.

The old idea that periods of massive destruction of medullary bone alternate with periods of rapid bone formation dies hard. Thus, Castillo *et al.* (1979) present a histogram showing the amount of medullary bone observed in the femurs of laying hens killed at 2 h intervals after ovulation. Huge differences

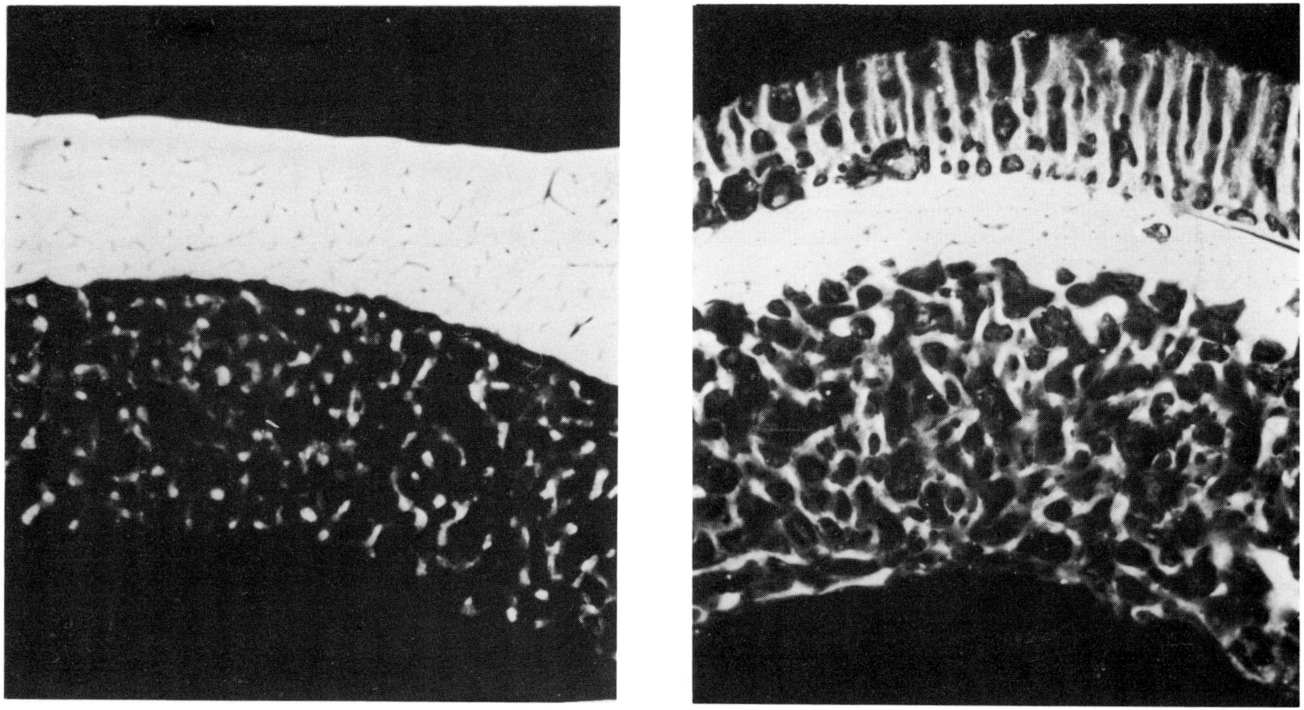

Fig. 12. Microradiographs of ground undecalcified sections through the tibia of laying hens: (left) control bird that had been in lay for 5 weeks on a high-calcium diet; (right) experimental bird that had been fed on a low-calcium diet ($0{\cdot}3$ g Ca kg^{-1}) for 9 weeks and that had ceased egg production for about 8 weeks. In the control section, note particularly the smooth, uneroded endosteal surface which is in marked contrast to the rough, highly eroded surface of the calcium-deficient bone. The loosely-packed columns of sub-periosteal bone in the section on the right are completely absent from the control bone section. Note also that the cortex of the control bone is about twice as thick as in the experimental section (magnification ×40). (From Luck, 1978.)

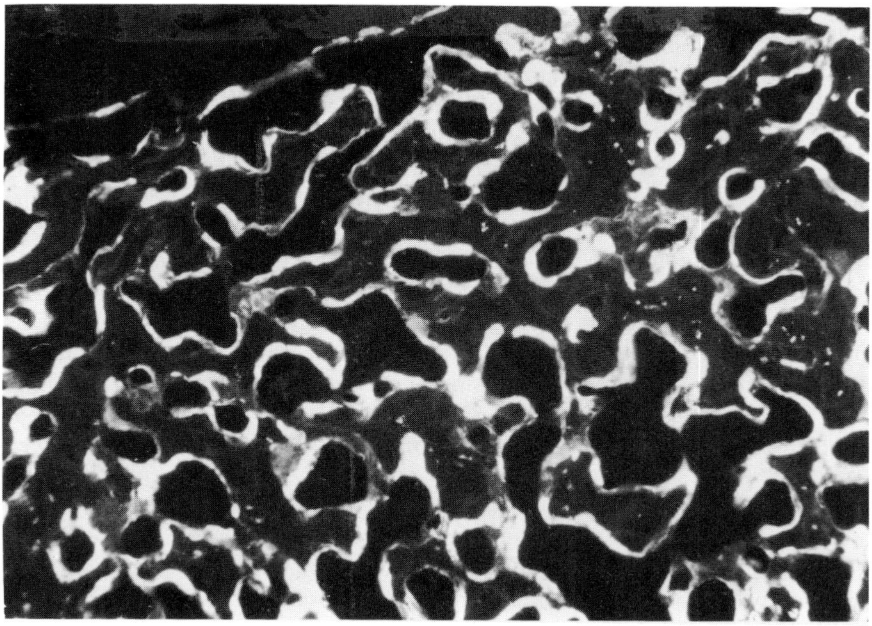

Fig. 13. Photomicrograph of a ground, undecalcified section of medullary bone from the femur of a laying hen injected with tetracycline immediately after laying and killed 24 h later, taken with a fluorescent microscope. Newly-formed bone surfaces exhibit a yellow fluorescence, showing clear white on the photograph: inactive surfaces and those undergoing resorption are dark or mottled. Intense black areas are occupied by marrow tissue. Central regions of bone show background fluorescence, similar in intensity to inactive and resorbing surfaces (which cannot be distinguished by this technique). Note that bone formation proceeds in discrete areas during eggshell formation, while adjacent areas are either inactive or undergoing resorption. (Section prepared by Miss Jean Kirkley and photographed by Dr. Walter Siller.)

are apparent at successive time intervals. In the period 5–7 h after ovulation, for example, approximately 50% of the medullary cavity is occupied by bony tissue, whereas in the succeeding 2-h period only 5% or so of medullary bone is present. Such great changes in the amount of medullary bone are totally unrealistic, and the differences observed from period to period are almost certainly a result of the individual variability of the experimental birds. It is inconceivable that medullary bone could be destroyed at this rate. In the pigeon it takes about 6 days for the medullary bone, which fills the entire marrow cavity, to be completely resorbed after the second egg of the clutch is laid (Bloom *et al.*, 1941). It is, therefore, pointless to look for changes in the *amount* of medullary present over short intervals of time.

Additional support for the view that PTH is responsible for the resorption of medullary bone during shell formation is provided by Miller (1978), who demonstrated that PTH induces morphological changes in the quiescent osteoclasts of the medullary bone of Japanese quail identical to those observed during active shell calcification (Miller, 1977). Similar observations had earlier been made for the domestic fowl (Taylor and Belanger, 1969). The latter authors suggested that osteocytic osteolysis may play an important part in the resorption process, but Candlish (1971), in an electron microscopic study, could not confirm this suggestion and observed only osteoclastic resorption in preparations of medullary bone.

PTH-induced bone resorption requires the participation of $1{,}25(OH)_2D_3$, and it is worthy of note that Abe *et al.* (1981) observed an increase in the circulatory concentration of this hormone about midnight, a time in the laying cycle when PTH secretion would be expected to be at or near a maximum and when provision of calcium for shell formation is known to be great (Tyler, 1954).

The effects of exogenous PTH on bone metabolism and on egg shell formation have been studied in Japanese quail (Dacke, 1976). When the hormone was injected within 2 to 6 h of oviposition, mobilization of ^{45}Ca from the skeleton for shell formation was increased, but shell thickness, measured as weight/unit area of shell, was significantly decreased. Neither of these actions of PTH was observed when the hormone was injected 12 to 16 h after oviposition, possibly because the endogenous level of PTH in the plasma was high at this time, saturating the target organ receptors. There is no obvious explanation for the decrease in shell thickness brought about by the PTH administered in the early stages of egg formation, particularly since shell calcification would not have begun. (Even in birds injected 6 h after oviposition, the egg would still have been only at the "plumping" stage). Whatever the mechanism, it would appear that the PTH was exerting an action, direct or indirect, on the oviduct and this action deserves to be investigated further.

C. The Organic Components of Bone

The organic matrices of medullary and cortical bone tissue differ in a number of respects. Candlish (1971) observed that, relative to cortical tissue, medullary bone was low in collagen (determined as hydroxyproline), high in proteoglycans ("mucopolysaccharides", determined as uronic acids) and low in calcium. As a result of a more detailed study of the proteoglycans present in the bone of laying hens, Candlish and Holt (1971) tentatively identified the major proteoglycan of medullary bone as keratosulphate and that of cortical bone as chondroitin sulphate. Medullary bone is also rich in glycoproteins (Stagni *et al.*, 1980).

D. Prostaglandins

Much of the interest in PGs in reproductive physiology of birds relates to their role in ovulation, ovum transport and oviposition. In Section V we have reviewed the evidence linking PGs with calcium and bone metabolism in both mammals and immature birds, and the possibility that PGs play a role in resorption of medullary bone and perhaps even in calcium secretion in the shell gland must now be accepted. There is no direct evidence for an involvement of PGs in these processes, but a number of observations are consistent with such a possibility. Hammond and Ringer (1978) showed that a single injection of indomethacin reduced the plasma calcium concentration in laying hens by 30%. Hammond *et al.* (1980) observed a broad peak of both PGE and PGF in the plasma of hens between 6 and 16 h after ovulation but thereafter, there was a sharp fall in both PGs at a time when shell calcification was still proceeding actively, so that the correspondence between circulating concentrations of PGs and presumed bone resorption is far from perfect. However, since PGE and PGF are local hormones, their concentration in the medullary bone tissue itself is of greater relevance than the plasma concentrations but these measurements have not yet been reported.

E. Calcitonin

The accepted physiological roles for CT are two-fold, namely to combat hypercalcaemia and to protect the skeleton against excessive resorption. In the laying hen, there is clearly a conflict between the need to provide calcium for the egg shell and the need to protect the skeleton, but there is a period between the time when the calcification of one shell is completed and that of the next egg is begun (i.e. during the period 0 to 4 h after oviposition) when CT might be expected to exert a protective influence on the skeleton.

In the present context, "hypercalcaemia" means an increased concentration of Ca^{2+} rather than of total calcium. The only time during the egg cycle when this situation is likely to arise is immediately before or after oviposition, when calcium is still being absorbed from the intestines and mobilized from the bone at a high rate without being removed from the blood by the shell gland. Figure 11 illustrates the changes in ionized calcium that occur during the egg cycle (no changes were observed in the mean concentrations of total calcium 0 to 3 h and 15 to 18 h after oviposition). In a preliminary study of the circulating concentrations of CT during the egg cycle using 10 laying hens (Baimbridge and Taylor, 1981), CT was not detectable in any bird during active shell formation, but in six of the hens CT was present in the plasma shortly after oviposition at a mean concentration of 1·54 ng ml^{-1}, assayed in terms of synthetic salmon CT. In the four birds that laid a second egg within 48 h of the first, CT was detectable until about the time of the next ovulation, but in the birds laying the last egg of a sequence CT could not be detected between 4 and 20 h after oviposition. Using the values for Ca^{2+} reported by Luck and Scanes (1979), the authors concluded that CT is secreted when the plasma concentration exceeds 1·5 mmol $litre^{-1}$. Dacke *et al.* (1972) had earlier shown that the mean level of CT in the plasma of Japanese quail was almost 40% lower during active shell formation than when shell calcification was not taking place.

According to Mueller and Leach (1974), intramuscular injection of porcine CT (10 MRC U kg^{-1}) into hens at the onset of eggshell calcification has no effect on shell thickness. Similarly, Dacke (1979) found no effect of salmon CT (3 MRC U kg^{-1}) on shell thickness when injected intraperitoneally into quail hens either 6 or 14 h after ovulation. There seems to be no evidence, then, to indicate an effect of CT on calcium secretion by the avian oviduct.

The only satisfactory way of determining whether or not CT protects the skeleton of laying birds is by studying the effects of ultimobranchialectomy (UBX). This has been done by Speers *et al.* (1970). Chicks were operated on when aged 1 to 2 days and were reared in the normal manner. The UBX birds were slightly slower in coming into lay than the sham-operated controls and their food consumption, egg production and egg weight were significantly reduced. Shell thickness was slightly less in the UBX birds than in the controls, but the difference was significant only during the first two weeks of egg production. No differences between the bones from the two groups could be detected and the authors concluded that no major impairment of growth, egg production, eggshell calcification or calcium metabolism due to ultimobranchialectomy occurred. Neither did UBX induce any significant changes in the skeletons of growing chickens (Brown *et al.*, 1969). Belanger and Copp (1972) studied the effect of chronic CT administration on the skeletons of laying hens. The birds were injected intramuscularly with 2 MRC U salmon CT d^{-1} for 4 months, after which their bones were taken for histological examination. The total amount of medullary bone was reduced, but the cortical bone was more dense and it is not possible to draw any meaningful conclusions from this experiment. The work of Baimbridge and Taylor (1981) has shown that CT is secreted for short periods at specific stages of the egg cycle and single daily injections of CT at fixed times of the day cannot be expected to mimic the physiological situation.

The combating of hypercalcaemia and the protection of the skeleton are two sides of the same coin, since the former function is achieved by the inhibition of bone resorption. Since there is now overwhelming evidence that CT is secreted in response to hypercalcaemia and that it is effective in restricting the rise in plasma calcium concentration, it follows inevitably that the hormone must prevent excessive loss of bone tissue whenever its concentration in the blood is elevated. Whether its major target is the cortical or medullary bone is a matter for speculation. Calcitonin is known to inhibit all bone-destroying cells and its quantitative effect on any particular area of bone is the product of the number of these cells present and the rate of blood flow through the area; for these reasons CT is likely to exert its major action on medullary bone. It is to be hoped that the experiments of Speers *et al.* (1970) will be repeated with the primary object of comparing the detailed histology and chemistry of the bones of the experimental and control birds. In any such experiment the plasma CT concentrations should be monitored to determine whether or not accessory C-cells are producing CT in the UBX birds.

F. Eggshell Formation

Losses to the poultry industry that result from cracked and broken eggs are very considerable, and a great deal of research has been directed towards ameliorating this problem. Shell strength is largely, but not entirely, dependent on shell thickness and shell thickness increases markedly as the daily intake of calcium rises from 2 to 4 g d^{-1} in laying hens. With dietary intakes above 4 g d^{-1} the increase is quite marginal, and above 5 g d^{-1} negligible (Agricultural Research Council, 1975). It is a common practice to include in the diet of laying hens the full estimated requirement of calcium in the form of finely-ground limestone. Scott *et al.* (1971) showed that eggshell strength was significantly increased when some or all of the ground limestone was replaced by oyster shell grit. The preferred combination was 25 g ground limestone and 50 g oyster shell per kg diet. Other reports (Kuhl *et al.*, 1977; Watkins *et al.*, 1977) have confirmed that both oyster shell and limestone grit improve shell strength and thickness when contributing 67–75% of the total supplementary calcium. The calcareous grit remains in the gizzard and provides a steady supply of calcium for absorption throughout the 24 h of each day, whereas, when finely-ground limestone is given as the sole source of calcium, there is a period in the middle of the night when supplies of dietary calcium are exhausted and when the rate of mobilization of skeletal calcium may not be great enough to enable shell calcification to proceed at the maximum rate (Scott *et al.*, 1971).

Laying hens appear to have a specific appetite for calcium which enables them to adapt their intake to their requirements and Taylor (1970b) showed that, when hens were fed on a low-calcium diet, the mean intake of calcareous grit was 10·6 g on egg-forming and 2·8 g on non-egg-forming days. Hughes (1972) demonstrated that calcium intake showed a marked circadian rhythm that reached a peak just before the onset of shell calcification. This rhythm persisted when the laying of soft-shelled eggs was induced by placing a thread in the oviduct. The author suggested that the increased intake of calcium was stimulated by either a nervous or an endocrine mechanism associated with ovulation, but the specific mechanism has not yet been identified.

It is recognized that shell thickness declines when hens are fed on diets deficient in vitamin D, but there is no benefit to be obtained from increasing the dietary concentration beyond the recommended requirement level. For this reason, work in this area has concentrated on studying the effects of feeding metabolites of vitamin D, in the belief that one factor limiting the ability of laying birds to absorb calcium may be their ability to convert vitamin D into $1,25(OH)_2D_3$. No convincing evidence has been obtained to indicate that shell thickness increases when $25(OH)D_3$ replaces D_3 in the diet (Ronald and Harms, 1976; Cohen *et al.*, 1978; Hamilton, 1980), but Morris *et al.* (1977) observed that the dietary inclusion of $1,25(OH)_2D_3$ (in the form of the calcinogenic plant *Solanum malacoxylon*) significantly increased shell thickness within 48 h in hens that had been in lay for nine months. It is well known that shell strength decreases towards the end of the laying season and Abe *et al.* (1981) observed that *in vitro* production of $1,25(OH)_2D_3$ by kidney tissue taken from birds during the most active period of shell calcification was markedly less in old than in young hens, and that the activity of the 1-hydroxylase was restored in old birds after a forced moult. These observations strongly suggest that one factor responsible for the reduced breaking strength of the shells of eggs laid by old hens is a defect in the production of $1,25(OH)_2D_3$.

References

Abe, E., Tanabe, R. and Yoshiki, S. (1979). *Biochem. biophys. Res. Commun.* **88**, 500–507.

Abe, E., Horikawa, H., Masumura, T., Sugahara, M., Kubota, M. and Suda, T. (1981). *In* "Hormonal Control of Calcium Metabolism" (D. V. Cohn, R. V. Talmage and J. L. Matthews, eds) Excerpta Medica, Amsterdam.

Agricultural Research Council (1975). "The Nutrient Requirements of Farm Livestock: No. 1, Poultry". Agricultural Research Council, London.

Baimbridge, K. G. and Taylor, T. G. (1980). *J. Endocr.* **85**, 171–185.

Baimbridge, K. G. and Taylor, T. G. (1981). *Comp. Biochem. Physiol.* **68A**, 647–651.

Baksi, S. N. and Kenny, A. D. (1977). *Endocrinology* **101**, 1216–1220.

Baksi, S. N. and Kenny, A. D. (1978a). *Am. J. Physiol.* **234**, E622–628.

Baksi, S. N. and Kenny, A. D. (1978b). *Biochem. Pharmac.* **27**, 2765–2768.

Baksi, S. N. and Kenny, A. D. (1979). *Pharmacology* **18**, 169–174.

Bannister, D. W. and Candlish, J. K. (1973). *Br. Poult. Sci.* **14**, 121–125.

Bar, A. and Hurwitz, S. (1975). *Poult. Sci.* **54**, 1325–1327.

Bar, A. and Norman, A. W. (1981). *Endocrinology* **109**, 950–955.

Bar, A. and Wassermann, R. H. (1973). *Biochem. biophys. Res. Comm.* **54**, 191–196.

Bar, A., Hurwitz, S. and Edelstein, S. (1975). *Biochim. biophys. Acta* **411**, 106–112.
Bar, A., Eisner, U., Montecuccoli, G. and Hurwitz, S. (1976). *J. Nutr.* **106**, 1336–1342.
Bar, A., Cohen, A., Edelstein, S., Shemesh, M., Montecuccoli, G. and Hurwitz, S. (1978). *Comp. Biochem. Physiol.* **59B**, 245–249.
Bates, R. F. L., Bruce, J. and Care, A. D. (1969). *J. Endocr.* **45**, xiv–xv (abs.).
Bates, R. F. L., Care, A. D., Peacock, M., Mawer, E. B. and Taylor C. M. (1975). *J. Endocr.* **64**, 6*P* (abs.).
Baxter, L. A. and De Luca, H. F. (1976). *J. biol. Chem.* **251**, 3158–3161.
Belanger, L. F. and Copp, D. H. (1972). *In* "Proceedings of 4th Parathyroid Conference, Chapel Hill, 1971" (R. V. Talmage and P. L. Munson, eds), pp. 41–50. Excerpta Medica, Amsterdam.
Bhattacharyya, M. H. and De Luca, H. F. (1974). *Biochem. biophys. Res. Comm.* **59**, 734–741.
Bikle, D. D., Spencer, E. M., Burke, W. H. and Rost, C. R. (1980). *Endocrinology* **107**, 81–84.
Bikle, D. D., Morrissey, R. L., Zolock, D. T. and Rasmussen, H. (1981). *Rev. Physiol. Biochem. Pharmac.* **89**, 63–142.
Bloom, W., Bloom, M. A. and McLean, F. C. (1941). *Anat. Rec.* **81**, 443–475.
Boelkins, J. N. and Kenny, A. D. (1973). *Endocrinology* **92**, 1754–1760.
Boelkins, J. N., Mazurkiewicz, M., Mazur, P. E. and Mueller, W. J. (1976). *Endocrinology* **98**, 403–412.
Bouillon, R., Van Baelen, H., Tan, B. K. and De Moor, P. (1980). *J. biol. Chem.* **255**, 10925–10930.
Boyle, I. T., Omdahl, J. L., Gray, R. W. and De Luca, H. F. (1973). *J. biol. Chem.* **248**, 4174–4180.
Brown, D. M., Perey, D. Y. E., Dent, P. B. and Good, R. A. (1969). *Proc. Soc. exp. Biol. Med.* **130**, 1001–1004.
Candlish, J. K. (1971). *Br. Poult. Sci.* **12**, 111–117.
Candlish, J. K. and Holt, F. J. (1971). *Comp. Biochem. Physiol.* **40B**, 283–293.
Candlish, J. K. and Taylor, T. G. (1970). *J. Endocr.* **48**, 143–144.
Canterbury, J. M., Lerman, S., Claflin, A. J., Henry, H., Norman, A. and Reiss, E. (1978). *J. clin. Invest.* **61**, 1375–1383.
Care, A. D. and Bates, R. F. L. (1972). *Gen. comp. Endocr. Suppl.* **3**, 448–458.
Care, A. D., Bates, R. F. L. and Gitelman, H. J. (1969). *J. Endocr.* **43**, lv–lvi (abs.).
Care, A. D., Bruce, J. B., Boelkins, J. N., Kenny, A. D., Conaway, H. H. and Anast, C. S. (1971). *Endocrinology* **89**, 262–271.
Castillo, L., Tanaka, Y., Wineland, M. J., Jowsey, J. O. and De Luca, H. F. (1979). *Endocrinology* **104**, 1598–1601.
Castillo, L., Tanaka, Y., De Luca, H. F. and Sunde, M. L. (1977). *Archs Biochem. Biophys.* **179**, 211–217.
Chen, P. S. and Bosmann, H. B. (1964). *J. Nutr.* **83**, 133–139.
Chen, T. C., Castillo, L., Korycka-Dahl, M. and De Luca, H. F. (1974). *J. Nutr.* **104**, 1056–1060.
Chertow, B. S., Baylink, D. J., Wergedal, J. E., Su, M. H. H. and Norman, A. W. (1975). *J. clin. Invest.* **56**, 668–678.
Clark, N. B. and Mok, L. (1981). *Calc. Tiss. Int.* **33**, 319 (abs.).
Cohen, A., Bar, A., Eisner, U. and Hurwitz, S. (1978). *Poult. Sci.* **57**, 1646–1651.
Common, R. H., Rutledge, N. A. and Hale, R. W. (1948). *J. agric. Sci.* **38**, 64–80.

Cooper, C. W., Schwesinger, W. H., Mahgoub, A. M. and Ontjes, D. A. (1971). *Science, N.Y.* **72**, 1238–1240.
Copp, D. H., Cockcroft, D. W. and Kuek, Y. (1967). *Can. J. Physiol. Pharmac.* **45**, 1095–1099.
Copp, D. H., Brooks, C. E., Low, B. S., Newsome, F., O'Dor, R. K., Parkes, C. O., Walker, V. and Watts, E. G. (1970). *In* "Calcitonin" (S. Taylor and R. Frazer, eds), pp. 281–294. Heinemann, London.
Corradino, R. A. (1973). *J. Cell Biol.* **58**, 64–78.
Corradino, R. A. and Wasserman, R. H. (1974). *Nature, Lond.* **252**, 176–718.
Corradino, R. A., Taylor, A. N. and Wasserman, R. H. (1969). *Fedn Proc. Fedn Am. Socs exp. Biol.* **28**, 760 (abs.).
Crooks, J. R. and Simkiss, K. (1974). *J. exp. Biol.* **61**, 197–202.
Crooks, J. R. and Simkiss, K. (1975). *Q. Jl exp. Physiol.* **60**, 55–63.
Cutler, G. B., Habener, J. F., Dee, P. C. and Potts, J. T. (1974). *FEBS Letts* **38**, 209–212.
Dacke, C. G. (1976). *J. Endocr.* **71**, 239–243.
Dacke, C. G. (1979). "Calcium Regulation in Sub-Mammalian Vertebrates", pp. 164–182. Academic Press, London and New York.
Dacke, C. G. and Kenny, A. D. (1973). *Endocrinology* **92**, 463–470.
Dacke, C. G. and Kenny, A. D. (1982). *In* "Aspects of Avian Endocrinology: Practical and Theoretical Implications" (C. G. Scanes, M. A. Ottinger, A. D. Kenny, J. Balthazart, J. Cronshaw and I. Chester Jones, eds). Texas Technical University Press, Lubbock.
Dacke, C. G. and Willins, S. A. (1982). *J. Physiol., Lond.* **322**, 9*P* (abs.).
Dacke, C. G. and Willins, S. A. (in press). *Proc. 9th Int. Symp. comp. Endocr.*
Dacke, C. G., Boelkins, J. N., Smith, W. K. and Kenny, A. D. (1972). *J. Endocr.* **54**, 369–370.
Dacke, C. G., Furr, B. J. A., Boelkins, J. N. and Kenny, A. D. (1976). *Comp. Biochem. Physiol.* **55A**, 341–344.
De Luca, H. F. (1979a). "Vitamin D. Metabolism and Function". Springer-Verlag, Berlin.
De Luca, H. F. (1979b). *Nutr. Rev.* **37**, 161–193.
De Luca, H. F. (1980). *Nutr. Rev.* **38**, 169–182.
Dietal, M., Dorn, G., Montz, R. and Altenahr, E. (1979). *Endocrinology* **105**, 237–245.
Dietrich, J. W., Goodson, J. M. and Raisz, L. G. (1975). *Prostaglandins* **10**, 231–240.
Edelstein, S., Lawson, D. E. M. and Kodicek, E. (1973). *Biochem. J.* **135**, 417–426.
Edelstein, S., Harell, A., Bar, A. and Hurwitz, S. (1975). *Biochim. biophys. Acta* **385**, 438–442.
Feinblatt, J. D. and Raisz, L. G. (1972). *In* "Calcium, Parathyroid Hormone and the Calcitonins" (R. V. Talmage and P. L. Munson, eds), p. 51. Excerpta Medica, Amsterdam.
Franklin, R. B. and Tashjian, A. H. (1975). *Endocrinology* **92**, 240–243.
Fraser, D. R. and Emtage, J. S. (1976). *Biochem. J.* **160**, 671–682.
Fraser, D. R. and Kodicek, E. (1970). *Nature, Lond.* **228**, 764–766.
Fraser, D. R. and Kodicek, E. (1973). *Nature, New Biology* **241**, 163–166.
Friedlander, E. J., Henry, H. L. and Norman, A. W. (1977). *Fedn Proc. Fedn Am. Socs exp. Biol.* **36**, 1096 (abs.).
Fritsch, H. A., Van Noorden, S. and Pearse, A. G. E. (1979). *Cell Tiss. Res.* **202**, 263–274.

Galan, F. G., Rogers, R. M., Girgis, S. I. and MacIntyre, I. (1981). *Brain Res.* **212**, 59–66.
Galante, L., Colston, K. W., Macauley, S. G. and MacIntyre, I. (1972). *Nature, Lond.* **238**, 271–272.
Garabedian, M., Holick, M. F., De Luca, H. F. and Boyle, I. T. (1972). *Proc natn. Acad. Sci. U.S.A.*, **69**, 1673–1676.
Girgis, S. I., Galan, F. G., Arnett, T. R., Rogers, R. M., Bone, Q., Ravazzola, M. and MacIntyre, I. (1980). *J. Endocr.* **87**, 375–382.
Gonnerman, W. A., Breitenbach, R. P., Erfling, W. F. and Anast, C. S. (1972). *Endocrinology* **91**, 1423–1429.
Habener, J. F. (1981). *A. Rev. Physiol.* **43**, 211–223.
Hamilton, R. M. G. (1980). *Poult. Sci.* **59**, 598–604.
Hammond, R. W. and Ringer, R. K. (1978). *Poult. Sci.* **57**, 1141 (abs.).
Hammond, R. W., Olsen, D. M., Frenkel, R. B., Biellier, H. V. and Hertelendy, F. (1980). *Gen. comp. Endocr.* **42**, 195–202.
Hay, A. W. M. and Watson, G. (1976). *Comp. Biochem. Physiol.* **53B**, 167–172.
Henry, H. L. (1981). *In* "Hormonal Control of Calcium Metabolism" (D. V. Cohn, R. V. Talmage and J. L. Matthews, eds), pp. 202–211. Excerpta Medica, Amsterdam.
Henry, H. L., Midgett, R. J. and Norman, A. W. (1974). *J. biol. Chem.* **249**, 7584–7592.
Henry, H. L., Norman, A. W., Taylor, A. N., Hartenblower, D. L. and Coburn, J. W. (1976). *J. Nutr.* **106**, 724–734.
Hodges, R. D. (1970). *Annls Biol. anim. Biochim. Biophys.* **10**, 255–275.
Holick, M. F. and Clark, M. B. (1978). *Fedn Proc. Fedn Am. Socs exp. Biol.* **37**, 2567–2574.
Holick, M. F., Frommer, J. E., McNeill, S. C., Richtand, N. M., Henley, J. W. and Potts, J. T. (1977). *Biochem. biophys. Res. Comm.* **76**, 107–114.
Holtrop, M. E. and Raisz, L. G. (1979). *Calcif. Tissue Int.* **29**, 201–205.
Hoyt, R. F., Tashjian, A. H. and Hamilton, D. W. (1972). *Endocrinology* **91**, 770–783.
Hughes, B. O. (1972). *Br. Poult. Sci.* **13**, 485–493.
Hughes, M. R., Baylink, D. J., Jones, P. G. and Haussler, M. R. (1976). *J. clin. Invest.* **58**, 61–70.
Hurwitz, S. (1964). *Poult. Sci.* **43**, 1462–1472.
Hurwitz, S., Bar, A. and Cohen, I. (1973). *Am. J. Physiol.* **225**, 150–154.
Imrie, M. H., Neville, P. F., Snellgrove, A. W. and De Luca, H. F. (1967). *Archs Biochem. Biophys.* **120**, 525–532.
Johnston, P. M. and Comar, C. L. (1955). *Am. J. Physiol.* **183**, 365–370.
Kenny, A. D. and Dacke, C. G. (1974). *J. Endocr.* **62**, 15–23.
Kimberg, D. V., Baerg, R. D., Gershon, E. and Grandusius, R. T. (1981). *J. clin. Invest.* **50**, 1309–1321.
Klein, D. C. and Raisz, L. G. (1970). *Endocrinology* **86**, 1436–1440.
Kowarski, S. and Schachter, D. (1975). *Am. J. Physiol.* **229**, 1198–1204.
Kowarski, S. and Schachter, D. (1980). *J. biol. Chem.* **255**, 10834–10840.
Kream, B. E., Jose, M., Yamada, S. and De Luca, H. F. (1977). *Science, N.Y.* **197**, 1086–1088.
Kuhl, H. J., Holder, D. P. and Sullivan, T. W. (1977). *Poult. Sci.* **56**, 605–611.
Lawson, D. E. M. (1978). "Vitamin D". Academic Press, London and New York.
Lawson, D. E. M., Charman, M., Wilson, P. W. and Edelstein, S. (1976). *Biochim. biophys. Acta* **437**, 403–415.
Le Van, L. (1980). *Ph.D. thesis, University of Wisconsin.*

Lewis, P. E. and Taylor, T. G. (1972). *J. Endocr.* **53**, xlv (abs.).
Lorence, R., Tanaka, Y., De Luca, H. F. and Jones, G. (1977). *Endocrinology* **93**, 718–722.
Luck, M. R. (1978). *Ph.D. thesis, University of Leeds.*
Luck, M. R. and Scanes, C. G. (1979). *Comp. Biochem. Physiol.* **63A**, 177–181.
Luck, M. R., Sommerville, B. A. and Scanes, C. G. (1980). *Comp. Biochem. Physiol.* **65A**, 151–154.
Luckert, B. P., Stanbury, S. W. and Mawer, E. B. (1973). *Endocrinology* **93**, 718–722.
McChesney, E. W. (1943). *J. Nutr.* **26**, 81–94.
MacGregor, R. R., Chu, L. L. H., Hamilton, J. W. and Cohn, D. V. (1973). *Endocrinology* **92**, 1312–1317.
McNeilly, A. S., Etches, R. J. and Friesen, H. G. (1978). *Acta endocr., Copenh.* **89**, 60–69.
Midgett, R. J., Speilrogel, A. M., Coburn, J. W. and Norman, A. W. (1973). *J. clin. Endocr. Metab.* **36**, 1153–1161.
Miller, S. C. (1977). *J. Cell Biol.* **75**, 104–118.
Miller, S. C. (1978). *J. Cell Biol.* **76**, 615–618.
Montecuccoli, G., Hurwitz, S., Cohen, A. and Bar, A. (1977). *Comp. Biochem. Physiol.* **57A**, 335–339.
Moriuchi, S. and De Luca, H. F. (1974). *Archs Biochem. Biophys.* **164**, 165–171.
Morris, K. M. L., Jenkins, S. A. and Simonite, J. P. (1977). *Vet. Rec.* **101**, 502–504.
Mueller, W. J. and Leach, R. M. (1974). *A. Rev. Pharmac.* **14**, 289–303.
Mueller, W. J., Hall, K. L., Maurer, C. A. and Joshua, I. G. (1973). *Endocrinology* **92**, 853–856.
Murdoch, G. H. and Rosenfeld, M. G. (1981). *J. biol. Chem.* **256**, 4050–4055.
Narbaitz, R. (1972). *Gen. comp. Endocr.* **19**, 253–258.
Narbaitz, R. (1975). *Gen. comp. Endocr.* **27**, 122–124.
Narbaitz, R. (1979). *Gen. comp. Endocr.* **37**, 440–442.
Narbaitz, R., Stumpf, W., Madhabananda, S., De Luca, H. F. and Tanaka, Y. (1980). *Gen. comp. Endocr.* **42**, 283–289.
Nicholson, R. A., Akhtar, M. and Taylor, T. G. (1979). *Biochem. J.* **182**, 745–750.
Nieto, A., Fando, J. J. L. and Candela, J. L. R. (1975). *Gen. comp. Endocr.* **25**, 259–263.
Norman, A. W. (1965). *Science, N.Y.* **149**, 184–186.
Norman, A. W. (1979). "Vitamin D: the Calcium Homoestatic Hormone". Academic Press, New York and London.
Norman, A. W. and Henry, H. L. (1974). *Clin. Orthop. Res.* **98**, 258–286.
Norman, A. W., Miller, B. E. and Putkey, J. A. (1980). *Prog. Biochem. Pharmac.* **17**, 160–167.
Oku, T., Shimura, F., Moriuchi, S. and Hosoya, N. (1975). *Proc. 10th Int. Cong. Nutr., Kyoto.*
Omdahl, J. L., Gray, R. W., Boyle, I. T., Knutson, J. and De Luca, H. F. (1972). *Nature, New Biology* **237**, 63–64.
Parsons, J. A., Reit, B. and Robinson, C. J. (1973). *Endocrinology* **92**, 454–462.
Pearse, A. G. E. (1976). *In* "Handbook of Physiology" (R. O. Greep, E. B. Astwood and G. D. Aurbach, eds), Vol. 7, pp. 411–422. Williams and Wilkins, Baltimore.
Perez Cano, R., Girgis, S. I., Galan Galan, F. and MacIntyre, I. (1982). *J. Endocr.* **92**, 351–355.
Potts, J. T. and Aurbach, G. D. (1976). *In* "Handbook of Physiology" (R. O. Greep. E. B. Astwood and G. D. Aurbach, eds), Vol. 7, pp. 423–430. Williams and Wilkins, Baltimore.

Rasmussen, H., Wong, M., Bikle, D. and Goodman, D. B. P. (1972). *J. clin. Invest.* **51**, 2502–2504.
Reynolds, J. J., Holick, M. F. and De Luca, H. F. (1973). *Calc. Tiss. Res.* **12**, 295–301.
Reynolds, J. J., Pavlovitch, H. and Balsan, S. (1976). *Calc. Tiss. Res.* **21**, 207–212.
Ribovich, M. L. and De Luca, H. F. (1975). *Archs Biochem. Biophys.* **170**, 529–535.
Roland, D. A. and Harms, R. H. (1976). *Poult. Sci.* **55**, 1982–1985.
Rost, C. R., Bikle, D. D. and Kaplan, R. A. (1981). *Endocrinology* **108**, 1002–1006.
Schneider, L. E., Nowosielski, L. and Schedl, H. P. (1977a). *Endocrinology* **100**, 67–73.
Schneider, L. E., Schedl, H. P., McCain, T. and Haussler, M. R. (1977b). *Science, N.Y.* **196**, 1452–1454.
Scott, M. L., Hull, S. J. and Mullenhoff, P. A. (1971). *Poult. Sci.* **50**, 1055–1063.
Sebrell, W. H. and Harris, R. S. (1954). *In* "The Vitamins", pp. 131–266. Academic Press, London and New York.
Sedrani, S. (1979). *Ph.D. thesis, University of Southampton.*
Sedrani, S. and Taylor, T. G. (1977). *J. Endocr.* **72**, 405–406.
Sedrani, S., Taylor, T. G. and Akhtar, M. (1981). *Gen. comp. Endocr.* **44**, 514–523.
Seyberth, H. W. Segre, G. V., Morgan, J. L., Swatman, B. J., Potts, J. T. and Oates, J. A. (1975). *N. Engl. J. Med.* **293**, 1278–1283.
Simkiss, K. (1967). *In* "Calcium in Reproductive Physiology", pp. 198–213. Chapman and Hall, London.
Simkiss, K. (1975). *Symp. Zool. Soc. Lond.* **35**, 307–337.
Simkiss, K. and Dacke, C. G. (1971). *In* "Physiology and Biochemistry of Domestic Fowl (D. J. Bell and B. M. Freeman, eds), Vol. 1, pp. 481–488. Academic Press, London and New York.
Somerville, B. A., Swaminathan, R. and Care, A. D. (1978). *Br. J. Nutr.* **39**, 411–414.
Spanos, E. and MacIntyre, I. (1977). *In* "Vitamin D, Biochemical, Chemical and Clinical Aspects related to Calcium Metabolism" (A. W. Norman, K. Schaefer, J. W. Coburn, H. F. De Luca, D. Fraser, H. G. Grigoleit and D. V. Herrath, eds), pp. 191–195. Walter de Gruyter, Berlin.
Spanos, E., Pike, J. W., Haussler, M. R., Colston, K. W., Evans, I. M. A., Goldner, A. M., McCain, T. A. and MacIntyre, I. (1976a). *Life Sci.* **19**, 1751–1756.
Spanos, E., Colston, K. W., Evans, I. M. S., Galante, L., MacAuley, S. J. and MacIntyre, I. (1976b). *Mol. Cell. Endocr.* **5**, 163–167.
Spanos, E., Barrett, D., MacIntyre, I., Pike, J. W., Lafilian, E. F. and Haussler, M. R. (1978a). *Nature, Lond.* **273**, 246–247.
Spanos, E., Barrett, D. I., Chong, K. T. and MacIntyre, I. (1978b). *Biochem. J.* **174**, 231–236.
Spanos, E., Brown, D. J., Stevenson, J. C. and MacIntyre, I. (1981). *Biochim. biophys. Acta* **672**, 7–15.
Speers, G. M., Perey, D. Y. E. and Brown, D. M. (1970). *Endocrinology* **87**, 1292–1297.
Spencer, E. M. and Tobiassen, O. (1977). *In* "Vitamin D, Biochemical, Chemical and Clinical Aspects related to Calcium Metabolism" (A. W. Norman, K. Schaefer, J. W. Coburn, H. F. De Luca, D. Fraser, H. G. Grigoleit and D. V. Herrath, eds), pp. 431–438. Walter de Gruyter, Berlin.
Spencer, R., Charman, M., Wilson, P. and Lawson, E. (1976). *Nature, Lond.* **263**, 161–163.
Stagni, N., de Bernard, B., Liut, G. F. and Zanetti, M. (1980). *Connect. Tiss. Res.* **7**, 121–125.
Steele, T. H. and De Luca, H. F. (1976). *J. clin. Invest.* **57**, 867–874.

Stern, P. H. (1980). *Pharmac. Rev.* **32**, 47–80.
Sunde, M. L., Turk, C. M. and De Luca, H. F. (1978). *Science, N.Y.* **200**, 1067–1069.
Talmage, R. V. (1970). *Am. J. Anat.* **129**, 467–476.
Tanaka, Y., Castillo, L. and De Luca, H. F. (1976). *Proc. natn. Acad. Sci., U.S.A.* **73**, 2701–2705.
Tanaka, Y., Castillo, L., Wineland, M. J. and De Luca, H. F. (1978). *Endocrinology* **103**, 2035–2039.
Tashjian, A. H., Voelkel, E. F., Levine, L. and Goldhaber, P. (1972). *J. exp. Med.* **136**, 1329–1343.
Taylor, A. N. and Wasserman, R. H. (1972). *Am. J. Physiol.* **223**, 110–114.
Taylor, T. G. (1970a). *Annls Biol. anim. Biochim. Biophys.* **10**, 83–91.
Taylor, T. G. (1970b). *In* "Proceedings 4th Nutrition Conference for Feed Manufacturers" (H. Swan and D. Lewis, eds), pp. 108–117. Churchill, London.
Taylor, T. G. and Belanger, L. F. (1969). *Calcif. Tissue Res.* **4**, 162–173.
Taylor, T. G. and Kirkley, J. (1967). *Br. Poult. Sci.* **8**, 289–295.
Taylor, T. G. and Moore, J. H. (1954). *Br. J. Nutr.* **8**, 112–124.
Taylor, T. G. and Moore, J. H. (1958). *Br. J. Nutr.* **12**, 35–42.
Taylor, T. G., Lewis, P. E. and Balderstone, O. (1975). *J. Endocr.* **66**, 297–298.
Trechsel, U., Bonjour, J.-P. and Fleisch, H. (1979). *J. clin. Invest.* **64**, 206–217.
Tucker, G., Gagnon, R. E. and Haussler, M. R. (1973). *Archs Biochem. Biophys.* **155**, 47–57.
Turner, R. T., Rader, J. I., Eliel, L. P. and Howard, G. A. (1979). *Gen. comp. Endocr.* **37**, 211–219.
Tyler, C. (1954). *J. Sci. Fd Agric.* **5**, 335–339.
Vanderwiel, C. J. and Talmage, R. V. (1979). *Endocrinology* **105**, 588–594.
Voelkel, E. F., Tashjian, A. H., Franklin, R., Wasserman, E. and Levine, L. (1975). *Metabolism* **24**, 973–986.
Wasserman, R. H. and Taylor, A. N. (1966). *Science, N.Y.* **152**, 791–793.
Watkins, R. M., Dilworth, B. C. and Day, E. J. (1977). *Poult. Sci.* **56**, 1641–1647.
Weber, J. C., Pons, V. and Kodicek, E. (1971). *Biochem. J.* **125**, 147–153.
Wilson, P. W. and Lawson, D. E. M. (1977). *Biochim. biophys. Acta* **497**, 805–811.
Wilson, P. W. and Lawson, D. E. M. (1978). *Biochem. J.* **173**, 627–631.
Wilson, P. W. and Lawson, D. E. M. (1981). *Nature, Lond.* **289**, 600–602.
Wong, R. G., Myrtle, J. F., Tsai, H. C. and Norman, A. W. (1972). *J. biol. Chem.* **247**, 5728–5735.
Ziegler, R., Delling, G. and Pfeiffer, E. F. (1970). *In* "Calcitonin 1969" (S. Taylor, ed.), pp. 301–310. Heinemann, London.
Zull, J. E., Czarnowska-Misztal, E. and De Luca, H. F. (1965). *Science, N.Y.* **149**, 182–184.

Note Added in Proof

The concentration of PTH in the plasma during the egg cycle has now been measured (R. Singh *et al.*, unpublished). The mean values were 0·64 pg ml^{-1} before shell calcification began, 3·4 pg ml^{-1} during active calcification and 1·2 pg ml^{-1} two to three hours before oviposition. There was a marked inverse relationship between plasma PTH and the Ca^{2+} concentrations reported by Luck and Scanes (1979) at the different stages of the egg cycle. It is clear, therefore, that PTH is actively secreted during the rapid phase of shell formation.

7 The Cardiovascular System

A. R. AKESTER

Sub-department of Veterinary Anatomy, University of Cambridge, England

PHYSIOLOGY BIOCHEMISTRY DOMESTIC FOWL, VOL. 5 ISBN 0-12-267105-8

I. Introduction

Although there are differences between the avian cardiovascular system and that of mammals, it is probable that, overall, there are more similarities. This is worth emphasizing, because the enthusiasm with which some comparative anatomists and physiologists stress the differences between the organ systems of different species may make one forget their overriding similarities.

Both birds and mammals have demonstrated a remarkable evolutionary versatility and, apart from the ability to live permanently under water, have managed to exploit virtually every environment. All this has been dependent on the efficiency and responsiveness of their cardiovascular system. It operates to provide nutrients, to remove metabolic waste material, to carry chemical messengers from one part of the body to another and to control body temperature.

Structural and organizational characteristics of blood vessels in different organs can be recognized as being directly related to the function of the organ. The kidney is a good example of this, with end arteries delivering blood, at high pressure, to fenestrated capillaries which are surrounded by a particularly well developed basement membrane.

Thermoregulation is very largely dependent on fluctuations of blood flow to specific regions, and whilst the central body (core) temperature in birds is maintained at about 41°C, parts of the periphery may be 30°C lower, with a vascular heat exchanger between the two.

The total blood volume in any animal is normally more or less constant and is about 240 ml in a 2·5-kg fowl. The basal metabolic rate in active (skeletal) muscle can be up to 300 times more than in the same tissue at rest (Gibbs,

1974). To permit this change in basal metabolic rate, blood flow through the tissue must be increased many times, whilst flow elsewhere must be reduced by about the same amount. Local dilator metabolites, autonomic nerves and specific vasoactive hormones cooperate to make this possible.

This chapter attempts to present a balanced view of the cardiovascular system in the domestic fowl. However, where important information is lacking (or not known to the author) reference is made to other avian species and occasionally to mammals.

II. Position of the Heart

One of the most profound differences between birds and mammals is the complete absence of a mammalian-type muscular diaphragm in the bird, so that there is no separate thorax and abdomen with alternating pressure regimes. It is therefore better to refer to the "body cavity" of birds rather than to "thorax and abdomen", as these latter terms inevitably carry with them an implication of the mammalian organization.

The heart of the domestic fowl, within its pericardium, lies in the cranial part of the body cavity, ventral to the lungs, at an angle of about 45° to the horizontal, and rests in a shallow depression at the cranial end of the sternum (Fig. 1). Between the heart and the ribs, on each side, is an anterior thoracic air sac. Between the base of the heart and the ventral surface of the lungs are the syrinx, two primary bronchi and part of the oesophagus. After the primary bronchi have entered the lungs the oesophagus lies immediately above the caudal aspect of the heart and joins the proventriculus between the left and right lobes of the liver. The pericardium covering the caudal aspect of the heart is in direct contact with the peritoneal covering of the liver.

III. Pericardium

The pericardium in birds is similar to that in mammals, being a bag of simple squamous epithelial cells (serous membrane) into which the heart has been invaginated. The visceral layer of the bag is intimately attached to the outer surface of the myocardium (Fig. 2a), whilst the parietal layer is free standing. Between the two layers is a thin film of pericardial fluid.

The serous pericardium is delicate and must be supported. The visceral layer is supported by the heart itself. The parietal layer is supported by an outer layer of tough collagen fibres (about 10 μm thick), which is called the fibrous pericardium (Fig. 2b). The visceral layer of the serous pericardium extends beyond the heart and covers the first part of the great vessels. It is then

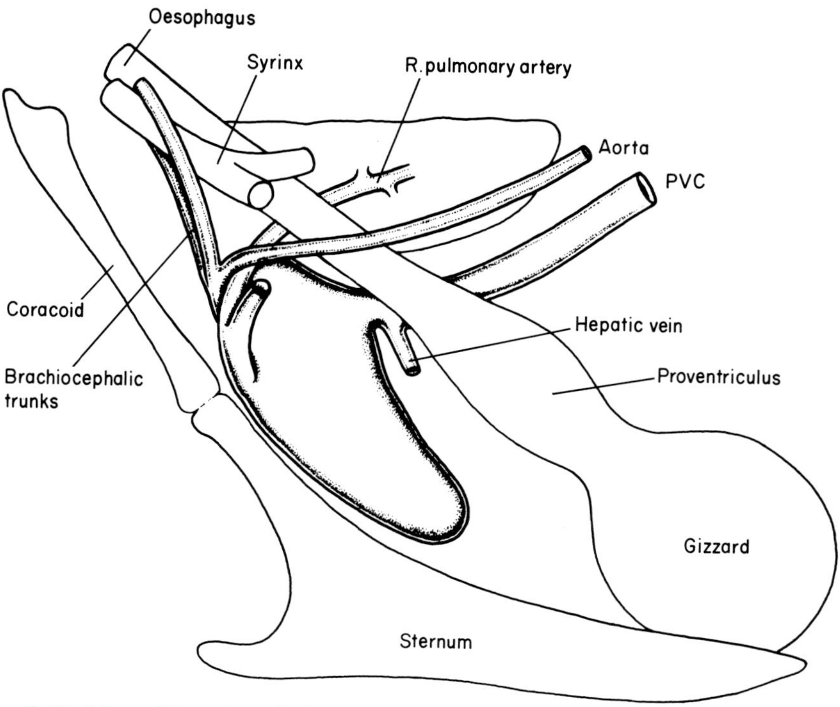

Fig. 1. Position of heart in relation to neighbouring structures. PVC, posterior vena cava.

reflected off these vessels as the parietal layer which lines the fibrous pericardium. The collagen fibres of the fibrous pericardium blend with the collagen fibres of the adventitia of the great vessels. At the caudoventral end of the heart, over the apex, the fibrous pericardium is continuous with the ventral ligament. This anchors the heart to the floor of the body cavity between the lobes of the liver, at about the centre of the sternum. On each side the pericardium is attached to the oblique septum.

The pericardium helps to protect the heart by isolating it from neighbouring structures. The serous layer provides lubrication for the movements which occur during cardiac contraction and relaxation. The fibrous layer probably helps to prevent over-distension. The effects of pericardectomy in birds are

---

Fig. 2. The pericardium (*a*) Shows visceral layer of serous pericardium attached to surface of myocardium. There is only a very thin layer of collagen fibres between the pericardium and the outermost layer of myocytes. (*b*) Part of the fibrous layer of the perietal pericardium to show the many alternating bands of dense collagen fibres.

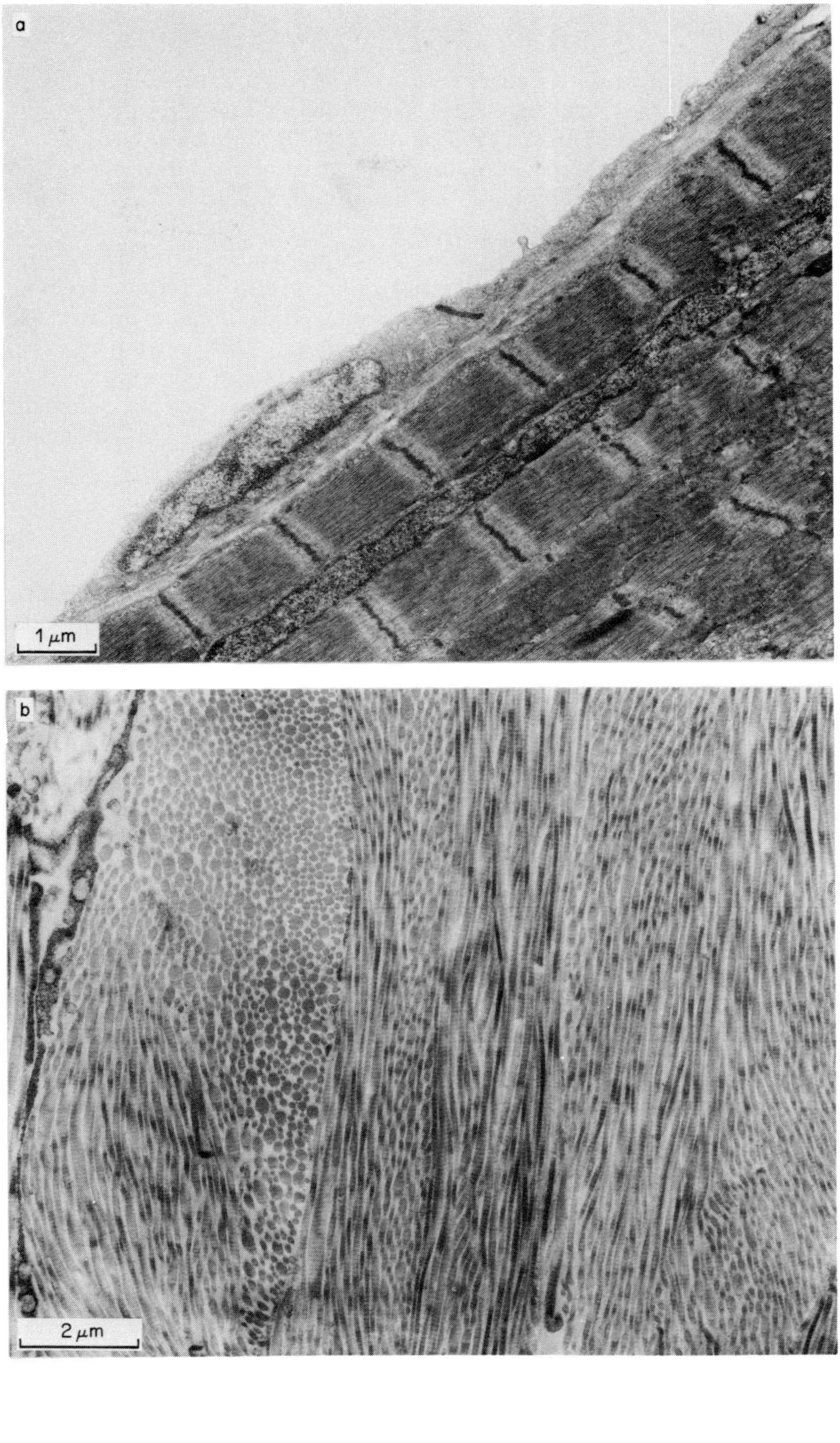
a
1 μm
b
2 μm

unknown, but in dogs it causes cardiac hypertrophy and an inability to respond to exercise (Nelemans, 1940). Congenital absence of the pericardium has been recorded in humans (Hering *et al.*, 1960), but not in birds.

It is possible that the pericardium assists atrial filling during ventricular systole, when the atrioventricular junction is pulled down by contraction of ventricular muscles. Ejection of blood from the ventricles (particularly the left) may contribute further to this downward movement. The pressure gradient between the venae cavae and right atrium and also between the pulmonary veins and left atrium increases, thus assisting venous inflow to the atria. No observations of this type have been made in birds, but it has been reported that opening the pericardium in the dog reduces the rate of filling of the right atrium (Holt *et al.*, 1960). The outer pericardium receives blood direct from the aorta and also from the internal thoracic arteries. It receives autonomic vasomotor and sensory nerves.

IV. Gross Structure of the Heart

In most major respects the avian heart closely resembles that of the mammal. Perhaps the most obvious difference is to be found in the right atrioventricular valve (Fig. 3). In birds it is a thick muscular fold applied to the interventricular septum and is completely different from its fibrous counterpart in mammals. No explanation for this difference has ever been given.

Venous blood returns from all parts of the body (except the myocardium) by way of the three venae cavae (Fig. 4). The right cranial vena cava and the single posterior vena cava enter the roof of the right atrium opposite one another (Fig. 5a). Their blood flows along a groove or gutter between two prominent muscular flaps or folds, which constitute the venous valves (Fig. 6b). They merge at their mid-point, so that the vascular groove becomes more shallow and the opposing currents of venous blood are deflected downwards towards the right atrioventricular aperture. The centre part of the groove thus functions in a way similar to the intervenous crest in mammals.

Whether these flaps should be called venous or sinus valves depends on one's ability to recognize a sinus venosus. Owen (1886), Quiring (1933), Simons (1960), Jones and Johansen (1972) and Baumel (1975, 1979) have claimed that it does exist in the domestic fowl, whilst Rose (1890), Kern (1926), Goodrich (1930), Akester (1971) and Vassal-Adams (1979) have been equally convinced that it does not. In the opinion of the present author, no sinus

Fig. 3. (*a*) Heart of domestic fowl (cranial view). Right side of heart has been partly detached from left side. (*b*) Section through heart. Note how the right antrioventricular valve (RAVV) is formed by atrial (above and thin) and ventricular (below and thick) muscle, being folded inwards towards the interventricular septum.

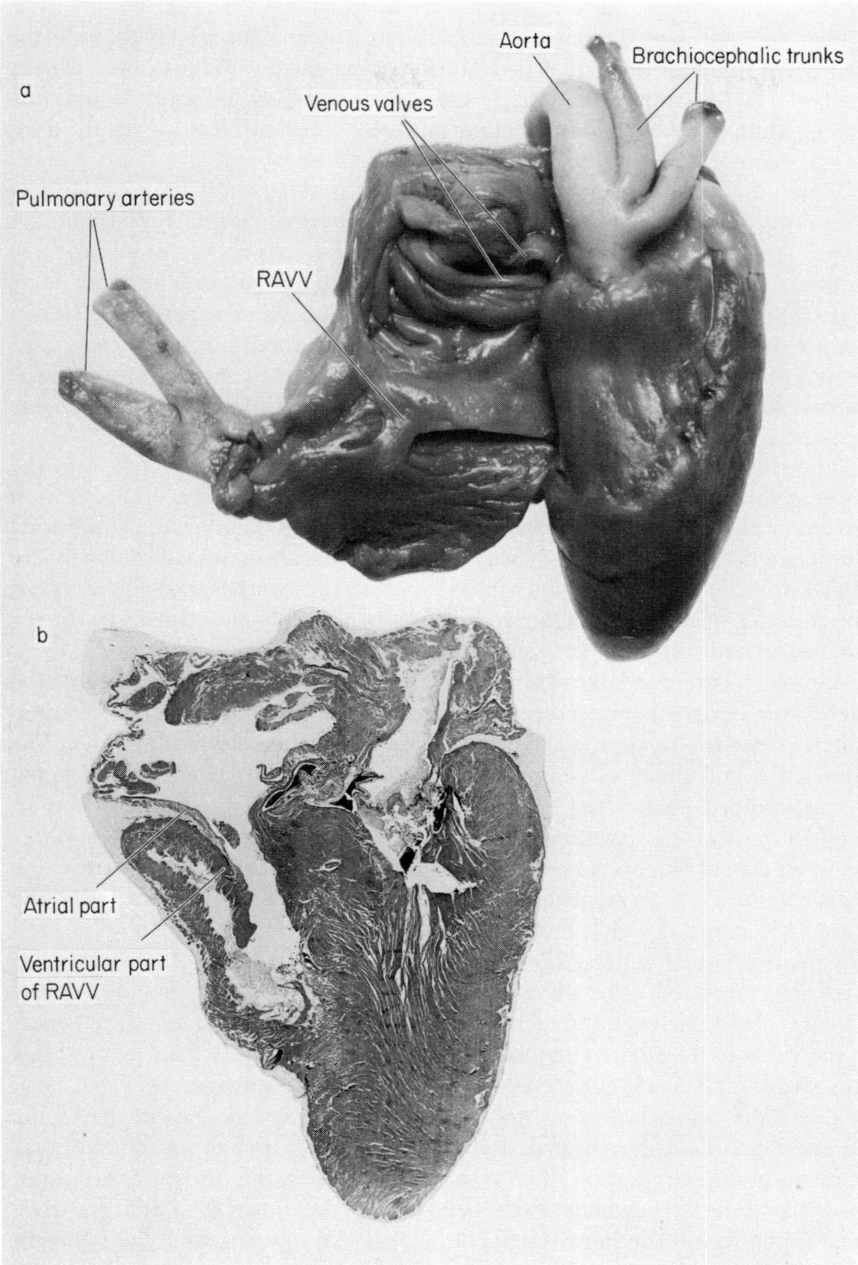
a
Aorta
Brachiocephalic trunks
Venous valves
Pulmonary arteries
RAVV
b
Atrial part
Ventricular part
of RAVV

venosus can be recognized in the mature domestic fowl, so that these valves, which are attached to the roof of the right atrium and which encircle the orifices of the posterior and right anterior vanae cavae, are best called venous valves. The left anterior vena cava discharges its blood, by way of a separate orifice, slightly to the left of that of the posterior vena cava but outside the flaps of the venous valve.

The right atrium is much larger than the left, and they both have a relatively thin muscular wall strengthened by muscular bars or ridges (Figs 4b, 6c). A particularly prominent bar of muscle arches across the dorsocranial aspect of both atria and has the interatrial septum attached to its lower surface. At its right hand end it divides into about six smaller bars which spread over the free wall of the right atrium to unite with a crescent-shaped shelf in its floor. This shelf forms the lateral margin of the right atrioventricular aperture and is extended to form the atrial part of the right atrioventricular valve. Similar muscular ridges spread over the free wall of the left atrium.

The interatrial septum is displaced to the left by a large pouch from the right atrium (Fig. 4), which spreads across the midline between the aortic arch (in front) and the pulmonary veins (behind). Venous blood from the myocardium enters the right atrium by way of several separate coronary veins so there is no coronary sinus. A fossa ovalis is not detectable either, possibly because the foramen ovale in the embryo consists of several small apertures in the interatrial septum.

Venous blood enters the roof of the right atrium and falls down through the right atrioventricular aperture into the right ventricle (Fig. 5a). This aperture is crescent-shaped and can be closed by contraction of a unique valve. The right atrioventricular valve in birds is a powerful muscular structure formed by an infolded part of the right atrial free wall being superimposed on an infolded part of the right ventricular free wall, with a layer of collagen fibres between them (Fig. 3). As one might expect, the bulk of the valve is provided by the ventricle. The resulting double layer of muscle is thus attached to the right atrium and ventricle laterally and directs its free edge in a spiral fashion downwards towards the interventricular septum. The ends of this valvular flap are connected cranially and caudally to the interventricular septum. There is also a narrow band of muscle which attaches the cranioventral corner of the valve to the right ventricular free wall (Figs 3, 5a). By contracting, this valve will apply itself closely to the interventricular septum.

The right ventricle lies on the cranial aspect of the heart and drives the pulmonary circulation, the pressure of which only reaches about one sixth that of the systemic circulation. The right ventricular wall is thus much thinner than that of the left ventricle. In the dead animal the thin-walled right ventricle is wrapped round the interventricular septum, so that the cavity of the right ventricle is crescent-shaped in cross section. The inflow tract lies caudal and to

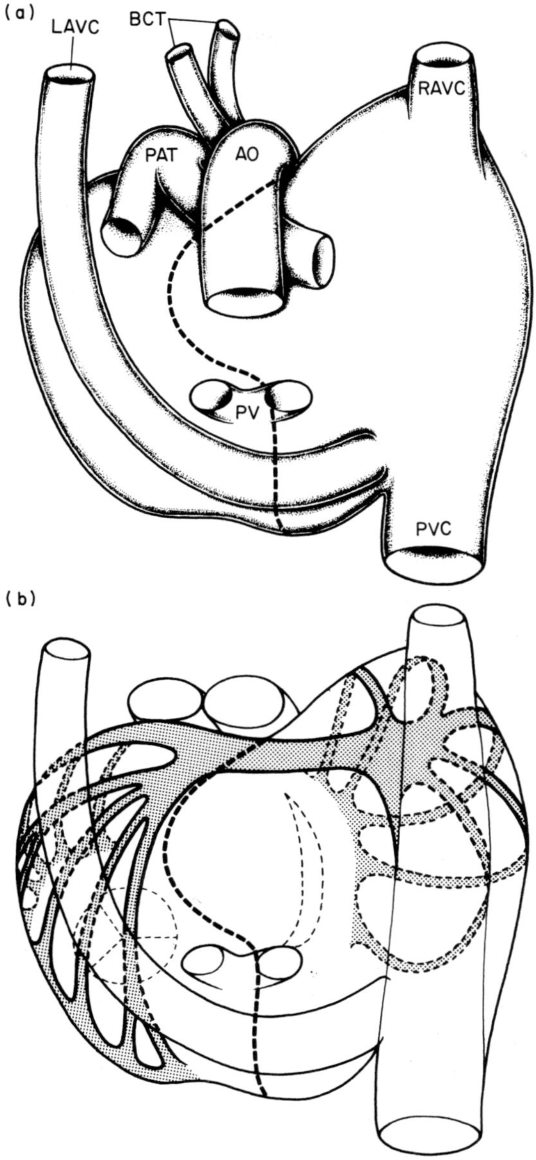

Fig. 4. Heart (dorsal view). Shows (*a*) connections of right and left anterior venae cavae (RAVC, LAVC), posterior vena cava (PVC), aorta (AO), brachiocephalic trunks (BCT), pulmonary arterial trunk (PAT), pulmonary vein (PV). The dashed line indicates the position of the inter-atrial septum. Note the right atrium is about twice the size of the left. And shows (*b*) position of large transverse muscular bar in roof of atria with smaller bars spreading round the atrial free walls. Positions of left and right atrioventricular values shown by fine dashed line. Heavy dashed line indicates position of interatrial septum.

the right of the aortic arch, whilst the outflow tract (conus arteriosus) lies to the left of the aorta. The pulmonary valve has three pocket-shaped cusps similar to those in mammals. The pulmonary trunk arches over the left atrium where it bifurcates to form left and right pulmonary arteries (Fig. 4).

Oxygenated blood returns from each lung by a single pulmonary vein. Immediately above the roof of the left atrium these two veins unite to form a single vessel which penetrates the left atrium and protrudes into its lumen. This vessel directs oxygenated blood through the left atrioventricular valve and into the left ventricle (Fig. 5b). The left atrioventricular valve in the domestic fowl more closely resembles its counterpart in mammals. It consists of rather irregular fibrous cusps supported by chordae tendinae, which are attached to the left ventricular wall either directly or by small papillary muscles. The valve itself does not contain muscle.

The left ventricle provides the power for the high pressure systemic circulation and so has a wall three to four times thicker than the right ventricle. The interventricular septum seems to be functionally associated more with the left than with the right ventricle. The apex of the heart consists entirely of left ventricular myocardium. Much of the inner surface of the left ventricle is trabeculated but the outflow tract to the aorta is perfectly smooth. The aortic valve cusps resemble those of the mammal but do not have a prominent fibrous nodule at the centre of their free border (Figs 6d, e).

V. Coronary Circulation

The whole of the myocardium, the visceral layer of the pericardium, the upper part of the parietal pericardium and the vasa vasorum of those parts of the great vessels adjacent to the heart, are supplied with oxygenated blood by branches from one or other of the left and right coronary arteries. The more ventral part of the parietal pericardium is supplied by branches from the internal thoracic artery.

There are normally two coronary arteries in the fowl, although one or two additional but smaller vessels have been reported (Lindsay and Smith, 1965), which are probably transposed branches of the major vessels. Dominance by one or other of the coronary arteries is usual, although they may be of equal size. In the fowl (and human), the right one is usually dominant. Each coronary artery branches from the aorta at a point level with the attachment of an aortic valve cusp (Fig. 6e). The orifice is thus just outside (distal to) the aortic sinus (of Valsalva). Each coronary artery soon divides into a smaller superficial branch and a larger deep branch.

The right superficial coronary artery (right circumflex) lies in the fat-filled groove between the right atrium and ventricle, sending branches to the walls of

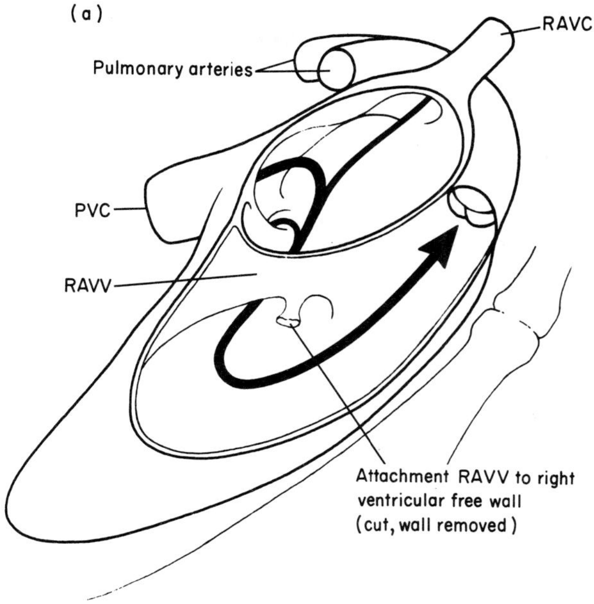

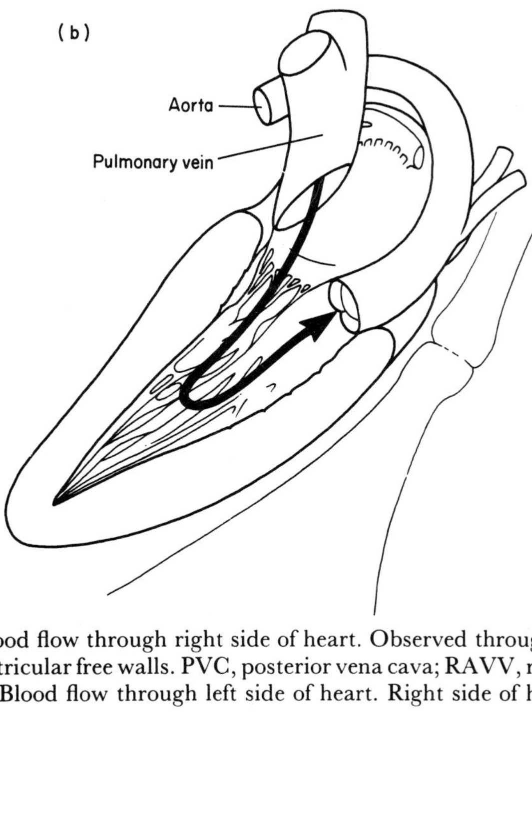

Fig. 5. (*a*) Blood flow through right side of heart. Observed through openings cut in atrial and ventricular free walls. PVC, posterior vena cava; RAVV, right atrioventricular valve. (*b*) Blood flow through left side of heart. Right side of heart removed.

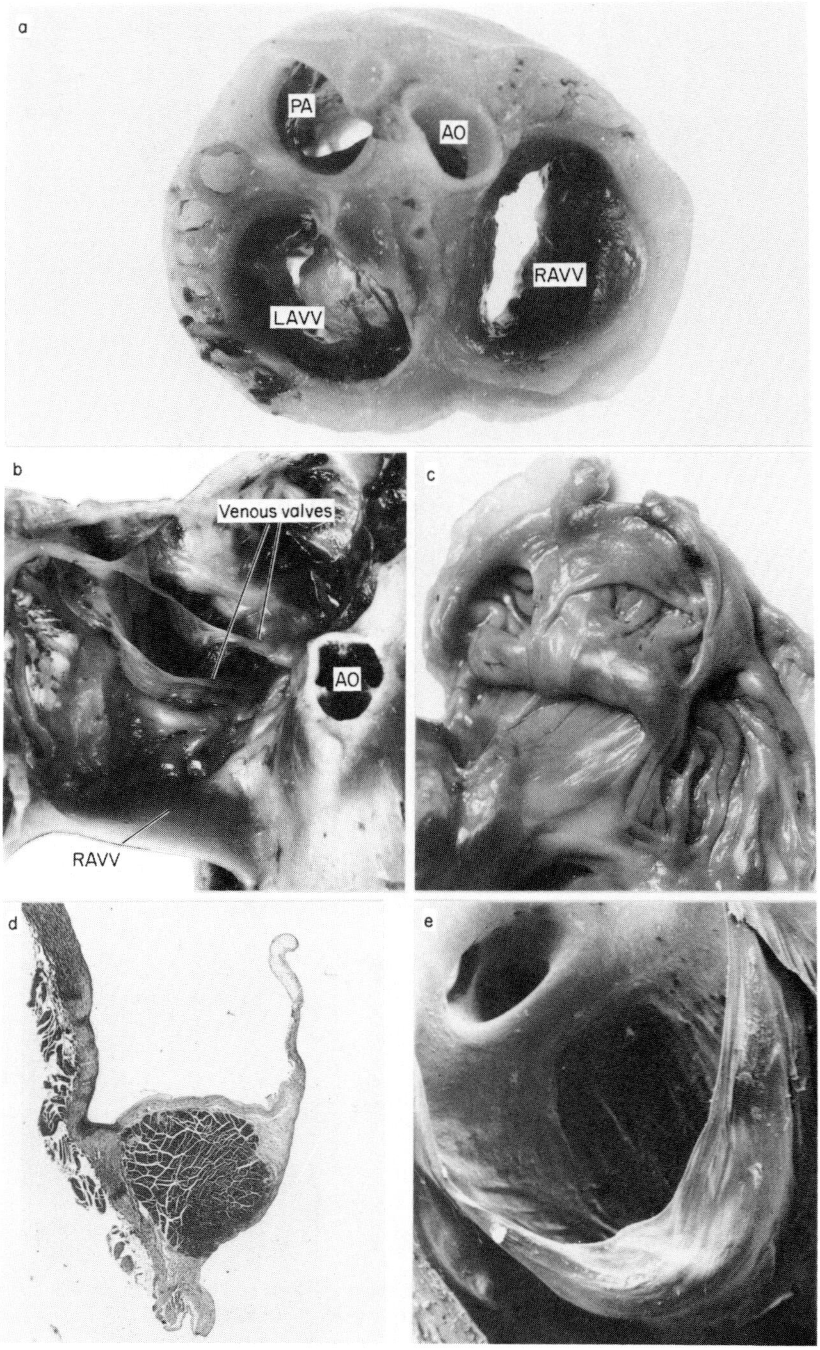
a
PA
AO
RAVV
LAVV
b
Venous valves
AO
RAVV
c
d
e

these cavities, the lateral part of the muscular right atrioventricular valve and the conus arteriosus (outflow tract of right ventricle). The right deep coronary artery runs largely in the interventricular septum, supplying it, the apex of the heart (left ventricle) as well as part of the right ventricle, the more medial part of the right atrioventricular valve and parts of both atria.

The left superficial coronary artery (left circumflex) lies in the fat-filled groove between the left atrium and ventricle. An interatrial branch supplies both atria, whilst the parent vessel sends branches to left atrium and ventricle. The left deep coronary artery supplies the left ventricular wall and the interventricular septum. There is also a small contribution to the right ventricle.

There are said to be significant anastomoses between superficial and deep branches of the same coronary artery and also between branches of different coronary arteries (Lindsay and Smith, 1965). If this is so, then there must be a reasonable collateral supply to the bird's heart, which is in marked contrast to the human, where there is virtually none, and the dog where it is very small.

Four major veins return venous blood from the myocardium to the right atrium. The dorsal cardiac vein is the largest, and provides the principal drainage for the left ventricle, although it also receives branches from adjacent parts of the right ventricle and from the interventricular septum. Its proximal part runs in the dorsal longitudinal groove and it joins the right atrium at a point slightly ventral to and to the right of the opening of the left superior vena cava. The left cardiac vein is the second largest. It drains part of the interventricular septum, parts of both ventricles and parts of both atria before joining the right atrium close to the left superior vena cava.

The left circumflex vein runs in the left coronary groove, parallels the left superficial coronary artery (left circumflex) and drains part of the left ventricle and atrium. It opens into the right atrium slightly ventral to and to the left of the left superior vena cava. On the ventral (anterior) aspect of the heart several small veins provide the main drainage for the right ventricle. Some of them also receive blood from the left ventricle, the interventricular septum and the right atrioventricular valve. They remain largely independent, take the place of a right circumflex vein, and join the right atrium as a group of three or four separate vessels.

Anastomoses between tributaries of the four major veins are common, but as

Fig. 6. (*a*) Section through heart just above the cardiac skeleton. AO, aorta; PA, pulmonary artery; LAVV, left atrioventricular valve; RAVV, right atrioventricular valve. (*b*) Shows venous valves attached to roof of right atrium. (*c*) A large muscular bar runs across the roof of both atria and divides into smaller bars to strengthen the atrial walls. The interatrial septum is attached to the ventral surface of the main muscular bar at about its mid point. (*d*) Section through one cusp of aortic valve. (*e*) A scanning electronmicrograph of cusp of aortic valve, aortic sinus (behind cusp) and entry to coronary artery.

the major vessels usually make independent junctions with the right atrium a coronary sinus, in the mammalian sense, is said not to exist (McKibben and Christensen, 1964; Lindsay, 1967).

In mammals, additional routes for the return of venous blood from the myocardium are well established. They include arteriosinusoidal, arterioluminal and Thebesian veins. These are all small communications from the inner part of the myocardium direct to the lumen of each chamber of the heart. It is not known (in the mammal or bird) exactly what proportion of the total drainage they provide, but it is likely to be small. In the domestic fowl, both Thebesian (Uchiyama, 1929) and luminal veins (Lindsay, 1967) have been described.

Blood flow through the coronary circulation is entirely dependent on left ventricular systole, but can only take place through the left ventricular myocardium during ventricular diastole. During systole the intramural pressure of the left ventricle is such as to prevent any flow into the left coronary artery, and to squeeze all the blood out of those coronary veins which drain the left ventricular wall and interventricular septum.

As blood is ejected from the left ventricle past the cusps of the aortic valve and into the aorta, eddy currents hold these cusps away from the wall of the aortic sinus. The first part of the elastic aorta expands to receive the bolus of blood. The aortic valve closes, probably simultaneously with the termination of systole, and the elastic recoil of the aorta forces blood in both directions. Most of it passes peripherally along the aorta, but some passes back towards the closed aortic valve and aortic sinus and as a result enters the coronary arteries. Between 5 and 10% of the total left ventricular output enters these arteries and as the heart only represents about 1% of total body weight its metabolic activity must be high.

Control of coronary blood flow is complicated, and poorly understood. Sympathetic stimulation of the heart increases myocardial activity and hence the concentration of metabolites. These cause relaxation of arteriolar smooth muscle and so increase coronary blood flow. Post ganglionic sympathetic noradrenergic neurones are distributed to all coronary blood vessels, except the capillaries (Akester *et al.*, 1969), but the balance of α (constrictor) and β (dilator) receptors on the vascular smooth muscle, which responds to the noradrenaline, is not known.

VI. Architecture of Ventricular Myocardium

A continuous, though fluctuating, stream of venous blood enters the atria at the top of the heart. It is sucked, or pushed down into the ventricles, turned round and pumped back up again, to leave by apertures very close to those by which it entered. For this sequence of events to continue throughout the life of the animal, a complicated organization of the musculature is likely to be required. Exactly what that organization is has been the subject of uncertainty for centuries. A useful summary of this work for the bird has been provided by Shaner (1923) and for the mammal by Brecher and Galletti (1963).

The fact that text-books, both for birds and mammals still use illustrations copied from descriptive work carried out by Mall (1911) suggests that little progress has been made. The original work was based on a doubtful procedure by which the collagenous framework of the heart was softened and weakened by prolonged exposure to acid. On the assumption that the sheets of cardiac muscle which remained could be separated from each other, in a physiologically meaningful way, they were "unwrapped" and appeared to indicate an extremely complicated system of muscle sheets and bundles.

One should remember that cardiac muscle, however it may be organized, consist of individual myocytes about 60 to 100 μm long and 7 to 12 μm wide in birds. These cells are connected together end-to-end by intercalated discs and side-to-side by desmosomes. They are also surrounded in small groups, by thin layers of collagen fibres. Larger groups or sheets of muscle are surrounded by thicker layers of collagen, which eventually provides a continuous framework throughout the entire heart. This supports the muscle, gives it something to pull on and also provides access to all parts of the heart for blood vessels, nerves and lymphatics, whilst causing minimal disturbance to the cardiac muscle itself.

Using the technique of acid maceration Shaner (1923) claimed that there are superficial and deep layers of ventricular muscle in the bird which originate in the cardiac skeleton, follow a spiral course round each ventricle, create a vortex at the apex and finally attach once more to the cardiac skeleton. Individual sheets of muscle are said to surround each ventricle and so must contribute to the interventricular septum, whilst more superficial layers are wrapped round both ventricles together. Obviously these could not contribute to the interventricular septum. If ventricular contraction starts at the apex, the spiral distribution of the muscle may contribute to a "wringing" action on the ejected blood.

Whilst the unwrapping procedure mentioned above was dependent on the destruction of all fibrous septa between the muscle sheets, a completely different approach has been suggested by Rodbard (1976). He maintained that, because of the intimate relationship between the muscle and its surrounding collagen, an understanding of one would automatically provide an understanding of the other. By injecting resin into the heart wall he claimed that it spread by way of all the collagenous septa and so formed a cast of those septa. These casts appeared to show that the ventricular myocardium consisted of three distinct regions (sub-organs), each of which was subdivided into four compartments, separated from each other by thick layers of connective tissue (super-capsules). Functional integration between the compartments was said to be provided by the conducting system. The three sub-organs were associated with:

(i) A short inflow tract surrounding the two atrioventricular valves.
(ii) The main pump, comprising the free walls of each ventricle and the interventricular septum.
(iii) A short outflow tract associated with the roots of the aorta and pulmonary trunk.

It is probably wise to conclude that the exact architectural arrangement of muscle cells within the ventricular myocardium has still to be clarified.

VII. Cardiac Skeleton

This refers to all the collagenous connective tissue that is distributed throughout the heart, which the earlier anatomists (Shaner, 1923) tried to destroy in their efforts to unravel the layers of muscle and which Rodbard (1976) tried to cast in resin so as to demonstrate the muscular architecture. Some of it supports the cusps of the four valves, whilst the rest is distributed widely throughout the myocardium to support the contractile cells and to provide routes of access for coronary blood vessels, nerves, lymphatics and the larger bundles of conducting cells. Frequently the term "cardiac skeleton" is restricted to the collagen which supports the valves, but the present author thinks it is better to use the term in a wider sense.

A large concentration of collagen forms a complicated support for the cusps of the aortic, pulmonary arterial and left atrioventricular valves, as well as for their inflow and outflow channels. A detailed study of this valvular support has never been published for any bird, but it is clear that it must be particularly well developed around the aortic valve. Here collagen fibres of the "skeleton" are probably continuous and interwoven with other collagen fibres within the cusps themselves, so that they can withstand the force of left ventricular systole tending to push them one way, and the force of aortic recoil tending to push them in the opposite direction.

Similarly, with the left atrioventricular valve there is a continuity of interlocking collagen bundles spreading from the annulus, which surrounds the aperture, into the substance of the valve leaflets, through them into the chordae tendinae and finally a link will be established with the collagen bundles which surround the muscle cells of the small papillary muscles to which the chordae tendinae are attached.

The muscular right atrioventricular valve, which is formed by an infolding of part of the right atrial and ventricular free walls, has a layer of collagen between the two layers of muscle, each of which is penetrated by supporting collagenous septa. The irregular sheet of collagen which supports the valve apertures and their cusps also ensures a complete muscular discontinuity between the atrial muscle and that of the ventricles. The only functional link between the two muscular regions is provided by the specialized conducting system. In addition to its widespread distribution throughout the entire heart, there will be continuity around the bases of the great vessels where collagen of the myocardium becomes confluent with collagen in the adventitia of these vessels.

Fat is deposited in association with various parts of the cardiac skeleton, its distribution varying with age, size and metabolism. There is usually a prominent pad of sub-epicardial fat, around the origins of the aorta and pulmonary trunk. This is extended round the coronary grooves between the atria and ventricles and also down the interventricular groove. There is an isolated patch of fat at the apex.

VIII. Ultrastructure of Cardiac Muscle

A. Myocyte

Myocytes are the contractile muscle cells of the heart (Fig. 7). They are arranged in bundles, or sheets, and are supported by collagen fibres, although their precise orientation and organization throughout the heart is uncertain. However, some are branched and they are all connected together into a three-dimensional mesh. It was once believed that they formed a true syncytium, but electron microscopy clearly demonstrated that they were discrete cells in contact with one another, although they were still separated by a thin layer of basement membrane (glycoprotein) and a very small amount of extracellular space.

"Contact" occurs at a number of different types of localized specializations on the cell membrane. It has been demonstrated that, at one type of membrane specialization (nexus), there are likely to be small cytoplasmic channels providing actual protoplasmic continuity from one cell to the next, so that the old idea of a syncytium may have returned in a more subtle way.

There are few reports on the length of avian myocytes. By disaggregating chicken cardiac muscle in hyaluronidase, Scott (1971a) found them to be about 60 μm long. Mammalian myocytes are usually said to be about 100 μm long. The diameter of avian cardiac muscle cells varies from 2 to 11·5 μm. The difficulty here is that different people, using different fixatives, have used different parts of the heart taken from different species. A diameter of 5 to 10 μm might be a reasonable range to have in mind. This suggests that avian myocytes, for the most part, are about half the size of those in mammals,

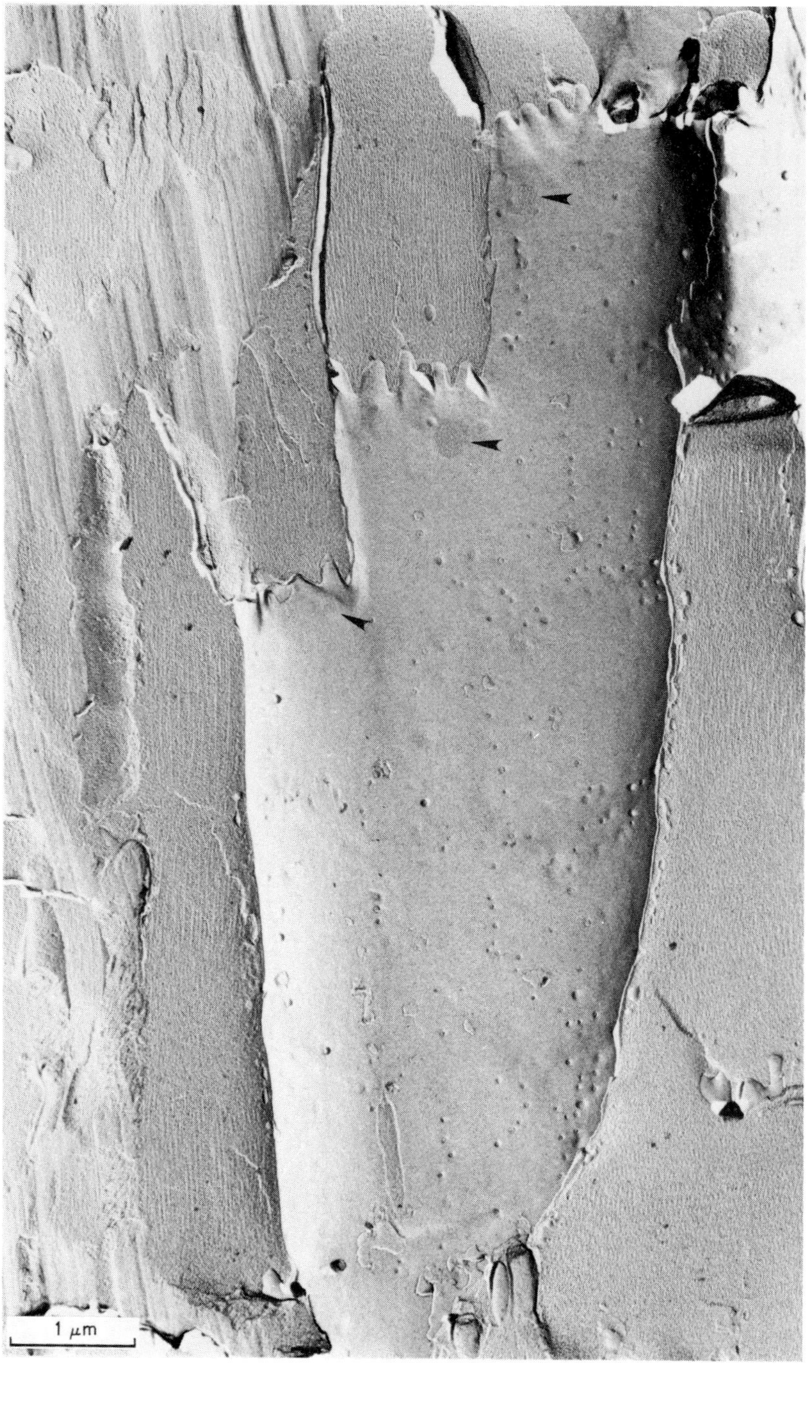
1 μm

although there is at least a strong possibility that the largest avian myocyte (12 μm?) is larger than the smallest to be found in mammals.

It is easy to distinguish between contractile cardiac muscle and non-muscle cells in the myocardium, using stained sections cut from dead and fixed material, in the electron microscope. However, it is sometimes difficult to distinguish between transitional cells (see Section X) and contractile cells. When it comes to distinguishing between cardiac muscle and non-muscle cells, which are alive in tissue culture, on pure morphological grounds, Marvin *et al.* (1979) have pointed out that it is impossible. It can only be done by using functional criteria, although Massons's trichrome stain appears to correlate well with them. Spontaneous contractions will obviously distinguish muscle from non-muscle, but non-contracting muscle can only be distinguished from non-muscle by recording its membrane potential or by its responsiveness to noradrenaline. In the latter case, contracting muscle contracts more rapidly, non-contracting muscle starts to contract whilst non-muscle will not respond at all.

B. Sarcolemma

Each cell is surrounded by a membrane or sarcolemma which forms a protective and selective barrier between the contents of the cell and the extracellular fluid. The sarcolemma carries receptors to neurotransmitters which respond to nervous activity and it is also important in triggering the onset of a contraction. The membrane is thought to consist of a double layer of oriented lipid molecules, with their fat-soluble (hydrophobic) ends directed towards one another at the centre of the membrane. Scattered throughout this double layer are large protein molecules, many of which are enzymes. They are free to move laterally within the membrane, forming what has been called a "fluid mosaic" (Singer and Nicolson, 1972). There is a resting potential across the membrane of −90 mV, with the inside negative to the outside. This is largely due to the high concentration of Na^+ associated with the outside of the membrane. Several specialized regions can be recognized on the sarcolemma which play a vital part in the normal activity of the cell. Differences in the enzyme activity of the sarcolemma isolated from the myocardium of newly hatched chicks, and from others 9 to 10 days old, suggests that some functional change may occur during early life (Hosey, 1980).

Fig. 7. Terminal part of a cardiac myocyte. Three transverse steps of an intercalated disc can be seen. There is a nexus on the flat cell membrane (arrows) just before each folded transverse step.

C. Intercalated Disc

This refers to the complicated interdigitation of terminal processes which takes place at the ends of each cell and by which one cell is "attached" to the next (Figs 7, 8). The sarcolemma terminates in such a way that localized parts of it are thrown into groups of transversely-oriented, finger-like folds. These folded regions occur at different levels and are connected together by flat, unfolded longitudinal parts of the membrane. In longitudinal section, under the electron microscope, an intercalated disc is seen as a series of steps across the width of two contiguous cells. The localized folded regions of one cell membrane interdigitate with similar regions from the next. An intercalated disc includes both the transverse folded parts of the two interlocking membranes and the flat longitudinal parts that connect them together.

There may be about six of these transverse folded regions in a single intercalated disc. It is unusual to see more than parts of two or three of them in a single longitudinal electron micrograph, but complete folded zones can be seen by freeze-fracturing across the long axis of the fibre (Akester, 1981). As a result of this, the fracture (cleavage) passes through the centre of one of the interlocking cell membranes so that the resultant surface replica is sometimes difficult to interpret but the number, position and size of the processes is obvious. In the domestic fowl, between 15 and 20 processes are grouped in an area about 3 μm long by 1 μm wide (Fig. 8a). The larger processes are usually about 0·5 μm long and are arranged in one or two rows with smaller processes on either side. The larger ones frequently branch into two near their tips. Folded zones are joined together by 3 to 4 μm of unfolded, longitudinal cell membrane. If a single myocyte has six folded zones on the terminal part of its membrane, it may associate four of them with similar zones on a second cell and the remaining two with a third cell. This will help to spread the contractile response widely and quickly through the "functional syncytium" of the myocardium.

D. Cell Membrane Specializations

Several localized regions of cell membrane are specialized for a particular role

---

Fig. 8. (*a*) Group of processes forming transverse part of intercalated disc (freeze-fractured replica, transverse fracture). (*b*) Group of processes similar to (*a*) seen in stained section. (*c*) Processes on transverse part of intercalated disc (freeze-fractured replica, longitudinal fracture). Note circular nexus (arrow) close to base of processes. (*d*) Processes similar to (*c*) seen in stained section. (*e*) Detail of nexus in (*c*). (*f*) Interlocking processes from contiguous cells form transverse part of intercalated disc. There are two nexuses (arrows). (After Akester, 1981, with permission).

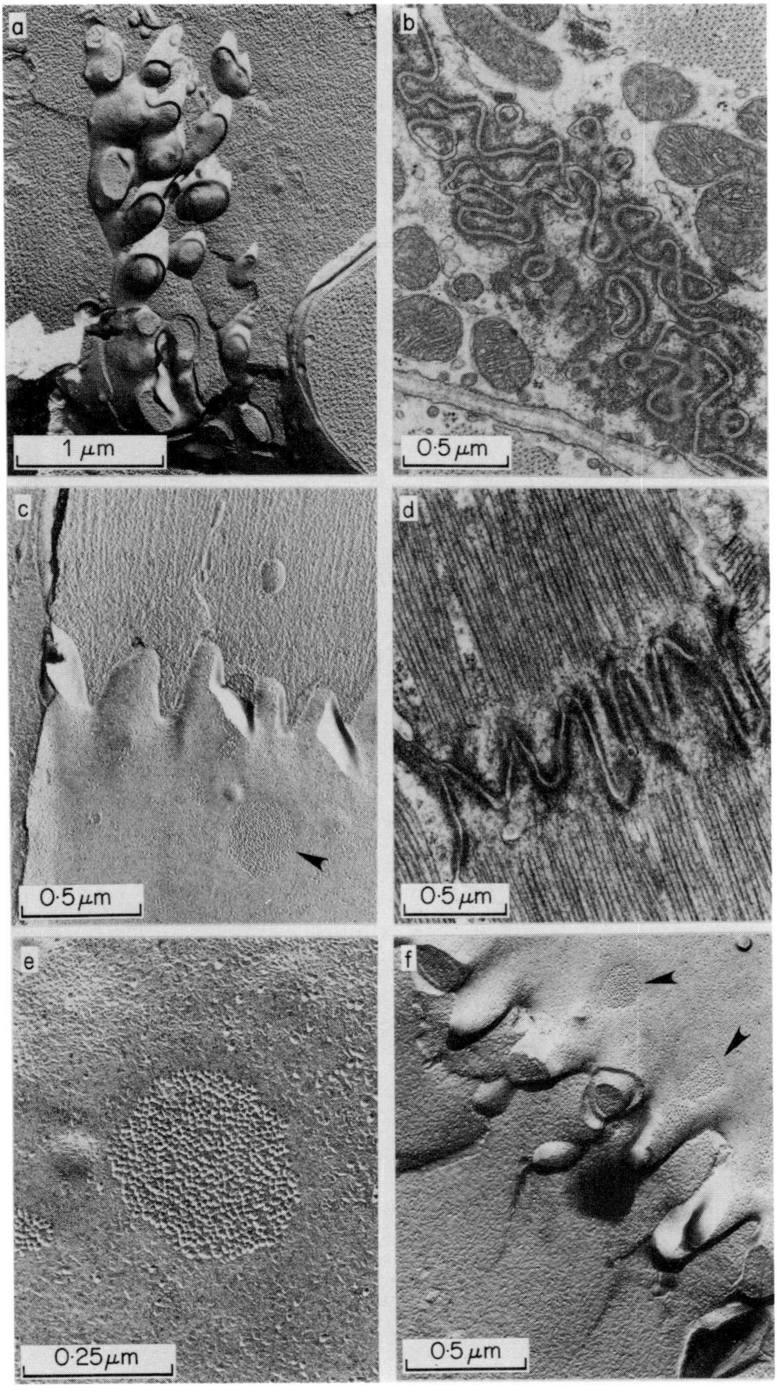
a
1 μm
b
0·5 μm
c
0·5 μm
d
0·5 μm
e
0·25 μm
f
0·5 μm

in the overall activity of the cell. Some of them are only found at intercalated discs, whilst others may be found on any part of the membrane, including the intercalated disc.

1. Macula Adherens (Desmosome)

These are very common, may occur at any place on the membrane, and consist of small plaques of membrane thickening which develop opposite one another on adjacent cells. They have been likened to "spot welds" and are concerned with holding cells together. In the domestic fowl, they are usually about 0·3 μm long (on a conventional 2-dimensional electron micrograph), but ones up to 5 μm have been seen (Akester, 1981). The small ones are probably circular or elliptical plaques whilst the long ones are more likely to be ribbon-shaped.

2. Fascia Adherens (Myofibrillar Insertion Plaque)

These are only found on the part of the cell membrane which forms the transverse, folded zones of an intercalated disc. They appear as elongated patches of increased electron density to which the actin myofilaments attach. In normal cardiac muscle cells, sarcomeres are always complete and stretch from one Z-disc to the next along the length of the myofibril. At the end of the cell, the cell membrane takes the place of a Z-disc.

It is important for the actin filaments to be strongly attached to the sarcolemma at an intercalated disc, and also to a Z-disc. They always attach at an acute angle to the folded cell membrane, but at right angles to the Z-disc. At both sites there may be some interlocking of the actin filaments to provide a solid base for contraction. Some information about how the actin filaments may be joined to the sarcolemma at the intercalated disc and to the Z-disc in the chicken myocardium has been presented by Tokuyasu *et al.* (1981). They attached recognizably different electron-dense labels (ferritin and iron dextran) to α-actinin and vinculin respectively, in very thin frozen sections of ultrastructurally intact chicken myocardium. They demonstrated that both these proteins were present at the fascia adherentes of intercalated discs but that only α-actinin was present in the Z-discs. As the iron dextran (marking vinculin) was found to be closer to the membrane than ferritin (marking α-actinin) at the intercalated disc, they suggested that the protein vinculin was directly involved in attaching actin filaments to the sarcolemma at the fascia adherens of the intercalated disc.

It is interesting that smooth muscle cells from the gizzard contain both α-actinin and vinculin in the dense plaques on the cell membrane, but only α-actinin in the dense bodies of the cytoplasm. This indicated that the fascia adherens on the intercalated disc of the cardiac myocyte and the dense plaque on the membrane of the smooth muscle cell had some structural similarities, as did the Z-disc of the cardiac myocyte and the dense body of the smooth muscle cell. However, it also made clear that the two membrane structures (containing vinculin) did not have the same structure as the two cytoplasmic structures (Z-disc and dense body) which did not contain vinculin. Neither of these proteins was found to be associated with desmosomes in the chicken myocardium.

3. Nexus (Gap Junction)

The most complicated and controversial of the various membrane specializations at the present time is the nexus. It consists of a group of particles (each about 8 nm in diameter) on the membrane of one cell apposed to a similar group on the membrane of an adjacent cell (Figs 7, 8c,e,f). The number of particles in a nexus and its overall size varies considerably. A detailed analysis of the nexus has been published (Loewenstein, 1981), but very little work has been done on birds.

There is widespread agreement that nexuses provide the site for low-resistance electrical conductivity between cardiac myocytes, but the evidence is not totally convincing. They are numerous and large (1 to 3 μm^2) in mammals, whereas, in birds, they are small and few (Scott, 1971b; Akester, 1981). In ventricular muscle of the dog, Spira (1971) has calculated that up to 40% of the intercalated disc may be occupied by nexuses. No such calculation has been made for any bird, but it is certain that the value will be very much smaller.

The particles of a nexus appear to be arranged in pairs, with one protruding from each cell, and contacting each other across the narrow extracellular space. In terms of space travel, one particle could be said to "dock" with the other. Such a pair of particles has been called a "connexon" (Caspar *et al.*, 1977). Each particle may consist of a group of protein sub-units which can be arranged either to form an open, or a closed channel. When open, the channel in each particle would be in continuity with the internal cytoplasm of its own cell. If the channel in each of a pair of apposed membrane particles were open, then a through channel would exist joining the two cells together. There could be one channel for each connexon.

A wide range of substances (dyes, amino acids, peptides, sugars) up to a size of 2000 Daltons have been injected into one cell and detected inside the next, without any leakage into the extracellular space. These experiments provide strong evidence for the existence of cell-to-cell cytoplasmic continuity, and suggest that the channels have a diameter of about 1·6 nm. It is likely that each cell contributes half of each channel (through its own membrane particle) and thus retains control over the patency of its own half-channel. By closing its own half it would, of course, seal off the whole channel and this may be important in protecting a healthy cell from the breakdown chemicals of an injured or dying neighbour.

The cell-to-cell communication provided by connexons at a nexus is very widely distributed throughout the animal kingdom and may represent a fundamental type of homeostatic or communication system based on a common structure of protein sub-units. This could explain why it is possible for connexon channels to develop between cells from different organs and species. Functional channels have developed between hampster kidney and human skin cells (Michalke and Loewenstein, 1971) and also between avian and mammalian cells (Epstein and Gilula, 1977).

In the adult domestic fowl, small nexuses have been demonstrated on the transverse folded parts of the intercalated disc (Scott, 1971b) and on the longitudinal straight parts by freeze-fracture replication (Akester, 1981). In the latter situation they occur a short distance (0·5 μm) away from the base of the processes which form the folded zone (Figs 7, 8c,e,f).

It may be assumed that membrane particles are free to move in the "fluid mosaic" of each sarcolemma and that in some way they are attracted together into groups or clusters to form a nexus. However, there is no information as to how stable they are, whether they move about, or how frequently they may be replaced during the life of the cell.

Because avian nexuses are small, it is easy to count the particles. This has shown that the packing density varies from one nexus to another. In the domestic fowl packing densities ranging from 6078 to 9112 particles μm^{-2} have been reported, with nexus areas from 0·0069 μm^2 to 0·0872 μm^2. The largest nexus so far described in the heart of the domestic fowl contained 530 membrane particles (Fig. 8e) (Akester, 1981). If each carried a channel approximately 2 nm diameter, there would be a total area of cytoplasmic continuity of about 0·0017 μm^2.

In support of the claim that the nexus constitutes a low-resistance channel for ionic flow, is the finding that electrical coupling between cells persists after desmosome and fascia adherentes have been separated by a Ca^{2+}-free medium, but is lost when nexuses are disrupted by a hypertonic medium (Barr *et al.*, 1965). If these connexons are really so important, one might expect electrical conductivity between adjacent cells to be largely independent of the resistance of the extracellular fluid. Sperelakis (1979), however, found that increased extracellular resistance considerably increased the longitudinal resistance of cardiac muscle.

Nexuses are also considered to be responsible for electrotonic coupling between smooth muscle cells. In the rat uterus, there is evidence which suggests that this coupling is hormone-dependent. In castrated females, uterine smooth muscle became unexcitable and showed a lack of nexuses. With oestrogen treatment, both excitability (Melton and Saldivar, 1964) and the number of nexuses (Bergman, 1968) returned to normal. It would be of great interest to know if hormones have any influence over electrical conductivity and nexus morphology in cardiac muscle. A theoretical possibility might be that noradrenaline (or some other hormone) could stimulate nexus development at an intercalated disc and so increase its conductivity. However, before this possibility could seriously be considered it would be necessary to know how rapidly nexuses can form or be expanded. Some information on this subject, for mammalian cardiac muscle in tissue culture, has been provided by Rush and Fambrough (1973) which suggests that they may develop in a few minutes. Presumably this would be too slow for a noradrenaline-induced response in the heart.

4. *Surface Vesicles*

These are numerous and are scattered, in an irregular fashion, over all parts of the sarcolemma except at the intercalated discs (Fig. 9a,b). Presumably, their role is to fill with extracellular fluid containing various nutrient molecules, some of which may be macromolecules, round off and then detach from the cell membrane (pinocytosis). They may then be moved around inside the cell to unite with other vesicles or with the sarcolemma on the other side of the cell.

Surface vesicles on cardiac myocytes in the domestic fowl have narrow necks (about 50 nm diameter) and expand to about 90 nm diameter in the surface layers of the cytoplasm. Their total depth from the sarcolemma is about 100 nm (Fig. 9a). In freeze-cleaved preparations, because of the splitting of the membrane (Branton *et al.*, 1975), many of the surface vesicles are broken at the neck but some seem to survive.

Surface vesicles develop from the cell membrane of many types of cell. Endothelial cells of blood capillaries have even greater numbers than cardiac muscle cells, which they closely resemble but their function may be different. Although there is no information on this subject in the bird, Essner *et al.* (1965) have shown, in the mammal, that myocyte surface vesicles have ATP-ase activity, whilst those on endothelial cells do not. In blood capillary endothelial cells surface vesicles are absent from a band of cell membrane either side of the line of contact between adjacent cells (Fig. 9c).

5. *Absence of T-tubules in Avian Cardiac Myocytes*

The lack of T-tubules is probably the most obvious difference between avian and mammalian cardiac myocytes and may be important in understanding the precise mechanism of excitation–contraction coupling in both mammals and birds. It is generally accepted that T-tubules, in mammalian cardiac myocytes, are essential for carrying the action potential from the sarcolemma,

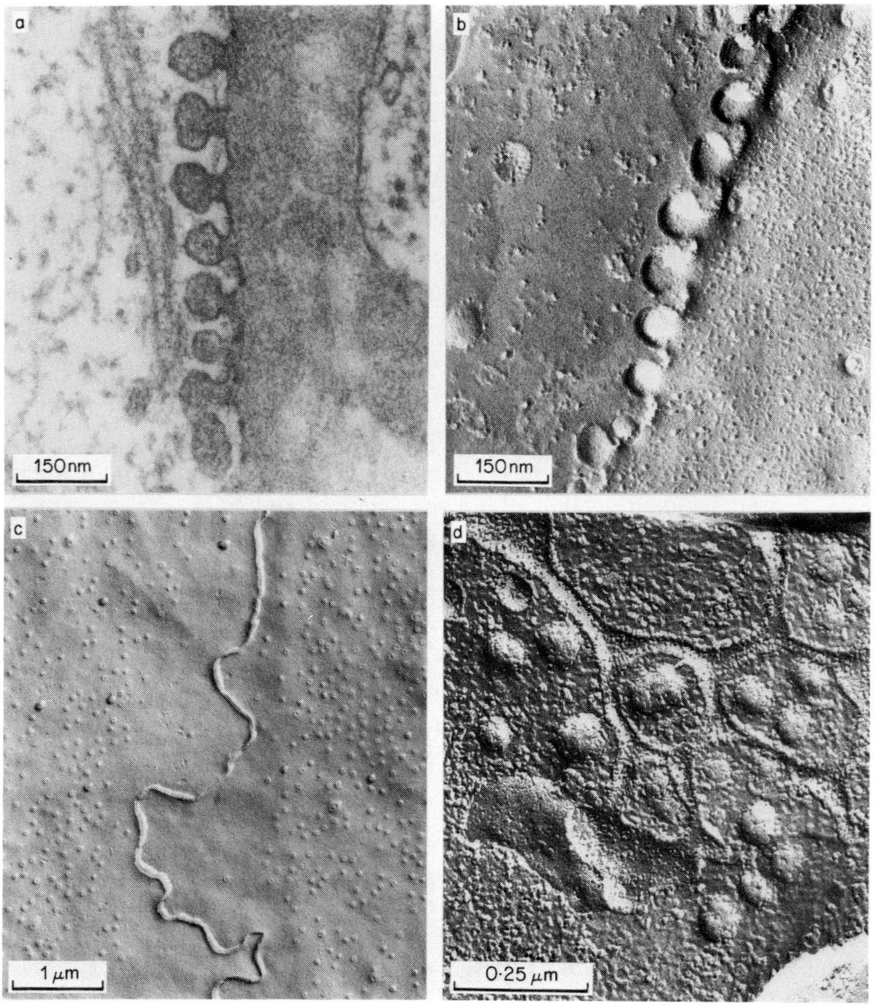

Fig. 9. (*a*) Surface vesicles on cardiac myocyte cell membrane. (*b*) Surface vesicles on cardiac myocyte (freeze-fractured replica). (*c*) Blood capillary endothelial cells. Note surface vesicle-free zone either side of cell junction. (Freeze-fractured replica). (*d*) Close association between sarcoplasmic reticulum and surface vesicles (freeze-fractured replica of cardiac myocyte from interventricular septum). (From Akester, 1981, with permission).

on the outside of the cell, into its depths in order to activate the Ca^{2+}-release mechanism in the sarcoplasmic reticulum. The mammalian cell is thought to be too big to do without this internal extension of the sarcolemma. The avian cardiac myocyte, in contrast, is presumed to be small enough not to require them. Unfortunately, this explanation is not wholly convincing. It has been suggested (Akester, 1981) that there is likely to be an overlap in the sizes of avian and mammalian myocytes, so that it is at least possible that the largest avian myocyte (without T-tubules) is larger than the smallest mammalian myocyte (with T-tubules).

As we have seen, the diameter of avian myocytes probably ranges from about 6 to 12 μm, whilst that of mammals is from about 12 to 25 μm, but all these figures are very small compared with the diameter of skeletal muscle fibres (100 μm). Perhaps we should be seeking an explanation for the presence of T-tubules in mammals, rather than one for their absence in birds.

Myocardial hypertrophy is a common response to hypertension. Again no information on the bird is available, but hypertrophic mammalian cardiac myocytes enlarge to a diameter of 200 μm (McNutt and Fawcett, 1974). It would obviously be of great interest to know if avian myocytes could hypertrophy to the same degree and if, with a hypertrophied diameter of about 100 μm, they could still function without developing T-tubules. In this context, it is interesting to note that Kelly and Chacko (1977) demonstrated the ability of avian cardiac myocytes in tissue culture to form tubular invaginations of the sarcolemma, which even developed internal coupling with the sarcoplasmic reticulum.

E. Myofilaments

Filaments of interlocking actin and myosin are organized into chains of sarcomeres which stretch from one end of the cell to the other (Fig. 10a,b). Although the mechanism of contraction has not been worked out on avian muscle, it is almost certain to be the same as in the mammal.

Actin filaments are attached to either side of the Z-discs and interdigitate with the thicker myosin filaments. In the absence of Ca^{2+}, two regulator proteins (troponin and tropomyosin) inhibit the actin–myosin reaction. In the presence of Ca^{2+}, the troponin sub-unit, troponin C, changes its form and as a result releases the inhibition, so that the actin–myosin reaction can take place and the sarcomere shortens. If this happens throughout the ventricle as a whole, we have systole.

The longitudinal alignment of the bundles of myofilaments, and the fact that they occupy most of the space inside the cell, imposes a similar alignment on many of the other organelles (Fig. 10b). This is demonstrated most markedly

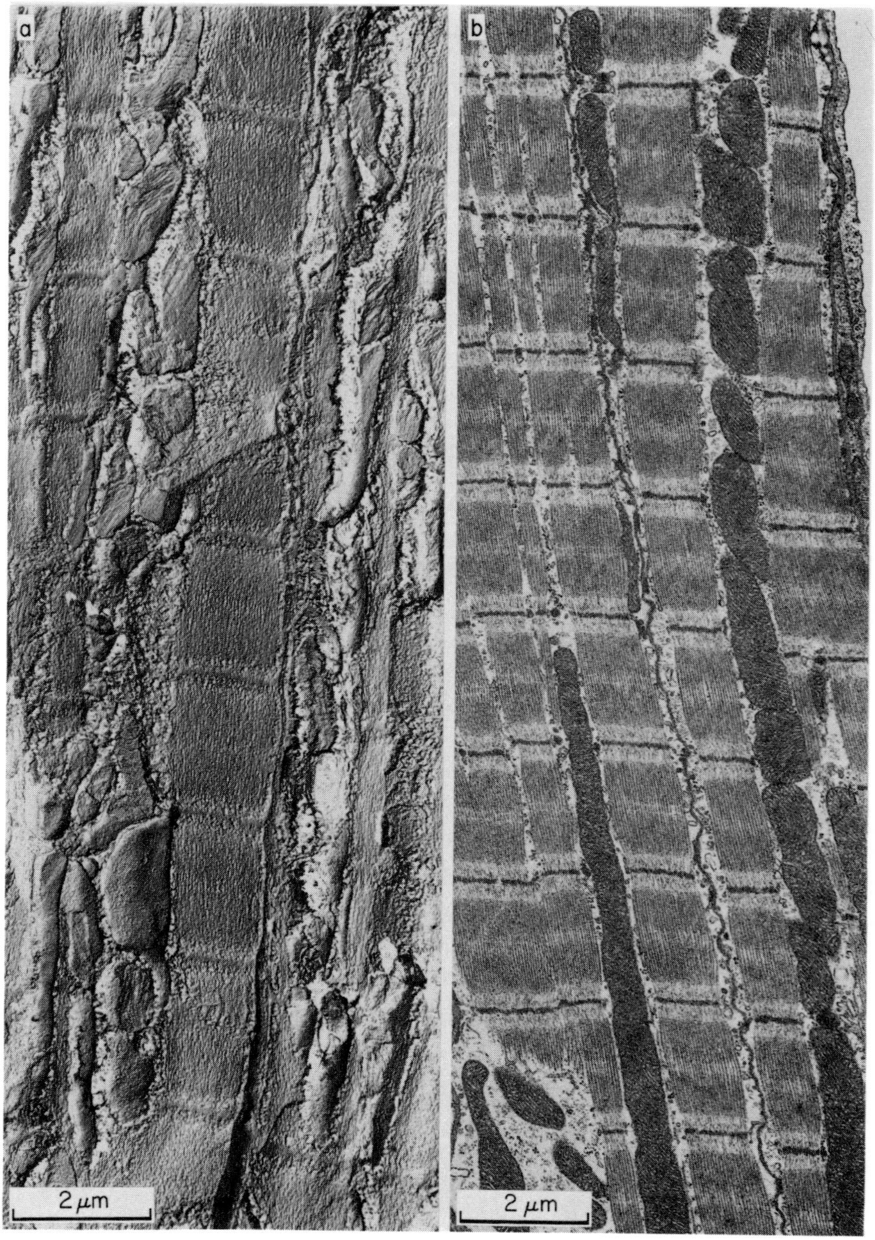

Fig. 10. Myofibrils in cardiac muscle cells by freeze-fractured replication (*a*) and by stained section (*b*).

by the mitochondria, which are present in many forms (Fig. 11). Myofilament bundles, or sarcomere chains are often called myofibrils, but it should be stressed that these collective structures, although they will all have the same length, need not have the same diameter. Similarly, each sarcomere will have the same length as all the others, but what that length will be will depend on its state of contraction or relaxation. In the domestic fowl, it is about 2 μm in the relaxed state.

Z-discs consist predominantly of protein, and will also vary in size according to the number of actin filaments in the bundles which insert into them. When a Z-disc lies immediately beneath the sarcolemma, one is attached to the other, so that in a contracted cell there may be a puckering of the cell membrane at the level of each Z-disc. Apart from stabilizing the cell membrane with respect to the underlying myofibrils, it is not easy to see what advantage this fusion has.

Suzuki *et al.* (1980) have demonstrated the inter-changeability of Z-disc protein and myofilaments between chicken and rabbit skeletal muscle, so that hybrid sarcomeres were formed and observed by electron microscopy. It seems likely that had heart muscle been used a similar result would have been obtained.

With constant rhythmic contraction and relaxation of the heart, some 300 times a minute throughout the life of a domestic fowl, there is likely to be considerable wear and tear on the contractile filaments. For this reason they are changed approximately every month.

F. Sarcoplasmic Reticulum

A delicate mesh of fine tubules surrounds each bundle of myofilaments. These meshes are interconnected so that the tubules are distributed throughout the entire cell. This system of tubules is the sarcoplasmic reticulum (Fig. 12). It is the equivalent in muscle of the smooth endoplasmic reticulum in other cells. In the domestic fowl the sarcoplasmic reticulum is extremely regular, with a tubular diameter of about 70 nm and an internal mesh diameter of about 200 nm (Akester, 1981). It probably spreads, as a continuous mesh, from one end of the cell to the other. It does not appear to have any localized dilatations (cisternae) or fenestrations in its wall, nor does it form any "diad" or "triad" relationships with non-existent T-tubules.

It is now well established that Ca^{2+} is essential for the regulator protein, troponin, to change its conformation and so remove the tropomyosin inhibition of the actin-myosin reaction, thus permitting contraction to occur. There are several sites from which this Ca^{2+} might come. The sarcolemma, basement membrane, sarcoplasmic reticulum and mitochondrial membranes have all been considered (Dhalla *et al.*, 1978). The sarcolemma may be the main site

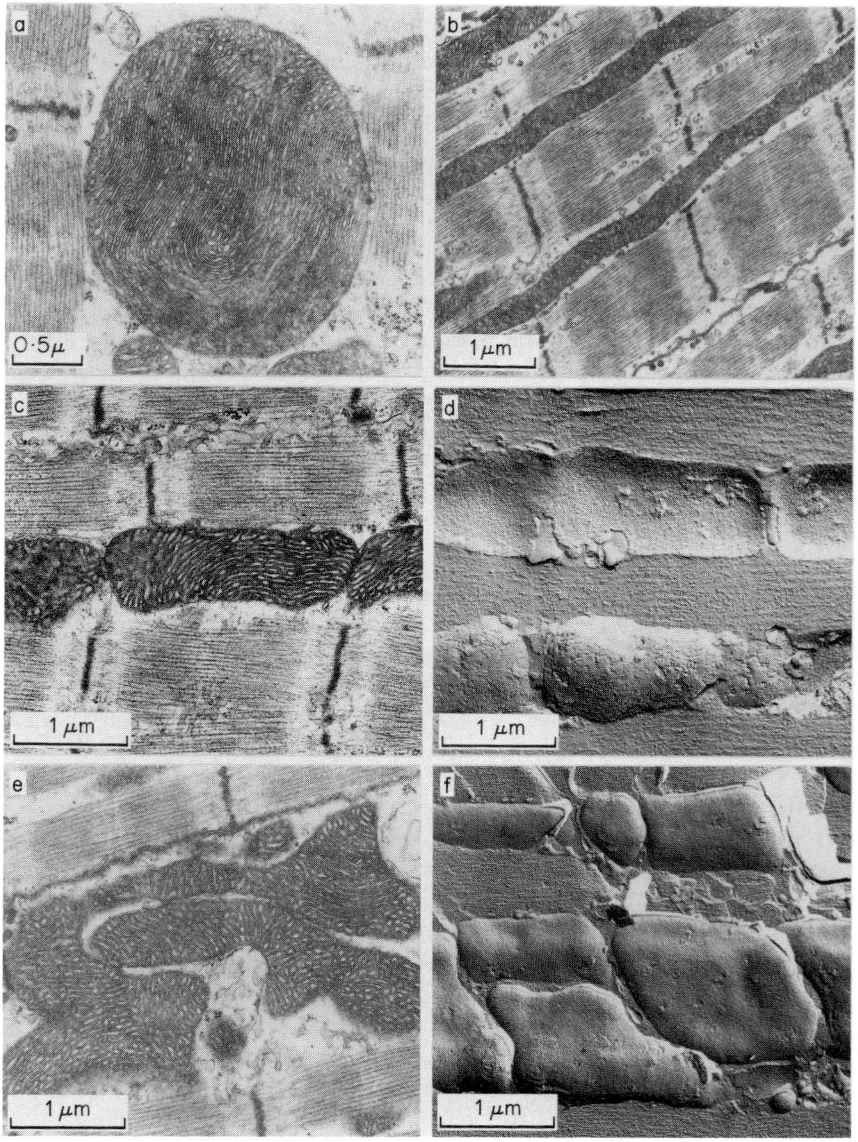

Fig. 11. The different sizes and shapes of mitochondria from cardiac muscle. (*a*) Appears to be spherical, diameter about 2 μm. (*b*) Mitochondrion about 8 μm long and 0·5 μm wide. (*c*) Mitochondrion about 2 μm long and 0·56 μm wide. (*d*) Freeze-fractured replica. (*e*) Branched mitochondria. (*f*) Freeze-fractured replica.

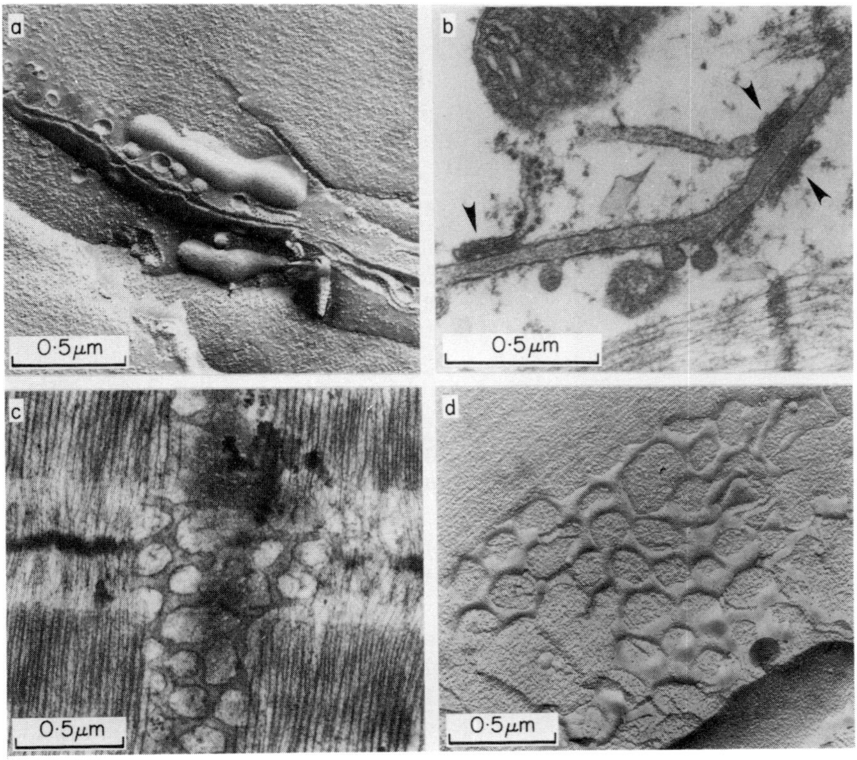

Fig. 12. (*a*) Part of sarcoplasmic reticulum immediately deep to surface vesicles in cardiac myocyte (freeze-fractured replica). (*b*) Peripheral couplings between sarcoplasmic reticulum and cell membrane form junctional complexes. Three are illustrated (arrows). (*c*) The sarcoplasmic reticulum appears to form a continuous mesh around the myofibrils and does not form dilatations or cysternae at the level of the Z-band. (*d*) Sarcoplasmic reticulum beside myofilaments in cardiac myocyte (freeze-fractured replica). (From Akester, 1981 with permission).

and the arrival of an action potential may increase its permeability to Ca^{2+}. A further possibility is that Ca^{2+} released from the sarcolemma may then stimulate Ca^{2+} release from the sarcoplasmic reticulum (Fabiata and Fabiata, 1975; Reuter, 1979; Loewenstein, 1981), but there is no information on this subject in the bird.

Relaxation follows contraction, with supreme regularity in the heart, and for this to occur the Ca^{2+}, which has flooded around the myofilaments during contraction, must be removed quickly. It is likely that the sarcoplasmic reticulum is the main site for Ca^{2+} uptake as well as being an important site for its release. A Ca^{2+}-binding protein, calsequestrin, has been identified in the sarcoplasmic reticulum (MacLennan and Wong, 1971). Ca^{2+}-ATP-ase (calcium pump protein) activity is associated with the sarcolemma and with the membrane of the sarcoplasmic reticulum. Both release and uptake of Ca^{2+} are likely to be energy-dependent processes. In fact, it has been estimated that the energy requirement for cardiac relaxation (diastole) in the mammal may consume about 15% of the total energy output of the heart (Langer, 1974).

Although there is a basic similarity in the mechanism of Ca^{2+} binding by the sarcoplasmic reticulum in both cardiac and skeletal muscle, the calcium pump protein (Ca^{2+}-ATP-ase) responsible for moving calcium into the sarcoplasmic reticulum is chemically different in the two sites. DeFoor *et al.* (1980) examined the calcium pump protein, from skeletal and cardiac muscle sarcoplasmic reticulum of several different species and found that there were greater differences between the calcium pump protein from the sarcoplasmic reticulum of cardiac muscle and that from skeletal muscle in the same species, than there were between the protein from the sarcoplasmic reticulum of cardiac muscle in one species and the same protein from the same site in another species. Thus, pigeon cardiac sarcoplasmic reticulum is antigenically closer to rabbit sarcoplasmic reticulum than to its own skeletal sarcoplasmic reticulum.

During systole, the force of contraction depends both on the concentration of Ca^{2+} which develops around the myofilaments and on the length of the sarcomere. The Ca^{2+} concentration will determine how many actin filaments are released from their tropomyosin inhibition and the sarcomere length will determine the extent of actin–myosin overlap, and thus the number of reactive sites that will be accessible to myosin crossbridges. The optimal length for sarcomere contraction is probably a little over 2 μm. If the sarcoplasmic reticulum is mainly concerned with Ca^{2+} uptake and if its release occurs mainly from or through the sarcolemma, then there must be some mechanism by which sequestered Ca^{2+} in the sarcoplasmic reticulum can be voided periodically from the cell. Occasional fusion of the sarcoplasmic reticulum with the sarcolemma has been suggested (Sommer and Johnson, 1970), but whilst there is no evidence for this, a close relationship between the subsarcolemmal sarcoplasmic reticulum and individual surface vesicles or even groups of these vesicles has been found (Akester, 1981) (Fig. 9d).

In mammals, an even closer relationship (coupling) develops between the sarcoplasmic reticulum and the sarcolemma at the surface of the cell (peripheral or external coupling) and also between the sarcoplasmic reticulum and the T-tubular extensions of the sarcolemma deep inside the cell (internal couplings). In birds, without T-tubules, there can only be peripheral couplings and it is possible that they are relatively more numerous than in mammals.

In the domestic fowl, that part of the sarcoplasmic reticulum which lies immediately beneath the sarcolemma approaches it at intervals, runs parallel for a short distance (about 0·25 μm) and then separates from it. Where the sarcoplasmic reticulum and sarcolemma are closely associated a junctional complex is formed. These are the sites where excitation–contraction coupling takes place. At these sites, the sarcoplasmic reticulum develops electron-dense granules in its lumen and electron-dense processes which appear to link it with the sarcolemma. It is not clear exactly what role these junctional granules and processes play in excitation–contraction coupling, but they are not normally found in other parts of the sarcoplasmic reticulum (Fig. 12b).

The only exception, to be reported in birds, is by Jewett *et al.* (1971, 1973) who have described, in the finch and hummingbird, a so-called "extended junctional sarcoplasmic reticulum", in which all the features of a junctional complex are present except for the sarcolemma. If the purpose of a junctional complex is to couple the sarcolemma to the sarcoplasmic reticulum, then it is hard to see what advantage this "extended junctional sarcoplasmic reticulum" can provide when it is remote from the sarcolemma.

Peripheral couplings are widespread over the sarcolemma in the domestic fowl and have been observed opposite one another in adjacent cells (Fig. 12b). Whether this is a device by which contraction in neighbouring cells can be synchronized, is not known. Various other modifications of the uniform mesh of sarcoplasmic reticulum that is found in the fowl, have been reported for different avian species. Cisternae have been described in the pigeon at the level of the Z- and H-discs (Saetersdal and Myklebust, 1975; Myklebust *et al.*, 1980) and fenestrations are said to occur in the chicken (Sommer and Waugh, 1976), although this was not confirmed by Akester (1981) and appears to be contradicted by Fig. 12c. In spite of these inter-species differences in the form taken by the sarcoplasmic reticulum, it is reasonable to assume that its role in the cardiac myocytes of all species is much the same.

IX. Impulse Generating and Conducting System

It is widely accepted that the general arrangement of sinoatrial and atrioventricular nodes, the atrioventricular bundle with its right and left bundle branches and their terminal ramifications throughout the myocardium in birds, broadly resembles the counterpart system in mammals. There is no doubt that there is a well developed interventricular bundle (Vassel-Adams, 1978). Conducting cells can be recognized in the connective tissue septa of the myocardium, being distributed with branches of the coronary arteries. In many parts of the heart, groups of conducting cells can be found immediately deep to the endocardium.

There have been many descriptions of the sinoatrial and atrioventricular nodes and even a third node (truncobulbar), but none has been carried out with the electron microscope. Photomicrographs of histological sections may convince their authors, but readers may be more sceptical. Nevertheless, parts of the impulse generating and conducting system have been convincingly "sighted" in many parts of the hearts of several different avian species (Fig. 13a,c). The problem is to fit them together into a convincing and cohesive whole, and unfortunately this has still to be done.

Virtually any sample of myocardium, when studied under the electron microscope, will show a few conducting cells scattered amongst the contractile cells (Akester, 1971; Akester and Akester, 1971a). The problem lies in demonstrating how these conducting cells are distributed. R. Mathur and Shrivastava (1979) believe they form continuous tracts which follow precise routes from sinoatrial to atrioventricular node, whilst Kim and Yasuda (1979) do not (both studies were based on the domestic fowl). Again, it is not known whether ramifications of the interventricular bundle are continuously distributed to groups of contractile cells, or whether these tracts become discontinuous as they approach the cells they are going to influence, so that they function like small "booster stations" scattered amongst the contractile cell.

Presumably there is a precise order of muscular contraction within the myocardium, possibly starting at the apex with successive groups of cells contracting sequentially upwards towards the outflow tract and inwards from the outer layers of the myocardium towards the sub-endocardial layer. This suggests that the muscle cells which will contract first are furthest away from the nodal source of their excitation. For this to happen there might be a greater frequency of conducting cells scattered amongst the contractile cells leading to these more distal parts of the myocardium. Alternatively the conducting cells might form continuous chains, though they have yet to be adequately demonstrated.

A possible development in this respect may lie in the discovery that conducting cells contain a greater concentration of the intermediate-sized filament protein, skeletin, than do contractile cells (Eriksson *et al.*, 1979). By treating frozen sections of myocardium with a fluorescent skeletin antiserum, conducting cells were shown to fluoresce with greater brightness than contractile cells. Several species were tested, including the domestic fowl. In addition to demon-

---

Fig. 13. (*a*) Conducting cell (light) amongst contractile muscle cells. Mitochondria are packed in rows between the bundles of myofilaments in the contractile cells, but are scattered at random in the conducting cell. (*b*) Transitional cell. Left hand side contains myofilaments organised as in a contractile cell. Right hand side is indistinguishable from the conducting cells in (*a*). (*c*) Transverse section through conducting cell. (*d*) Bundle of nerve fibres embedded in Schwann cell cytoplasm. The fibre packed with mitochondria may be sensory. The smallest fibre is only about 0·3 μm in diameter.

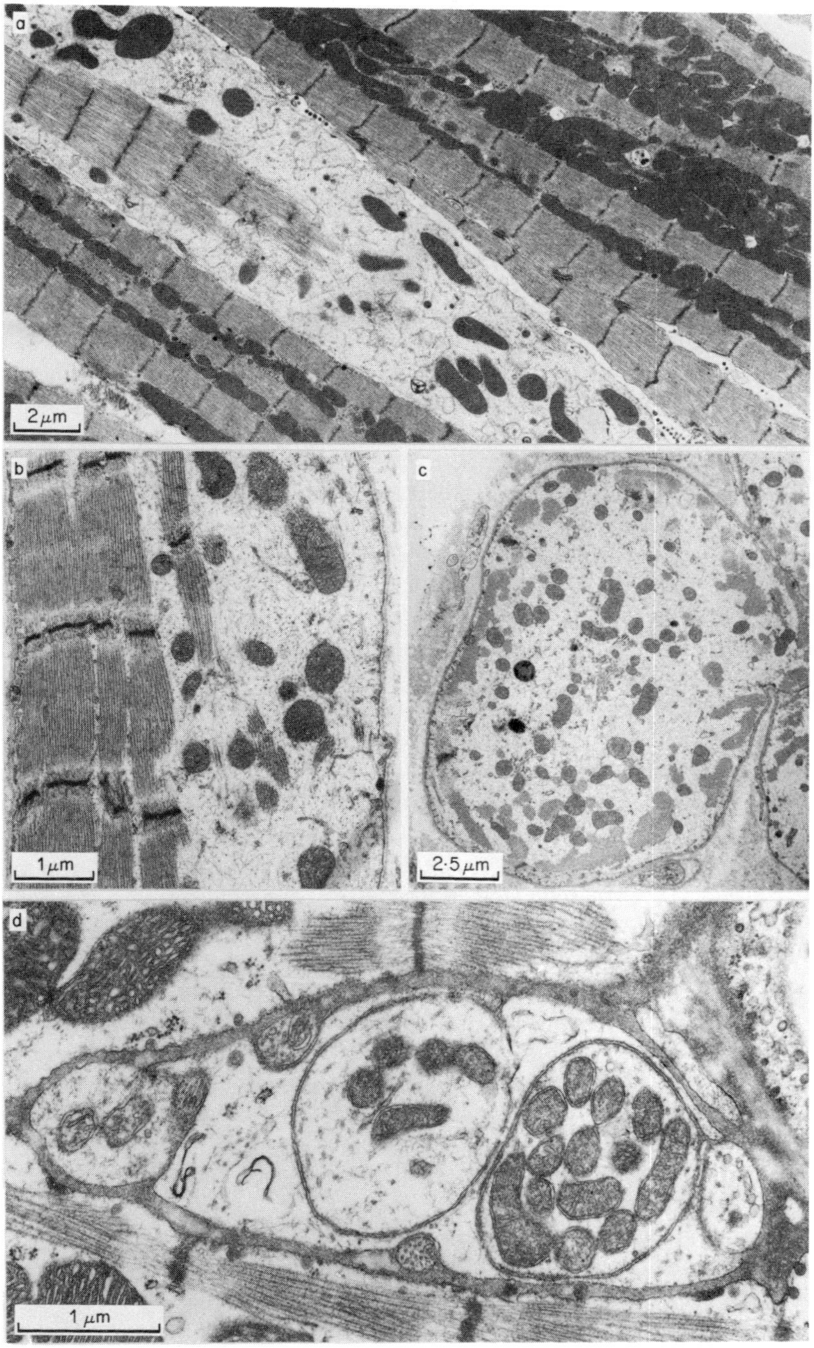
a
2 μm
b
1 μm
c
2·5 μm
d
1 μm

strating a high concentration of skeletin fibres in conducting cells, this method of immunofluorescence showed them to be present in both Z-discs and intercalated discs. It is thought that skeletin may provide a transverse linkage between Z-discs and the sarcolemma and also between adjacent Z-discs in contractile cells, as well as providing a cytoskeleton for conducting cells.

One of the oldest and still most frequently quoted accounts of the impulse generating the conducting system in the domestic fowl is by Davies (1930). He claimed that the sino-atrial node was situated at the base of the right venous valve in the wall of the right atrium and that the atrioventricular node lay in the caudal part of the interatrial septum close to the cardiac skeleton. As in mammals, the atrioventricular node leads directly into the atrioventricular bundle, which enters the interventricular septum and soon divides into left and right bundle branches for distribution throughout the ventricular myocardium. Davies (1930) also described a third branch (recurrent branch) which doubled back in the interventricular septum to loop round the root of the aorta and join a ring of conducting tissue situated in the base of the right atrioventricular valve. This right atrioventricular ring bundle originated in the sino-atrial node. No such ring has been described in the mammal and one must presume that its main function is to control the powerful muscular atrioventricular valve which is such a distinctive (but still unexplained) feature of the avian heart.

R. Mathur and Shrivastava (1979) described the sino-atrial node in the domestic fowl as being horse-shoe shaped and lying in the wall of the right atrium beside the opening of the left anterior vena cava. They claimed to have identified three internodal tracts which they called right, middle and left atrial bundles. In contrast, Kim and Yasuda (1979) claimed that the sino-atrial node of domestic fowl lies in the right atrial wall, between the right anterior vena cava and the posterior vena cava, at the base of the right sino-atrial (venous) valve and that there are no internodal tracts. Murakami *et al.* (1981) dealing with several birds (but not the domestic fowl) placed the node in the right atrial wall close to the opening of the right anteria vena cava. They also denied the existence of internodal tracts within the atrial muscle. They claimed that in the duck, heron and budgerigar the sino-atrial node is well developed and spreads into the flaps of the sino-atrial (venous) valve.

An atrioventricular node is said to be present in some avian species but absent in others (Table 1). It is unfortunate that practically all the accounts quoted in Table 1 refer to different species and that there is very little confirmation by independent workers about the position of the atrioventricular node in the same species. The difficulty in finding the node, or even of knowing exactly what to look for, was stressed by Vassall-Adams (1981). Starting with the easily recognizable interventricular bundle in the upper part of the interventricular septum, he followed it

Table 1.
Claimed presence or absence of atrioventricular node in different avian species

Present	Absent
Davies (1930): Pigeon	Drennan (1927): Ostrich
Prakash (1956): Indian fowl	Adams (1937): Kiwi
Khanna (1957): Domestic pigeon	De Meyer (1952): Sparrow
T. Singh (1958): Sparrow	Khan and Qayyum (1975): Jungle bush quail
Prakash *et al.* (1960): Domestic fowl	
Yousuf (1965): Sparrow	
R. Mathur (1971): Duck, pigeon	
Baumel (1975): Domestic fowl	
Kim and Yasuda (1979): Domestic fowl	
G. B. Mathur and Mathur (1979): Spotted mannikin	
R. Mathur and Shrivastava (1979): Domestic fowl	
Kim and Yasuda (1980): Domestic fowl	
Murakami, *et al.* (1981): Duck, pigeon. Japanese quail, makaw, budgerigar, jungle crow (by implication)	

back towards its origin. Whilst still in the interventricular septum, the bundle broke up into many strands which he called its "dispersal area". These scattered branches of the bundle passed through the cardiac skeleton to disperse into atrial muscle and also to unite with the ring of conducting cells that surround the right atrioventricular valve. As the direction of conduction is from atrium to ventricle it would have been better to call the "dispersal area" a "concentration area". However, if this description is correct, it is possible that the avian atrioventricular node is not a compact structure from the lower end of which a large atrioventricular bundle detaches itself. Instead it may be a diffuse region in the lower interatrial septum from which several small scattered bundles of conducting cells penetrate the cardiac skeleton and enter the upper end of the interventricular septum where, by merging together, they are concentrated into a well developed interventricular bundle. This may explain why many workers have considered the node to be absent (Table 1). On the other hand, what were those people describing who have been convinced of its presence? Unfortunately, no one has provided convincing illustrative proof. It is the opinion of this author that all birds will eventually be shown to have some sort of nodal tissue in positions broadly similar to those in the mammal. The most urgent requirement in this respect is for the ultrastructure of avian nodal tissue to be clearly described.

We seem to be on firmer ground with the main part of the interventricular bundle and its principal branches. This is probably the easiest part of the system to identify and has been described in many different species: Davies (1930), domestic fowl; Prakash (1956), common Indian fowl; Khana (1957), Indian blue rock pigeon; Yousuf (1965), sparrow; Vassal-Adams (1978), ostrich and turkey; G. B. Mathur and Mathur (1979), spotted mannikin; and Kim and Yasuda (1979), domestic fowl. The interventricular bundle is a broad, flat ribbon of conducting cells which originates in the "atrioventricular node", on the atrial side of the cardiac skeleton. In the domestic fowl it is said not to be surrounded by a fibrous sheath (Kim and Yasuda, 1979), whilst in the common Indian fowl a fibrous sheath is said to be present (G. B. Mathur and Mathur, 1979). The main bundle runs within the interventricular septum towards the apex. According to Davies (1930), about a quarter of the way down a recurrent branch is given off which runs back in the interventricular septum, passing to the left of, and then caudal to the root of the aorta. It helps to form a ring of conducting cells surrounding the right atrioventricular aperature (right atrioventricular ring bundle) and finally unites with the "atrioventricular node". Quite how this reputedly continuous ring of conducting cells functions, has not been explained. Soon after giving rise to the recurrent branch, the main bundle divides into right and left bundle branches, which are distributed to the myocardium of the right and left ventricles.

These two branches divide continuously as they penetrate the myocardium, along the connective tissue septa which lie between bundles of cardiac muscle. They follow branches of the coronary arteries, which are being distributed along the same septa. Eventually the terminal ramifications of these bundles will become single conducting cells in direct contact with contractile cells, and possibly forming intercalated discs with them. However, it must be stressed that there is no clear information as to whether these conducting cells form a continuous link from atrioventricular node to contractile cell, or whether this link becomes discontinuous in its terminal ramifications.

Kim and Yasuda (1979) have described a third node (truncobulbar), which they say is situated in the fibrous tissue of the aortic ring, ventral to the origin of the left coronary artery. This node is said to connect, by way of a truncobulbar bundle, to the main inter-ventricular bundle and to the atrioventricular node by way of the right atrioventricular ring bundle. It would appear that this "truncobulbar bundle" is the same as the "recurrent branch of the interventricular bundle" of Davies (1930).

There is reasonable agreement that the right atrioventricular ring bundle runs between the ventricular and atrial muscular components of the right atrioventricular valve. If, as seems most likely, this bundle sends small branches into the ventricular component of the valve (Fig. 3) then there would appear to be two functional links between atrial and ventricular muscle (even if one of them goes no further than the right atrioventricular valve).

According to Kim and Yasuda (1979) there appears to be an inverse ratio in the sizes of the atrioventricular and truncobulbar nodes. If the atrioventricular node was large, the truncobulbar node would be small or absent. Whether this suggests that the latter is a displaced part of the former or not has still to be clarified. There have been claims that a similar third node exists in mammals (Anderson, 1972), but it has not been widely accepted, nor has the truncobulbar node been confirmed in the bird.

X. Transitional Cells

Contractile and conducting cells can easily be distinguished, mainly on their content of highly organized and oriented myofibrils (Section IX: Fig. 13a). About half of the contractile cell contents are myofibrils, which dominate the appearance of the cell. The conducting cell contains no normal myofibrils, but a few scattered and rather disorganized fragments, perhaps two or three sarcomeres long. It has been suggested that, between these two extremes, there may be a complete spectrum of "transitional cells" (Akester, 1971, 1981), beginning with cells which resemble conducting cells but contain a somewhat greater number of slightly better organized sarcomere chains, and ending with cells in which their myofibrils are so well organized that they are virtually indistinguishable from contractile cells (Fig. 13b). The difficulty lies in recognizing these cells. One half of a transitional cell might be packed with fully developed myofibrils, whilst the other half might show all the characteristics of a conducting cell. Depending on how the specimen was cut for study in the electron microscope such a cell could be interpreted in two completely different ways.

It is known that contractile cells can hypertrophy, mainly by laying down more myofibrils. It is also known that, within a normal contractile cell, there is a steady turnover of myofibrils (their life span is about a month). If this is so, then it would seem at least reasonable to suggest that conducting cells, via the intermediary of transitional cells, may be transformed into contractile cells and *vice versa* (Akester, 1981). It must be stressed that there is no evidence for this speculation, but at least it serves to suggest how complicated the conducting system may be.

XI. Ultrastructure of Conducting (Purkinje) Cells

Conducting cells in the heart of the domestic fowl are easily recognised with the light microscope when they occur in tracts or bundles, but individual conducting cells scattered amongst contractile cells are less easy to find. With the electron microscope, however, an isolated conducting cell is easily distinguished (Fig. 13a,c). Its main distinctive feature is the relative lack of electron density (and thus a light appearance), due to the absence of highly organized myofibrils.

Conducting cells are much wider than contractile cells (diameter about 30 μm) and usually contain two nuclei. Compared with contractile cells, they exhibit "internal disorganization", with a mass of short, delicate microfilaments scattered, apparently at random, throughout the cell cytoplasm (Hirakow, 1966; Gossrau, 1968; Akester and Akester, 1971a; Scott, 1971a), although Bogusch (1974) claims to have recognized a meaningful organization.

Short chains of reasonably well organized sarcomeres frequently occur, but as they peter out into the cytoplasm the myofilaments and the Z-discs to which they are attached are reduced, respectively, in numbers and in size. Sometimes the bundles of actin filaments, which occur at the end of a few poorly developed sarcomeres, insert obliquely into the under surface of the sarcolemma. Mitochondria are fewer than in contractile cells, but are widely distributed throughout the cell. They take on many shapes and in life would replicate periodically and be in a state of constant movement. The sarcoplasmic reticulum is less well developed in the conducting cell, but still makes peripheral couplings with the sarcolemma.

When seen from the outside, the sarcolemma of a conducting cell is not significantly different from that of a contractile cell: neither has T-tubules and both have large numbers of surface vesicles. Conducing cells form intercalated discs with each other and probably with contractile cells. An intercalated disc between contiguous conducting cells is less complicated than one between contractile cells. In the former case the intercalated disc tends to cross the whole cell at the same level, without the stepwise arrangement which is such a feature of the latter (Akester, 1981).

If the nexus is the site of low-resistance electrical conductivity between cells, then one might expect them to be more numerous, or better developed, at an intercalated disc between conducting cells than at one between contractile cells. The best way to demonstrate a nexus is by replication of the freeze-fractured sarcolemma (Akester, 1981). In this respect, it should be remembered that with all freeze-fracturing it is the cell membrane itself that is being split, so that we are usually making a replica of an abnormal internal surface (Branton *et al.*, 1975). In the deep-frozen specimen, the hydrophobic (lyophilic) centre of the sarcolemma, between its inner and outer leaflets, is probably the weakest part and this is why it splits. As yet, no comparison of nexuses on conducting and contractile cells in the avian heart has been made by freeze-fractured replication or by any other method.

XII. Innervation of the Heart

Nerve fibres and cell bodies can be recognized by an increasing number of staining techniques, but very few of them indicate what type of nerve it is. The exception lies in the noradrenergic, postganglionic sympathetic neurones and other neurones (in the brain), the transmitters of which are catecholamines (adrenaline, noradrenaline, dopamine). When exposed to formaldehyde gas in the presence of dried protein these substances react to produce intensely fluorescent substances called isoquinolines (Falck *et al.*, 1962; Falk, 1962). In the context of the cardiovascular system, these will be noradrenergic postganglionic sympathetic nerves (Akester *et al.*, 1969).

This highly specific technique, which identifies the transmitter substance, has been supported by an equally specific procedure which identifies the enzyme responsible for producing the transmitter (dopamine β-hydroxylase which converts dopamine to noradrenaline) and can therefore be used to recognize noradrenergic neurones (Hartman, 1973). Paraformaldehyde-induced fluorescence has been applied widely to avian tissue, dopamine β-hydroxylase immunofluorescence has not.

Neither of these techniques can be used with the electron microscope and it is only at this level of magnification that the relationship between axon terminal and effector cell (usually smooth muscle) can adequately be appreciated. When noradrenaline is released by an axon terminal (swelling, varicosity) and crosses the narrow intercellular space to react with specific receptors on the effector cell membrane, there is always some surplus to requirement. Most of this surplus noradrenaline is taken back into the axon from which it came, incorporated into vesicles, and may be released again as part of the next burst of axonal activity. In the same way, noradrenergic terminals will take up false transmitters like 5- and 6-hydroxydopamine and also radioactive noradrenaline. These substances can be recognized in the axons under the electron microscope, and thus provide a method for identifying postganglionic sympathetic fibres, which tend to be characterized by a high concentration of dense-core vesicles (Fig. 14c). In the heart and blood vessels (and also in other viscera) cholinergic axons are usually taken to be those that are obviously not noradrenergic (Fig. 14d). Whilst acetylcholinesterase (the enzyme which breaks down acetylcholine) can be demonstrated histochemically, at the level of both the light and the electron microscope, it is so widely distributed that its presence does not necessarily indicate a cholinergic nerve. Indeed, noradrenergic nerves may themselves carry acetylcholinesterase. Unfortunately, there is still no adequate technique to demonstrate choline acetyltransferase, which synthesizes the transmitter substance of cholinergic nerves (Burt and Narayanan, 1976).

It is easy to show nerves in cardiac tissue. Depending on the technique, one

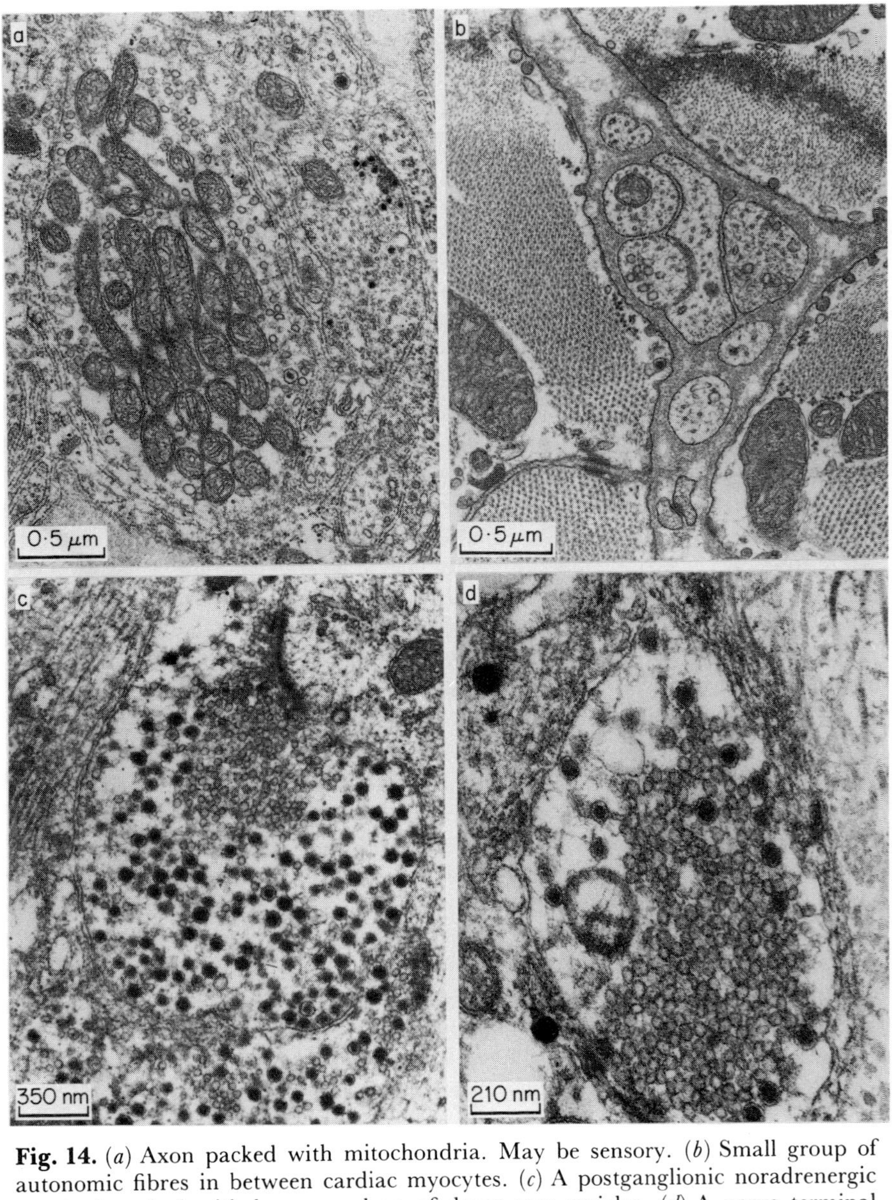

Fig. 14. (*a*) Axon packed with mitochondria. May be sensory. (*b*) Small group of autonomic fibres in between cardiac myocytes. (*c*) A postganglionic noradrenergic terminal packed with large numbers of dense-core vesicles. (*d*) A nerve terminal containing many small clear vesicles and a small number of dense-core vesicles. Possibly a cholinergic nerve.

may or may not be able to say what kind of nerve is being demonstrated, and it is only with the electron microscope that one can say with confidence which effector cell is being innervated. Using paraformaldehyde-induced fluorescence, noradrenergic postganglionic sympathetic axons have been identified in all the major parts of the heart (Akester *et al.*, 1969; Akester and Akester, 1971b). They appear to be innervating cardiac muscle, and may be innervating conducting cells directly. They are said to innervate the impulse generating cells situated in the nodes (Bennett and Malmfors, 1970) and are distributed to all branches of the coronary arteries (Akester, 1971, 1979).

Although the mature, isolated and perfused avian or mammalian heart will continue to beat rhythmically for a considerable time, it will not be as responsive as the intact heart. The heart of both birds and mammals receives a double innervation (primarily to the nodes) of parasympathetic and sympathetic fibres. However, they do not behave in exactly the same way. In the resting mammal, parasympathetic tone appears to be dominant with only a small sympathetic influence, whilst in resting birds, the influences of the two parts of the autonomic nervous system are more equally balanced (Johansen and Reite, 1964).

Bilateral vagotomy causes a 65% increase in heart rate in the duck (Johansen and Reite, 1964) and a 100% increase in the pigeon (Knoll, 1897). In contrast, Sturkie (1965) found that total removal of all vagal tone in the chicken caused only an 8% increase, from 288 to 312 beats min^{-1}. Experimental stimulation of the peripheral end of the cut vagus in the duck does not have the same effect on each side. The right side is more effective in causing bradycardia than the left (Johansen and Reite, 1964).

Preganglionic sympathetic axons, which will influence the heart of the pigeon, leave the spinal cord in the last cervical and first three thoracic spinal nerves (MacDonald and Cohen, 1970). They synapse in the appropriate paravertebral ganglia with postganglionic noradrenergic nerves. These are collected together to form the prominent cardiac nerve, which passes, on both sides, along the external jugular vein and cranial vena cava to the heart. Here it is joined by branches from the vagus and by sensory fibres coming from the heart to form an extensive cardiac plexus. Nerve fibres from this plexus then spread throughout the heart, pericardium, aortic arch, pulmonary trunk and the terminal parts of the three venae cavae. The cardiac nerve may also provide autonomic fibres to the primary bronchi, lungs and pleurae. Preganglionic axons associated with the cardiac nerve in the domestic fowl are said to be restricted entirely to the first thoracic segment (Hsieh, 1951), whilst in the mammal they have a much wider origin, from the first to the sixth thoracic segment (Saccomanno, 1943). For some (unexplained) reason autonomic fibres from the right side of the animal seem to have a dominant influence on the heart. The right cardiac sympathetic nerve is more effective than the left at causing cardiac acceleration and we have seen that the right vagus is more effective than the left at causing bradycardia.

After cutting both cardiac (sympathetic) and both vagus nerves (i.e. complete denervation) to the heart in domestic fowl, duck and pigeon, Tummons and Sturkie (1968) showed that stimulation of the peripheral end of the right cardiac nerve caused a 48% increase in heart rate (235 to 345 beats min^{-1}), whilst stimulation on the left side increased heart rate by about 32%.

Acknowledging the difficulty of understanding the individual functions of cardiac muscle, nodal cells, conducting cells, sympathetic and parasympathetic nerves, when they are all functioning simultaneously in the adult heart. Kirby *et al.* (1980) have suggested that this might be done in the embryonic heart where each component develops at a different time in a precise sequence.

It would appear that parasympathetic fibres from the vagus enter the heart, in association with postganglionic parasympathetic neurones (ganglion cells), at 3·5 d of incubation, before the arrival of any sympathetic nerves. It is possible that this may be related to the fact that the vagus nerves play a dominant role in cardiac control throughout the whole vertebrate series. The most primitive fish (cyclostomes) have no effective innervation of the heart, adjustments being carried out by direct myocardial responses to changes in stretch and pressure. In all other fish there is a parasympathetic but no sympathetic supply, so that cardiac responses must be dependent on variation in the level of vagal inhibitory activity. Amphibians receive a sympathetic as well as a parasympathetic supply, although the latter is dominant. The vagus may also dominate the heart in resting mammals, but in resting birds sympathetic and parasympathetic influences are about equally balanced (Tummons and Sturkie, 1969). It would appear reasonable to assume that the totally denervated heart, thanks to its inherent contractile nature and the ability of the impulse generating and conducting system to impose upon it an appropriate sequence of contraction, is capable of maintaining an adequate resting circulation around the body. Some measure of response is provided by fluctuations of vagal inhibitory activity, but the development of a sympathetic innervation was essential before the avian heart could reach the remarkable level of versatility that it has now achieved. This permits an Arctic tern to migrate 17 500 km from the Arctic to the Antarctic, geese to fly at 9000 m (Dorst, 1974), and the sparrow to remain active and alert at a simulated altitude of 6100 m whilst its mammalian companion of comparable size was lying moribund (Tucker, 1968).

Small groups of acetylcholinesterase-positive cell bodies (ganglia) have been found scattered widely over the surfaces of both atria and ventricles and also in association with branches of the coronary artery in the domestic fowl (Smith, 1971). They were interpreted as being parasympathetic and may be the same as the ganglion cells which Kirkby *et al.* (1980) recognized in the early chick embryo.

A dense plexus of varicose noradrenergic fibres together with what appear to be their cell bodies has been demonstrated in the fibrous flaps of the left A-V valve in chickens, in the chordae tendinae and also in the papillary muscle of the left ventricle. Some (or all) of these cell bodies may be small intensely fluorescent cells (SIF cells), which are dopaminergic. It has been suggested that SIF cells may release dopamine which influences the tension applied to the chordae tendinae by the papillary muscle (Strinskaya *et al.*, 1980).

Undoubtedly, there is a widespread innervation of the avian heart by parasympathetic (inhibitory) and sympathetic (excitatory) nerves, but a knowledge of their precise distribution is not yet available. It is not known how many cardiac myocytes are innervated by a single axon, whether all myocytes are directly innervated or not, whether those that are innervated always receive a double innervation, or if some are only innervated by one or other division of the autonomic nervous system. There is also much scope for an increased understanding of factors which modulate the effect of autonomic nervous activity. These may include hormones from distant sites, and prostaglandins released by the effector cells.

Sensory nerves will also be present, but their precise distribution is not known. They will probably be associated with coronary blood vessels and with the pericardium. They may be scattered throughout the myocardium (angina pectoris is painful in the human). There have been suggestions that they may be characterized by a high concentration of mitochondria (Fig. 14a).

XIII. Blood Volume, Blood Pressure, Heart Rate, Cardiac Output

A. Blood Volume and Distribution

Although total blood volume remains virtually constant, under normal conditions, at about 240 ml in a 2·5-kg fowl and 117 ml in a 1·8-kg fowl, the distribution of this blood through the body varies considerably, according to the metabolic activity of each tissue. The left side of the heart is concerned more with responding to fluctuations of peripheral resistance by changing the pressure at which it ejects arterial blood, than with volume change. It is sometimes called a "pressure pump". On the other hand, the right side is concerned more with handling a variable volume of blood and has little need to respond to major changes in pulmonary resistance, because they do not normally occur. It can be regarded as a "volume pump". Veins have a greater (collective) capacity (venous reservoir) than arteries. At any time, about 70%

of the circulating blood is contained within them. The ability to vary the volume of this reservoir and to allow more or less blood to return to the heart will be an important function of the larger veins.

Blood can only flow from a point of relatively high pressure to one of lower pressure, and the pulsatile nature of this flow is progressively reduced as the blood passes from the aorta and large distributing arteries to the capillary plexuses. The power to produce the pressure which propels the blood around the body is generated by the left ventricular myocardium. The peripheral resistance is caused mainly by the extent to which the arterioles are constricted. Capillaries are simple tubes of endothelial cells with no contractile ability of their own. If an arteriole is open then those capillaries connected directly to it will be open as well and blood will flow through both. Of course, many arterioles normally supply a particular capillary plexus, so that many of them would have to be constricted before the blood flow through that tissue as a whole would be affected.

Blood flow through an active tissue may be ten times greater than through the same tissue at rest (Falkow, 1960). The increased flow is caused by relaxation (vasodilation) of a greater number of arterioles so that many more capillaries carry blood. Vasodilation in the active tissue must be counterbalanced by vasoconstriction in some other tissue. One of the most dramatic illustrations of vasomotor closure of blood vessels occurs when a duck dives under water. In these conditions it is obviously an advantage to reduce oxygen consumption to a minimum. There is an intense sympathetic vasoconstriction of blood vessels in all the tissues except the heart, brain and certain endocrine glands. Virtually no blood flows through the constricted vessels of the skeletal muscles, even though they are physically active, so that high concentrations of lactic acid accumulate. Heart rate slows markedly (from 186 to 21 beats min^{-1}) as a result of increased vagal and reduce sympathetic activity. Cardiac output drops to about 25% of normal (Jones and Holeton, 1972a) and the total energy metabolism (and hence oxygen requirement) falls to about 10% of normal (Pickwell, 1968). Stroke volume usually increases slightly and blood pressure to the brain is maintained at near normal levels. After the dive, autonomic influences are reversed. The heart rate and stroke volume increase and peripheral vasoconstriction is changed to vasodilatation. Accumulated lactic acid (oxygen debt) is washed out of the muscles into the blood, where it may reach ten times the pre-dive level (Scholander, 1940). A similar compensatory vasodilatation can be demonstrated experimentally. If the main artery supplying blood to the hind limb is clamped the peripheral vessels will constrict. After release of the clamp the peripheral vessels dilate and blood flow through the limb (for a short time) will be about twice the pre-clamp rate. This has been demonstrated for the duck (Butler and Jones, 1969) and fowl (Akester and Brackenbury, 1973).

B. Blood Pressure

Blood pressure in the domestic fowl varies with age, sex, breed, state of health and the conditions under which the recordings are made. A considerable range of pressures has been reported (see Sturkie, 1976). A reasonable figure for the adult fowl would be about 165 mmHg (systolic) and 135 mmHg (diastolic), with a pulse pressure of about 30 mmHg. However, 191/154 mmHg (Ringer *et al.*, 1957a) and 130/85 mmHg (Woodbury and Abreu, 1944) show the upper and lower limits of those quoted. An even greater range of systolic pressures from 175 to 350 mmHg has been reported for the turkey (Speckmann and Ringer, 1964). Perhaps about 190 mmHg (systolic) and 150 mmHg (diastolic) with a pulse pressure of 40 mmHg would be sensible figures to have in mind for the normal adult turkey. It seems most improbable that the considerable range of "normal" systolic pressures quoted above (130 to 191 mmHg in the fowl and 175 to 350 mmHg in the turkey) can apply to the truly resting state. Nevertheless systolic blood pressures in birds (about 165 mmHg in chicken and duck, 190 mmHg in turkey) are certainly higher than in mammals of comparable size, though pulmonary pressures in birds and mammals are roughly the same.

A relationship between hormones and blood pressure has been established, with pressure in the mature male fowl being about 20% higher than in the female. Castration in male and female birds resulted in both having blood pressures similar to that of the normal male, suggesting that blood pressure is not increased by androgens in the male, but is reduced by oestrogens in the female.

A genetic link has been established with blood pressure, and hypertensive as well as hypotensive strains have been established (Sturkie, 1976). Hypertensive birds were said to have a greater peripheral resistance but lower cardiac output and stroke volume, whilst those from a hypotensive strain had a lower peripheral resistance but higher cardiac output and stroke volume. The heart rate of the two strains was virtually the same. There is a suggestion that hypertension may have some survival advantage over hypotension under experimental conditions. When subjected to stress caused by submersion in cold water (20°C), to treadmill exercise and even disease, hypertensive animals survived longer than hypotensive ones.

C. Heart Rate

Attempts to establish normal heart rate in birds handled experimentally have resulted in a wide range of results. In general, larger animals have a heart rate slower than smaller ones and males beat slower than females. Heavy breeds of domestic fowl have slower rates than light ones. Heart rate increases in a cold environment and with exercise. The adult fowl heart beat frequency is said to range from 350 to 450 beats min^{-1} (Ringer *et al.*, 1957b), although Tummons and Sturkie (1969) put it at 280 to 290 beats min^{-1}. The turkey is said to range from about 160 to 280 beats min^{-1} (Ringer and Rood, 1959), although Speckmann and Ringer (1963) have recorded the Broad Breasted Bronze turkey at 149 beats min^{-1}. The resting rate in the duck has been given as 174 beats min^{-1} by Bech and Nomoto (1982), 186 beats min^{-1} by Jones and Holeton (1972b) and as 219 beats min^{-1} by Langille and Jones (1975). Some small birds have remarkably high beat frequencies. The American tree sparrow and the canary have been recorded at 1000 beats min^{-1} (Slautterback, 1965) but whether this should be regarded as a true resting rate is not clear.

The "psychological" effect of being subjected to experimental conditions creates a sense of "apprehension" or "fear" in a bird, which has a marked effect on its heart rate. This is obviously stimulated by an intense sympathetic and adrenal medullary response associated with reduced vagal tone. Tummons and Sturkie (1969) allowed a cockerel 15 min to "settle down" (out of sight of the operators) after having ECG electrodes attached to both sides of the sternum and to both legs. The animal was then "excited" by a sudden grasping and shaking of its comb for 2 to 3 min. This resulted in the animal's heart rate increasing from about 280 to 380 beats per min. A similar response has been demonstrated by Jones *et al.* (1981) who used radiotelemetry to monitor heart rate. Under carefully controlled conditions, a bird was exposed to the slow approach of a person wearing a white coat, who finally opened the cage door and held the bird for about 2 min. Heart rate and behaviour changed progressively as the person approached (303 beats min^{-1} with mild agitation) and then opened the cage door (645 beats min^{-1} with total panic). These experiments were an attempt to relate an animal's behaviour and heart rate to a sense of fear, which the authors defined as "the psychophysiological response to perceived danger'.

This kind of cardiac response is dependent on an intact sympathetic innervation. After sympathectomy resting heart rate drops by about 20%. When excited (afraid?) heart rate in the sympathectomized bird increases to the resting pre-sympathectomized level but never above it. This was due to a reduction in vagal tone and could also be caused by vagotomy. A normal resting heart rate can be maintained after total denervation, but such an animal cannot increase its heart rate in response to an external stimulus (excitement/fear). It would appear that vagal slowing and sympathetic speeding of the heart in the resting state are about equally balanced in birds (Tummons and Sturkie, 1969).

D. Cardiac Output

Cardiac output has been measured by dye-dilution techniques and by electromagnetic flowmeters which form a cuff around the vessel. Some values of output in the duck are: 286 (Sturkie, 1966), 394 (Jones and Holeton, 1972a) and 560 ml kg^{-1} min^{-1} (Folkow *et al.*, 1967). Cardiac output in the male chicken (286 ml kg^{-1} min^{-1} is said to be significantly higher than in the female (253 ml kg^{-1} min^{-1}) (Sturkie and Vogel, 1959). Sapirstein and Hartman (1959), however, found a common value of 218 ml kg^{-1} min^{-1}. In the mature male turkey cardiac output was given as 231 ml kg^{-1} min^{-1} (Speckmann and Ringer, 1963).

Jones and Holeton (1972b) have reported (for the duck) that in a cuffed pulmonary artery, blood flow stopped altogether after 8 weeks due to its total occlusion, but cardiac output (measured by dye dilution) remained normal (385 ml kg^{-1} min^{-1}). Presumably this was because the entire right ventricular output went to the other lung.

Distribution of cardiac output to the various tissues will depend on their respective metabolic activities. In the resting animal, some idea of the relative proportion to reach different organs has been given by Sapirstein and Hartman (1959), using a radioactive indicator dilution technique in the fowl. They found that the kidneys received about 15% and the coronary supply to the heart about 5% of the total cardiac output (218 ml kg^{-1} min^{-1}). Under conditions of reduced oxygen tension, as would occur in flight at high altitude, birds increase their cardiac output and ventilation volume per minute (Jones and Holeton, 1972a). Grubb (1981) studied the responses of blood flow through skeletal muscles in the resting duck under similar conditions (hypoxia, 35–40 Torr) and found that there was no increase in flow, although there was an increase in oxygen extraction. The main reason for this was considered to be the existence of an extremely high resting flow rate under normoxic conditions. In the duck this was found to be 45 ml 100 g^{-1} tissue min^{-1}, whch is more than four times the comparable rate in the dog (10 ml 100 g^{-1} tissue min^{-1}). Even then hypoxic, sympathetic vasomotor tone was considerable. Denervation increased blood flow by about 50%. It is possible that the generous level of blood flow through the resting limb may reduce the amount by which flow needs to increase in active muscle, particularly under hypoxic conditions (high altitude). Presumably a bird's hind limb muscles are relatively inactive in flight. It would have been more interesting if these studies had been carried out on the subclavian artery which supplies (via the pectoral artery) the large flight muscles, which would have been very active under these conditions.

Observations have also been made on cardiovascular responses to exercise in ducks trained to walk on a treadmill (Bech and Nomoto, 1982). The extent of the exercise was indicated by a 3·5 times increase in oxygen consumption. Under these conditions cardiac output increased from 540 ml kg^{-1} min^{-1} to 870 ml kg^{-1} min^{-1}. Blood flow in the ischiadic artery increased 3·7 times and in the internal carotid artery by 2·3 times. Increased cardiac output was due entirely to an increase in heart rate (from 174 to 328 beats min^{-1}). If anything there was a small reduction in stroke volume.

Blood pressure, cardiac output and peripheral resistance are all interrelated in such a way that an appropriate flow of blood takes place through capillary plexuses all over the body. The main factor in determining the rate of fluid transfer from capillary lumen to extracellular space is the ratio of pre- to post-capillary resistance to blood flow. This depends on the respective diameters, or degree of vasoconstriction/dilatation, of the small vessels either side of the capillary plexus and is controlled by a combination of autonomic vasomotor activity, the concentration of vasoactive metabolites and hormones. If pre-capillary resistance is increased (by sympathetic constriction of arterioles) then mean capillary pressure and trans-capillary flow would be reduced. If pre-capillary resistance becomes more than post-capillary resistance then tissue fluid flows back into the capillaries. This enables an animal to make good lost blood volume at the expense of tissue fluid after severe haemorrhage, and in this respect birds appear to be more efficient than mammals. Pigeons are able to recover after loss of 70% of their total blood volume (Kovach and Szasz, 1968). α-Receptor blockade of arteriolar smooth muscle slows this recovery, indicating the importance of sympathetic vasoconstriction (Djojosugito *et al.*, 1968).

XIV. Distribution and Structure of the Major Arteries and Veins

In birds, the aorta is the persistent right branch of the embryonic paired dorsal aortae. Almost immediately beyond the cusps of the aortic valve, just distal to the top of the left and right coronary sinuses, are the openings of left and right coronary arteries (Fig. 6e). Soon after this, left and right brachiocephalic trunks leave the ascending aorta, each of which terminates in a large subclavian and a smaller common carotid artery (Figs 3, 15). The subclavian artery supplies mainly, the flight muscles (pectoral artery), wing (brachial artery), cranial floor of body cavity and ventral parts of intercostal spaces (internal thoracic artery). The short common carotid artery supplies structures in the head and neck. Its branches include the vertebral, vagus, oesophagotracheobronchial and thyroid arteries. The ascending branch of the vertebral (in the arterial canal of the cervical vertebrae) and the vagus artery (beside the jugular vein), after supplying structures in the neck (spinal cord, muscles, vertebrae, oesophagus, crop, trachea, thymus, skin, etc.) anastomose at the top of the neck with descending branches of the occipital artery, and so help to form arterial loops in the neck (Figs 15, 16). In birds, the vertebral artery does not contribute directly to the brain or meninges.

The common carotid artery is continued as the internal carotid. Left and right internal carotid arteries pass up the neck buried under sub-vertebral muscles. In some species (not the fowl) these vessels are so close together that the fuse into a single trunk, but always separate again as they approach the

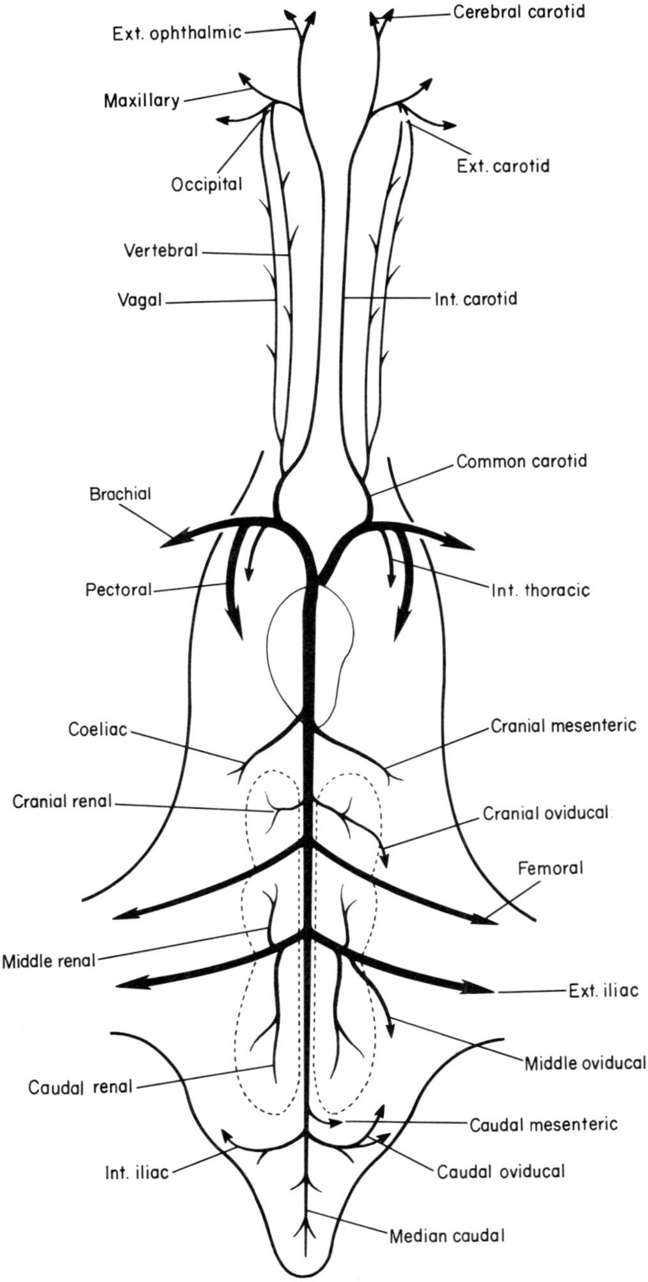

Fig. 15. Diagram of principal arteries in body cavity and neck of fowl.

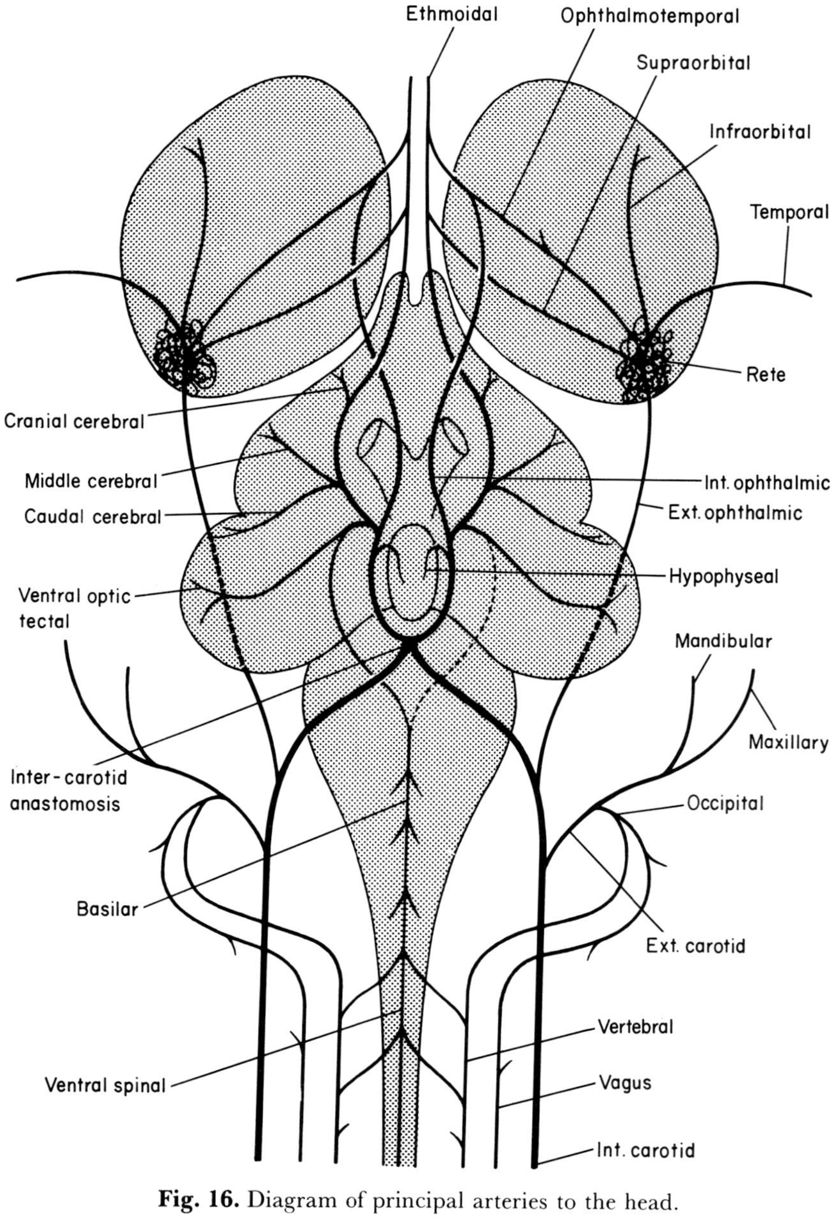

Fig. 16. Diagram of principal arteries to the head.

head. At the top of the neck, each internal carotid artery gives off an external carotid artery which supplies external structures of the head (jaw muscles, tongue, palate, lower jaw, skin, feathers, etc.), whilst descending branches supply structures in the upper part of the neck.

Each internal carotid terminates in an external ophthalmic (which supplies extracranial structures and forms the ophthalmic rete) and cerebral carotid artery, which passes through the carotid canal in the base of the skull to supply brain and meninges. There are anastomoses between arteries outside the cranial cavity and also between intracranial and extracranial arteries. Immediately caudal to the pituitary gland, the cerebral carotid artery from each side unite to form the intercarotid anastomosis. This is the avian counterpart of the mammalian circle of Willis and so provides a major collateral blood supply to the brain. The precise form of this intercarotid anastomosis varies in different avian species, but its function is the same in all. The (intracranial) internal ophthalmic artery, which leaves the cerebral carotid artery beside the pituitary gland, enters the orbit with the optic nerve, where it anastomoses with the (extracranial) ophthalmotemporal artery. Together they supply all structures in the orbit.

After the intercarotid anastomosis the cerebral carotid arteries separate to surround the pituitary gland (which they supply) and then divide into caudal and cranial branches. One or other of the two caudal branches (usually the right one) is dominant, the opposite branch being much smaller or nonexistent. These two caudal branches (if there are two) unite to form the single basilar artery which supplies cerebellum, pons, medulla, inner ear and continues through the foramen magnum as the ventral spinal artery. The cranial branch provides caudal, middle and cranial cerebral arteries and then leaves the cranial cavity to enter the orbit as the ethmoidal artery. This artery receives anastomoses from the supra-orbital and ophthalmotemporal arteries and leaves the orbit beside the olfactory nerve to enter the roof of the nasal cavity.

Ligation of the internal carotid and vertebral arteries causes the animal to die in about 1 min (Richards and Sykes, 1967). An anastomosis is provided between the vertebral and external carotid arteries by the deep occipital artery, the importance of which has been demonstrated by selective arterial ligation. The domestic fowl can tolerate ligation of any three of the four principal arteries in the neck. The fourth one apparently maintains an adequate supply *via* the occipito-vertebral and intercarotid anastomoses. However, when both internal carotid arteries and both occipito-vertebral anastomoses are ligated the small anastomoses which connect vertebral and basilar arteries are unable to maintain an adequate cerebral blood flow, so the animal dies. Cerebral arteries and veins receive what appears to be a dual innervation of noradrenergic (sympathetic) and acetylcholinesterase-positive (presumed parasympathetic) nerves (Tagawa *et al.*, 1979).

The descending aorta arches over the atria of the heart, above the division of the pulmonary trunk into left and right pulmonary arteries, and continues along the roof of the body cavity until it terminates in the tail (Fig. 15). Along its course it provides branches which supply all those parts of the body not provided for by the brachiocephalic trunks and coronary arteries. Thus it supplies: a series of paired segmental arteries to the vertebral column and spinal cord, which also supply intercostal arteries in the cranial part of the body cavity; a single coeliac artery, which supplies the lower end of oesophagus, proventriculus, gizzard, liver, spleen, duodenum, pancreas and caeca; a single cranial mesenteric artery, which suppplies the jejunum, ileum and caeca; paired renal arteries direct to cranial division of each kidney, adrenals, gonads, oviduct or vas deferens; paired external iliac arteries which continue as femoral arteries into hind limb; paired ischiadic arteries, which are the largest branches of the descending aorta and the main supply to the hind limbs, and also provide renal arteries to middle and distal divisions of kidneys (the left ischiadic artery also provides middle oviducal artery); a single caudal mesenteric artery, which supplies the distal part of ileum, parts of caeca, rectum and cloaca; and paired internal iliac arteries, which supply the ureters, vas deferens or caudal part of oviduct, cloacal bursa (bursa of Fabricius), tail, skin, feathers, and brood patches on ventrocaudal abdominal wall.

In birds, the structure of the cranial (thoracic) aorta is significantly different from that of the caudal (abdominal) aorta. The change occurs at the level of the coeliac and cranial mesenteric arteries. In the cranial part, where there is much more elastic tissue and relatively little smooth muscle, the concentric sleeves of compact elastic fibres are connected together by smooth muscle cells which insert into them. Running between the smooth muscle cells are additional elastic fibres together with bundles of collagen fibres (Berry *et al.*, 1974). This provides an extremely efficient arrangement for resisting over-distension, by distributing the force of ventricular systole uniformly throughout the wall. It also appears to create conditions in which atherosclerosis does not normally occur (Stout and Thrope, 1980).

There are from about 15 to 30 concentric elastic lamellae in the cranial aortae of adult birds. The structural integrity of these lamellae is dependent on the cross-linkage of their elastic fibres, which is controlled by a copper-dependent enzyme, lysyl oxidase. There is evidence that this enzyme is also vitamin B_6-dependent, so that vitamin B_6 (pyridoxin) deficiency might predispose an animal to atherosclerosis. Pyridoxin-deficient chicks show a degree of structural disorganization of the elastic lamellae and a 50% reduction in lysyl oxidase activity in their aorta (Levene and Murray, 1977).

Caudal to the cranial mesenteric artery the aorta becomes less elastic, more muscular and more prone to atherosclerosis. Distributing arteries, which are the main vessels carrying blood to the organs and tissues, have a tunica media consisting almost entirely of smooth muscle cells, with bundles of collagen fibres scattered amongst them. Close to the endothelial lining is an internal elastic lamella and outside the muscular media are two or three layers of elastic fibres comprising the outer elastic lamella (Fig. 18c).

An unusual feature of arterial wall construction is found in the cranial mesenteric artery in the fowl, turkey (Ball *et al.*, 1963) and, presumably, in other birds. Outside the outer elastic lamella is a longitudinal layer of smooth muscle, which runs the whole length of the artery until it divides into its terminal branches. Longitudinal muscle also occurs in mammalian pulmonary arteries, pulmonary veins and pulmonary arterio-venous anastomoses (Bader, 1963), but in none of these sites is it as well developed as in the avian cranial mesenteric artery. No satisfactory explanation has been offered. It is said to enable the vessel to cope with "longitudinal stress", but it is difficult to see why the avian cranial mesenteric artery (with longitudinal muscle) should be subjected to any more stress than its mammalian counterpart (without longitudinal muscle).

Isolated preparations of this muscle, in an organ bath, contract strongly in response to acetylcholine whilst the contracted muscle is made to relax by noradrenaline. Relaxation was unaffected by α-blockade but was prevented by β-blockade (Bolton, 1968). If a cholinergic mechanism (postganglionic parasympathetic) causes contraction and a noradrenergic mechanism (postganglionic sympathetic) causes relaxation of the longitudinal muscle in the cranial mesenteric artery, then it has much in common with the unique renal portal valve (see Section XVII) and also with smooth muscle of the alimentary canal.

In general terms, veins parallel the arteries. The entire length of the alimentary canal caudal to the oesophagus drains into the hepatic portal vein, as does venous blood from the pancreas, spleen and gall bladder. The caudal mesenteric (coccygeomesenteric) vein, as well as draining the colorectum and cloaca, provides a unique major anastomosis between hepatic portal and renal portal systems (see Sections XVII and XVIII). Large hepatic veins join the posterior vena cava a short distance caudal to the heart (Fig. 17).

Veins have thinner walls and a greater capacity than arteries. At any time, about 70% of the total blood volume of an animal is contained within the veins so that their importance as a blood reservoir, to help control fluctuations of flow and demand by different tissues, is considerable. Venous blood pressures are very low and may be about 12 mmHg in the smaller veins, 5 mmHg in the hepatic portal vein as it enters the liver, 1 mmHg in the venae cavae and about 0 or -1 mmHg in the right atrium. Veins have basically the same structure as arteries with an endothelial lining (interna) muscular layer (media) and outer layer of connective tissue (adventitia). Veins have a much greater innervation than arteries and the nerves penetrate the entire thickness of the muscular

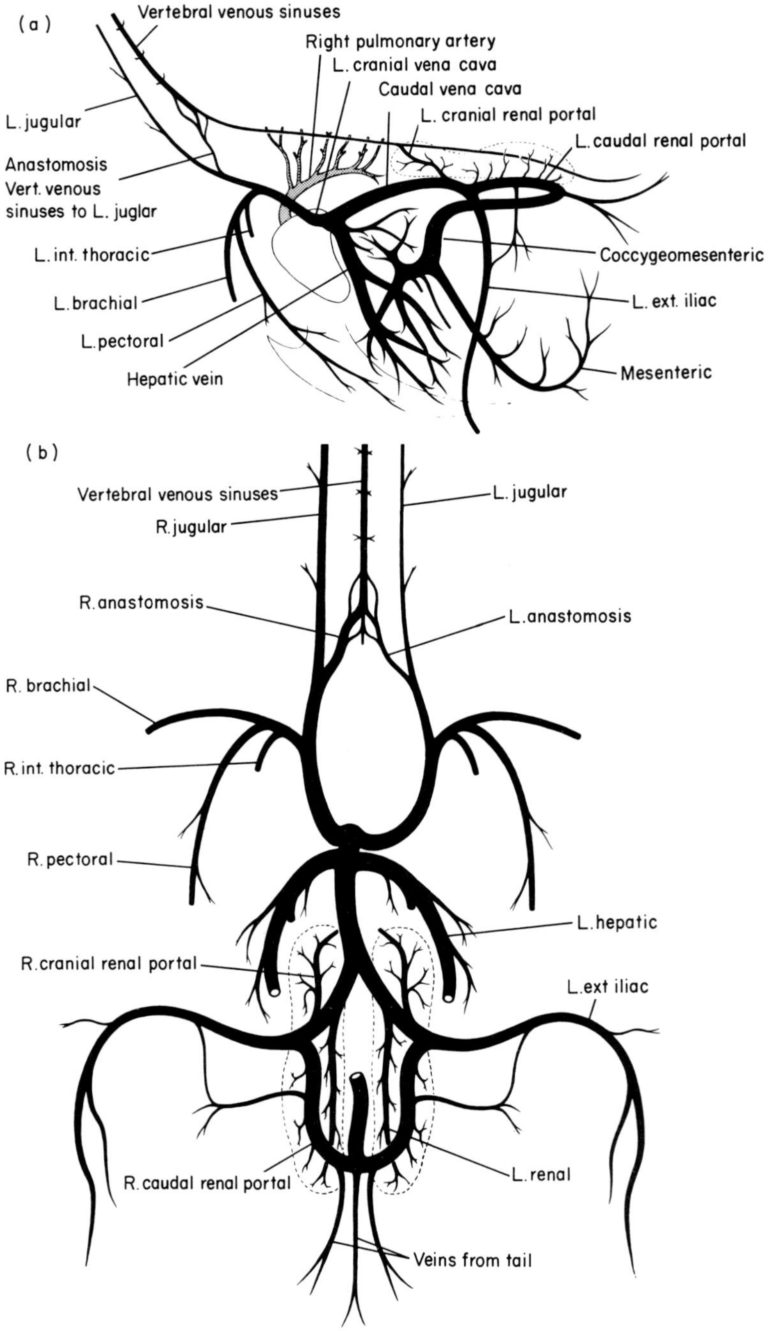

Fig. 17. (*a*) Principal veins of domestic fowl (lateral view). (*b*) Principal veins (ventro-dorsal view). The hepatic portal system and most of the coccygeomesenteric vein has been removed.

layer. In arteries, the nerves only rarely penetrate the muscle and are usually confined to the adventitia outside the outer elastic lamella (Fig. 18) (Akester, 1978).

Cardiac muscle extends along both anterior venae cavae to their junction with the jugular veins, and also along the posterior vena cava to its junction with the hepatic veins. There are conducting cells associated with this striated muscle and it is quite likely that rhythmic contractions in the three venae cavae contribute to the flow of venous blood into the right atrium.

XV. Thermoregulation

Birds maintain their deep (core) body temperature close to 41°C, compared with 39°C in most domestic mammals and 37°C in the human. This near constant body temperature is maintained in spite of considerable fluctuations of heat production inside the animal and environmental temperature immediately outside the animal. Heat is produced internally mainly as a by-product of metabolism. The principal site is the large flight muscles which comprise about 25% of the total body weight. Because muscular activity is only about 25% efficient, approximately 75% of the energy consumption is converted to heat. This may be an advantage in a cold environment, but will be a disadvantage in a hot one. As a direct result of the increased activity of the flight muscles during flight there may be a sevenfold increase in heat production. Some of this will be lost by convection and radiation to the air flowing over the skin covering the flight muscles (Hart and Roy, 1967). However, the bulk of this heat (as much as 80% of the total produced by the animal in flight) is eliminated by way of the lower legs as a result of their greatly increased blood flow (Baudinette *et al.*, 1976). An indication of the remarkable magnitude of this blood flow has been provided by direct measurement in the Giant Fulmar (Johansen and Millard, 1973), where a flow rate of 10 litre m^{-2} min^{-1} was calculated for the foot. This is about twice the maximum flow rate to the skin of man during heat stress (Folkow and Neil, 1971).

Temperature changes in the bird's immediate environment will result in appropriate responses, which are directed either towards increasing heat retention and minimizing heat loss or vice versa. In either case, the cardiovascular system will play an essential part. Recognition of temperature change must be by thermosensitive neurones, (probably free nerve endings) presumably in the skin, but also in the spinal cord and brain.

Overall control of temperature regulation lies in the hypothalamus, where thermosensitive neurones respond to local changes in temperature caused largely by the temperature of the inflowing arterial blood. This blood comes from the intercarotid anastomosis (which is regarded as being the avian counter-

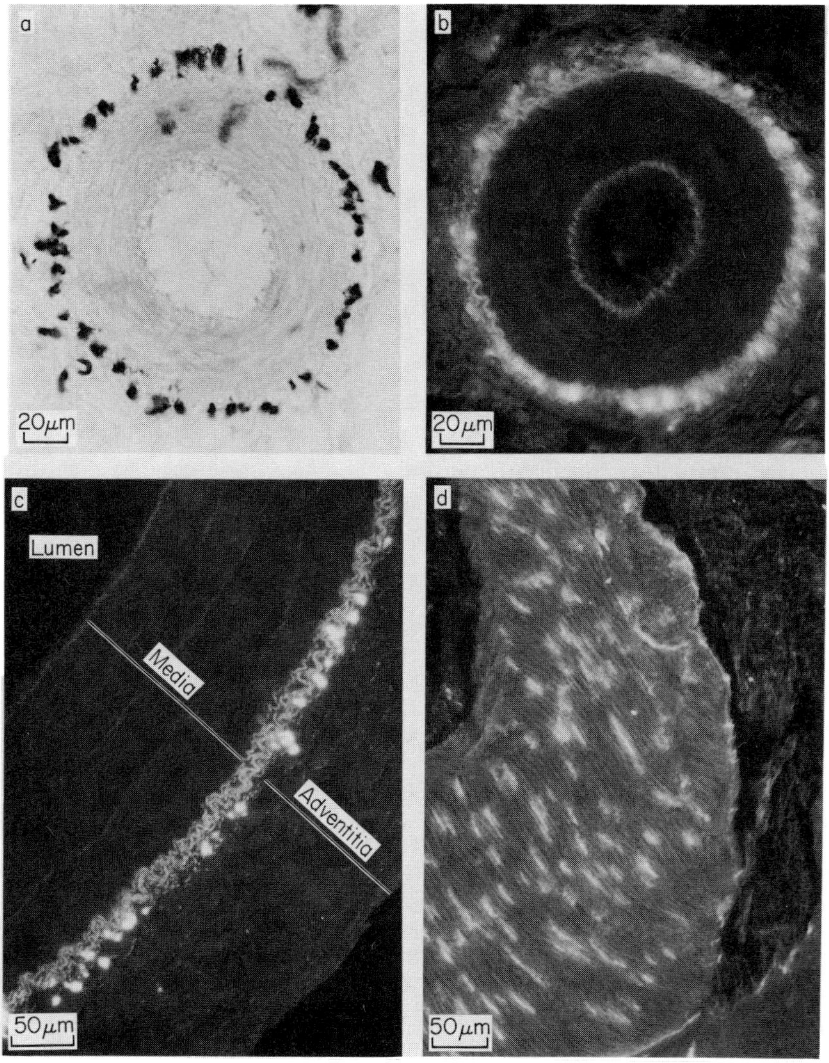

Fig. 18. (*a*) Arteriole showing acetylcholinesterase-positive (black) nerves in the adventitia. None enters the muscular tunica media. (*b*) Arteriole, adjacent section to the one shown in (*a*), with fluorescent noradrenergic nerves restricted to the adventitia. (*c*) Femoral artery (domestic fowl). Noradrenergic nerves (bright fluorescent dots) are outside (to the right of) the outer elastic lamina. There are no nerves within the tunica media. (*d*) Caudal vena cava with noradrenergic (postganglionic sympathetic) nerves distributed throughout the entire muscular layer.

part of the mammalian circle of Willis) and which is surrounded by the cavernous sinus. In the resting domestic fowl the temperature of the hypothalamus is normally about 1°C below that of the deep body cavity (Scott and van Tienhoven, 1971). It has been suggested by Richards (1970a) that cool blood returning from the skin of the head and the nasal cavities to the cavernous sinus may be responsible for cooling the arterial blood which flows from the intercarotid anastomosis to the hypothalamus. A second possible site for heat exchange between arterial blood flowing to the brain and cooled venous blood, is the vascular rete (Fig. 16) on the external ophthalmic branch of the internal carotid artery (Richards, 1970b; Kilgore and Boggs, 1976; Kilgore *et al.*, 1979; Pettit *et al.*, 1981). The importance of the ophthalmic rete in pigeons, in this respect, has been demonstrated by blocking the arterial branches which supply it. When this is done, the hypothalamic temperature rises slightly (0·36°C) above deep body temperature instead of being about 1°C below it.

Any increase in hypothalamic temperature resulting from greater metabolic heat production or an increased environmental temperature, will stimulate regulatory mechanisms which get rid of surplus heat. The most important of these for the bird in a high environmental temperature, where loss of heat by conduction, convection and radiation is ineffective, is by panting. The relationship between panting and blood flow to the upper respiratory tract (trachea, larynx, pharynx and mouth) has been demonstrated in the duck by Beck and Johansen (1980). In panting there is a 10 to 20 times increase in the rate of (rather shallow) respiration, as a result of which considerable quantities of water are evaporated from the mucous membranes lining the upper respiratory tract. To provide this water for evaporation, blood flow to the region is more than doubled (measured in the carotid artery), whilst blood to some other parts of the body (measured in the ischiadic artery) is reduced

Under less extreme conditions, loss of surplus heat occurs without the need for evaporative cooling, by increasing the blood flow to, and thus the heat loss from, those parts of the body which are not feathered. Whilst this includes the comb and wattles (Whittow *et al.*, 1964; Fujii *et al.*, 1979), the legs are more important. Indeed a bird which is panting in a high ambient temperature, will stop panting immediately its legs are cooled. A practical illustration of this is provided by storks which urinate on to their long legs so that they may be cooled by evaporation of the water in the urine. Underlying all these procedures are important adjustments to the blood flow in the legs. They include the nervous control of vascular shunts, a heat exchange system in the vascular rete at the lower end of the tibiotarsus and adjustments to the blood flow in the feet, particularly in birds with webbed feet which habitually spend long periods of time standing in water. The Glaucous-winged Gull in a cold environment (−16°C) maintains a marked temperature gradient in its legs, by operating a heat exchange at its tibiotarsal rete: temperatures of 37·8°C at the top, 7°C in the middle and 0 to 4°C at the bottom of the leg have been recorded (Irving and Krog, 1955). A similar mechanism exists in the mallard (Midtgard, 1980). When these birds wish to eliminate surplus heat, vascular shunts bypass the tibiotarsal rete and a large flow of blood (far greater than its metabolic requirements) enters the legs to dissipate heat *via* the superficial vessels in the feet and lower part of the legs. To conserve heat vasoconstriction greatly reduces the flow to the legs. The bulk of the blood that does enter the legs passes through the heat exchanger at the tibiotarsal rete thus permitting the arterial blood to transfer much of its heat to the returning venous blood. That part of the cranial tibial artery which constitutes the arterial shunt was found to have a thicker muscular wall and greater noradrenergic innervation than did the rest of this vessel. No sphincter-like adaptation was found in the venous shunt but it also received a greater noradrenergic innervation than did other parts of the same vein.

Radiant heating, which was restricted to the head of pigeons, caused a rapid increase in blood flow to the feet, which reached a temperature about 12°C above that of the environmental air (25°C), so that heat loss could occur by convection, conduction and radiation. In the absence of artificial heating (of the head) foot and air temperatures were the same. These responses were unaffected by systemic cholinergic blockade and so were assumed to have been caused by noradrenergic sympathetic neurones (Bernstein, 1974).

When a bird's requirement is to conserve maximum heat (e.g. when standing on ice) the intense vasoconstriction which minimizes blood flow to the lower part of the legs must not be so prolonged as to cause frostbite, for this reason the vasoconstriction is released at intervals and then reapplied (Johansen and Tonnesen, 1969). This protective cold-induced vasodilatation has been observed in several species, including man (Brown and Page, 1952) and the domestic fowl (Grant and Bland, 1931). There can be no doubt that vasomotor adjustments to blood flow in the legs of all birds (Steen and Steen, 1965) are of supreme importance in thermoregulation and will always be employed so long as an adequate heat gradient can be maintained between the skin and the surrounding air. However, when the ambient temperature rises to about that of the body, evaporative cooling by panting becomes inevitable.

XVI. Lung

There are several important differences between the respiratory systems of birds and mammals and they have a direct influence on blood flow to the lungs. Because birds lack a mammalian-type muscular diaphragm, respiratory movements in birds cause pressure changes which are simultaneously uniform throughout the entire body cavity. There can be no "waterfall effect" between abdomen and thorax in the venous return to the heart in birds (Folkow and Neil, 1971).

Outside the avian lungs is a series of air sacs which act like bellows. The cranial sacs are mainly concerned with "driving" inspiration (intercostal muscles), thus sucking air through the lungs. Stale air enters the expanding cranial sacs from the lung, and fresh air, as well as passing through the lungs, enters the expanding caudal sacs. The caudal sacs are mainly concerned with "driving" expiration (abdominal muscles). Thanks to a complicated routing system the fresh air stored in the caudal sacs passes into the lungs by the same route that was followed by fresh air during inspiration. This means that during both inspiration and expiration a stream of fresh air passes through the lungs, in the same direction (caudocranial), providing a continuous, unidirectional flow along the tertiary bronchi.

Essentially, an avian lung consists of a large number of tertiary bronchi (about 1 mm in diameter in the fowl) along the hollow centres of which passes a current of air. Surrounding the central lumen and connected to it is a very large number of closely packed pouches (diameter about 100 μm), which in turn connect with a mass of air capillaries (diameter about 6 μm). The air capillaries spread outwards towards the periphery of the tertiary bronchus forming a three-dimensional mesh. This means that a mass of intercommunicating air capillaries forms a continuous plexus in the wall of every tertiary bronchus. Oxygen perfuses peripherally from the central lumen along which a unidirectional flow of air is maintained (Fig. 19).

Running in between the tertiary bronchi are branches of the pulmonary artery and vein. At intervals the pulmonary artery gives off terminal branches which spread out over the peripheral surface of the tertiary bronchi (Fig. 20). Each branch supplies a limited zone of those tertiary bronchi which lie within its reach. These vessels (about 15 μm in diameter) give rise to blood capillaries (diameter about 6 μm) which form a plexus throughout the tertiary bronchial wall and along its length (Akester, 1975).

Immediately outside the central airway of the tertiary bronchus, at the level of the air pouches, the blood capillaries drain into the first rudiments of the pulmonary veins (Figs 19a, 20b,c). These pass through the capillary zone to the periphery of the tertiary bronchus, where they drain into larger branches. These drain oxygenated blood from all parts of the lung into a single large pulmonary vein which leaves the lung at the hilus in close association with the primary bronchus. This vessel, from each lung, unites immediately above the left atrium and a large single vessel enters its roof (Fig. 5b).

A mesh of blood capillaries interlocks with that of the air capillaries in a most intimate way so that a capillary zone, occupying about half the thickness of the wall spreads along every tertiary bronchus. This zone constitutes the gaseous exchange surface of the lung. When seen under the electron micro-

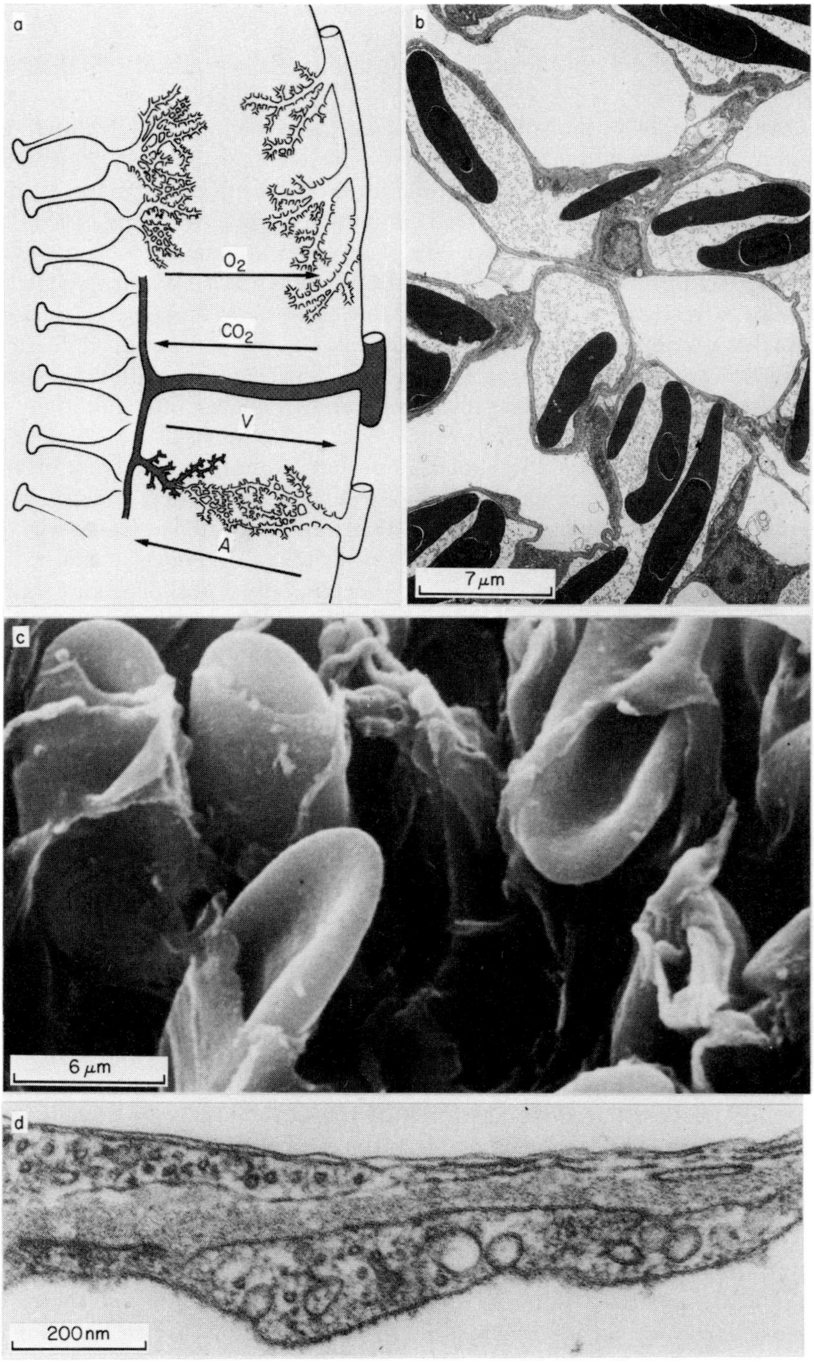
a
O_2
CO_2
V
A
b
7 μm
c
6 μm
d
200 nm

scope the extreme delicacy of the inter-locking capillary plexuses becomes apparent (Fig. 19b). There is virtually no collagenous support tissue amongst the capillaries and only a tenuous basement membrane (60 to 80 nm wide) lies between blood capillary endothelium (80 nm thick) and air capillary epithelium (40 nm thick). This constitutes the diffusion barrier and the distance between red blood cells and air capillary lumen is about 200 nm. The comparable barrier in man is said to be about 350 nm (Weibel, 1972).

Pulmonary blood capillaries (diameter 6 μm) are amongst the smallest in the body and several times smaller than those in the kidneys and liver. This might be expected as it is desirable for the haemoglobin in the red cells to come as close as possible to the oxygen in the air capillaries, thus minimizing the diffusion distance. In fact, the capillaries are so narrow that red cells are forced into single file and are even rolled up sideways in order to pass through (Akester, 1974). This raises an interesting point about the flow of cells and plasma. In large vessels the haematocrit is about 40%, so that 60% of the total blood volume is occupied by plasma. Scanning electronmicrographs suggest that, in the pulmonary capillaries, the rolled up and overlapping red cells occupy at least 60% of the available volume (Fig. 19c). Plasma is therefore confined to a narrow film between red cells and endothelial cells and to what is left of the groove on the inner aspect of each red cell, which is already partly filled by the overlap of the red cell immediately behind. This means, either that the electronmicrograph is misleading, or that plasma flows along the capillaries faster than red cells, or that there are preferential channels which only carry plasma. The third possibility has never been demonstrated. A blend of the first and second is most likely.

There has been much discussion as to whether blood and air flow in the avian lung is counter-current or not. At first sight, with blood obviously flowing in one direction and the unidirectional flow of air experimentally established (Bouverot and Dejours, 1971; Brackenbury, 1971; Bretz and

---

Fig. 19. (*a*) To illustrate what happens in the capillary zone of a tertiary bronchus. Air enters the pouches (ostia) at left. O_2 diffuses peripherally through air capillaries. Deoxygenated blood is delivered by pulmonary artery (white) at periphery and flows centrally through blood capillary plexus (A). CO_2 diffuses centrally through air capillaries. Oxygenated blood is collected by venules at base of pouches and passes through capillary zone (V) to periphery of tertiary bronchus. (*b*) Stained section transmission EM of part of capillary zone. Shows interlocking blood and air capillaries. (*c*) Red blood cells rolled up sideways to pass through very small blood capillaries. (From Akester, 1974, with permission.) (*d*) Diffusion barrier consists of blood capillary endothelium (below) and air capillary epithelium (above) with a small amount of basement membrane between them. (Endothelium about 80 nm thick; epithelium about 40 nm thick; basement membrane about 60 nm; total barrier may be less than 200 nm.)

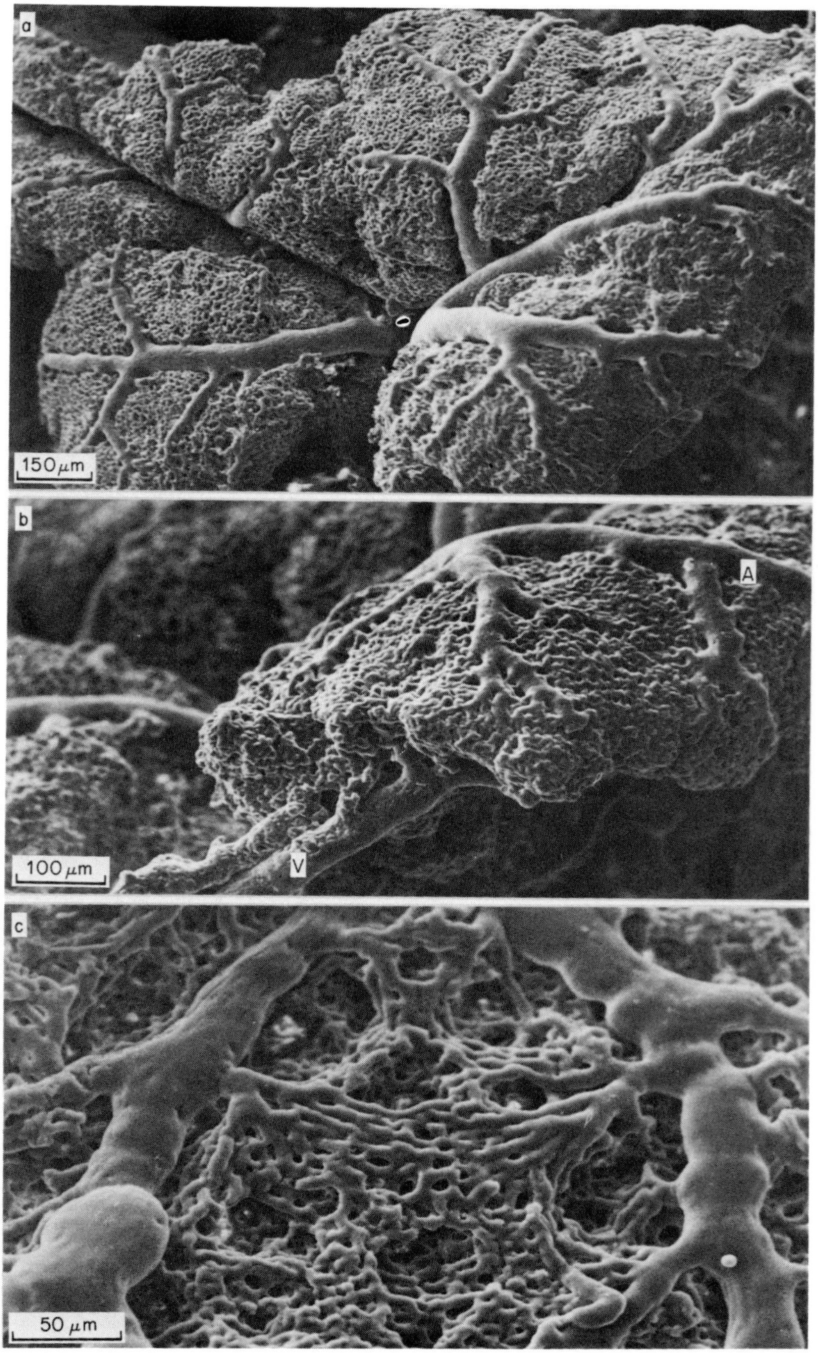

a
150 μm
b
A
V
100 μm
c
50 μm

Schmidt-Nielsen, 1971; Scheid and Piiper, 1971) it was tempting to assume that there was a counter current relationship (Schmidt-Neilsen, 1971). However, a consideration of the way in which the air and blood capillary plexuses interlock should make it obvious that neither could run counter to the other for a distance much greater than about twice their own diameter, so frequent is their branching. On anatomical grounds counter-current and co-current relationships are out of the question. A cross-current system is the only one that could exist. This was shown by Scheid and Piiper (1972), who measured the oxygen loading of the blood during uni-directional ventilation of the lung (air entered by the trachea and left by the posterior thoracic air sac). In this situation, air flowed through the tertiary bronchi of the lung in a caudocranial direction (as normal). They then blocked the primary bronchus by inflating a small balloon at a point between the connections of anterior and posterior groups of secondary bronchi. Air was no longer able to flow along the primary bronchus to enter the tertiary bronchi via the posterior group of secondary bronchi, instead, it entered by the anterior group and left by the posterior group and thus flowed through the tertiary bronchi in a cranio-caudal direction (opposite to normal). However, although they had reversed the direction of air flow in the tertiary bronchi, and obviously the direction of blood flow had remained the same, there was no difference in the oxygenation of the blood. The effective relationship between blood and air flow in the wall of the tertiary bronchi is cross-current, in spite of various claims to the contrary (Abdalla and King, 1975).

All major tissues of the body require a supply of oxygenated blood and the lungs are no exception. In the mammal, a broncho-oesophageal artery leaves the right fifth intercostal artery, a branch from which sends a bronchial artery into each lung. In birds, a broncho-oesophageal artery branches from the base of the right common carotid artery. As it runs towards the lungs it gives off branches to the oesophagus and syrinx, behind which it divides into left and right bronchial arteries.

In the domestic fowl, each bronchial artery becomes closely associated with its own primary bronchus, around which it forms a vascular plexus. Venous drainage from this plexus is by way of an oesophageal vein. At the hilus of the lung the bronchial artery anastomoses with the pulmonary artery. Apparently, the intrapulmonary part of the primary bronchus in the fowl does not receive a

---

Fig. 20. Scanning electronmicrographs of the pulmonary circulation. (*a*) Latex cast of pulmonary artery. Terminal branches arching over parts of adjacent tertiary bronchi. (*b*) Latex cast of part of capillary zone in wall of tertiary bronchus. Terminal branch of pulmonary artery (A) delivers blood at periphery (top). Rudiment of pulmonary vein (V) collects blood near centre (bottom). (*c*) Blood capillaries draining into first rudiments of pulmonary vein. (Reproduced from Akester, 1975, by permission.)

blood supply from the bronchial artery, but from the pulmonary artery instead. Drainage of this blood is by the pulmonary veins (Abdalla and King, 1976a). One can only assume that there is sufficient oxygen left in the pulmonary arterial (venous) blood for the limited metabolic requirements of the primary bronchus. There may even be a very small diffusion of oxygen directly through the epithelium.

The possibility has been raised (Abdalla and King, 1976b) that the direction of blood flow in the bronchial artery may be from pulmonary artery (pressure about 25 mmHg) to common carotid (pressure about 145 mmHg). In view of these pressure differences, this possibility might be hard to accept. However, it has received some support from experiments with isotope-labelled microspheres (diameter 15 ± 5 μm). These were injected into the brachial vein, and most were presumed to be too big to pass through pulmonary capillaries. About 0·3% of the total (i.e. the smallest) did pass through the lungs and reached kidney, spleen and brain, but 0·6% of the total was found in the extra-pulmonary primary bronchial vessels (plexus from bronchial artery). This indicated a perfusion (of microspheres) per gram of primary bronchial tissue two hundred times greater than that received by kidney, spleen or brain (Parry and Yates, 1978).

In some species (goose, duck, turkey), the broncho-oesophageal artery arises symmetrically from both common carotids, and supplies the entire length of the primary bronchus. However, venous drainage resembles the fowl. The extrapulmonary part drains to the oesophageal vein, whilst the intrapulmonary part drains to the pulmonary veins. Small anastomoses were found between bronchial and pulmonary arteries (Abdalla and King, 1977).

Burger and Estavillo (1977) have demonstrated veno-venous anastomoses between the pulmonary (presumably venous) and systemic venous systems. Ligation of the main pulmonary artery and vein entering and leaving a lung might have been expected to isolate the lung from the systemic circulation. It did not. Indian ink injected into the lung by way of the ligated pulmonary artery reached all parts of the animal, even though it could not leave the lung by the pulmonary vein. The anastomoses were also demonstrated in reverse. With pulmonary artery and vein still ligated, a systemic injection of indian ink reached the "isolated" lung. The anastomoses were shown to be small but numerous, between the pulmonary veins and vertebral venous sinuses and also with intercostal veins. No adequate explanation for this has yet been offered, nor has it been clarified in which direction the blood normally flows. Could it be a method of protecting the left side of the heart? If too much blood is returning to the left atrium, perhaps some of it could be shunted into systemic veins.

The efficiency of respiration in a bird depends on the total surface area which is available for gaseous exchange between the red blood cells and the lumen of the air capillaries. Surprisingly, few attempts have been made to measure this area. One of them (Akester and Brackenbury, 1977; Brackenbury and Akester, 1978) was based on the ultrastructural appearance of the interwoven blood and air capillary plexuses which comprise the bulk of the capillary zone in the wall of every tertiary bronchus (Fig. 19b). The zone is remarkably uniform with blood and air capillaries of more or less equal size. In an attempt to provide a basis for calculating the total surface area, it was suggested that each capillary plexus (because of the frequency of its three-dimensional branching) could be regarded as consisting of a basic repetitive unit, like a six-pointed star (Fig. 21c–e), made up from seven hollow cubic sub-units. Obviously capillaries have a rounded and not a square cross-section, but the square was chosen for convenience and had no influence on the general calculation. The six-pointed star was only intended to be a generalization. Some could be four or five-pointed and would easily fit into a six-pointed system.

An adult chicken's lung contains about 500 tertiary bronchi each about 2 cm long and 1 mm diameter (branching was ignored). As the capillary zone was about 200 μm wide its internal diameter would be 600 μm ($1000 - 200 \times 2$). With an external diameter of 1000 μm the mean diameter would be 800 μm. Each tertiary bronchus was then cut (notionally) along its length to form a slab of exchange tissue with a quadrilateral cross section (Fig. 21a). By transferring the triangular strip from one side to the other, the cross section became rectangular. To calculate the area of exchange surface (capillary wall) the slab of tissue was divided into sections 6 μm thick (the diameter of the capillaries) along three series of parallel planes intersecting each other at right angles. These are represented by A–A, B–B, C–C in Fig. 21b. Each of these many planes would be a chequer board of (blood and air) capillary walls (black) and (blood and air) capillary lumens (white). These areas would be arranged in such a way that where the plane of the wall was indicated in black the adjacent white part of the plane would indicate a transverse section through a (blood or air) capillary lumen (Fig. 21c). The direction of blood or air flow within this lumen would be at right angles to this plane. This showed that half the total area of each plane was occupied by capillary wall and half by capillary lumen.

When a vascular "six-pointed hollow star" is interlocked with an air capillary "hollow star" an arrangement like that shown in Fig. 21d would occur. Theoretically, the route that red blood cells might take through such a mesh could either be almost infinitely tortuous (route B in Fig. 21e) or almost direct along a series of near parallel tubes (route A in Fig. 21e). However, in reality the mesh would be distorted, so that the theoretically direct channels would themselves be tortuous.

The total surface area of each series of planes parallel to A–A, B–B, or C–C

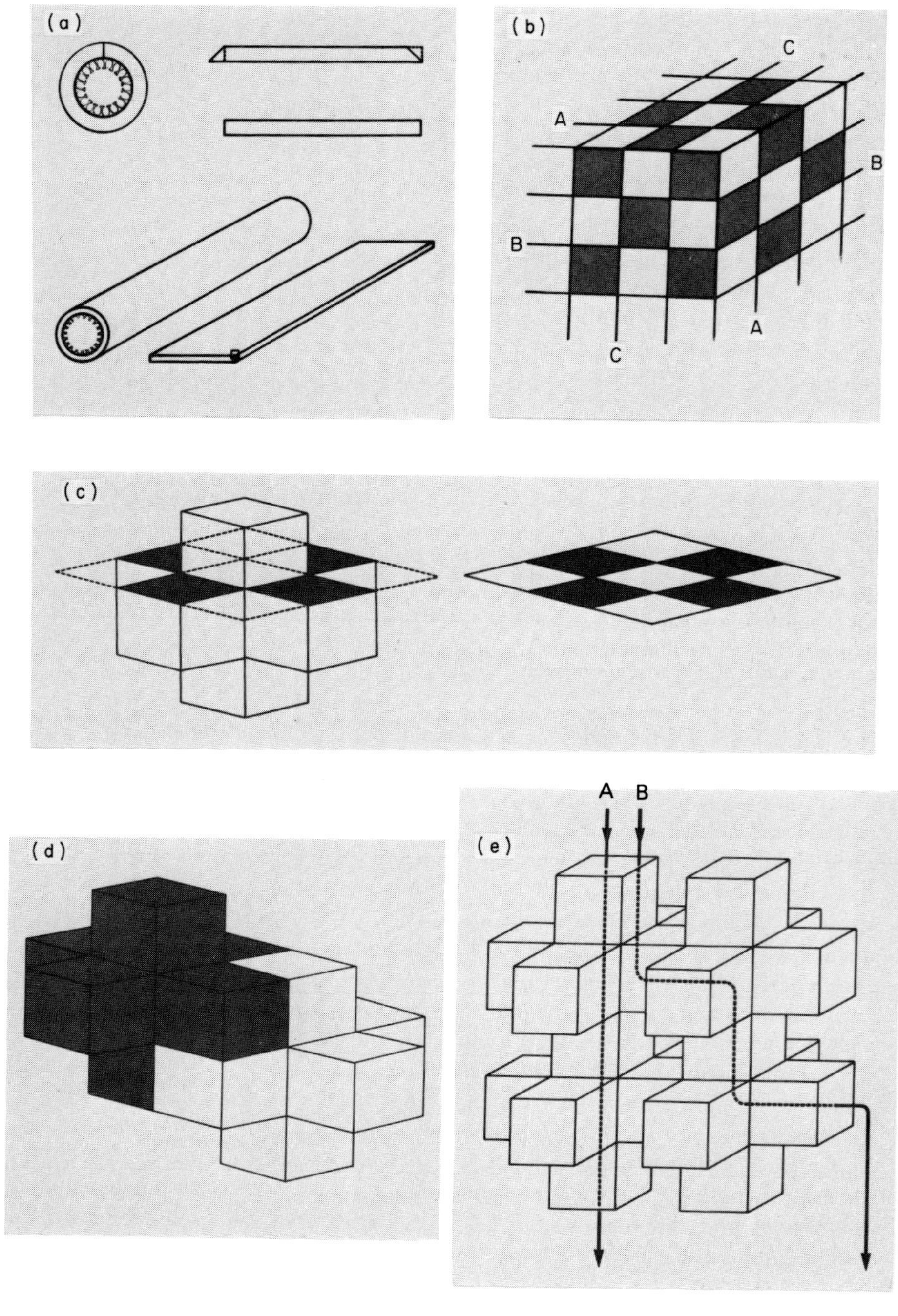

(a)
(b)
C
A
B
B
A
C
(c)
(d)
A
B
(e)

in Fig. 21b throughout the entire slab of exchange tissue in a single tertiary bronchus was 16·7 cm^2 or 50 cm^2 for all three series of planes added together. With only half of this area devoted to capillary wall (where gaseous exchange would take place) and with 500 tertiary bronchi in each lung, the total area of exchange surface (capillary wall) would be about 2·5 cm^2. In a 2·3-kg fowl this gave about 11 cm^2 g^{-1} body tissue, which was less than the 17·9 cm^2 g^{-1} proposed by Duncker (1972) but similar to that of 12·8 cm^2 g^{-1} (90 m^2 for 70-kg man) estimated for the human (Weibel, 1972).

It is quite possible that the lung of a 2·3-kg fowl is no larger than that of a 2-kg bird. The extra weight simply being due to fat or muscle. By applying the general calculation outlined above to a 2-kg fowl a figure of 14 cm^2 g^{-1} body tissue is obtained. Birds may have a somewhat greater gaseous exchange area per unit weight of body tissue than mammals, but more accurate measurements are required to prove it.

Fig. 21. An interpretation of the capillary zone in a tertiary bronchus and a suggested method of calculating the surface area available for gaseous exchange. (From Brackenbury and Akester, 1978, with permission). (*a*) The capillary zone occupies that part of the tertiary bronchus which lies between the base of the pouches and the periphery. It is about 200 μm wide. The external diameter of the tertiary bronchus is about 1 mm. The internal diameter of the capillary zone is thus 600 μm (1000–200 × 2). The mean diameter is, therefore, about 800 μm. Because the internal diameter of the capillary zone is less than the outside diameter, when the tertiary bronchus is (notionally) cut open along its (2 cm) length and laid out flat, the capillary zone would have a quadrilateral cross-section. By transposing a triangular strip from one side to the other, the cross section would become rectangular. (*b*) To illustrate how the entire capillary zone could be cut into three series of planes (A-A, B-B, C-C) 6 μm apart (the capillary diameter), each series being at right angles to the other two. The part illustrated here is the small corner of the slab of capillary zone in (*a*). The total surface area of the series of planes parallel to A-A is the same as the area of the series parallel to B-B and also to the area of the series parallel to C-C. Black represents (blood or air) capillary wall. White represents (blood or air) capillary lumen. Half of each plane is occupied by capillary wall and half by capillary lumen. The direction of (blood or air) flow in the white areas would be at right angles to the plane of the (blood or air) capillary wall (black). (*c*) To show how the proposed basic unit, represented by a six-pointed hollow star, fits into the concept of cutting the exchange tissue into 6 μm thick slices to provide equal area of capillary wall (black) and capillary lumen (white). (*d*) A six-pointed hollow star (black) representing the basic unit of the blood capillary plexus, interlocking with a similar unit (white) representing the basic unit of the air capillary plexus. (*e*) Four basic units of the same type (blood or air) linked together. Theoretically the fluid (blood or air) could take a direct route "A" or a tortuous route "B". In reality, the theoretical precision of the model would be distorted so that all routes taken by blood and air through the capillary zone would be tortuous and so would resemble route "B".

XVII. Kidney

There can be no doubt that the blood supply to the avian kidney provides one of the most complicated vascular situations of any organ in any vertebrate. This complication, which is poorly understood, is due largely to the existence of a renal portal system. A renal portal system is a fundamental feature of the vertebrates, being present in fish, amphibians, reptiles, birds and in the mesonephros of embryonic, but not adult, mammals (Mossman, 1948). Whilst it is present in birds, they are the only group known to be able to switch it on or off, but the circumstances under which this happens remain almost a complete mystery (Akester, 1967).

Venous blood is collected from both hind limbs, pelvis, tail and caudal part of the gut (colorectum and cloaca) and is delivered to the kidneys as renal portal blood. The main source of this blood is most likely to be the musculature of the hind legs (Fig. 22a). Renal portal blood (when it enters kidney tissue) is applied to the proximal and distal tubules of all the nephrons but not to the glomeruli. Avian glomeruli only receive arterial blood (which is obviously a pre-requisite for ultrafiltration), but the capillaries (or sinusoids) which are associated with the proximal and distal tubules carry both postglomerular (arterial) and renal portal (venous) blood (Fig. 23b–e).

Renal plasma flow (RPF) is about 40 ml kg^{-1} min^{-1} (Skadhauge, 1964). However, the RPF will consist of both arterial and renal portal venous blood, and whilst these two sources of blood are independently variable, they are not independently measurable by this technique.

Fig. 22. (*a*) Principal veins associated with the avian kidneys: EIV, external iliac vein; CaRPV, caudal renal portal vein; CrRPV, cranial renal portal vein; RV, renal vein; CMV, coccygeomesenteric vein; VVS, vertebral venous sinuses; PVC, posterior vena cava. (*b*) Radiograph of simultaneous injection of 1·5 ml radiopaque dye into each external iliac vein. Radiopaque blood enters all lobes of each kidney via caudal and cranial renal portal veins. Some of the blood by-passes the kidney via the open renal portal valve and also via the cranial renal portal vein and the vertebral venous sinuses. This was the experimental justification for (*c*) V. (*c*) Different patterns of blood flow through the kidneys, demonstrated by injecting radiopaque dye into both external iliac veins. Each of these is different, but in every case left and right kidneys are the same. On about 25% of cases blood flow through one kidney was different from that through the other (not illustrated) (*d*) Different routes by which blood can by-pass the kidneys: (1) through open renal portal valve and posterior vena cava; (2) via caudal renal portal vein and coccygeomesenteric vein to liver; (3) via cranial renal portal vein and vertebral venous sinuses to right jugular vein and right anterior vena cava. (*e*) Renal portal valve (longitudinal section). Treated with paraformaldehyde to induce fluorescence in catecholamines. Note intense innervation of fluorescent noradrenergic nerves. (*f*) Isolated renal portal valve. (*a–d*) from Akester, 1967; (*e*) from Akester and Mann, 1969, with permission.

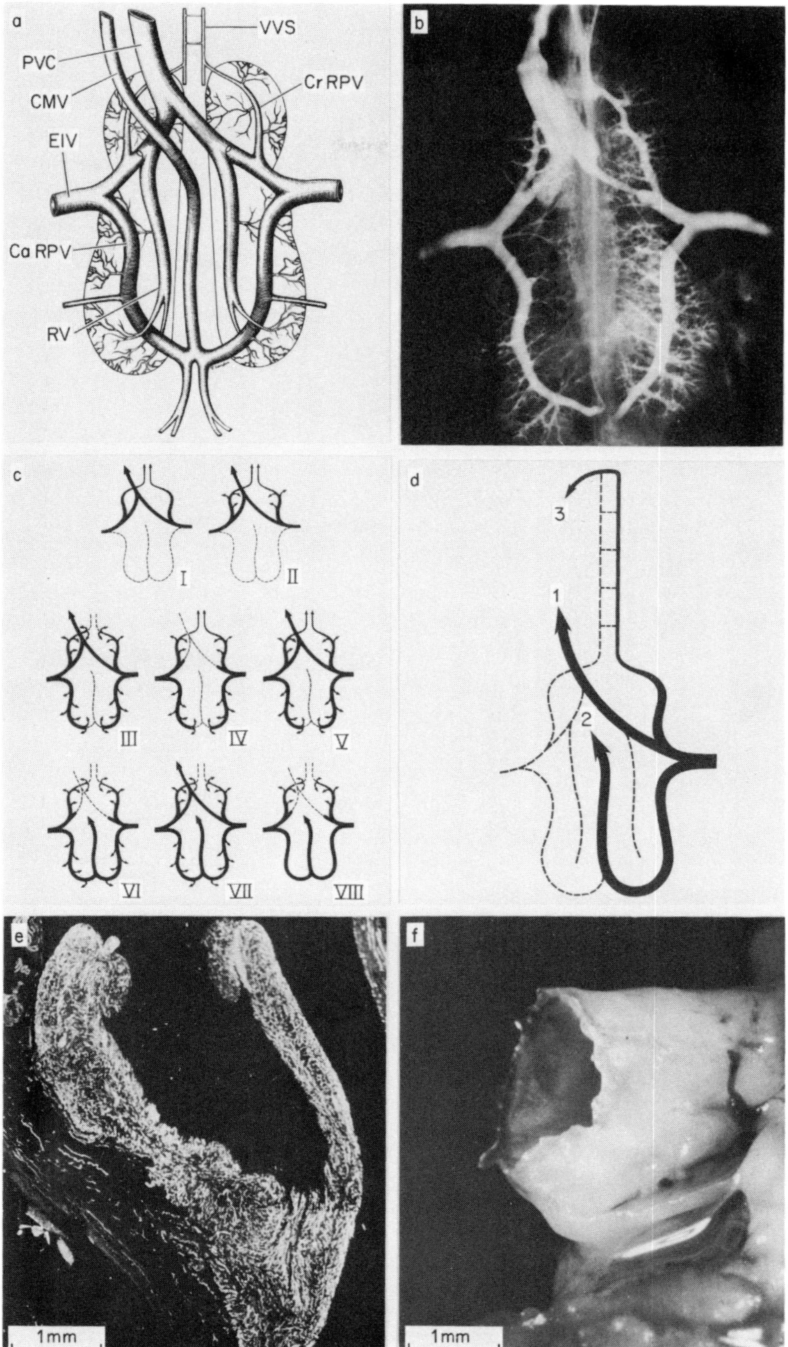
a
VVS
PVC
Cr RPV
CMV
EIV
Ca RPV
RV
b
c
I
II
III
IV
V
VI
VII
VIII
d
3
1
2
e
1mm
f
1mm

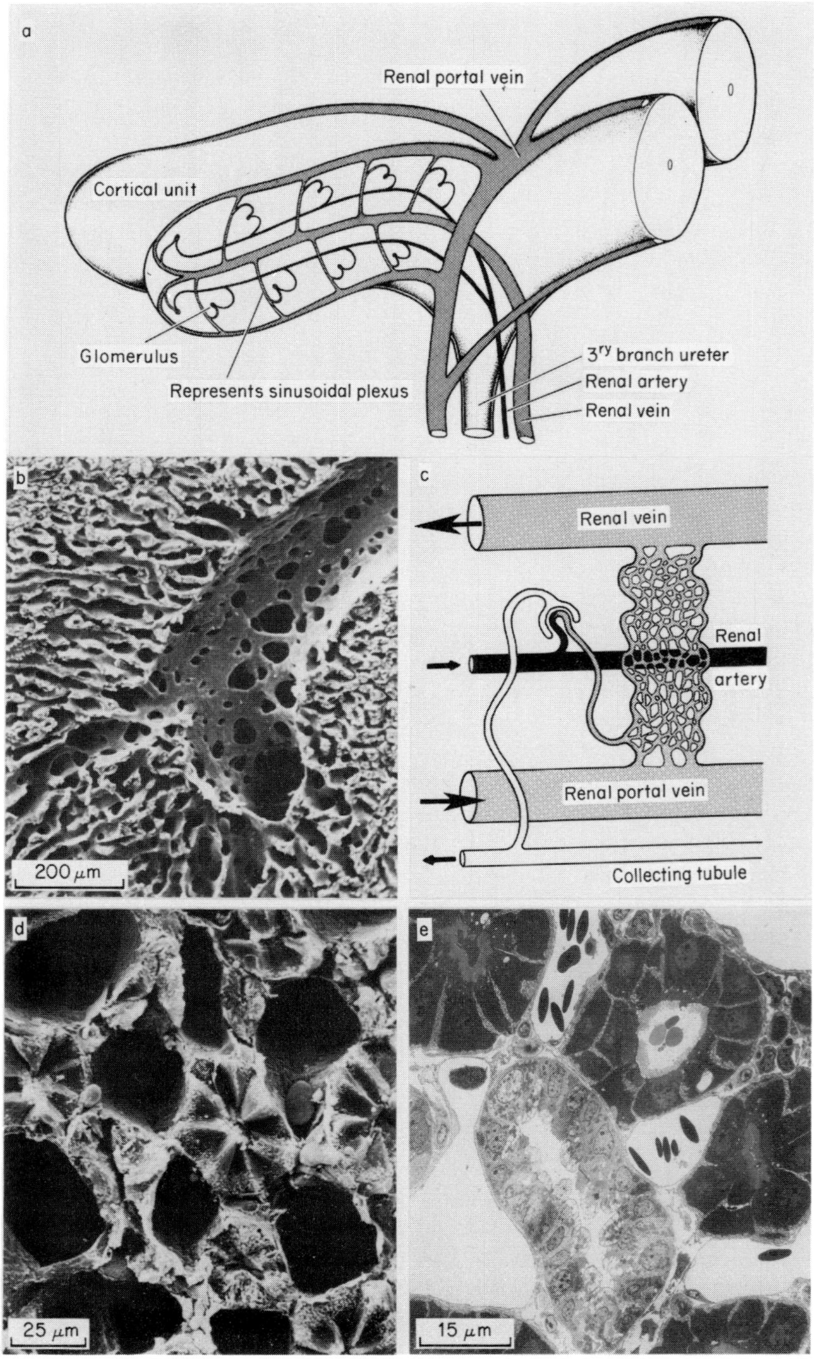
a
Renal portal vein
Cortical unit
Glomerulus
Represents sinusoidal plexus
3ry branch ureter
Renal artery
Renal vein
b
200 μm
c
Renal vein
Renal
artery
Renal portal vein
Collecting tubule
d
25 μm
e
15 μm

The relationship between blood capillaries and nephron tubules in the kidney (Fig. 23d,e) is very similar to that between blood sinusoids and cords of hepatocytes in the liver. Both capillaries and sinusoids are the smallest blood vessels in their respective organs, and both have a lumen diameter of about 30 μm. In each organ, the smallest blood vessels form a three-dimensional mesh which interlocks with a similar mesh of branching and anastomosing tubules (kidney) or hepatocyte cords (liver). The similarity can be taken further and includes the interlocking meshes of blood and air capillaries in the lung (Fig. 19b). However, lung capillaries are amongst the smallest in the body (diameter 6 μm), whilst those in the liver and kidney are amongst the largest. It would be better if the liver and kidney vessels were both called sinusoids. A renal artery enters the cranial division of each kidney directly from the aorta. The middle and caudal divisions of the kidney receive their arterial blood by renal branches from the ischiadic artery, which supplies the hind limb (Fig. 15).

It is essential to be clear about the lay-out of all the veins associated with the kidneys before one can appreciate their functional role (Fig. 22a). A large vein (external iliac), draining most of the blood from the hind limb, approaches the lateral border of each kidney where it bifurcates. The caudally directed branch passes through the middle and caudal divisions of the kidney and anastomoses with its counterpart from the other side immediately behind the kidneys. This vessel is the caudal renal portal vein and as it passes through the kidney gives off branches which penetrate the tissue. The cranially directed branch continues on the ventral surface of the kidney and gives off a major branch to the cranial division of the kidney. This is the cranial renal portal vein, branches, from which enter the tissue of the cranial division. The parent vessel finally unites with the vertebral venous sinuses. The caudal renal portal veins are also joined by the coccygeomesenteric vein, so there is a three-way anastomosis of large veins immediately caudal to the kidneys.

The external iliac vein merges with the renal vein and the resultant vein is called the common iliac. These veins, from each side, unite to form the

---

Fig. 23. (*a*) Blood supply to cortical units of kidney lobule. Renal portal blood is delivered at the periphery, flows through the sinusoids and is collected by the central vein of each cortical unit. Arteries (black) supply glomeruli. (*b*) Central vein of cortical unit with associated sinusoids as shown in a scanning electronmicrograph. The "walls" of the sinusoids are the tubules. (*c*) Detail of blood flow through cortical unit. Sinusoids (only small part shown) connect peripheral branch of renal portal vein to central rudiment of renal vein. Artery (black) supplies glomeruli. Efferent arteriole joins sinusoids at periphery. Distal tubule of nephron connects with peripheral collecting tubule (white). (*d*) Mesh of sinusoids interlock with proximal tubules. Sinusoids (black) and tubules are approximately the same size. (*e*) Sinusoids (white) amongst proximal and distal tubules.

posterior vena cava which runs along the dorsal edge of the liver to the right atrium (Figs 17a, 22a). Within the external iliac vein, just before it unites with the renal vein, is a unique valve (Fig. 22f). Excluding the heart, the renal portal valve is the only intravascular smooth muscle valve known throughout the vertebrates. It varies slightly in appearance from one species to another and also between different individuals, but in the fowl it is usually a short sleeve-like structure with some degree of papillation around the aperture. It is heavily innervated by noradrenergic (postganglionic sympathetic) and also by acetylcholinesterase-positive (presumed parasympathetic) nerves (Fig. 22e) (Akester and Mann, 1969). Acetylcholine causes the valve to contract (close), whilst noradrenaline causes the contracted valve to relax (open) (Rennick and Gandia, 1954).

Whilst Sperber (1949) was the first to show that the renal portal system was active, Akester (1964, 1969) demonstrated the complexity of the renal portal system to blood flowing into it. By injecting a radiopaque dye into the external iliac vein, or (preferably) one of its tributaries, a great variety of vascular flow patterns was shown to occur in the kidneys of the healthy, anaesthetized adult fowl lying on its back or side (Fig. 22c). At one extreme, all the potentially renal portal blood was seen to enter kidney tissue, traverse the sinusoids and leave by way of the renal veins. At the other extreme, none of this blood entered the kidney, but by-passed it instead, using one or other of the following three routes: (i) via the open renal portal valve and posterior vena cava; (ii) via the caudal renal portal vein and coccygeomesenteric vein to the hepatic portal vein and liver; and (iii) via the cranial renal portal vein and vertebral venous sinuses to the right jugular vein and anterior vena cava (Fig. 22d). The most common arrangement seemed to be for the shunts to operate partially, so that a variable proportion of renal portal blood by-passed the kidney, whilst the remainder entered the sinusoids. An extremely versatile system has thus evolved. The by-pass route involving the coccygeomesenteric vein is particular interesting as it means that potentially renal portal blood can be diverted to the liver, although the circumstances under which this may happen are not understood. There is a further complication in that the coccygeomesenteric vein appears to be able to reverse its flow and, on occasions, carry potentially hepatic portal blood to the kidneys (Akester, 1967; Purton, 1970).

These findings have been confirmed by Shimada and Sturkie (1973), who made direct, continuous recordings of blood flow in the coccygeomesenteric vein and in the posterior vena cava. With an electromagnetic flowmeter placed at the centre of the coccygeomesenteric vein, out of a total of 36 recordings, 23 showed a flow towards the kidneys and 13 showed a flow towards the liver. Blood flow in the posterior vena cava, just before the heart was about 222 ml min^{-1}.

It might seem reasonable to assume that two similar organs like the kidneys would receive the same pattern of blood flow at the same time. Whilst this did appear to happen on most occasions, on about 25% of other occasions the experimental flow through one kidney was totally different from that through the other (Akester, 1967).

In some respects, avian kidneys can be regarded as being predominantly of a reptilian type, with a small amount of mammalian-type tissue "grafted on". The cortex contains reptilian-type nephrons with small glomeruli (40 μm diameter), has no loops of Henle and does not have the ability to create an osmotic gradient by counter-current osmotic multiplication. The cortex is subdivided into roughly cylindrical units, each one of which contains a single, large central vein (first rudiment of renal vein), whilst terminal branches of the renal portal vein are distributed around the periphery. The peripheral veins are connected to the central vein by a three-dimensional plexus of sinusoids which interlock with a similar mesh made of (proximal and distal) nephron tubules (Figs 23b–e). Terminal branches of the renal arteries lie between the peripheral and central veins and send afferent arterioles into the small cortical (reptilian-type) glomeruli. Only two or three capillaries are contained in these glomeruli (Figs 24a–c). They have been seen to branch or anastomose (A. R. Akester, unpublished) and closely resemble their mammalian counterparts, being fenestrated and associated with a thick basement membrane, on the other side of which are placed the pedicels of the podocytes which constitute the visceral layer of the glomerular capsule (Figs 24d–f).

Efferent arterioles leave the glomeruli, pass to the periphery of the cortical unit, and join the plexus of sinusoids which connect the peripheral branches of the renal portal vein to the central branch of the renal vein. Blood in the sinusoids is thus mixed renal portal (venous) and postglomerular (arterial), and is directed centrally as it flows around the proximal and distal tubules (Fig. 23).

Nephrons deliver urine to collecting ducts at the periphery of cortical units. From here the ducts enter a conical-shaped medullary zone, and by progressive union form larger collecting ducts until, finally, a single duct is formed at the tip (ureteral end) of a medullary cone. This duct is a tertiary branch of the ureter (Fig. 23a). At the base (cortical end) of a medullary cone and beneath the cortical units is a region containing a small number of larger (mammalian-type) glomeruli (100 μm diameter). These are associated with nephrons which do have a loop of Henle, vasa recta and the ability to maintain an osmotic gradient throughout the medullary cone, by counter-current osmotic multiplication. These mammalian-type nephrons also have a mixture of renal portal and postglomerular blood flowing through their tubular sinusoids. However, the vasa recta, which are associated with their loops of Henle, only receive blood from the postglomerular efferent arteriole (Wideman *et al.*, 1981).

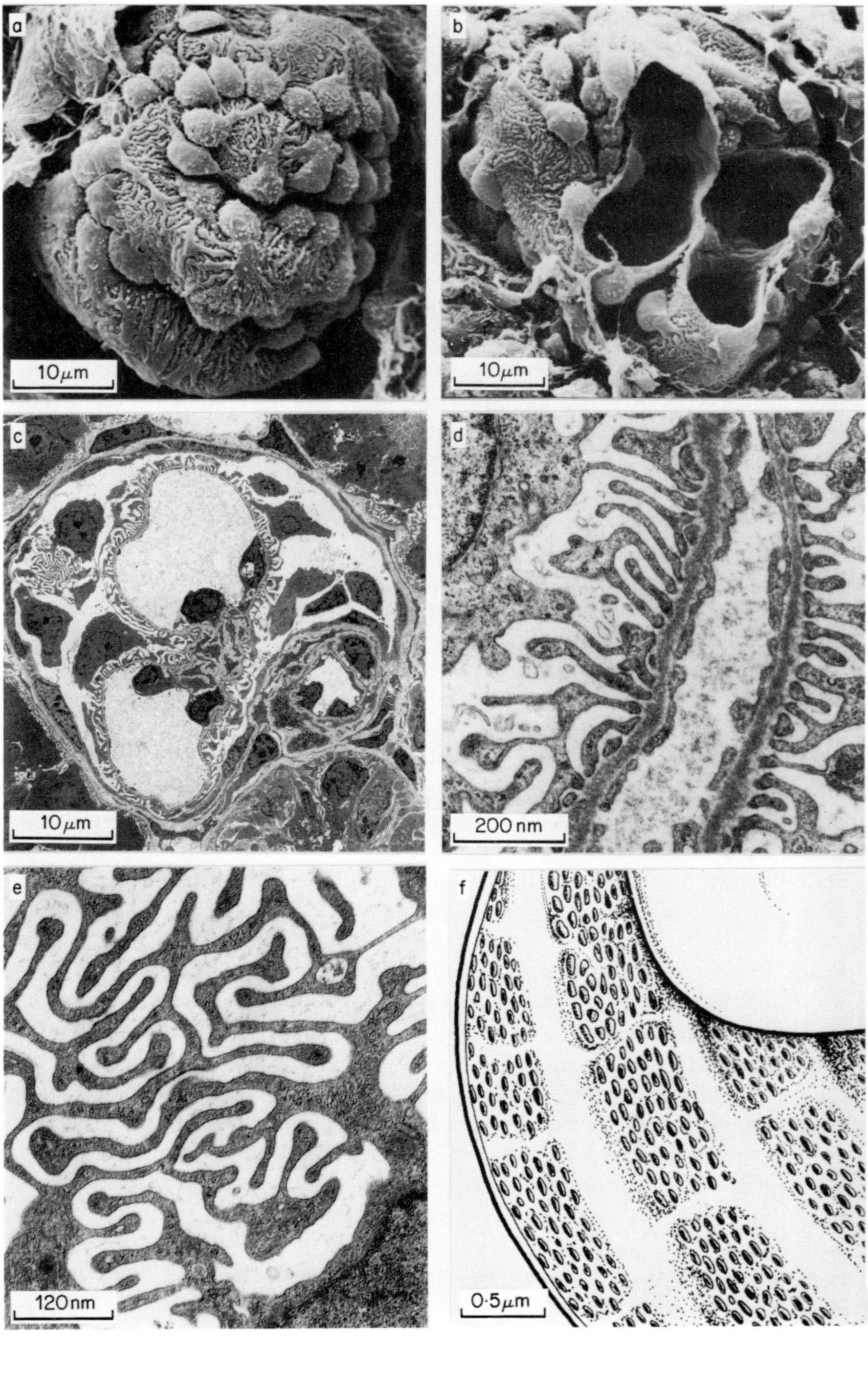
a
10 μm
b
10 μm
c
10 μm
d
200 nm
e
120 nm
f
0·5 μm

Birds which have adapted to a desert environment have a higher proportion of mammalian-type nephrons (about 22%) than non-desert birds (7%) (Johnson and Mugass, 1970). This is virtually the same proportion as that between juxtamedullary nephrons (with loops of Henle and vasa recta) and outer cortical nephrons (without loops of Henle or vasa recta) which is found in desert and non-desert mammals. During conditions of water shortage a bird is said to be able to close down the blood supply to its outer cortical (reptilian-type) glomeruli, whilst maintaining the supply to the relatively small number of mammalian-type nephrons capable of operating a counter-current osmotic multiplier (Braun and Dantzler, 1972).

In the avian kidney, all those cortical units (containing reptilian-type glomeruli) the urine from which drains into a single medullary cone, together with the associated group of mammalian-type nephrons, is considered to be a renal lobule. A lobe is regarded as being all that kidney tissue the urine from which drains into a secondary branch of the ureter. Terminal branches of the renal portal veins which pass between cortical units and finally spread out over their surface are therefore interlobular, whilst the first rudiment of the renal vein, at the centre of each cortical unit, is probably best called the central vein of a cortical unit. As several cortical units are contained in a lobule there can not be a central lobular vein in the sense that it is found in the mammalian liver. Interlobular (renal portal) veins, as they reach the surface of the kidney and spread out over the cortical units, have a star-shaped pattern and so have been called stellate veins.

XVIII. Liver

In the domestic fowl the liver has two main lobes. They partly surround the heart cranially, the proventriculus dorsally and the gizzard caudally. The liver receives blood from a large right, and a smaller left, portal vein. The former receives venous blood from proventriculus, gizzard, duodenum, pancreas, jejunum, ileum, caeca, colorectum and spleen, and distributes it to both lobes

---

Fig. 24. (*a*) Reptilian-type glomerulus in cortical part of kidney. Three or four capillary loops can be seen in this scanning electronmicrograph, covered with podocytes and their processes. (*b*) Similar glomerulus to (*a*) with two capillaries (or different parts of the same capillary) broken open. (*c*) Glomerulus (stained section). Parts of three capillaries are shown surrounded by podocytes. (*d*) Podocyte processes in contact with thick basement membrane surrounding glomerular capillary. Only a small number of fenestrations are seen in a transverse section. (*e*) To show complexity of podocyte branching. (*f*) To illustrate the quantity and uniformity of the fenestrations. Non-fenestrated cell cytoplasm form bands round the endothelial cell. A small part of a red blood cell is shown at top right.

of the liver. The latter receives blood mainly from the proventriculus and gizzard, and delivers it to the left lobe.

The coccygeomesenteric (caudal mesenteric) vein is of particular interest because, in addition to collecting blood from the colorectum and cloaca, it forms a major venous anastomosis with the caudal renal portal veins immediately behind the kidneys. Under experimental conditions, using intravenous injections of radiopaque material, the blood flow in the coccygeomesenteric vein has been visualized and shown to flow (on different occasions) in opposite directions. When radiopaque material is introduced into the external iliac vein it may flow caudally into the kidney, or it may flow cranially into the liver (Akester, 1964, 1967). The same results have been obtained by making similar injections into one of the mesenteric veins. On these occasions the radiopaque material usually entered the liver (which one would expect), but sometimes it flowed caudally along the coccygeomesenteric vein to the kidneys (which one might not have expected) (Purton, 1970).

Hepatic portal blood is distributed by terminal branches of the portal vessels into the great plexus of sinusoids which ramifies throughout the liver in intimate association with the branching cords of hepatocytes. A transverse section through a cord of hepatocytes shows four or five, somewhat wedge-shaped cells, pointing towards a small hole at the centre. This hole is a bile canaliculus, and is simply a space between the surrounding cells whose micro-villi protrude into it. The canaliculus runs in the centre of the cord, so that when the cord branches or unites with another cord the canaliculus branches or unites with another canaliculus.

A longitudinal section through a length of cord shows two row of hepatocytes facing each other across the small central cavity of a bile canaliculus, with a blood sinusoid closely applied to the other side of each line of hepatocytes. It is this view of a liver cord which has given rise to the belief that cords (sheets) of avian hepatocytes are two cells thick. In fact, each cord consists of four or five cells arranged circumferentially around a small central canaliculus and which are extended in sequence along the length of the cord. The branching cords form a three-dimensional mesh which interlocks with a similar mesh of sinusoids. This means that a significant part of the surface area of every hepatocyte is closely associated with a sinusoid and extends its microvilli into the space of Diss. The sinusoidal plexus unites with the first rudiments of the hepatic vein. A large hepatic vein leaves each lobe of the liver and unites to form a single vessel which joins the posterior vena cava immediately caudal to the right atrium of the heart. As the posterior vena cava is embedded in the dorsal part of the liver a few small hepatic veins drain into it directly.

By recording hepatic portal venous and hepatic venous pressures, in the adult anaesthetized fowl, the pressure drop across the liver has been shown to be about 4 mmHg (Purton, 1975). The mean pressure in the hepatic portal vein was about 5·2 mmHg whilst the mean pressure in the hepatic vein was about 1·4 mmHg.

The rate of portal venous blood flow into the liver will obviously vary with metabolic activity, physical activity and the direction in which blood is flowing in the coccygeomesenteric vein. Under experimental conditions, with an anaesthetized adult fowl lying on its back, the hepatic portal blood flow rate was found to be 32 ml kg^{-1} min^{-1} in the fowl and 25 ml kg^{-1} min^{-1} in the goose. Blood flow in the coccygeomesenteric vein was found to vary from 26 to 33 ml kg^{-1} min^{-1} (Purton, 1975).

There is also a hepatic artery (branch of the coeliac), which enters the liver and follows the general pattern of branching of the right hepatic portal vein. In the mammal, the hepatic artery terminates in arterioles which discharge high-pressure blood directly into the sinusoids at the periphery of the classical lobules. These arterioles are under autonomic vasomotor control, which intermittently opens and closes them. When open, brief jets of high pressure blood are injected into the slow-flowing hepatic portal venous blood. No such observations have yet been made on a bird's liver, but it seems reasonable to assume that there is a similar arrangement. Hepatic portal and hepatic veins, as well as branches of the hepatic artery, receive an autonomic innervation (Akester, 1971). It is likely that these large veins will provide a variable reservoir for venous blood returning from the alimentary canal, pancreas and spleen.

XIX. Hypophyseal Portal System

Hypothalamic control of the adenohypophysis is by the production of (as yet only partly identified) releasing factors, which are produced in the hypothalamus and then passed down to the adenohypophysis by way of a portal system. In mammals there is only one hypophyseal portal system, in birds there are two (Vitums *et al.*, 1964).

An anterior group of portal vessels originates in the anterior capillary plexus of the median eminence, whilst a posterior group of portal vessels originates in the posterior capillary plexus of the median eminence. Both capillary plexuses in the median eminence are supplied by branches of the hypophyseal artery, which is a branch of the cerebral carotid artery. It would appear that in some species the two capillary plexuses in the median eminence remain distinct, whilst in others they are connected together. However, in all cases so far studied, the two sets of portal vessels originating from them remain distinct and unconnected (Dominic and Singh, 1969, 1971).

It is possible that the anterior group of portal vessels provides a route by which the anterior part of the median eminence (supraoptic and paraventricular nuclei) could control the anterior part (lobe) of the adenohypophysis, and in a similar way the posterior part of the adenohypophysis could be controlled by the posterior part of the median eminence (infundibular nuclei). There are well established cytological differences between the anterior and posterior parts of the adenohypophysis (Rahn and Painter, 1941; Wingstrand, 1951; Mikami, 1958, 1960; Farner *et al.*, 1967; Singh and Dominic, 1968), and it would appear that each part of the adenohypophysis might be controlled by a specific region of the median eminence, each having its effect by way of a specific set of portal vessels. However, as yet there is no physiological evidence to support this.

The veins of each portal system lead into a plexus of fenestrated capillaries within the adenohypophysis. From this plexus venous blood is delivered, by several connections, to the cavernous sinus which surrounds the hypophysis. It finally reaches the jugular vein by way of the cerebral carotid vein.

XX. Blood–Brain Barrier

Certain dyes, when injected into the cerebral blood vessels, do not reach the tissues of the brain. This suggests that a barrier exists between the capillary endothelium and the surrounding tissue, and has been confirmed by the fact that substances which do not reach brain tissue from the capillaries are able to do so when injected into the ventricles. Tight junctions are said to run continuously along the entire capillary endothelial junction, and may prevent large molecules from passing through (Delormé *et al.*, 1970; Stewart and Wiley, 1981).

The blood–brain barrier, which appears to be caused primarily by a relatively impermeable capillary endothelium, develops progressively in the embryo and from hatching to maturity. The first indication of an effective barrier in the chick can be found at day 16 *in ovo* when horseradish peroxidase in the cerebral blood vessels does not leave the capillaries to enter the brain (Wakai and Hirokawa, 1978). Intravenous injections of nicotine caused adrenaline release from the adrenal medulla, which had a direct influence on the electrical activity of the brain (increased slow wave and sleep). This was more marked in the young bird (immature blood–brain barrier) than in the adult (mature barrier) (Key and Marley, 1962).

A relatively small number of surface (micropinocytotic) vesicles is a feature of cerebral capillary endothelial cells. This may reduce the amount of bulk transfer that can occur in these capillaries, and so contribute to a barrier between the blood and brain. There is a suggestion that endothelial cells of cerebral capillaries are metabolically more active than those in the capillaries of muscle. In the former, mitochondria occupy about 6% of the cell volume compared with only about 3·5% in the latter (Stewart and Wiley, 1981). This difference is even more marked in mammals where mitochondria occupy about 10 to 11% of the cerebral capillary endothelial cell volume.

In the mammal, various enzymes have been shown to be present in much larger concentrations in the endothelial cells of cerebral capillaries than in those of other issues. These include: alkaline phosphatase and butyril cholinesterase, the roles of which (if any) in the blood-brain barrier are not known; aromatic amino acid decarboxylase, which may prevent L-dopa entering the brain (Bertler *et al.*, 1966); and gamma-glutamyl transpeptidase, which may be involved in the transportation of amino acids across the endothelial cell (Orlowski and Meister, 1965). In the cerebral capillary endothelial cells of the adult fowl, with the exception of alkaline phosphatase (the function of which is unknown), none of the above enzymes has been found.

Whilst the precise nature of the avian blood–brain barrier remains obscure, it seems to be associated with extensive tight junctions, a higher proportion of mitochondria, a relatively small number of surface vesicles and possibly a relatively high concentration of certain enzymes.

XXI. Pecten

The pecten is a pigmented, highly vascular, pleated structure attached to the retina which protrudes into the vitreous body of the eye (Fig. 25). Although many functions have been attributed to it (including that of providing a stroboscopic effect), its most likely role is one of nutrition. There is no retinal artery in birds and it is generally agreed that the pecten takes its place. This means that nutrients and oxygen must leave blood capillaries in the pecten and diffuse through the vitreous body to reach the cells of the retina. Carbon dioxide and waste products must diffuse in the opposite direction (Akester, 1973).

The pecten is supplied by a branch of the ophthalmotemporal artery (terminal branch of external ophthalmic). Blood capillaries ramify in the pleats of the pecten amongst melanocytes which occupy the spaces between them. The structure of the capillary endothelium is most dramatic. A narrow central cytoplasmic zone, which contains mitochondria, Golgi and other organelles, expands to house the nucleus. Either side of this zone the cytoplasm is extended in the form of a layer of microprocesses. Some are microvilli but the majority are microplates, which protrude into the capillary lumen on one side and away from it on the other. These plates overlap one another and so are oriented, for the most part, parallel to the long axis of the capillary. The plates are about 50 to 60 nm thick and 1·5 μm long (Fig. 25f). They were first recognized by Semba (1962). More recently, they have been demonstrated by freeze-fractured replication (A. R. Akester, unpublished). There can be no

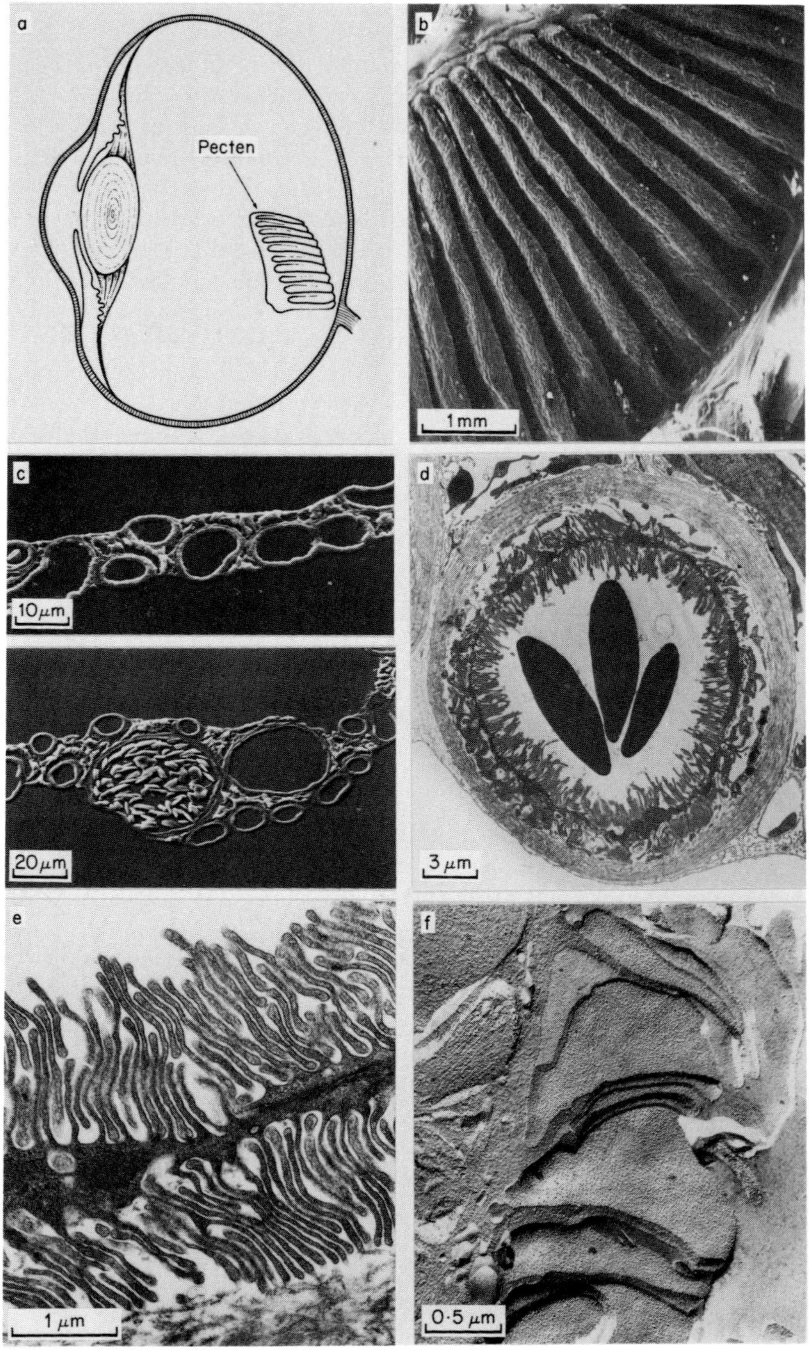
a
Pecten
b
1 mm
c
10 μm
20 μm
d
3 μm
e
1 μm
f
0·5 μm

doubt that they increase considerably the surface area available for diffusion purposes. At intervals the capillaries are surrounded by pericytes which have a very thin cytoplasm, and no microprocesses. Their nuclei are similar in size and appearance to those of the capillary endothelium. Surrounding every capillary is a well developed basal laminar (about 0·6 μm thick), which has a certain amount of structural organization in the form of randomly scattered fibres. It is chemically similar to basement membrane, being PAS-positive, but much thicker and more solid in appearance (Fig. 25d).

In different species the number of pleats varies from 3 to 30 (Fig. 25b). In the domestic fowl there are about 18. At its inner end each pleat is attached to the retina, whilst at its outer end the pleats are embedded in a terminal structure called the bridge. In an adult fowl the pecten extends about 5 mm into the vitreous body of the eye. However, its shape and size varies considerably in different species and in some it extends as a gentle curve from the retina as far as the caudal surface of the lens (Wood, 1917). Surprisingly little experimental work has been carried out on this unique organ. When it was surgically destroyed by coagulation, the retina degenerated (Wingstrand and Munk, 1965). The same authors also demonstrated an oxygen gradient across the vitreous body from pecten to retina. Bawa and Yash Roy (1972) have shown that alkaline phosphatase activity in the pecten is increased during light adaptation and reduced during dark adaptation. This may be associated with an increased movement of metabolites through pecten capillaries during light adaptation. These findings, together with the fact that dyes can be transferred from the pecten to the vitreous body (Fielding, 1972) comprise the scant evidence for its nutritional role.

The pecten is most probably responsible for maintaining intra-ocular pressure and any major interference with its blood supply causes intra-ocular pressure to drop to that of peripheral venous pressure (12 mmHg).

It has been shown in the section on the head that arterial anastomoses provide a collateral supply to important structures if their normal supply is upset. However, there would appear to be limitations in the effectiveness of these anastomoses. Intra-ocular pressure has been measured at 26 mmHg in the domestic fowl (Akester and Brackenbury, 1976). If the internal carotid and vertebral arteries are clamped on one side of the neck there is a dramatic and

---

Fig. 25. (*a*) Position of pecten. (*b*) Vascular pleats of pecten are attached to the retina (right) and to the bridge (top left). There are usually 18 pleats in the fowl, 13 are shown. (*c*) Transverse section through parts of two pleats showing capillaries and venules. (*d*) Transverse section through single capillary. (*e*) Transverse section through capillary endothelial cell. Note narrow central zone of cytoplasm with microprocesses on each side. (*f*) Freeze-cleaved replica demonstrating that most of the processes are flat, overlapping plates.

almost immediate fall in intra-ocular pressure on the same side, to that of peripheral venous pressure (about 12 mmHg). In spite of the various anastomoses which are said to exist, intra-ocular pressure is only restored by about one third of its fall. In contrast, if internal carotid and vertebral arterial clamps are placed on the opposite side to the eye being studied, then the fall in intra-ocular pressure is less. Clamping both arteries on both sides simultaneously caused an immediate fall in intra-ocular pressure, to that of peripheral venous pressure. This was followed by a partial restoration of intra-ocular pressure by about one third, which took 20 s to occur (Fig. 26).

During the time when all four clamps were applied (90 s), systemic arterial pressure increased from 255 mmHg to 325 mmHg, and dropped back to

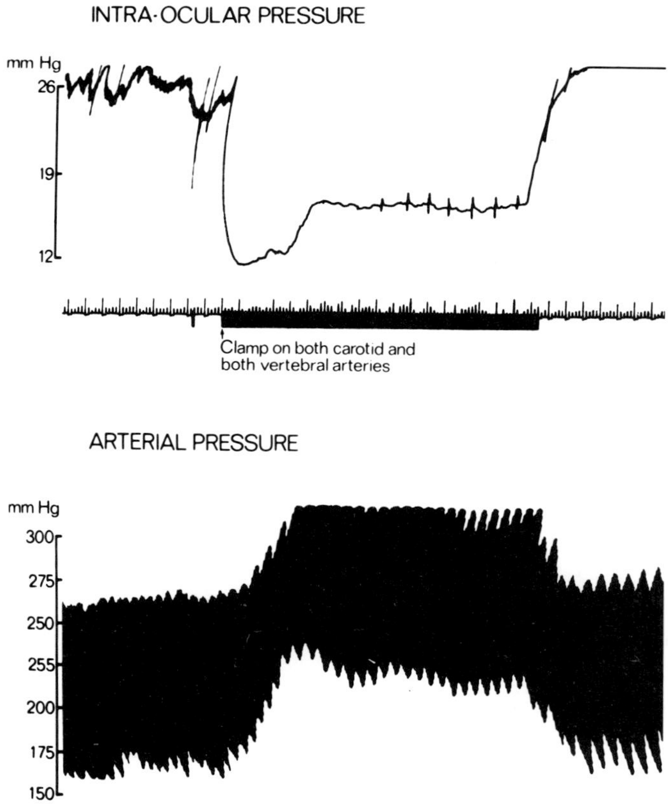

Fig. 26. The effect of clamping both internal carotid arteries and both vertebral arteries on intra-ocular pressure. (From Akester and Brackenbury, 1976, with permission).

255 mmHg on release of the clamps. The vagus artery (Fig. 17) anastomoses with the deep occipital at the top of the neck and may provide the collateral supply to the ophthalmotemporal, which enabled the latter to restore part of the lost intra-ocular pressure. Vasodilation in the spinal arteries, which anastomose with the basilar, may also have made a contribution. However, if a bird can survive with any three of the four major arteries in the neck clamped (Richards and Sykes, 1967), why, with only two of them clamped, could it not maintain its intra-ocular pressure on the ipsilateral side?

XXII. Other Structures

Every organ and tissue in the body is totally dependent on its blood supply if it is to continue functioning normally. An adequate consideration of the cardiovascular system should, therefore, include all parts of the body. Unfortunately, neither time nor space allows this. However, brief reference should be made to a number of additional structures which have something distinctive about their blood supply.

Flight is obviously the most distinctive feature of birds as a class. The huge flight muscles receive an appropriately large blood supply (via the pectoral arteries), which may be increased four to five times in flight. The muscle contains both "red" and "white" fibres. The former are more numerous, small (30 μm), contain many mitochondria, much myoglobin and are loaded with fat. The latter are larger (70 μm), contain fewer mitochondria, little myoglobin and are loaded with glycogen. Twice as much energy can be obtained by oxidizing fat as can be obtained from the same weight of glycogen. The "red" fibres are therefore the ones which provide the bulk of the work in steady prolonged flight, and they receive a rather better blood supply than the white ones. The white fibres may be more concerned with producing a lot of energy in a short time for "take-off". In addition to a three or four-fold increase in blood flow, which is mainly caused by an increased heart rate, the amount of oxygen removed from the blood by active muscle cells is also increased.

The blood supplies to both male and female gonads show distinctive features. Testicular arteries arise from the cranial renal artery and break up into small vessels amongst the seminiferous tubules. In birds, with abdominal testes, there is no pampiniform plexus to provide a heat exchanger between outflowing (warmer) arterial blood and returning (cooler) venous blood.

The pedunculated ovarian follicle receives three or four arteries by way of its narrow stalk. As they spread throughout the follicle wall they leave a relatively avascular band (the 3 mm wide stigma), which runs in a meridional fashion almost completely round the follicle. Ovulation takes place by a split developing, by some unknown mechanism, around the follicle at the stigma.

Splitting of the stigma and release of the ovum will occur *in vitro,* but only if the follicle is removed from the ovary within about 2 h of the normal time of ovulation. This suggests that some change in the stigma may be initiated an hour or two before it ruptures (Olsen and Neher, 1948).

An erectile phallus is present in birds. In some (including ducks and geese) it is a truly intromittent organ, whilst in the domestic fowl it is not. However, in all birds the erectile tissue consists of cavities which can be filled with lymph produced by associated vascular bodies. In the duck elongated lymph cavities lie on either side of the proctodeum. Each surrounds a vascular structure from which small glomerulus-like clusters of blood capillaries invaginate the wall of the lymph cavity. Lymph diffuses into a lymph cavity from the blood capillaries and then, by contraction of the cloacal sphincter, the lymph is forced into the erective tissue of the phallus.

In the domestic fowl (with a non-intromittent phallus) there is a similar association of vascular and lymph structures in the floor of the proctodeum. Discharge of lymph from the vascular body engorges the lymph folds (or pads) which protrude through the vent. The vas deferens on each side discharges semen into a groove between left and right swollen, lymph-filled pads.

There is said to be an adrenal portal system in birds by which venous blood, collected from the neighbouring part of the abdominal body wall, is delivered to the adrenal gland (Goodchild, 1969, for domestic fowl; Holmes and Phillips, 1976, for duck and gull), but its significance is unknown.

On the ventral surface of the skin of birds is an area specially concerned with providing warmth for the eggs during incubation. The incubation (brood) patch develops in whichever sex is responsible for incubating the eggs. In the domestic fowl it is only the female. In phalaropes (small marine birds) the male is concerned with incubation and only he develops the brood patch. Both male and female quail develop a patch and share the responsibility of incubation. The skin of this area undergoes a localized moult in some species or the feathers are plucked out by others. The blood vessels undergo a marked hypertrophy, which is stimulated, at the appropriate time, by the synergistic activity of oestrogen or testosterone, prolactin and progesterone.

Transplantation of skin from the incubation patch to the animal's back does not result in an incubation patch developing in the wrong place (Jones, 1971). This makes an interesting comparison with the development of feather germs experimentally transplanted to a follicle at a different site. The feather germ develops true to the follicle from which it came and not true to the recipient follicle at the new site.

An incubation patch has been induced experimentally by hormone injections in female sparrows and also in male sparrows where one would not normally develop (Selander and Yang, 1966). The response was impressive, with a five-fold increase in epidermal thickness, a seven-fold increase in the number of dermal blood vessels and a six-fold increase in the diameter of the principal vessels. The whole area became markedly oedematous.

We have seen how different organs exhibit distinctive features in their blood supply. In some there are end arteries with no collateral supply, others have a good collateral supply. The smallest capillaries in different organs vary considerably in size and in their relationship to the cells of the organ. Capillaries may be fenestrated or not. Some have more surface vesicles than others and their enzyme activity varies. Some carry a few scattered microvilli, some have none, whilst others have masses of microprocesses, some of which are microvilli but the majority are microplates. If we knew enough about it we might find that the blood supply to each organ was unique and "tailor-made" to suit its functional requirements.

Acknowledgements

It is a pleasure to acknowledge the considerable help given by Ian Edgar and Ken Thurley in the preparation of the illustrations, Wendy Roberts for a computer search of the literature and Shirley Kirkwood for her help in typing the manuscript.

References

Abdalla, M. A. and King, A. S. (1975). *Resp. Physiol.* **23**, 267–290.
Abdalla, M. A. and King, A. S. (1976a). *J. Anat.* **121**, 537–550.
Abdalla, M. A. and King, A. S. (1976b). *Resp. Physiol.* **27**, 187–191.
Abdalla, M. A. and King, A. S. (1977). *J. Anat.* **123**, 697–704.
Adams, W. E. (1937). *Proc. Zool. Soc. Lond.* **B107**, 417–441.
Akester, A. R. (1964). *J. Anat.* **98**, 365–376.
Akester, A. R. (1967). *J. Anat.* **101**, 569–594.
Akester, A. R. (1971). *In* "Physiology and Biochemistry of the Domestic Fowl" (D. J. Bell and B. M. Freeman, eds), Vol. 2, pp. 783–839. Academic Press, London and New York.
Akester, A. R. (1973). *Biorrheology* **10**, 491.
Akester, A. R. (1974). *J. Anat.* **117**, 657–658.
Akester, A. R. (1975). *J. Anat.* **119**, 417–418.
Akester, A. R. (1978). *In* "Microcirculation" (G. Kaley and B. M. Altura, eds). University Park Press, Baltimore.
Akester, A. R. (1979). *In* "Form and Function in Birds" (A. S. King and J. McLelland, eds), Vol. 1, pp. 381–441. Academic Press, London and New York.
Akester, A. R. (1981). *J. Anat.* **132**, 161–179.
Akester, A. R. and Akester, B. V. (1971a). *J. Anat.* **108**, 616–617.
Akester, A. R. and Akester, B. V. (1971b). *J. Anat.* **108**, 618–619.
Akester, A. R., Akester, B. V. and Mann S. P. (1969). *J. Anat.* **104**, 591.

Akester, A. R. and Brackenbury, J. H. (1973). *J. Anat.* **115**, 144–146.

Akester, A. R. and Brackenbury, J. H. (1976). *J. Anat.* **122**, 742–743.

Akester, A. R. and Brackenbury, J. H. (1977). *J. Anat.* **124**, 255.

Akester, A. R. and Mann, S. P. (1969). *J. Anat.* **104**, 241–252.

Anderson, R. H. (1972). *J. Anat.* **111**, 453–468.

Bader, H. (1963). *In* "The Anatomy and Physiology of the Vascular Wall" (W. T. Hamilton and P. Dow, eds). Chap. 26. Handbook of Physiology. Sect. 2: Circulation Vol. II. American Physiology Society, Washington, D.C.

Ball, R. A., Sautter, J. H. and Katter, M. S. (1963). *Anat. Rec.* **146**, 251–255.

Barr, L., Dewey, M. M. and Berger, W. (1965). *J. gen. Physiol.* **48**, 797–823.

Baudinette, R. V., Loveridge, J. P., Wilson, K. J., Mills, C. D. and Schmidt-Nielsen, K. (1976). *Am. J. Physiol.* **230**, 920–924.

Baumel, J. J. (1975). *In* "Sisson and Grossman's The Anatomy of the Domestic Animals" (R. G. Getty, ed.), Vol. 2, Saunders, Philadelphia.

Baumel, J. J. (1979). *In* "Nomina Anatomica Avium" (J. J. Baumel, A. S. King, A. M. Lucas, J. E. Breazile and H. E. Evans, eds), pp. 343–407. Academic Press, London and New York.

Bawa, S. R. and Yash Roy, R. C. (1972). *Expl. Eye Res.* **13**, 92–97.

Bech, C. and Nomoto, S. (1982). *J. exp. Biol.* **97**, 345–358.

Bech, C. and Johansen, K. (1980). *Acta physiol. scand.* **110**, 351–355.

Bennett, T. and Malmfors, T. (1970). *Z. Zellforsch. mikrosk. Anat.* **106**, 22–50.

Bergman, R. A. (1968). *J. Cell Biol.* **36**, 639–648.

Bernstein, M. H. (1974). *Am. J. Physiol.* **226**, 1350–1355.

Berry, C. L., Germain, J. and Lovell, P. (1974). *Atherosclerosis,* **19**, 47–59.

Bertler, A., Falck, B., Owman, Ch. and Rosengrenn, E. (1966). *Pharmac. Rev.* **18**, 369–385.

Bogusch, G. (1974). *Cell Tiss. Res.* **150**, 43–56.

Bolton, T. B. (1968). *J. Physiol. Lond.* **196**, 273–281.

Bouverot, P. and Dejours, P. (1971). *Resp. Physiol.* **13**, 330–342.

Brackenbury, J. H. (1971). *Resp. Physiol.* **13**, 319–329.

Brackenbury, J. H. and Akester, A. R. (1978). *In* "Respiratory Function in Birds, Adult and Embryonic" (J. Piiper, ed.). Springer-Verlag, Berlin, Heidelberg.

Branton, D., Bullivant, S., Gilula, N. B., Karnovsky, M. A., Moor, H., Muhlenthaler, K., Northcote, D. H., Packer, L., Satir, B., Speth, V., Staehlin, L. A., Steere, R. L. and Weinstein, R. S. (1975). *Science, N.Y.* **190**, 54–56.

Braun, E. J. and Dantzler, W. H. (1972). *Am. J. Physiol.* **222**, 617–629.

Brecher, G. A. and Galletti, P. M. (1963). *In* "Handbook of Physiology" (W. F. Hamilton and P. Dow, eds), Sec. 2, Circulation, Vol. II. American Physiological Society, Washington, D.C.

Bretz, W. L. and Schmidt-Nielsen, K. (1971). *J. exp. Biol.* **54**, 103–118.

Brown, G. M. and Page, J. (1952). *J. appl. Physiol.* **5**, 221–227.

Burger, R. E. and Estavillo, J. A. (1977). *Anat. Rec.* **188**, 39–44.

Burt, A. M. and Narayanan, C. H. (1976). *Exp. Neurol.* **53**, 703–713.

Butler, P. J. and Jones, D. R. (1969). *In* "Avian Biology" (D. S. Farner and J. R. King, eds), p. 219. Academic Press, London and New York.

Caspar, D. L. C., Goodenough, D. A., Makowski, L. and Phillips, W. C. (1977). *J. Cell Biol.* **74**, 605–628.

Davies, F. (1930). *J. Anat.* **64**, 129–147.

Defoor, P. H., Levitsky, D., Biryukova, T. and Fleischer, S. (1980). *Archs. Biochem. Biophys.* **200**, 196–205.
Delormé, P., Gayet, J. and Grignon, G. (1970). *Brain Res.* **22**, 269–283.
De Meyer, R. (1952). *Arch. Biol.* **43**, 455–513.
Dhalla, N. S. Das, P. K. and Sharma, G. P. (1978). *J. mol. Cell Cardiol.*,**10**, 363–385.
Djojosugito, A. M., Folkow, B. and Kovách, A. G. B. (1968). *Acta physiol. scand.* **74**, 114–122.
Dominic, C. J. and Singh, R. M. (1969). *Gen. comp. Endocr.* **13**, 22–26.
Dominic, C. J. and Singh, R. M. (1971). *J. Endocr.* **49**, 355–356.
Dorst, J. (1974). "The Life of Birds," Vol. I, p. 35. Weidenfield and Nicholson, London.
Drennan, M. R. (1927). *Br. med. J.* **i**, 321–322.
Duncker, H. R. (1972). *Resp. Physiol.* **14**, 44–63.
Epstein, M. L. and Gilula, N. B. (1977). *J. Cell Biol.* **75**, 769–787.
Eriksson, A., Thornell, L.-E., and Stigbrand, T. (1979). *J. Histochem. Cytochem.* **27**, 1604–1609.
Essner, E., Novikoff, A. B. and Quintana, N. (1965). *J. Cell Biol.* **25**, 201–215.
Fabiata, A. and Fabiata, F. (1975). *J. Physiol., Lond.* **249**, 469–495.
Falck, B. (1962). *Acta physiol. scand.* **56**, Suppl. 197.
Falck, B., Millarp, N. A., Thieme, G. and Torp, A. (1962). *J. Histochem. Cytochem.* **10**, 348–354.
Farner, D. S., Wilson, F. E. and Oksche, A. (1967). *In* "Neuroendocrinology" (L. Martini and W. F. Ganong, eds), Vol. 2. pp. 529–582. Academic Press, New York and London.
Fielding, M. (1972). *J. Anat.* **113**, 295–296.
Folkow, B. (1960). *Circulation* **21**, 760–768.
Folkow, B. and Neil, E. (1971). "Circulation," p. 593. Oxford University Press, New York.
Folkow, B., Yonce, L. R. and Nilsson, N. J. (1967). *Acta physiol. scand.* **70**, 347–361.
Fujii, S., Tamura, T. and Okamoto, T. (1979). *J. Fac. appl. Biol. Sci. Hiroshima Univ.* **18**, 217–224.
Gibbs, C. L. (1974). *In* "The Mammalian Myocardium" (G. A. Langer and A. J. Brady, eds). Wiley, New York.
Goodchild, W M. (1969). *Br. Poult. Sci.* **10**, 183–185.
Goodrich, E. S. (1930). "Studies on the Structure and Development of Vertebrates." Macmillan, New York.
Gossrau, R. (1968). *Histochemie* **13**, 111–159.
Grant, R. T. and Bland, E. F. (1931). *Heart* **15**, 385–407.
Grubb, B. R. (1981). *J. appl. Physiol.* **50**, 450–455.
Hart, J. S. and Roy, O. Z. (1967). *Am. J. Physiol., Lond.* **213**, 1311–1316.
Hartman, B. K. (1973). *J. Histochem. Cytochem.* **21**, 312–332.
Hering, C. A., Wilson, S. J. and Ball, E. R. (1960). *J. thorac. cardiovasc. Surg.* **40**, 49–55.
Hirakow, R. (1966). *Arch. histol. jap.* **27**, 485–499.
Holmes, W. N. and Phillips, J. G. (1976). *In* "General, Comparative and Clinical Endocrinology of the Adrenal Cortex" (I. Chester Jones and I. W. Henderson, eds), Vol. 1, pp. 293–420. Academic Press, London and New York.
Holt, J. P., Rhode, E. A. and Kines, H. (1960). *Circ. Res.* **8**, 1171–1181.
Hosey, M. M. (1980). *J. Supramol. Struct.* **9**, (Suppl. 4), 74.

Hsieh, T. M. (1951). *Ph.D. thesis, University of Edinburgh.*
Irving, L. and Krog, J. (1955). *J. appl. Physiol.* **7**, 355–364.
Jewett, P. H., Sommer, J. R. and Johnson, E. A. (1971). *J. Cell Biol.* **49**, 50–65.
Jewett, P. H., Leonard, S. D. and Sommer, J. R. (1973). *J. Cell Biol.* **56**, 595–600.
Johansen, K. and Millard, R. W. (1973). *J. comp. Physiol.* **85**, 47–64.
Johansen, K. and Reite, O. B. (1964). *Comp. Biochem. Physiol.* **12**, 479–488.
Johansen, K. and Tonnesen, K. H. (1969). *Acta physiol scand.* **76**, 21A.
Johnson, O. W. and Mugass, J. N. (1970). *Condor* **72**, 288–292.
Jones, R. E. (1971). *Biol. Rev.* **46**, 315–339.
Jones, D. R. and Holeton, G. F. (1972a). *J. exp. Biol.* **56**, 657–666.
Jones, D. R. and Holeton, G. F. (1972b). *Comp. Biochem. Physiol.* **41A**, 639–645.
Jones, D. R. and Johansen, K. (1972). *In* "Avian Biology" (D. S. Farner and J. R. King, eds), Vol. 2, pp. 158–285. Academic Press, London and New York.
Jones, R. B., Duncan, I. J. H. and Hughes, B. O. (1981). *Behav. Proc.* **6**, 121–133.
Kelly, A. M. and Chacko, S. (1977). *J. mol. cell. Cardiol.* **9**, 419–424.
Kern, A. (1926). *Gegenbaurs morph. J.* **56**, 264–315.
Key, B. J. and Marley, E. (1962). *Electroenceph. clin. Neurophysiol.* **14**, 90–105.
Khan, M. A. and Qayyum, M. A. (1975). *Anat. Anz.* **137**, 1–11.
Khanna, R. K. (1957). *J. Anim. Morph. Physiol.* **4**, 33–42.
Kilgore, D. L., Jr. and Boggs, D. F. (1976). *Am. Zool.* **16**, 203.
Kilgore, D. L., Boggs, D. F. and Birchard, G. T. (1979). *J. comp. Physiol.* **129**, 119–122.
Kim, Y. and Yasuda, M. (1979). *Zentbl. Vet Med.* **8**, 138–150.
Kim, Y. and Yasuda, M. (1980). *Zentbl. Vet Med.* **9**, 7–20.
Kirby, M. L., Weidman, T. A. and McKenzie, J. W. (1980). *Devl. Neurosci.* **3**, 174–184.
Knoll, P. (1897). *Pflügers Arch. ges. Physiol.* **67**, 587–614.
Kovách, A. G. B. and Szász, E. (1968). *Acta physiol. hung.* **34**, 301.
Langer, G. A. (1974). *In* "The Mammalian Myocardium" (G. A. Langur and A. J. Brody, eds). Wiley, New York.
Langille, B. L. and Jones, D. R. (1975). *Am. J. Physiol.* **228**, 1856–1861.
Levene, C. I. and Murray, J. C. (1977). *Lancet*, **i**, 628–630.
Lindsay, F. E. F. (1967). *J. Anat.* **101**, 555–568.
Lindsay, F. E. F. and Smith, H. J. (1965). *Am. J. Anat.* **116**, 301–314.
Lowell, B. and Jones, D. R. (1975). *Am. J. Physiol.* **228**, 1856–1861.
Loewenstein, W. R. (1981). *Physiol. Rev.* **61**, 829–913.
MacDonald, R.-L. and Cohen, D. H. (1970). *J. comp. Neur.* **140**, 343–358.
McKibben, J. S. and Christensen, G. C. (1964). *Am. J. vet. Res.* **25**, 512–517.
MacLennan, D. H. and Wong, P. T. S. (1971). *Proc. natn. Acad. Sci. USA* **68**, 1231–1235.
McNutt, N. S. and Fawcett, D. W. (1974). *In* "The Mammalian Myocardium" (C. A. Langer and A. J. Brody, eds). Wiley, New York.
Mall, F. P. (1911). *Am. J. Anat.* **11**, 211–266.
Marvin, W. J., Jr., Robinson, R. B. and Hermsmeyer, K. (1979). *Circ. Res.* **45**, 528–540.
Mathur, G. B. and Mathur, P. K. (1979). *Indian J. Zool.* **20**, 59–66.
Mathur, R. (1971). *Thesis, Indore University.*
Mathur, R. and Shrivastava, A. (1979). *Acta morph. neerl. scand.* **17**, 181–189.
Melton, C. E., Jr. and Saldivar, J. T., Jr. (1964). *Am. J. Physiol.* **207**, 279–285.
Michalke, W. and Loewenstein, W. R. (1971). *J. Cell Biol.* **75**, 769–787.
Midtgard, U. (1980). *Acta zool., Stockh.* **61**, 39–49.
Mikami, S. (1958). *J. Fac. Agric. Iwate Univ.* **3**, 473–545.

Mikami, S. (1960). *J. Fac. Agric. Iwate Univ.* **4**, 359–379.
Mossman, H. W. (1948). *Biol. Rev.* **23**, 237–255.
Murakami, T., Saito, I. and Mochizuki, K. (1981). *Exp. Anim.* **30**, 263–268.
Myklebust, R., Dalen, H. and Saetersdal, T. S. (1980). *Cell Tiss. Res.* **207**, 31–41.
Nelemans, F. A. (1940). *Archs néerl. Physiol.* **24**, 337–390.
Olsen, M. W. and Neher, B. H. (1948). *J. exp. Biol.* **109**, 355–366.
Orlowski, M. and Meister, A. (1965). *J. biol. Chem.* **240**, 338–347.
Owen, R. (1866). "On the Anatomy of Vertebrates, Vol. II: Birds and Mammals." Longmans, London.
Parry, K. and Yates, M. S. (1978). *J. Anat.* **127**, 199.
Pettit, T. N., Whittow, G. C. and Grant, G. S. (1981). *Auk* **98**, 844–846.
Pickwell, G. V. (1968). *Comp. Biochem. Physiol.* **27**, 453–485.
Prakash, R. (1956). *Proc. natn. Inst. Sci. India* **22B**, 22–27.
Prakash, R., Bhatnagar, S. P. and Yousuf, N. (1960). *Anat. Rec.* **136**, 322.
Purton, M. D. (1970). *J. Anat.* **106**, 189P.
Purton, M. D. (1975). *Comp. Biochem. Physiol.* **51A**, 949–955.
Quiring, D. P. (1933). *J. Morph.* **55**, 81–116.
Rahn, H. and Painter, B. T. (1941). *Anat. Rec.* **79**, 297–311.
Rennick, B. R. and Gandia, H. (1954). *Proc. Soc. exp. Biol. Med.* **85**, 234–236.
Reuter, M. (1979). *A. Rev. Physiol.* **41**, 413–424.
Richards, S. A. (1970a). *J. Physiol., Lond.* **211**, 341–358.
Richards, S. A. (1970b). *Brain Res.* **23**, 265–268.
Richards, S. A. and Sykes, A. H. (1967). *Comp. Biochem. Physiol.* **21**, 39–50.
Ringer, R. K. and Rood, K. (1959). *Poult. Sci.* **38**, 395–397.
Ringer, R. K., Sturkie, P. D. and Weiss, H. S. (1957a). *Am. J. Physiol.* **190**, 54–56.
Ringer, R. K., Weiss, H. S. and Sturkie, P. D. (1957b). *Am. J. Physiol.* **191**, 145–147.
Rodbard, S. (1976). *Acta card.* **31**, 27–56.
Rose, C. (1890). *Morph. Jb.* **16**, 27–96.
Rush, J. E. and Fambrough, E. (1973). *Devl. Biol.* **30**, 166–186.
Saccomanno, G. (1943). *J. comp. Neur.* **79**, 355–378.
Saetersdal, T. S. and Myklebust, R. (1975). *J. mol. Cell. Cardiol.* **10**, 287–292.
Sapirstein, L. A. and Hartman, F. A. (1959). *Am. J. Physiol.* **196**, 751–752.
Scheid, P. and Piiper, J. (1971). *Resp. Physiol.* **11**, 308–314.
Scheid, P. and Piiper, J. (1972). *Resp. Physiol.* **16**, 304–312.
Schmidt-Nielsen, K. (1971). *Scient. Am.* **225**, 73–79.
Scholander, P. F. (1940). *Hvalräd, Skr. Nor. Vidensk. Akad.* **22**, 1.
Scott, T. M. (1971a). *Ph.D. thesis, University of Edinburgh.*
Scott, T. M. (1971b). *J. Anat.* **110**, 259–273.
Scott, N. R. and van Tienhoven, A. (1971). *Trans. Am. Soc. agric. Engrs* **14**, 1027–1033.
Selander, R. K. and Yang, S. Y. (1966). *Gen. comp. Endocr.* **6**, 325–333.
Semba, T. (1962). *Kynshu J. med. Sci.* **13**, 217–232.
Shaner, R. F. (1923). *J. Anat.* **58**, 59–70.
Shimada, K. and Sturkie, P. D. (1973). *Jap. J. vet. Sci.* **35**, 57–63.
Simons, J. R. (1960). *In* "Biology and Comparative Physiology of Birds" (A. J. Marshall, ed.), Vol. 1, pp. 345–362. Academic Press, London and New York.
Singer, S. J. and Nicolson, G. L. (1972). *Science, N.Y.* **175**, 720–731.
Singh, R. M. and Dominic, C. J. (1968). *Proc. 55th Indian Sci. Congr.* Part 3, 456–457.
Singh, T. (1958). *Proc. natn. Inst. Sci. India* **24**, 140–144.

Skadhauge, E. (1964). *Acta endocr., Copenh.* **47**, 321–330.
Slautterback, D. B. (1965). *J. Cell Biol.* **24**, 1–21.
Smith, R. B. (1971). *Acta anat.* **79**, 112–119.
Sommer, J. R. and Johnson, E. A. (1970). *Am. J. Cardiol.* **25**, 184–194.
Sommer, J. R. and Waugh, R. A. (1976). *Am. J. Path.* **82** 191–232.
Speckman, E. W. and Ringer, R. K. (1963). *Can. J. Biochem. Physiol.* **41**, 2337–2341.
Speckman, E. W. and Ringer, R. K. (1964). *Can. J. Physiol. Pharmac.* **42**, 553–562.
Sperber, I. (1949). *Zool. Bidr. Upps.* **27**, 429–448.
Sperelakis, N. (1979). *A. Rev. Physiol.* **41**, 441–457.
Spira, A. W. (1971). *J. Ultrastruct. Res.* **34**, 409–425.
Steen, I. and Steen, J. B. (1965). *Acta physiol. scand.* **63**, 285–291.
Stewart, P. A. and Wiley, M. J. (1981). *J. comp. Neurol.* **202**, 157–167.
Stout, L. C. and Thorpe, L. W. (1980). *Atherosclerosis,* **36**, 545–558.
Strinskaya, L. A., Leont'eva, G. R., Avakyan, O. M. and Govyrin, V. A. (1980). *J. evol. Biochem. Physiol.* **16**, 178–182.
Sturkie, P. D. (ed.), (1965). "Avian Physiology", 2nd edn, p. 127. Comstock, New York.
Sturkie, P. D. (1966). *Proc. Soc. exp. Biol. Med.* **123**, 487–488.
Sturkie, P. D. (ed.), (1976). "Avian Physiology", 3rd edn. Springer-Verlag, New York.
Sturkie, P. D. and Vogel, J. A. (1959). *Am. J. Physiol.* **197**, 1165–1166.
Suzuki, A., Saito, M. and Nonami, Y. (1980). *Agric. Biol. Chem.* **44**, 1553–1559.
Tagawa, T., Ando, K. and Wasano, T. (1979). *Cell Tiss. Res.* **198**, 43–51.
Tokuyasu, K. T., Dutton, A. M. Geiger, B. and Singer, S. J. (1981). *Proc. natn. Acad. Sci. USA* **78**, 7619–7623.
Tucker, V. A. (1968). *J. exp. Biol.* **48**, 55–66.
Tummons, J. L. and Sturkie, P. D. (1968). *Life Sci.* **7**, 377–380.
Tummons, J. L. and Sturkie, P. D. (1969). *Am. J. Physiol.* **216**, 1437–1440.
Uchiyama, T. (1929). *Morph. Jb.* **60**, 296–322.
Vassal-Adams, P. R. (1978). *J. Anat.* **127**, 196–198.
Vassal-Adams, P. R. (1979). *J. Anat.* **128**, 427.
Vassal-Adams, P. R. (1981). *J. Anat.* **133**, 677.
Vitums, A., Mikami, S.-O., Oksche, A. and Farner, D. S. (1964). *Z. Zellforsch. mikrosk. Anat.* **64**, 541.
Wakai, S. and Hirokawa (1978). *Cell Tiss. Res.* **195**, 195–203.
Weibel, E. R. (1972). *Resp. Physiol.* **14**, 26–43.
Whittow, G. C., Sturkie, P. D. and Stein, G., Jr (1964). *Am. J. Physiol.* **207**, 1349–1353.
Wideman, R. F., Jr., Braun, E. J. and Anderson, G. L. (1981). *J. Morph.* **168**, 249–267.
Wingstrand, K. G. (1951). "The Structure and Development of the Avian Pituitary." Gleerup, Lund.
Wingstrand, K. G. and Munk, O. (1965). *Biol. Skr.* **14**, 1–64.
Wood, C. A. (1917). "The Fundus Oculi of Birds especially as Viewed by the Ophthalmoscope." Landside Press, Chicago.
Woodbury, R. A. and Abreu, B. E. (1944). *Am. J. Physiol.* **142**, 114–120.
Yousuf, N. (1965). *Anat. Rec.* **152**, 235–250.

8 Blood Groups

D. G. GILMOUR

Laboratoire de Médecine Expérimentale, Collège de France, Paris, France

I. Introduction

The term blood group was originally used to describe inherited antigenic properties of erythrocytes. Some blood group loci also code for antigens on other tissues, especially *B* (see below). The A and C antigens, like B, have been found on lymphocytes (Schierman and Nordskog, 1962; Wong *et al.*, 1972), and the *C* locus determines variable histocompatibility responses (Schierman and Nordskog, 1965). Although single letters were used to designate chicken blood group antigens and loci, a more precise terminology was needed, because most letters had been used for other genes.

PHYSIOLOGY BIOCHEMISTRY DOMESTIC
FOWL, VOL. 5 ISBN 0–12–267105–8

At a symposium on "Mutant Nomenclature and Gene Symbolism" during the 1977 meeting of the US Poultry Science Association, it was agreed that the prefix *Ea-* should be proposed, standing for erythrocyte alloantigen as in the mouse. The blood group systems and loci would be Ea-A, Ea-B . . . and *Ea-A*, *Ea-B* . . . This terminology was used in a tabulation of blood groups by Gilmour (1979) and in a list of genes by Somes (1980). These lists contain thirteen Ea systems: A, B, C, D, E, H, I, J, K, L, N, P, and R, but only twelve independent (unlinked) loci, because *Ea-A* and *Ea-E* are closely linked with a recombination fraction of about 0·005 (Briles, 1968).

II. Non-B Blood Group Systems

A. Ea-R and Viral Susceptibility

The only addition to the list in the previous edition is Ea-R, with one antigen R_1 detected by immune antisera and a "silent" allele *r* coding for no antigen or an antigen not detected. The *Ea-R* locus is independent of eleven other blood group loci (Briles and Crittenden, 1971). *N* was not tested. In segregating progeny, R_1 is closely associated with dominant susceptibility ($Tv\text{-}B^{sl}$) to subgroup B leukosis-sarcoma (L-S) viruses (Crittenden *et al.*, 1970). This finding gave promise that cell membrane receptors for L-S viruses might be detectable with immune sera against erythrocytes, or preferably against chick embryo fibroblasts which resemble the normal targets of infection. So far, there has been no success in numerous attempts to develop immune sera against other R antigens on erythrocytes, nor against other *Tv-B* allelic receptors or receptors for subgroup A or C viruses (W. E. Briles, personal communication).

B. Ea-K and Viral Haemagglutination

The vaccinia haemagglutinogen (Vh) system differs from other blood groups because it is not detected by immune antiserum. Agglutinability of chicken erythrocytes by extracts of vaccinia and some other viruses, and by phospholipids such as Wasserman antigen, is dominant over inagglutinability, with gene symbols *Vh* and *vh* (Gilmour, 1960), as confirmed by Mendelian testing (Gilmour and Allison, 1969). McPhee (1971) reported a similar system using Kahn antigen, another phospholipid. It was found that *Vh* is determined by the *Ea-K* locus (Brown *et al.*, 1973). Chickens segregating for twelve Ea systems (not including N) were tested for blood groups and agglutinability by vaccinia virus extract. Only K was correlated with Vh. The recessive genotype *kk*, determining absence of K antigen (Briles and Briles, 1972), was associated with inagglutinability by virus, thus corresponding with *vhvh*. Genotypes were quantitatively associated with vaccinia haemagglutination titre, with $K^1K^1 > K^1K^2 > K^2K^2 > K^2K^3$, and larger differences between these and $K^1k > K^2k > K^3k$. The *K* alleles presumably code for varying amounts of a receptor site on erythrocytes which reacts with phospholipids leading to agglutination, and the *kk* genotype for absence of an active receptor, and absence of blood group antigen.

III. The *B* Major Histocompatibility Complex

A. Introduction

1. *Structure*

Ea-B antigens are only some of the properties coded by a short chromosomal segment known as the *B* or major histocompatibility complex (MHC). This has three sub-loci, *B-G* coding for erythrocyte surface antigens only, *B-F* for histocompatibility antigens on most tissue cells, and *B-L* for antigens restricted to B lymphocytes, some monocytes and macrophages, and a few T-lymphocytes which may be suppressor cells. The *B* complex is analogous to mouse *H-2* and human *HLA*, with the B-F antigens corresponding to H-2D, K and HLA-A, B, C antigens, and the *B-L* antigens to the immune-response-associated (Ia) antigens coded by *H-2I* or *HLA-D/DR*. The B-G antigens are unique and there are no corresponding H-2 or HLA antigens.

2. *Functions*

Information on normal functions of the chicken MHC is scarce, but much can be inferred from knowledge of the mammalian MHC (see Dausset, 1981; Klein *et al.*, 1981; Benacerraf, 1981), which will now be outlined. Normal functions are distinguished here from functions which have been used in research on the chicken MHC. The latter concern histocompatability, and in humans are important to clinical medicine in matching donors and recipients for transplants of whole organs such as kidneys, or for bone marrow replacement in leukemia, radiation injury, and other conditions.

Normally the MHC antigens are concerned with discrimination by immune mechanisms between the body's self antigens and foreign (non-self) antigens occurring in the body either from viral or bacterial infection, or (perhaps) from malignant transformation of body cells. The major histo-antigens (H2-D, K, and presumably B-F) of body cells may be modified by viral infection (or, perhaps, malignant transformation) and then stimulate specific activation of cytolytic T-lymphocytes which initiate destruction of the altered cells. This inhibits viral replication, or provides immune surveillance of incipient tumours. The Ia antigens (and presumably B-L) regulate cooperation between antigen-presenting macrophages, helper T-cells, and B-lymphocytes. Stimulation of helper T-cells, by foreign antigens of invading bacteria or viruses in association with Ia antigens, leads to B-cell antibody responses against microbes and toxins or to delayed hypersensitivity (DH) responses against intracellular infections by parasites or bacteria. The non-self antigens in association with Ia may also generate specific suppressor T-cells. These suppress either helper T-cell responses, providing one mechanism of inherited immunological unresponsiveness, or cytolytic T-cell responses, leading to release of tumours from immune surveillance and hence to progressive growth.

In normal immune functions, it is crucial that the response of T-cells is to the animal's own syngeneic MHC antigen modified by, or in association with, non-self antigen. Conversely, histocompatibility responses of practical interest in research and medicine are directed against allogeneic MHC antigens of other individuals, and are unphysiological in that grafts or cell transfers do not occur naturally (except in pregnancy, where special inhibitor mechanisms apply). Non-self H2D, K or HLA-A, B, C antigens stimulate cytolytic T-cells and other host immune mechanisms, which then react against these antigens as targets causing graft rejection. Ia antigens are more important in stimulating T-cell proliferative responses, as in the mixed lymphocyte and graft-versus-host reactions. The role of such responses in graft rejection is sometimes small, sometimes large (Dausset, 1981). Ia antigens are also important in experimental or clinical induction of specific immune tolerance because they are involved in generation of suppressor T-cells. Dependent on the antigen and the method of tolerizing, these may suppress antibody formation or DH mediated by helper T-cells, or graft rejection by cytolytic T-cells (Klein *et al.*, 1981; Dausset, 1981). Some counterparts of these "unphysiological" MHC functions are described later for the corresponding B-F and B-L antigens in the chicken.

B. Breeding and Functional Analysis

The major contribution by Hala and his collaborators, with the immunochemical work described below, led to the three-locus model for the chicken MHC. It was known that histo-incompatibility between donor and recipient chickens was associated with differences in Ea-B antigens, reported for skin graft rejection by Schierman and Nordskog (1961), for graft-versus-host (GVH) splenomegaly by Jaffe and McDermid (1962) and for the mixed lymphocyte reaction (MLR) by Miggiano *et al.* (1974). Sublines developed in Prague from the highly inbred Reaseheath lines were used. Gilmour (1959,

1960) had reported that all four Reaseheath lines were still segregating for the *Ea-B* locus and for one or more other *Ea* loci after 20–25 generations of full-sib matings. With this information, the Prague group selected within three Reaseheath lines and developed pairs of sublines differing in Ea-B antigens and skin graft compatibility. Because of the high level of inbreeding, each pair was expected to be identical at all genetic loci except the *B* complex, and was thus *congenic*. Two *B* congenic lines, CB and CC, were developed (Hasek *et al.*, 1966) from the C line of Gilmour (1959), and the congenic pair WA and WB (Hala *et al.*, 1966) from the W line.

Tests were made for genetic recombination (crossing over) between sub-loci within *B*. Crosses between CB and CC congenic lines (respectively B^{12} and B^{4} in current terminology, see below) were backcrossed to the WB line (B^{10}). Among 1205 progeny tested with specific haemagglutinating antisera to B4, B12 and B10 antigens, 1204 reacted as expected, either 4/10 or 12/10, but one reacted with all three sera, as if 4/12/10 (Hala *et al.*, 1975, 1976). After exclusion of mismating or pedigree error by appropriate tests, it was concluded that recombination had occurred. The recombinant haplotype (short chromosomal segment) was designated B^{R1}, and was shown to code for a combination of two Ea-B antigens (4 + 12) which segregated allelically to the Ea-B10 antigen in progeny from the recombinant male and inbred females. This suggested that erythrocyte antigens were determined by both *B* sub-loci, which was confirmed by immunizations and absorptions.

Skin grafted on the recombinant chicken was accepted from CB and WB but rapidly rejected from CC donors, showing that B^{R1} coded for a histocompatibility antigen inherited from CB and not CC. It was postulated that the *B* complex was divided into two sub-loci, *B-F* determining Ea and histo-antigens and *B-G* determining Ea antigens alone (Hala *et al.*, 1975, 1976). Confirmation came from further functional tests of the recombinant male and its progeny, which showed that GVH and MLR responses as well as skin graft rejection were determined by differences at the *B-F* sub-locus as defined at that time (Vilhelmova *et al.*, 1977). B^{R1} is now designated B^{12r1} in the recently proposed terminology (Briles *et al.*, 1982), signifying the first reported recombinant originating from the haplotype containing the $B\text{-}F^{12}$ allele. An alternative descriptive term is $B(F^{12}.G^{4})$.

C. Immunochemistry of Antigens

In the initial work by Ziegler and Pink, immune antisera against Ea-B antigens were raised by reciprocal immunizations with blood between Prague WA and WB congenic lines and used for specific immunoprecipitation of radiolabelled surface antigens of peripheral blood leukocytes (PBL). In polyacrylamide gel electrophoresis of the antigens under non-reducing conditions, two main molecules were found with apparent molecular weights (MW) 42 000 and 11 500 from WA, or 45 000 and 11 500 from WB (Ziegler and Pink, 1975). This allelic MW difference was reproducible. By analogy with mammals, the larger molecule was presumed to represent the main histo-antigen of chicken, non-covalently linked to the smaller molecule, the polypeptide β_2-microglobulin. Analyses of leukocytes from Prague CB and CC and from an American line G-B1 (Schierman *et al.*, 1977) gave similar results (Ziegler and Pink, 1976). The leukocyte antigens of both CC and G-B1 were precipitated by antisera to CC and were thus crossreactive or identical, although their Ea-B antigens differed (B4 and B13 respectively). Later, antigens similar or identical to leukocyte B-F antigens were immunoprecipitated from erythrocytes (Kubo *et al.*, 1977; Ziegler and Pink, 1978).

One anti-B4 serum precipitated three molecules from CC or G-B1 leukocytes, the two B-F molecules and an extra molecule with MW 30 000. Only the last of these was precipitated by the B4 serum absorbed with B4 erythrocytes, showing that it was on leukocytes and not erythrocytes. In this distribution and in MW it resembled the Ia antigens of mammals. It was postulated that the *B-F* sub-locus of Hala and his co-workers coded for two distinct antigens, here named B and B-L, determined by sub-loci within *B-F* (Ziegler and Pink, 1976). This terminology was modified by Hala *et al.* (1977), who used *B-F* and *B-L* (instead of *B* and *B-L*, respectively) to refer to the supposed sub-loci within their original *B-F*. This change was agreed in correspondence between these authors and others, and was used in listings by Gilmour (1979) and Somes (1980). Because B-G and B-F were responsible for blood group reactions, they were both comprised within Ea-B.

D. The Three-locus Model

Evidence confirming the model came from immunochemical analyses of erythrocyte B-G antigens and functional studies (Pink *et al.*, 1977). Antibodies expected to be specific for B-G4 antigen and without reaction against B-F or B-L antigens were raised by immunizing WA × CB chickens (10/12) with blood from B^{R1}/B^{12} heterozygotes (F12.G4/F12.G12). These precipitated two molecules from CC or CB/R1 but not CB erythrocytes, with apparent MW of 160 000 and 135 000 under non-reducing, and 42 000 and 31 000 under reducing, conditions. These clearly differed from leukocyte B-F or B-L antigens, and made up the B-G antigen coded by B^{R1}, which differed from B-G12 of CB and was similar or identical to B-G4 of CC.

The immunochemical similarity between the leukocyte antigens (B-F + B-L) of CC and G-B1 was confirmed as functional identity by skin grafting and

MLC reactions (Pink *et al.*, 1977). These lines differed for Ea-B (Briles and Briles, 1982), but evidently only at B-G and not B-F. This was confirmed by direct immunofluorescent detection of antigen on line CC erythrocytes but not leukocytes with immune sera obtained by immunizing G-B1 × CB birds with CC blood. Similar sera specifically immunoprecipitated the characteristic B-G molecules from CC or CB/R1 erythrocytes, but not from CB erythrocytes or CC leukocytes. Thus, the *B* haplotypes of CC and G-B1 code for identical B-F and B-L, but different B-G antigens (Pink *et al.*, 1977). The CC haplotype can be described as $B^{(F4.G4)}$ and G-B1 as $B^{(F4.G13)}$, where F^n signifies $F^n.L^n$ unless there is specific evidence to the contrary (Briles *et al.*, 1982).

E. Cellular Distribution of B Antigens

Distribution of *B* antigens between erythrocytes and leukocytes was determined immunochemically and confirmed by immunofluorescence (IF). Restriction of B-L antigen to particular cell types was reported by Ewert and Cooper (1978). Antisera developed by reciprocal immunizations with bursal B cells between two RPRL inbred lines, 7_2 and $15I_5$ (respectively B2 and B15), were used in two-stage indirect IF labelling of lymphoid cells. In peripheral blood leukocytes (PBL) about 20% of mononuclear cells were labelled, in thymus about 4%, and bursa 88%. B-lymphocytes were discriminated from other mononuclear cells by simultaneous detection of B-L and surface immunoglobulin M (sIgM, characteristic of 99% of B cells) by double labelling with reagents conjugated to contrasting fluorochromes. In PBL most $B\text{-}L^+$ cells in PBL were also $sIgM^+$, but spleen, bone marrow, and bursal cortex had a considerable population of $B\text{-}L^+.sIgM^-$ cells, which were mostly monocytes or macrophages as identified morphologically and by tests of latex particle ingestion. These were rare in bursal medulla or PBL. The low incidence in PBL may have been an artifact of the method of isolation, slow speed (SS) centrifuging. We confirmed that $B\text{-}L^+.sIgM^-$ cells are rare in SS PBL, but they were more plentiful (6–9%) in PBL isolated by flotation on Ficoll-Hypaque at a specific gravity of 1·09 (T. L. Fredericksen and D. G. Gilmour, unpublished).

Antiserum absorbed with B-cells did not label macrophages, showing that B-cell and macrophage B-L antigens are identical (Ewert and Cooper, 1978). $B\text{-}L^+.sIgM^+$ cells were confirmed as B-cells by their absence in agammaglobulinaemic bursectomized chickens. The distribution of B-L resembles that of Ia in mammals, except that B-L was not detected on activated T-cells, perhaps because the mitogen doses used were sub-optimal. Using IF with double labelling, we found B-L on T-cells stimulated with larger doses of mitogens (Fredericksen and Gilmour, unpublished), as also reported by Crone *et al.*

(1981). B-L occurs on lymphoblastoid T-cell lines derived from virally-induced malignant lymphomas (Schat *et al.*, 1982).

A rosetting method was developed for histological identification of B-L antigens. This has advantages over IF in that rosettes can be separated on density gradients, allowing recovery of B-L$^+$ cells by erythrocyte lysis for studies of functions or detailed histology. Numerical results by counting rosettes from different tissues were similar to those obtained by IF, while additionally B-L antigens were found on a few unactivated T lymphocytes, since only 1% of thymus lymphoid cells were sIgM$^+$ at four weeks old, while 5% were B-L$^+$ (Nowak *et al.*, 1981). Using IF with double labelling, Hala *et al.* (1981) found that 0·5% of PBL were B-L$^+$ T-cells.

MHC determination of the above antigen detected by IF was established by tests of backcross progeny from the RPRL inbred lines 6_3 and 15_1. B-L and Ea-B antigens segregated in parallel, and no recombinants were found in 208 progeny (Ewert *et al.*, 1980). No recombinants between *Ea-B* and *B-L* were obtained in "over 1000 informative typings" (Crone *et al.*, 1981). Detection of 0/1208 recombinants is compatible statistically with close linkage of two sub-loci with a recombination fraction (RF) up to at least 0·003. This may be compared with an estimated RF between *B-G* and *B-F* of 0·0004 based on 4/10 252 (Hala *et al.*, 1981) and 3–4/8912 (Koch *et al.*, 1983). Recent evidence for recombination between *B-F* and *B-L* is discussed below in Section G.

F. Disease Resistance and Immune Responses

1. *Specific*

There are many reports of association of *Ea-B* with variation in immune responses, but mechanisms have been rarely studied. One example similar to specific immunological unresponsiveness as in mammals is the very low antibody response of an inbred line to the synthetic co-polymer GAT^{10} derived from glutamic acid, alanine, and tyrosine. "Nonresponse" segregated with *Ea-B*^{15} of California line UCD 007 in F2 progeny from crosses with high-responder lines (Benedict *et al.*, 1975). The mechanism was probably an inherited helper T-cell defect because GAT^{10} conjugated with an immunogenic carrier, methylated bovine serum albumin (MeBSA), elicited high responses in UCD 007 chickens (Benedict *et al.*, 1977). In contrast, very low response to GT (a co-polymer of glutamic acid and tyrosine), associated with *Ea-B*^{13} of line G-B1, was not converted to high response following conjugation of GT with MeBSA (Koch and Simonsen, 1977). Induction of specific suppressor cells was probably the mechanism in this case.

In auto-immune thyroiditis in Obese strain chickens, one or more loci determine development of antibodies to thyroglobulin, and of auto-immune cytotoxic T-cells probably mediated by suppressor T-cell defects (Boyd and Wick, 1982), but there is no evidence that these initial abnormal responses to self antigen are associated with the MHC (Wick *et al.*, 1979). Variations in antibody titre and in severity of symptoms are associated with *Ea-B* (Bacon *et al.*, 1974) and at least one other non-MHC immune response locus (Bacon and Rose, 1979; Wick *et al.*, 1979). Suppressor T-cells may be the mechanism of such variation, because the condition is exacerbated by thymectomy (Wick *et al.*, 1970).

Ea-B is associated with major variation in regression of tumours induced by Rous sarcoma virus (RSV) (Collins *et al.*, 1977; Schierman *et al.*, 1977), although non-MHC loci can affect lesser variation (Collins *et al.*, 1980; Gilmour *et al.*, 1983). Association with *B-F* (meaning *B-F* or *B-L*) rather than *B-G* was shown by Plachy and Benda (1981), comparing Prague CB and CC lines with congenic CB.R1 homozygous for the B^{R1} recombinant. Most evidence indicates that MHC-associated variation is highly specific. Lines G-B1 and G-B2 and the corresponding B^{13} and B^{6} homozygotes from F2 or backcross progeny show differing responses to strains within RSV subgroups. In an extreme example, line G-B1 or B^{13} chickens strongly regress sarcomas induced by B77 strain but not those induced by PR-RSV, both subgroup C, while G-B2 or B^{6} chickens react conversely (McBride *et al.*, 1981). Differences were even found in responses to tumours induced by separate clones of B77 (Cutting *et al.*, 1981a). High specificity was also indicated by the finding of genetic complementation for strong regression in F1 hybrids between two related lines G-B1 (B^{13}) and G-B3 (B^{15}), neither of which can regress sarcomas induced by subgroup B SR-RSV. The MHC and at least one non-MHC locus were involved, because only 50% of B^{13}/B^{15} heterozygotes in backcross progeny were high regressors (Cutting *et al.*, 1981b).

The association of *Ea*-B^{21} with resistance to Marek's disease (MD) appears to be mediated by rather specific high immune responsiveness (see Section III F.2). Association of *Ea-B* with resistance to the leukosis complex (later known to be mainly MD) was found for B^{14} *vs.* B^{13} by Allen and Gilmour (1962, cited by Gilmour, 1971), and for B^{21} *vs.* B^{19} and MD by Hansen *et al.* (1967). In both studies, comparisons were made within sire-families from heterozygous sires (*13/14* or *19/21*), thus avoiding stratification errors. Dam blood groups were not a source of variation. Two-way selection for resistance to MD within Cornell random-bred stock (51% MD incidence) led to marked differences between non-inbred lines (incidence 13% compared with 91%) after only two generations of selection (Cole, 1968), implying that resistance depended on very few genes of large effect. In later generations, *Ea*-B^{21} was in high frequency in the resistant line (Cornell N) and in low frequency in susceptible Cornell P (Briles and Stone, 1975; Pazderka *et al.*, 1975), suggesting association of B^{21} with resistance. This was confirmed by comparisons within families from heterozygous sires in backcross progeny from N × P and in backcross-type progeny within Cornell random-breds (Briles and Stone, 1975; Briles *et al.*, 1976, 1977). B^{21}-associated resistance was found in other populations, as shown by comparisons of B^{21} with other *B* alleles in F2 progeny (Longenecker *et al.*, 1976), although the differences were not as large as B^{21} compared with B^{19}.

2. General

The possibility that disease resistance may sometimes be general rather than specific came from a brief report that a line selected for high regression of RSV-induced tumours was also more resistant to Marek's disease, gave higher antibody responses to some antigens, and had greater amounts of immunoglobulin than unselected controls (Carte *et al.*, 1972). MHC association of general resistance was suggested by the finding in F4 and F5 progeny from lines 6_3 and 15_1 that B^5 homozygotes, which were low RS regressors (Collins *et al.*, 1977), also had lower resistance to MD and to tumours induced by lymphoid leukosis virus (especially erythroblastosis) than high regressor B^2 homozygotes or heterozygotes (Bacon *et al.*, 1981). On the other hand, Cornell N and P lines, with MHC-associated high or low resistance to MD, show no differences in Rous sarcoma regression (Calnek *et al.*, 1975), in immunoglobulin levels (Higgins and Calnek, 1975), or in antibody or DH responses to several antigens (D. G. Gilmour, unpublished). These findings argue for the specificity of the large MHC-associated differences in MD resistance between lines N and P.

There is one haplotype, *Ea-B*^{1}, which is associated with generalized low immune response. In the original inbred line H1 the B^1 homozygotes had high mortality and their matings together gave no progeny (Briles and Allen, 1961). In comparisons with B^2 and B^{19} in a population (S1) derived from crosses of inbred lines H1 and H45, B^1 has been consistently associated with high mortality (Nordskog *et al.*, 1973), low antibody responses to a variety of antigens (Pevzner *et al.*, 1975, 1978, 1979), low regression of Rous sarcomas (Gebriel *et al.*, 1979), low resistance to MD (Pevzner *et al.*, 1981), and low rate of development and low final levels of IgG (Rees and Nordskog, 1981). The genetics of this generalized low immune responsiveness (IR) was studied by tests of antibody response to one of the antigens, GAT^{10}, in a large sample of the S1 population. The majority of birds were classified as either B^1(*low*) or B^{19}(*high*), but a few reacted as B^1(*high*) or B^{19}(*low*), and these rare combinations then segregated as entities (Pevzner *et al.*, 1978). This suggests that the chromosomal region determining this generalized low IR is separate from *Ea-B* but closely linked with it, and that the new combinations were derived from past recombinational events. In all subsequent (1979–1981) studies cited above, the various other low responses were associated with low GAT^{10} response in both the original B^{1} (*low*) and the "recombinant" B^{19} (*low*) haplotypes. This general low responsiveness has no counterpart in mammals.

G. Present Status of the Three Sub-loci

Until recently, the genetic evidence for three sub-loci within *B* was incomplete, because recombination had not been observed between the postulated *B-F* and *B-L* sub-loci, but only between *B-G* and *B-F*. The discrimination of *B-L* from *B-F* was postulated on serological, immunochemical and histological evidence (see above, Sections IIIB–E) which indicated analogy with the mouse *H-2* complex. There was evidence, however, that recombination had taken place between *Ea-B* as detected by haemagglutination (i.e., *B-G* + *B-F*) and a chromosomal region coding for low IR to GAT^{10} (Pevzner *et al.*, 1978). The significance of this recombination was not clear until the so-called *Ir-GAT* sub-locus was more clearly specified, using antisera produced by reciprocal immunizations with lymphocytes between descendants of the original B^{19} (*low*) recombinant individuals and parental-type B^{19} (*high*). Such sera, which would be expected to react with the antigenic products of the *Ir-GAT* region only, specifically immunoprecipitated surface antigen from B lymphocytes (bursal cells) having the known characteristics of B-L antigen. Furthermore, the *Ea-B* antisera used in haemagglutination tests specifically immunoprecipitated characteristic B-G antigen from erythrocytes and B-F antigen from erythrocytes or leukocytes, but not B-L antigen (Birkmeyer and Nordskog, 1982, and personal communication).

These findings showed conclusively that the recombinational events detected by Pevzner *et al.* (1978) had occurred between *Ea-B* (*B-G* + *B-F*) and *B-L*. Because all previous recombinations had occurred between *B-G* and the rest of the MHC (*B-F* + *B-L*), it could be further concluded that the *Ea-B*/*Ir-GAT* recombinations had occurred between *B-F* and B-L.

References

Allen, C. P. and Gilmour, D. G. (1962). *Genetics, Princeton* **47**, 1711–1718.
Bacon, L. D. and Rose, N. R. (1979). *Proc. natn. Acad. Sci. USA* **76**, 1435–1437.
Bacon, L. D., Kite, Jr., J. H. and Rose, N. R. (1974). *Science, N.Y.* **186**, 274–275.
Bacon, L. D., Witter, R. L., Crittenden, L. B., Fadly, A. and Motta, J. (1981). *Poult. Sci.* **60**, 1132–1139.
Benacerraf, B. (1981). *Science, N.Y.* **212**, 1229–1238.
Benedict, A. A., Pollard, L. W., Morrow, P. R., Abplanalp, H. A., Maurer, P. H. and Briles, W. E. (1975). *Immunogenetics* **2**, 313–324.
Benedict, A. A., Pollard, L. W. and Maurer, P. H. (1977). *Immunogenetics* **4**, 199–204.

Birkmeyer, R. C. and Nordskog, A. W. (1982). *Proc. 18th Int. Conf. Anim. Blood Groups Biochem. Polymorphisms,* **14**, p. 71.

Boyd, R. L. and Wick, G. (1982). *Int. Archs Allergy appl. Immunol.* **69**, 286–295.

Briles, W. E. (1968). *Genetics, Princeton* **60**, 164.

Briles, W. E. and Allen, C. P. (1961). *Genetics, Princeton* **46**, 1273–1293.

Briles, W. E. and Briles, R. W. (1972). *Anim. Blood Groups Biochem. Genet.* **3** (Suppl. 1), 82–83.

Briles, W. E. and Briles, R. W. (1982). *Immunogenetics* **15**, 449–459.

Briles, W. E. and Crittenden, L. B. (1971). *Poult. Sci.* **50**, 1558.

Briles, W. E. and Stone, H. A. (1975). *Poult. Sci.* **54**, 1738–1739.

Briles, W. E., McGibbon, W. H. and Stone, H. A. (1976). *Poult. Sci.* **55**, 2011–2012.

Briles, W. E., Stone, H. A. and Cole, R. K. (1977). *Science, N.Y.* **195**, 193–195.

Briles, W. E., Bumstead, N., Ewert, D. L. Gilmour, D. G., Gogusev, J., Hala, K., Koch, C., Longenecker, B. M., Nordskog, A. W., Pink, J. R. L., Schierman, L. W., Simonsen, M., Toivanen, A., Toivanen, P., Vainio, O. and Wick, G. (1982). *Immunogenetics* **15**, 441–447.

Brown, K. S., Briles, W. E. and Brown, E. R. (1973). *Proc. Soc. exp. Biol. Med.* **142**, 16–18.

Calnek, B. W., Higgins, D. A. and Fabricant, J. (1975). *Avian Dis.* **19**, 473–482.

Carte, I. F., Smith, J. H., Weston, C. R. and Savage, T. F. (1972). *Poult. Sci.* **51**, 1792.

Cole, R. K. (1968). *Avian Dis.* **12**, 9–28.

Collins, W. M., Briles, W. E., Zsigray, R. M., Dunlop, W. R., Corbett, A. C., Clark, K. K., Marks, J. L. and McGrail, T. P. (1977). *Immunogenetics* **5**, 333–343.

Collins, W. M., Heinzelmann, E. W., Corbett, A. C., Zsigray, R. M. and Dunlop, W. R. (1980). *Poult. Sci.* **59**, 1172–1177.

Crittenden, L. B., Briles, W. E. and Stone, H. A. (1970). *Science, N.Y.* **169**, 1324–1325.

Crone, M., Jensenius, J. C. and Koch, C. (1981). *Scand. J. Immunol.* **14**, 591–597.

Cutting, J. A., Watanabe, D. H., Strebel, F. R., Vogt, P. K. and McBride, R. A. (1981a). *J. Immunogenetics* **8**, 297–305.

Cutting, J. A., Watanabe, D. H., Strebel, F. R. and McBride, R. A. (1981b). *J. Immunogenetics* **8**, 215–223.

Dausset, J. (1981). *Science, N.Y.* **213**, 1469–1474.

Ewert, D. L. and Cooper, M. D. (1978). *Immunogenetics* **7**, 521–535.

Ewert, D. L., Gilmour, D. G., Briles, W. E. and Cooper, M. D. (1980). *Immunogenetics* **10**, 169–174.

Gebriel, G. M., Pevzner, I. Y. and Nordskog, A. W. (1979). *Immunogenetics* **9**, 327–334.

Gilmour, D. G. (1959). *Genetics, Princeton* **44**, 14–33.

Gilmour, D. G. (1960). *Br. Poult. Sci.* **1**, 75–100.

Gilmour, D. G. (1971). *In* "Physiology and Biochemistry of the Domestic Fowl" (D. J. Bell and B. M. Freeman, eds), Vol. 2, pp. 883–896. Academic Press, London and New York.

Gilmour, D. G. (1979). *In* "Inbred and Genetically defined Strains of Laboratory Animals" (P. L. Altman and D. D. Katz, eds), Part 2, pp. 650–652. Federation of American Societies for Experimental Biology, Bethesda.

Gilmour, D. G. and Allison, A. C. (1969). *Virology* **37**, 237–242.

Gilmour, D. G., Collins, W. M., Fredericksen, T. L., Auclair, B., Clark, K. K. and Urban, W. E. (1983). *Immunogenetics* **17**, 43–54.

Hala, K., Hasek, M., Hlozanek, I., Hort, J., Knizetova, F. and Mervartova, H. (1966). *Folia biol., Praha* **12**, 407–422.

Hala, K., Vilhelmova, M. and Hartmanova, J. (1975). *Folia biol., Praha* **21**, 363.
Hala, K., Vilhelmova, M. and Hartmanova, J. (1976). *Immunogenetics* **3**, 97–103.
Hala, K., Vilhelmova, M. and Hartmanova, J. (1977). *In* "Avian Immunology" (A. A. Benedict, ed.), pp. 227–232. Plenum Press, New York.
Hala, K., Boyd, R. and Wick, G. (1981). *Scand. J. Immunol.* **14**, 607–616.
Hansen, M. P., Van Zandt, J. N. and Law, G. R. J. (1967). *Poult. Sci.* **46**, 1268.
Hasek, M., Knizetova, F. and Mervartova, H. (1966). *Folia biol., Praha* **12**, 335–342.
Higgins, D. A. and Calnek, B. W. (1975). *Infect. Immun.* **12**, 360–363.
Jaffe, W. P. and McDermid, E. M. (1962). *Science, N.Y.* **137**, 984.
Klein, J., Juretic, A., Baxevanis, C. N. and Nagy, Z. A. (1981). *Nature, Lond.* **291**, 455–460.
Koch, C. and Simonsen, M. (1977). *Immunogenetics* **5**, 161–170.
Koch, C., Skjodt, K., Toivanen, A. and Toivanen, P. (1983). *Tissue Antigens* **21**, 129–137.
Kubo, R. T., Yamaga, K. and Abplanalp, H. A. (1977). *In* "Avian Immunology" (A. A. Benedict, ed.), pp. 209–220. Plenum Press, New York.
Longenecker, B. M., Pazderka, F., Gavora, J. S., Spencer, J. L. and Ruth, R. F. (1976). *Immunogenetics* **3**, 401–407.
McBride, R. A., Cutting, J. A., Schierman, L. W., Strebel, F. R. and Watanabe, D. H. (1981). *J. Immunogenetics* **8**, 207–214.
McPhee, C. P. (1971). *Br. Poult. Sci.* **12**, 439–449.
Miggiano, V. C., Birgen, I. and Pink, J. R. L. (1974). *Eur. J. Immunol.* **4**, 397–401.
Nordskog, A. W., Rishell, W. A. and Briggs, D. M. (1973). *Genetics, Princeton* **75**, 181–189.
Nowak, J. S., Vainio, O., Lassila, O., Toivanen, P. and Gilmour, D. G. (1981). *J. Immunol. Methods* **42**, 325–335.
Pazderka, F., Longenecker, B. M., Law, G. R. J., Stone, H. A. and Ruth, R. F. (1975). *Immunogenetics* **2**, 93–100.
Pevzner, I. Y., Nordskog, A. W. and Kaeberle, M. L. (1975). *Genetics, Princeton* **80**, 753–759.
Pevzner, I. Y., Trowbridge, C. L. and Nordskog, A. W. (1978). *Immunogenetics* **7**, 25–33.
Pevzner, I. Y., Trowbridge, C. L. and Nordskog, A. W. (1979). *J. Immunogenetics* **6**, 453–460.
Pevzner, I. Y., Kujdych, I. and Nordskog, A. W. (1981). *Poult. Sci.* **60**, 927–932.
Pink, J. R. L., Droege, W., Hala, K., Miggiano, V. C. and Ziegler, A. (1977). *Immunogenetics* **5**, 203–216.
Plachy, J. and Benda, V. (1981). *Folia biol., Praha* **27**, 363–368.
Rees, M. J. and Nordskog, A. W. (1981). *J. Immunogenetics* **8**, 425–431.
Schat, K. A., Chen, C. H., Shek, W. R. and Calnek, B. W. (1982). *J. natn. Cancer Inst.* **69**, 715–720.
Schierman, L. W. and Nordskog, A. W. (1961). *Science, N.Y.* **134**, 1008–1009.
Schierman, L. W. and Nordskog, A. W. (1962). *Science, N.Y.* **137**, 620–621.
Schierman, L. W. and Nordskog, A. W. (1965). *Transplantation* **3**, 44–48.
Schierman, L. W., Watanabe, D. H. and McBride, R. A. (1977). *Immunogenetics* **5**, 325–332.
Somes, Jr., R. G. (1980). *J. Hered.* **71**, 168–174.
Vilhelmova, M., Miggiano, V. C., Pink, J. R. L., Hala, K. and Hartmanova, J. (1977). *Eur. J. Immunol.* **7**, 674–679.
Wick, G., Kite, Jr., J. H. and Witebsky, E. (1970). *J. Immunol.* **104**, 54–62.

Wick, G., Gundolf, R. and Hala, K. (1979). *J. Immunogenetics* **6**, 177–183.
Wong, S. Y., Pazderka, F., Longenecker, B. M., Law, G. R. J. and Ruth, R. F. (1972). *Immunol. Comm.* **1**, 597–613.
Ziegler, A. and Pink, J. R. L. (1975). *Transplantation* **20**, 523–527.
Ziegler, A. and Pink, J. R. L. (1976). *J. biol. Chem.* **251**, 5391–5396.
Ziegler, A. and Pink, J. R. L. (1978). *Immunochemistry* **15**, 515–516.

9 The Lymphoid System

L. N. PAYNE AND P. C. POWELL

Department of Experimental Pathology, Houghton Poultry Research Station, Huntingdon, England

PHYSIOLOGY BIOCHEMISTRY DOMESTIC FOWL, VOL. 5 ISBN 0-12-267105-8

I. Introduction

Much progress has been made in knowledge of the lymphoid system of the fowl during the 10 years that have elapsed since the previous review (Payne, 1971). Whereas delineation of the structure and function of the bursa- and thymus-dependent lymphoid systems was the major advancement during the 1960s, the subsequent decade has seen progress on several fronts, reflecting the great growth of immunology generally. Notable among the developments in avian immunology have been the studies on the origin of lymphoid stem cells, the ontogenesis of bursal and thymic lymphoid cells, the definition of the various types of T-cell function, the phenomenon of cloacal drinking and antigen uptake by bursal epithelium, and the structure and function of the Harderian gland.

In this review we have tried to include the major advances in knowledge of the lymphoid system of the fowl. The topics are presented in the same order as, and should be read in conjunction with, the earlier review (Payne, 1971). Further information can be obtained from other general reviews (Firth, 1977; Glick, 1978; Rose, 1981), collections of original or review papers (Benedict, 1977; Rose *et al.*, 1981), and reviews of specialized topics, including the bursa (Weber, 1975; Glick, 1977; Ivanyi, 1981), immunity to infectious diseases (Rose *et al.*, 1981), immunogenetics (Longenecker and Mosman, 1981a,b), immunoglobulins (Higgins, 1975; Benedict and Yamaga, 1976), lymphocyte markers (Higgins, 1981), ontogeny (Szenberg, 1976; Rose and Orlans, 1981; Seto, 1981; A. Toivanen *et al.*, 1981), phylogeny (Shields *et al.*, 1979; Manning, 1981), structure of lymphoid tissues (Hodges, 1974; White, 1981), and the thymus (Kendall, 1980; Chi *et al.*, 1981).

We have used the anatomical terms recommended in the *Nomina Anatomica Avium* (Baumel *et al.*, 1979).

II. Thymus

A. Structure

Earlier accounts of the morphology of the fowl thymus (*thymus*) have been supplemented by the descriptions of Hodges (1974) and Rose (1981). White (1981) described the blood vascular system within the organ. A network of arterioles runs along the corticomedullary junction from which capillaries are sent outwards into the cortex (*cortex thymicus*) as far as the capsule (*capsula thymica*). These drain into veins running with the arterioles between the cortex and the medulla (*medulla thymica*), thus forming arcades or loops with collateral anastomoses. Endothelial cells, connected by desmosomes and surrounded by a basement membrane, line the lumina of the capillaries (Frazier, 1973). In mice, the endothelial junctions of the cortical vessels are impermeable to a variety of macromolecular tracers, even of low molecular weight, thus forming a blood–thymus barrier (Raviola and Karnovsky, 1972); in addition to the endothelial barrier the vessels are continuously invested by reticular epithelial cells and macrophages associated with a second basement membrane (Frazier, 1973). The post-capillary venules and capillaries which descend to supply the medulla from the cortex and the cortico–medullary arterioles leak macromolecular peroxidase tracer. These post-capillary venules are lined by high endothelium and are the sites at which lymphocytes may travel between the medulla and the blood stream: lymphocytes may be observed infiltrating the vessel walls. The blood–thymus barrier therefore appears to protect cortical but not medullary thymocytes from contact with blood-borne substances. This would explain the lack of effect of experimentally administered anti-thymocyte serum on the thymic cortex (White, 1981).

The ultrastructure of the chick thymus has been described by Frazier (1973), who distinguished four main cell types: lymphoid cells, epithelial cells, macrophages and myoid cells. The epithelial cells were classified into four morphological and functional groups: reticular, undifferentiated, cystic and squamous. Reticular epithelial cells form a supporting network for the free cells of the thymus. They are characterized by the presence of long cytoplasmic processes, connected by desmosomes, which envelope and provide a micro-environment for the maturation of thymic lymphoid cells. Undifferentiated epithelial cells, without long thin cytoplasmic processes, are present in groups in the medulla. They possibly represent a reserve of epithelial cells which are able to differentiate and replace some of the other, more differentiated, types. Cystic epithelial cells are involved in the formation of intracellular and intercellular cysts in the medulla. Squamous epithelial cells, with many cytoplasmic fibrils and desmosomes, are found in groups in the medulla, where they are associated with the formation of Hassall's corpuscles (*corpuscula thymica*), consisting of concentric rings of squamous epithelial cells interconnected by many desmosomes. The centre of the corpuscles may contain sheets of osmiophilic material resembling the surface layers of the chick epidermis. Macrophages containing phagocytosed material are present in moderate numbers in the cortex and the medulla. Also in the medulla are a small number of large cells with pale cytoplasm containing few organelles. These cells increase markedly in number under certain circumstances in the thymi of chicks infected with Marek's disease virus (Frazier, 1974a). They lack desmosomal connections and are not phagocytic; they may be primitive reticulum cell precursors of macrophages. The fine structure of thymic epithelial vesicles has also been described by Isler (1976) and, in ducks, by Hashimoto *et al.* (1982). Post-natal structure and growth of the chick thymus are described by Hashimoto and Sugimura (1976a) and Bellamy and Mohamed (1982).

Differentiation antigens with specificity for thymus-derived cells have been characterized using heterologous antisera (Albini and Wick, 1974; Hudson and Roitt, 1973). About 65% and 80% of the mononuclear cells in the spleen and the peripheral blood, respectively, are T-cells (Chi *et al.*, 1981). The caecal tonsils contain about 35% T-cells, and the Harderian glands only 10% (Albini and Wick, 1974). T-cells may be separated from cell suspensions by standard methods such as nylon wool adherence (Stinson *et al.*, 1978; Lamont and Van Alten, 1981). In addition to xenoantigens, four systems of T-differentiation alloantigens have been recognized. Two occur in the East Lansing line 6 and 7 chickens which are identical at the major histocompatibility locus (B^2/B^2). Th-l (Gilmour *et al.*, 1976) antigens are expressed on 75% thymus cells and 25% peripheral T-cells. Ly-4 (Fredericksen *et al.*, 1977) alloantigens occur on 70% peripheral T-cells and on 15% thymocytes. The other alloantigen systems are CA1 (Galton and Ivanyi, 1977a) present in *B*-locus homozygous (B^{14}/B^{14}) chickens on erythrocytes, peripheral blood lymphocytes and thymocytes, but absent from bursa cells, and TA (Galton and Ivanyi, 1977b) in B^{14}/B^{14} chickens on 80% thymocytes, 45% spleen T-lymphocytes and 75% of peripheral T-lymphocytes.

B. Development

Moore and Owen (1967a,b,c) showed, using parabiotic pairs of embryos of opposite sex, that thymic lymphocytes are derived from blood-borne stem cells which invade the rudimentary thymus. These conclusions, based on the karyotyping of actively dividing cells, were confirmed by Le Douarin and Jotereau (1973, 1975) who showed, by making use of interspecies (chicken/quail) differences in the structures of interphase nuclei, that all T-cells originated from immigrant stem cells. Similar techniques, using interspecies hybrids (Dieterlen-Lievre *et al.*, 1979) or sex chromosome or immunoglobulin allotype markers in chick–chick chimaeras (Lassila *et al.*, 1978), have been used to show that the stem cells are originally located within the embryonic mesenchyme and that they move to the yolk sac when the circulation is established. Chick–chick yolk sac-embryo chimaeras have been hatched and the intra-embryonic origin of the stem cells for the thymus has been demonstrated functionally by the specific stimulation of T-lymphocytes (Lassila *et al.*, 1979a; Martin *et al.*, 1979). The exact nature and site of origin of the intra-embryonic pluripotential stem cells is not clear, although it appears that commitment to develop along the T-cell or B-cell lineage occurs at about day 12 or 13 of incubation (Brand *et al.*, 1978; Weber and Foglia, 1980). The stem cells are probably the haemocytoblastic "wandering cells" described by Danchakoff (1915–16), which form haematopoietic foci in the mesenchyme around the heart and dorsal to the pharynx and oesophagus, and in subcutaneous tissue and muscles. Haemocytoblasts that are competent to invade the thymus rudiment are present in the blood at least 60 h before the thymus itself is ready to be colonized (Le Douarin *et al.*, 1976, 1977).

When first visible, at 5 d of incubation, the thymus consists of epithelial tubular extensions of the pharyngeal pouches surrounded by a mesenchymal capsule. In contrast to the bursa, this mesenchyme can be replaced by the mesenchyme of the somatopleure (A. Toivanen *et al.*, 1981). According to Owen and Ritter (1969), the first stem cells invade the thymic anlage at 6 or 7 d. Le Douarin *et al.* (1975) demonstrated migration beginning on the second half of day 7 and continuing for 36 h. A second invasion of cells occurs at about the time of hatching, completely replacing the earlier cells which leave the thymus. The stem cells initially proliferate vigorously within the thymus, but later more slowly (Sällström and Alm, 1974a; Sugimoto *et al.*, 1977a) and the epithelial cells become compressed and stellate. The stem cells when they enter the thymus are large with intensely basophilic cytoplasm and large nuclei, but during differentiation the cell size reduces and at the same time the number of cells with T-cell surface markers increases to reach almost 100% at hatching (Albini and Wick, 1975; Sugimoto *et al.*, 1977a). The thymic lobes begin to be divided into lobules at 9 d by ingrowths of mesenchyme from the thymic stroma which become compressed to form the thin interlobular septa. These convey blood vessels to the thymus, the differentiation of which into cortical and medullary zones begins at 13 d. From about 14 d lymphocytes from the cortex appear to migrate into the more vascular medulla, and thence into the general circulation (Sugimoto *et al.*, 1977a,b).

Attempts to demonstrate functions characteristic of mature T-cells early in embryogenesis have been unsuccessful. Jankovic *et al.* (1975) reported the graft-versus-host reactivity of thymocytes at 14 d, but Droege (1976) found only extremely weak graft-versus-host reactivity at hatching. Responsiveness to T-cell mitogens has developed by 20 d (Sällström and Alm, 1974b), and helper T-cell activity is indicated by the vigorous IgG response following immunization during the first week after hatching.

The development of the lymphoid organs depends upon interactions between primitive progenitor cell populations, and it appears that B-cells perform an essential function in thymic development. B-cells can be detected in the thymus from about the 11th to the 17th d of incubation (Schauenstein and Wick, 1977). Treatment of the developing embryo with testosterone has effects on the thymus as well as on the bursa (Warner and Szenberg, 1964) and surgical bursectomy at 70 h results in severe atrophy of the thymic cortex (Fitzsimmons *et al.*, 1973, 1977). In a similar way, the normal development of the bursa also requires T-cells (Hirota *et al.*, 1981a). The collaboration between B- and T-cells required in the differentiation of B-cells was found not to be restricted by histoincompatibility, unlike the collaboration essential for effective function (P. Toivanen *et al.*, 1974a,b). A full account of the development of the thymus and of the origin and maturation of thymocytes is given by A. Toivanen *et al.* (1981).

C. Function

There is overwhelming evidence that the thymus is a maturation centre in which stem cells differentiate into T-lymphocytes. Experiments using antisera to surface antigen markers suggest that the cells pass through a sequence of maturation steps which might be related to the different micro-environments the thymic lymphocytes experience on their way to the medulla from the cortex (White, 1981). The functions of T-lymphocytes in the chicken are similar to those in mammals, and include helper and suppressor effects on antibody production, delayed hypersensitivity, graft-versus-host activity, macrophage activation and cytotoxicity. The role of T-lymphocytes in the immune response in the chicken has been comprehensively reviewed by Chi *et al.* (1981).

1. Helper Activity

Because of the ease of bursectomy, T-cell activity can be studied in the near absence of antibody or of B-lymphocytes; however, it is difficult to study the dependence of B-lymphocyte activity on T-cells because surgical thymectomy is difficult and T-lymphocytes may be seeded to the periphery before hatching (Hemmingsson, 1972a). Nevertheless, when combined with irradiation or with treatment with anti-lymphocyte serum, thymectomy does diminish antibody production (Cooper *et al.*, 1966; Ivanyi and Salerno, 1971; Rouse and Warner, 1972a). Cooperation between B- and T-lymphocytes in producing an antibody response apparently occurs as in the mouse. Cell transfer experiments have shown that a primary response to *Brucella abortus* can be transferred by bursa cells alone, but spleen cells are required to transfer responses to sheep erythrocytes and protein antigens. Thymus cells fail to transfer antibody responses to any antigen. The production of antibody to *B. abortus* by B-lymphocytes apparently does not require the cooperation of T-lymphocytes, the antigen being termed "T-independent"; other antigens are T-dependent

(Gilmour *et al.*, 1970; Thorbecke *et al.*, 1980). T-dependency has also been demonstrated by the treatment of spleen cell suspensions prior to adoptive transfer with specific antisera and complement. The transfer of responsiveness to sheep erythrocytes and to *B. abortus* was abolished by specific anti-B or anti-immunoglobulin antiserum, whereas anti-T antiserum reduced the response only to sheep erythrocytes (McArthur *et al.*, 1971). In response to haptens, specific priming of T-lymphocytes with a low dose of a carrier was shown to prepare for an enhanced antibody response to a hapten linked to that carrier (Sarvas *et al.*, 1974). However, when larger doses of carrier were given no enhanced response was observed; this was not apparently due to the stimulation of suppressor cells, but to antibody formation against the carrier which tended to suppress the primary anti-hapten response.

2. *Suppressor Activity*

Infections with certain viruses, e.g. those of Marek's disease or reticuloendotheliosis (Lee, 1979; Carpenter *et al.*, 1977) stimulate cells, probably macrophages, which suppress the *in vitro* proliferative response of T-lymphocytes to lectins. However, suppressor cells have been identified in the T-cell rich, macrophage-depleted, fraction of spleen cells from chickens with Marek's disease (Theis, 1977). Antigen-specific suppressor T-cells have been demonstrated after intravenous injection of sheep erythrocytes, both *in vitro* and by cell transfer experiments. Their activity is demonstrable when exposed to antigen immediately after explantation. After culturing for 2 d in the absence of antigen they seem to disappear and instead helper activity is expressed after exposure to antigen (Chi *et al.*, 1980). Chickens rendered agammaglobulinaemic by chemical or surgical bursectomy have splenic suppressor T-cells apparently active against immunoglobulin-secreting cells. These can be demonstrated by the transfer into irradiated recipients of lymphoid cells which induce "infectious agammaglobulinaemia" (Blaese *et al.*, 1974), and the splenic suppressor activity can be enhanced by intravenous injection of bursa cells.

3. *Delayed Hypersensitivity and Lymphocyte Proliferative Responses*

Chickens may be stimulated to produce good delayed hypersensitivity responses even in the absence of antibodies and of immunoglobulins (Jankovic *et al.*, 1963; Warner *et al.* 1971). Delayed hypersensitivity develops 2 to 3 weeks after sensitization with antigen in an appropriate adjuvant. Complete Freund's adjuvant, but not incomplete adjuvant, is adequate for protein antigens (Palladino *et al.*, 1978). Greater delayed responses may be obtained by manipulation of the antigens, e.g. of sheep erythrocytes by treatment with glutaraldehyde or of protein antigens by lipid conjugation. Contact hypersensitivity to oxazolone after application of the chemical to the wattle or comb skin has also been reported (Palladino *et al.*, 1977). Studies in bursectomized chickens on allergic contact dermatitis to low molecular weight contact allergens such as picryl chloride and oxazolone indicated that it is primarily a T-cell response which is modulated by B-cells (Weidanz *et al.*, 1976). The adoptive transfer of delayed hypersensitivity has been achieved with spleen cells and with peripheral blood leukocytes. Delayed hypersensitivity has been shown to be involved in experimentally induced immunity to syngeneic fibrosarcomas (Palladino and Thorbecke, 1978a,b) which follows the injection of the cells together with live BCG or killed *Corynebacterium parvum*. Peripheral blood leukocytes and spleen cells from immunized birds cause local inhibition of tumour growth when inoculated with the tumour cells into the wing webs of normal recipients. The cells responsible are T-lymphocytes, but their effect depends upon the recruitment and activation of macrophages. The stimulation of a delayed hypersensitivity reaction to an unrelated antigen such as human gammaglobulin can also cause the regression of fibrosarcomas, presumably owing to a bystander cytotoxic effect (Palladino and Thorbecke, 1978c). Delayed hypersensitivity is also involved in the regression of Rous sarcomas (see Payne, 1981).

Peripheral blood leukocytes and spleen cells from normal or agammaglobulinaemic chickens respond in culture to T-cell mitogens and alloantigens while those from thymectomized chickens do not (P. Toivanen and A. Toivanen, 1973a). The culture conditions used by different investigators have varied considerably (Kirchner and Oppenheim, 1972; Lee, 1974, 1978; Chi *et al.*, 1981).

The *in vitro* responsiveness of lymphocytes to T-cell mitogens is under genetic control. Concanavalin A responses may be controlled by a single (dominant) gene not linked to sex, the *B* complex or allotype loci, and are independent of phytohaemagglutinin responsiveness (Miggiano *et al.*, 1976). Compared with East Lansing line 6 chickens, line 7 birds show a greater lymphocyte proliferative capacity, as measured by graft-versus-host activity (Pazderka *et al.*, 1975), mixed lymphocyte reactivity and Concanavalin A-responsiveness (see Chi *et al.*, 1981), apparently associated with their greater susceptibility to Marek's disease, possibly owing to the higher reactivity of their suppressor T-cell population.

Graft-versus-host reactions are also the responsibility of T-lymphocytes, although the proliferative response involves both donor T-cells and host cells (Biggs and Payne, 1959; Weber, 1970) at least some of which are neither T-cells nor B-cells (Palladino and Thorbecke, 1978a).

4. *Cytotoxic Activity*

Cytotoxic cells have been described in the chicken although often the cells cannot be identified as T-cells. The reaction between sensitized T-cells and specific antigen results in cytotoxic activity *in vivo* (Palladino and Thorbecke, 1978b) and *in vitro* (Radwan *et al.*, 1975), attributable probably to macrophages. T-cells with cytotoxic activity directed against cells infected with Marek's disease virus were demonstrated by Ross (1977), and Sharma (1977) showed that the effectors of cell-mediated immunity to Marek's disease tumour antigens were also cytotoxic T-cells. The antiviral cytotoxic spleen cells which Wainberg *et al.* (1974) found in chickens with Rous sarcomas were apparently restricted in their activity by histocompatibility antigens, suggesting a role for these in the cytotoxic mechanism. Such restriction does not seem to operate in the killing of Marek's disease virus-infected cells by T-cells (Lee *et al.*, 1981). Schat and Calnek (1980) were unable to demonstrate *in vitro* cytotoxicity of spleen lymphocytes against syngeneic Marek's disease tumour cells although the same effector cells were active against allogeneic target cells.

5. *Lymphokine Production*

Much of the behaviour of lymphocytes, both *in vivo* and *in vitro*, may be explained on the basis of the release of soluble factors (lymphokines). For example, when sensitized cells are exposed to antigen *in vitro* a factor is released which inhibits cellular migration (Zwilling *et al.*, 1972; Vlaovic *et al.*, 1975; Rose and Hesketh, 1974). Other lymphokines that have been reported are a monocyte chemotactic factor (Kirchner *et al.*, 1974) and a mitogenic factor (Oates *et al.*, 1972). It is therefore appropriate to use the whole range of established tests for cell-mediated immunity in investigations in the chicken (Bloom and David, 1976). Production of thymic cell growth factor by mitogen-stimulated chicken spleen cells was reported by Schauenstein *et al.* (1982).

6. *Disease Resistance*

The role of cell-mediated immunity in resistance to Marek's disease has been clearly demonstrated by the abolition of the acquisition of age-related resistance by neonatal thymectomy (Sharma *et al.*, 1975). In contrast, Payne *et al.* (1976) reported that thymectomy increases the resistance of genetically susceptible chickens as might be expected of a malignancy of T-cells (by removing suitable target cells). T-cell immunity is also important in resistance to parasites such as coccidia (Davis, 1981).

7. *Antibody Production*

In addition to its role as a primary lymphoid organ, the thymus acts as a peripheral lymphoid organ and as a site of antibody formation. Newly-hatched chicks may have as many as 7% B-cells among the lymphocytes of the thymus and, later, immature and mature plasma cells are present in increasing numbers; after 4 weeks germinal centres may be seen in the medulla (Albini and Wick, 1974; Hudson and Roitt, 1973). Active antibody production has been demonstrated in the thymus, and thymus cells can be separated into two populations by density gradient centrifugation, one exhibiting graft-versus-host reactivity and the other antibody-forming capacity (Tamminen *et al.*, 1973).

8. Hormones

There have been persistent efforts to allocate an endocrine function to the thymus. Ultrastructurally, cystic epithelial cells shown cytoplasmic features suggestive of a secretory function (Frazier, 1973), although stronger candidates as a source of thymic hormone are the specialized secretory cells similar in appearance to those described by Olah and Glick (1978a, 1981) and Olah *et al* (1979) in the medulla of the bursa (A. M. Lawn, personal communication). Thymic factors are probably required in addition to contact with the epithelium for the differentiation of T-cells. Brand *et al.* (1976, 1978) demonstrated that a thymus extract, thymopoietin, could include embryonic, but not neonatal, bone marrow cells in differentiate into T-lymphocytes *in vitro* (as shown by Th-1 antigen expression). T-cell precursors are present in the bone marrow throughout ontogeny and occur transiently in the bursa.

9. Haematopoiesis

The thymus decreases in size with the onset of sexual maturity, and thereafter the parenchyma becomes replaced by fatty and fibrous tissue. In certain wild birds recrudescence of the thymus may occur following the annual breeding season, and at this stage the gland contains many immature erythrocytes and lymphocyte-like cells and may be performing an erythropoietic function (Kendal and Ward, 1974; Bacchus and Kendall, 1975). Occasionally there is a similar recrudescence in domestic chickens after the breeding season or after the administration of thyroxine (Brake *et al.*, 1981). Prolonged stress may lead to involution of the thymus.

III. Cloacal Bursa (Bursa of Fabricius)

A. Structure

A detailed account of the ultrastructure of the cloacal bursa (*bursa cloacalis*) is given by Frazier (1974b), with particular reference to the relative contributions of the various cell types to the cortex and medulla of the lymphoid follicles (*folliculi lymphatici*). Cells in the medulla were characterized by Naukkarinen and Sorvari (1982). A cell with secretory properties, possibly the source of bursal hormonal factors (see below), was described by Olah and Glick (1978a; 1981) and Olah *et al.* (1979). Niedorf and Wolters (1974) described a migration of macrophages from the cortex to the medulla where they are phagocytic, and morphologically distinguishable from the reticular-epithelial cells. The number of lymphoid follicles in the bursa has been estimated to be between 8000 and 12 000 (Olah and Glick, 1978b).

A specialized differentiation of bursal epithelium, with pinocytotic activity, where it overlies lymphoid follicles, has been described (Figs 1–5); this provides a mechanism for transport of antigens from the lumen of the bursa into the lymphoid follicle (Bockman and Cooper, 1973; Holbrook *et al.*, 1974; Olah and Glick, 1978b). Enzymic activities of bursal epithelium (and other lymphoid tissues) were described by Ruuskanen *et al.* (1977). Two types of bursal follicles, "button-like" and "projecting", were revealed in studies with the scanning electron microscope; these had the characteristic "follicle-associated epithelium" and were separated by "interfollicular surface epithelium" (Holbrook *et al.*, 1974; Naukkarinen *et al.*, 1978) (Fig. 3). Lymph vessels are present in the interfollicular and sub-epithelial connective tissue, but have not been demonstrated in the lymphoid follicles (Ekino *et al.*, 1979). An area of T-cell localization dorsal to the bursal duct was described by Odend'hal and Breazile (1979, 1980), and may play a role in B- and T-cell cooperation in the bursa. Post-natal development of the duck bursa is described by Ward and Middleton (1971) and Hashimoto and Sugimura (1976a) and of the chicken bursa by Bellamy and Mohamed (1982) and Romppanen (1982).

Bursa-specific non-immunoglobulin cell surface determinants can be detected on bursal and peripheral B-cells (Hudson and Roitt, 1973; Wick *et al.*, 1973; Albini and Wick, 1974). In the bursa, cells bearing B-determinants first appear at about 12 days of incubation, and increase to 90% after hatching. Boyd and Ward (1978) also detected a chicken B-lymphocyte specific antigen on cortical and medullary bursal lymphocytes, and a chicken mature B-lymphocyte antigen localized in the medulla. A chicken foetal-associated antigen was found in the cortex and characterized as a more immature feature of lymphoid cells. Chicken B-cells share an antigenic determinant with brain (Potworowsky and Forget, 1975). Alloantigens can also be used as B-cell markers (Donnelly *et al.*, 1976).

B. Development

Vasculogenesis of the bursa in embryos from 10 d old and in chicks up to 5 d old was described by Schoenwolf *et al.* (1981). The specialized follicle-

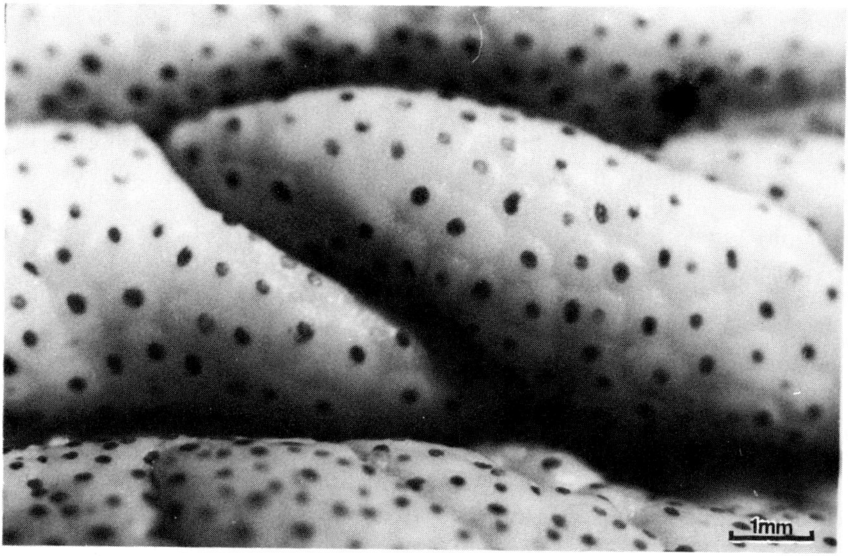

Fig. 1. Areas of uptake of carbon particles by follicle-associated epithelium on folds of the bursa of an 8-week-old chicken, 4 h after application of indian ink to the lips of the vent.

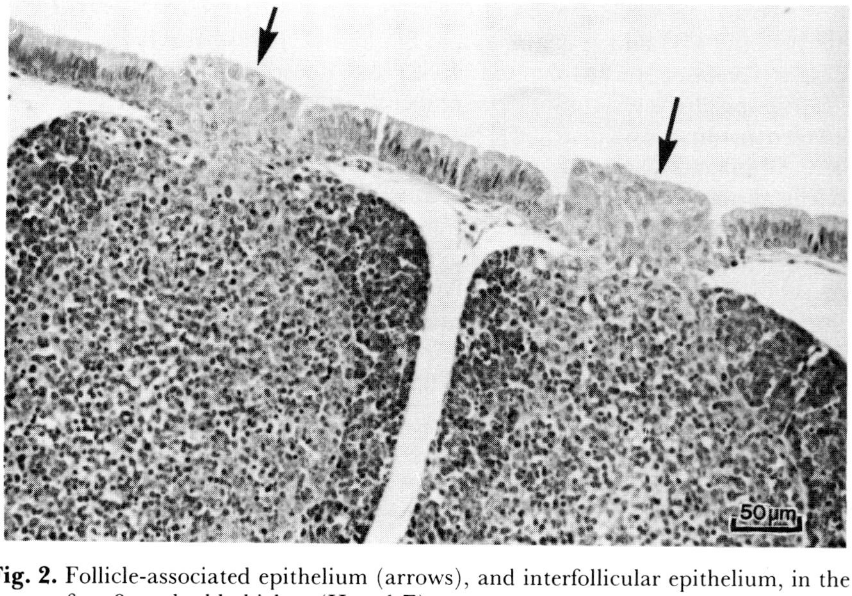

Fig. 2. Follicle-associated epithelium (arrows), and interfollicular epithelium, in the bursa of an 8-week-old chicken (H and E).

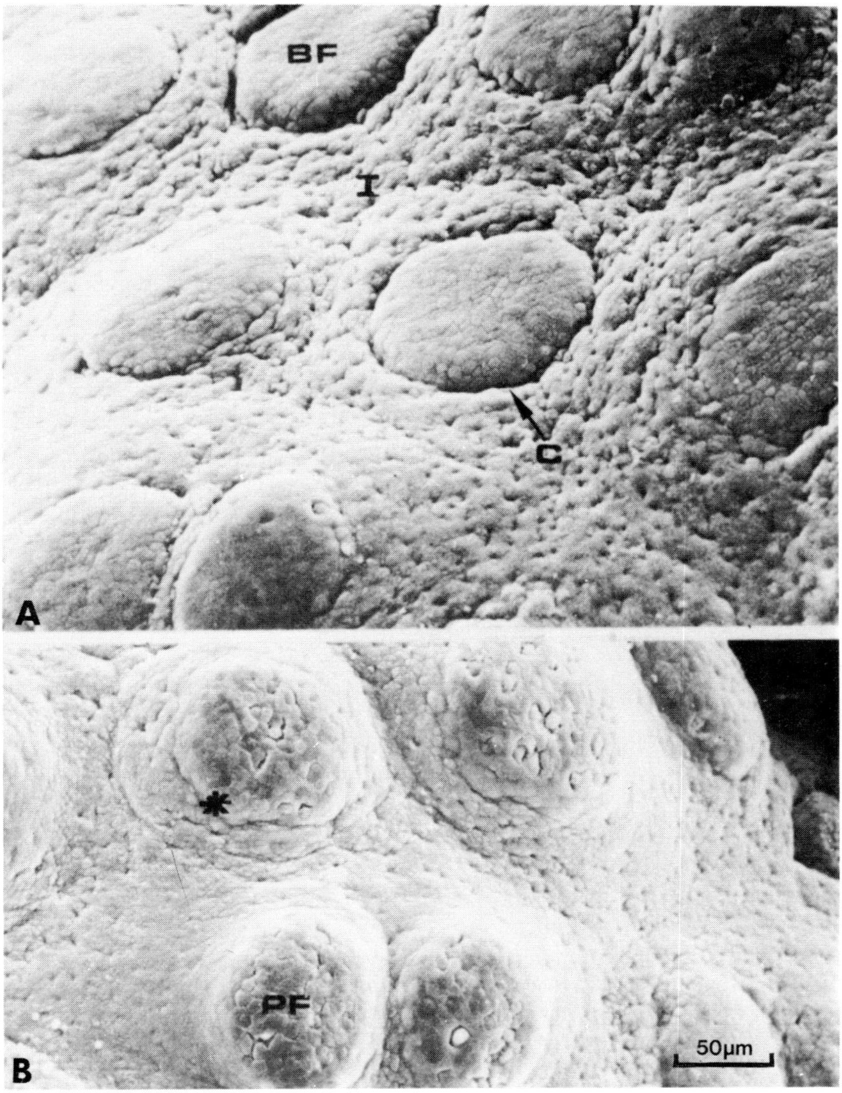

Fig. 3. Scanning electronmicrographs of: (*a*) button-like follicles (BF), showing a crypt (C) which separates the follicle from the surrounding interfollicular epithelium (I); and (*b*) projecting follicles (PF), showing point of transition (*) between follicular and interfollicular epithelium. (From Holbrook *et al.*, 1974, by kind permission).

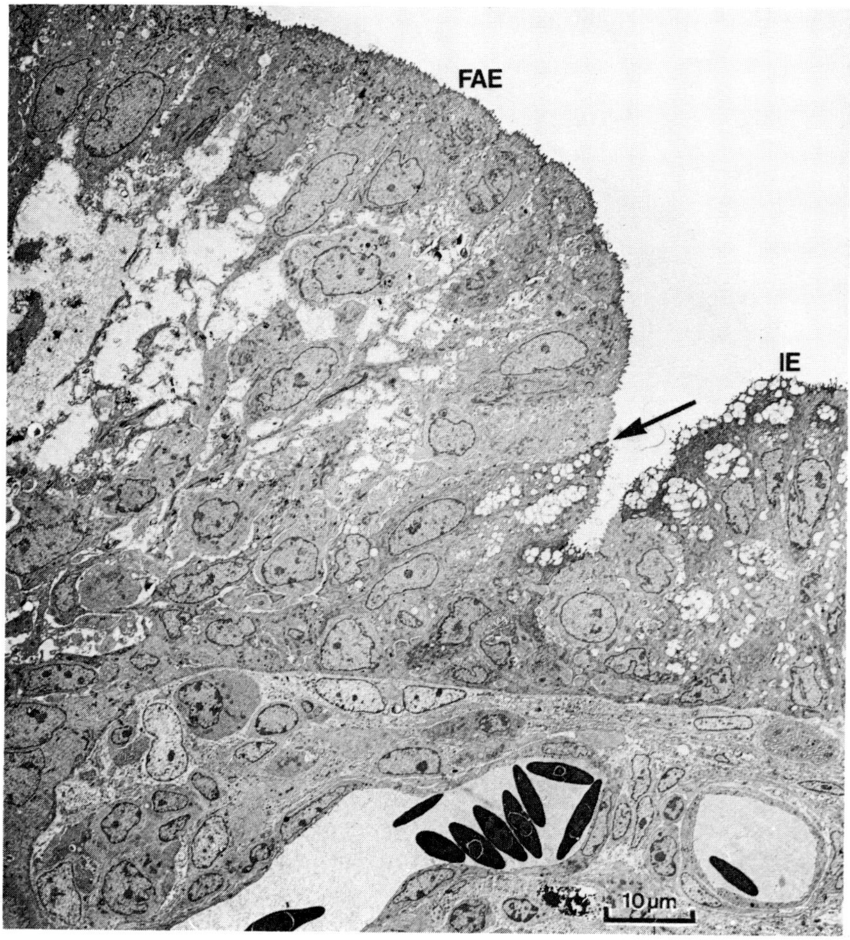

Fig. 4. Transmission electronmicrograph of bursa of an 8-week-old chicken, showing junction (arrow) between follicle-associated epithelium (FAE) and interfollicular epithelium (IE). Note the mucus-containing cells of the interfollicular epithelium. (Courtesy of Dr A. M. Lawn).

associated epithelium appears at the 13th day of incubation (Naukkarinen *et al.*, 1978). There is evidence that the adrenal gland influences bursal growth (Kilkarni *et al.*, 1971). Other studies on the development of the bursa have centred on the origin of lymphoid cells and their functional maturation. Using parabiotic embryos of opposite sex, and sex chromosome cell-markers, Moore and Owen (1966) showed that the stem cells of the bursal lymphoid system

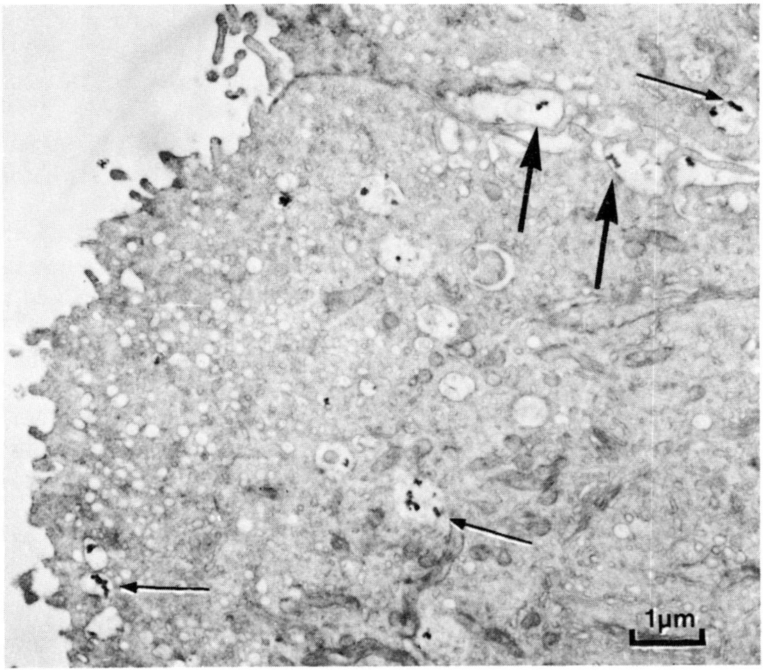

Fig. 5. Transmission electronmicrograph of the follicle-associated epithelium of the bursa of an 8-week-old chicken 4 h after application of indian ink to the lips of the vent. Carbon particles are present in pinocytotic vesicles (small arrows) and in the intercellular space (large arrows). (Courtesy of Dr A. M. Lawn).

arise in an extra-bursal site. Later these stem cells were shown to be present in the yolk sac at 7 d of incubation (Moore and Owen, 1967b; Metcalf and Moore, 1971). More recently, an earlier location of stem cells was identified within the embryo body at a stage before vascular connections have been established between the embryo and the yolk sac (Dieterlen-Lievre *et al.*, 1976, 1979; Martin *et al.*, 1978; 1979; Lassila *et al.*, 1978, 1979a). Studies of Lassila *et al.* (1979b, 1980) show that the stem cells are present in mesenchymal tissue of the 7-d-old chick embryo. These cells are termed "prebursal stem cells"; they start to enter the bursa at 8 d of incubation, but may remain pluripotent until about 12 to 13 d (A. Toivanen *et al.*, 1981).

The stem cells proliferate within the epithelial buds of the developing bursa, giving rise to the medullary part of the lymphoid follicles; the cortex of the follicle develops at the time of hatching (Cooper *et al.*, 1972; Houssaint *et al.*, 1976) by migration of more mature cells from the medulla via lymphoid vessels

(Ekino *et al.*, 1979). An account of follicular development is given by Edwards *et al.* (1975).

Functional differentiation of lymphoid stem cells in the bursa requires contact with the bursal epithelium (P. Toivanen and A. Toivanen, 1973b; Houssaint *et al.*, 1976). More recently, renewed interest has been shown in the existence of bursal hormones concerned with lymphoid cell differentiation. A small polypeptide, "bursopoietin", present in bursal extract, was shown to stimulate differentiation of primative bursal cells (Brand *et al.*, 1976, 1978; Goldstein *et al.*, 1976; Gilmour *et al.*, 1977) and another soluble factor may be concerned with late differentiation (Baba and Okuno, 1976; Baba and Kita, 1977; Heller and Friedman, 1979).

During late embryonic life and early post-hatching the bursa contains "bursal stem cells" (P. Toivanen *et al.*, 1972a,b,c; P. Toivanen and A. Toivanen, 1973b). These are themselves immunologically incompetent, but within the inductive environment of the bursa they will differentiate into competent B-cells. They can reconstitute functional and morphological integrity of the lymphoid cell-depleted bursae of newly-hatched chicks treated with cyclophosphamide (Lerman and Weidanz, 1970; Linna *et al.*, 1972) (Fig. 6). However, bursal stem cells cannot restore immunological competence of surgically bursectomized, cyclophosphamide-treated chicks, illustrating the importance of the bursal micro-environment. The ability of bursal cells to reconstitute the bursae of cyclophosphamide-treated chicks is lost at about six weeks of age, but at this time bursal cells can restore functional competence in the absence of the epithelial bursal rudiment; similarly competent cells are also present in the spleen, bone marrow and thymus, and are termed "post bursal cells" (A. Toivanen *et al.*, 1972; P. Toivanen and A. Toivanen 1973b; Ivanyi *et al.*, 1972; Matsuda *et al.*, 1975). Post-bursal cells have been subdivided into "early" and "late" categories, depending respectively on whether they can or cannot home to the bursa and form germinal centres in the spleen.

Full restorative properties of bursal stem cells in cyclophosphamide-treated chicks occurs only when donor and host are syngeneic; in allogeneic recipients, IgM production and antibody production to thymus-independent antigens is restored, but IgG production, responses to thymus-dependent antigens, and germinal centre formation are absent (P. Toivanen *et al.*, 1974a; A. Toivanen and P. Toivanen, 1975). Apparently, host T-cells recognize the allogeneic B-cells as foreign, even though they are not rejected.

The first cells in the bursa which express immunoglobulin appear at about day 12; they express IgM and increase in number during subsequent embryonic development. The first IgG-positive cells appear at 14 d and IgA-positive cells at 16 d (Kincade and Cooper, 1971; Tao-Wiedmann *et al.*, 1975; Lydyard *et al.*, 1976; Grossi *et al.*, 1977; Chen, 1978). These changes are believed to involve cellular switches in production from IgM → IgG → IgA,

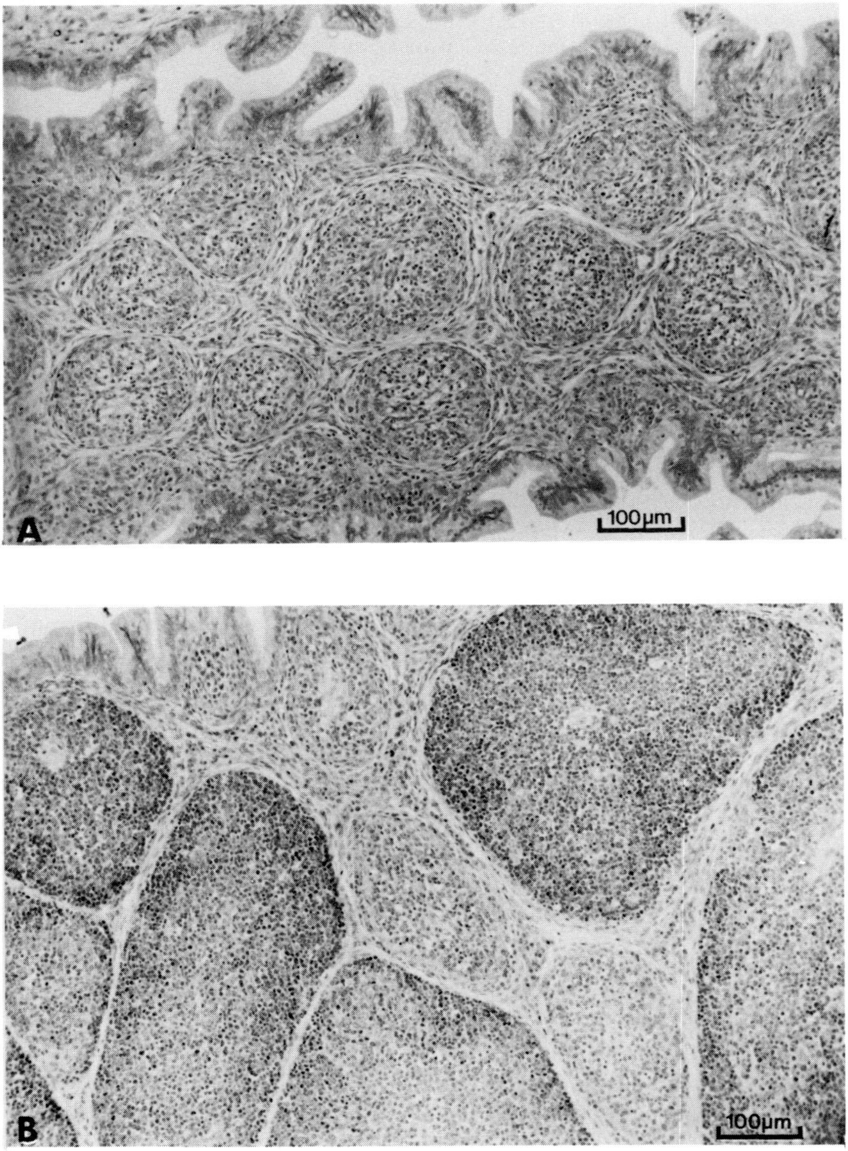

Fig. 6. (*a*) Bursa of 58-day-old chicken, following injection of 4 mg of cyclophosphamide daily for the first three days of life, showing loss of lymphoid tissue in the follicles. (*b*) As (*a*), but bird reconstituted by intravenous inoculation of 2×10^7 bursal cells from 7-day-old isogeneic donors, showing lymphoid cell repopulation of most follicles (H and E).

and seeding out of immunocompetent B-cells into the peripheral lymphoid tissue during the late stages of embryogenesis occurs in the same order. Evidence for these sequential changes is:

(i) Treatment of 13-d embryos with anti-IgM serum followed by bursectomy suppresses the development of all classes of immunoglobulin (Kincade *et al.*, 1970; Kincade and Cooper, 1973).

(ii) Bursectomy at 17 d reduces the levels of circulatory IgM and IgG and the number of plasma cells and germinal centres.

(iii) Bursectomy at 19 d often results in normal or enhanced amounts of IgM, but no other Ig classes (Cooper *et al.*, 1969).

(iv) Neonatal bursectomy, when IgM and IgG cells have seeded out into peripheral lymphoid tissues, results in a deficiency of IgA cells (Kincade and Cooper, 1973).

Antigen-binding cells are detected in the bursa from about the 14th day of incubation (Dwyer and Warner, 1971; Lydyard *et al.*, 1976; Moriya and Ichikawa, 1979). Cells binding a given antigen occur in several follicles and any one follicle contains cells binding several antigens. B-cell clones forming antibody to specific antigens arise at different times.

The capacity to respond to an antigenic challenge with antibody formation is not manifested until shortly after hatching. Immunization of 18- to 19-d-old embryos results in detectable antibody production from 2 days after hatching (see Seto, 1981). Availability of T-cells to interact with B-cells may be the limiting factor for neonatal humoral immunity. Germinal centre formation, which is dependent on such an interaction, cannot be induced before 4 d of age (Vainio *et al.*, 1978).

The question has been raised of whether B-cell differentiation can occur in the absence of the bursa. Following surgical removal of the bursal anlagen at 70 h of incubation, Ig-forming cells were observed in the spleen, and IgM in the serum, following repeated immunization (Fitzsimmons *et al.*, 1973; Jankovic *et al.*, 1977). Several candidates for extra-bursal sites of B-cell differentiation have been suggested, including bone marrow (Eskola, 1977; Eskola and Toivanen, 1977; Weber and Mausner, 1977), and intestinal lymphoid tissue (Bryant *et al.*, 1973).

C. Chemical Inhibition of the Bursa

Following the use of testosterone to cause bursal ablation, studies have been made with a synthetic androgen analogue, mibolerone, which when fed during the first few weeks of life, causes a slow but progressive involution of the bursa with retention of immunocompetence (Romero *et al.*, 1977), although absence of post-bursal stem cells in the spleen of mibolerone-treated chickens was reported (Romero *et al.*, 1978a). The bursal regression prevents development of lymphoid leukosis tumours (Romero *et al.*, 1978b). Antiserum against μ-chain has also been administered to embryos to abrogate lymphoid development (Kincade *et al.*, 1970). In recent years, however, increasing use has been made of cyclophosphamide to cause bursal ablation.

This drug, when administered to newly-hatched chicks, produces a severe, long-lasting, and according to some workers, permanent, destruction of B-cell function (Lerman and Weidanz, 1970; Glick, 1971; Linna *et al.*, 1972; Rouse and Szenberg, 1974; Eskola and Toivanen, 1974) (Fig. 6). Similar changes occur in the duck (Hashimoto and Sugimura, 1976b; Sigmura and Hashimoto, 1976). A severe, but transient, destruction of the thymus-dependent lymphoid system also occurs (Sharma and Lee, 1977). The bursa of a cyclophosphamide-treated chick shows loss of bursal lymphoid follicles, interfollicular fibrosis, but retention of reticuloepithelial tissue; later, limited follicular lymphoid recovery may occur (Hoffmann-Fezer *et al.*, 1977a). Treated birds show a marked deficiency of serum immunoglobulins and impaired antibody synthesis. The completeness of the depletion of B-cell structure and function varies according to the dose of drug and times of administration (Hirota and Bito, 1975).

Another method of chemical bursectomy has been described by Romppanen and Sorvari (1980a,b) and Romppanen *et al.* (1981) in which colchicine is applied to the anal lips of young chicks. This resulted in a transient loss of lymphoid cells from bursal lymphoid follicles, with limited repopulation later, no major effects on the spleen and thymus, and decreased serum IgG levels and antibody responses.

D. Function

From the studies reviewed by Payne (1971), and those described above, it is evident that the main functions of the bursa are the immunological education of prebursal stem cells to form immunoglobulin-producing cells, and the seeding of the resultant bursal stem cells to the peripheral, secondary, lymphoid tissues where they produce immunoglobulins and specific antibodies, and perform other immunological functions. Bursal cells have been shown to migrate to germinal centres and peri-ellipsoidal areas in the spleen (Hemmingsson, 1972b; de Kruyff *et al.*, 1975; Glick, 1977). In addition, evidence has accrued that the bursa may itself function as a peripheral lymphoid organ, involving the phenomenon of "cloacal drinking" discussed below.

New knowledge on the function of bursal lymphoid tissue and cells is reviewed in the following sections.

1. Immunoglobulin and Antibody Synthesis

A full account of immunoglobulin and antibody synthesis in the chicken and other birds is given by Higgins (1975) and Benedict and Yamaga (1976). Low molecular weight antibody, designated IgG, with sedimentation coefficient of 7S, occurs in fowl serum, as does a high molecular weight, 17S, antibody, IgM. As in mammals, the primary antibody response in the fowl consists chiefly of IgM, and the secondary response of IgG.

An IgA-like immunoglobulin, associated with local immunity, which probably binds with a secretory component, has been studied by several workers (Lebacq-Verheyden *et al.*, 1972; Orlans and Rose, 1972, Bienenstock *et al.*, 1972). It is found particularly in bile, lachrymal fluid, saliva, and secretions in the intestinal, respiratory and reproductive tracts and is thought to occur as a trimer of mol. wt. 500 000 and a monomer of mol. wt. 170 000 (Kobayashi and Hirai, 1980).

Evidence for the involvement of an IgE-like antibody in passive cutaneous anaphylaxis in the fowl has been conflicting (see Benedict and Yamaga, 1976), but recent work suggests IgE occurs (Burns and Maxwell, 1981). A homologue to mammalian IgD has been reported by Chen *et al.* (1982).

Allotypes of IgG and IgM, controlled at two closely linked loci, have been recognized in the chicken (see Ivanyi, 1981) and can be used as B-cell markers to identify donor cells in chimaeric or reconstituted recipients. In contrast to the mammal, the chicken shows only limited variation of antibody spectrotypes as revealed by isoelectric focusing or electrophoresis (Huang and Dreyer, 1978).

2. "Cloacal Drinking" and Immunological Responsiveness of the Bursa

When fluids are dropped onto the vent (cloacal orifice) of embryos or chickens, rhythmic contractions of the sphincter muscles cause the fluid to be sucked into the cloaca, bursa and lower part of the intestinal tract (Schaffner *et al.*, 1974; R. Sorvari *et al.* 1977); this phenomenon has been termed "cloacal drinking" (Figs 1 and 7). R. Sorvari and T. Sorvari (1977) found that carbon particles so administered were taken up from the bursal lumen by the specialized follicle-associated epithelium (Bockman and Cooper, 1973; Naukkarinen *et al.*, 1978; Naukkarinen and Sorvari, 1980) by endocytosis and passed into the medulla and cortex of the bursal follicle (Fig. 5). Killed bacteria administered in this way stimulated an agglutinin response, and it is suggested that this mechanism may be a way in which the fowl gains part of its immunity to environmental micro-organisms. Transport of carbon from the medulla to other parts of the bursa and to the bursal lumen is described by Naukkarinen (1982). Bursal lymphocytes bind, and produce antibodies against, *E. coli* (Van

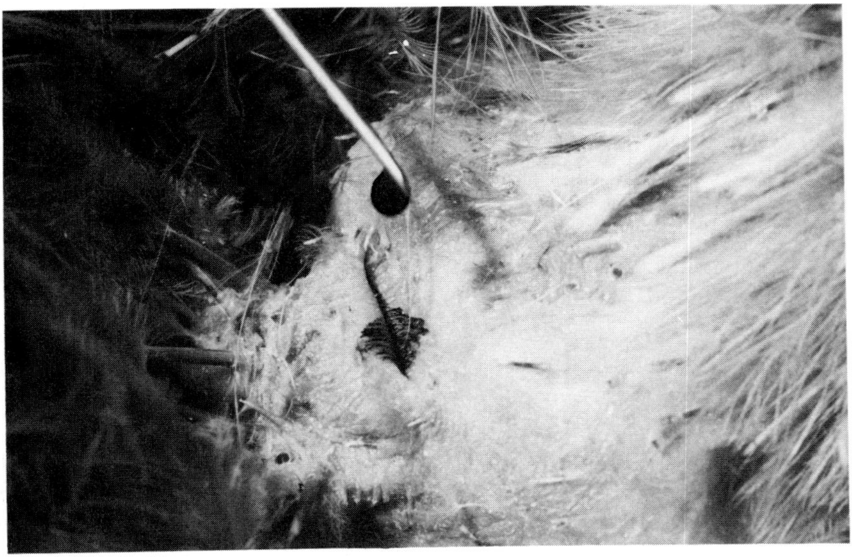

Fig. 7. Uptake of indian ink dropped onto the lips of the vent: so-called "cloacal drinking".

Alten and Meuwissen, 1972; Waltenbaugh and Van Alten, 1974). Bursectomy four to five days after intrabursal antigenic priming was found to enhance humoral responses, possibly due to removal of bursa-derived suppressor cells (Hirota *et al.*, 1981b). Isolation of the bursa from the cloacal environment by ligation of the embryonic bursal duct has been reported to retard bursal development and immune functions by Ekino *et al.* (1980), but not by others (Lupetti and Dolfi, 1980).

3. Disease Resistance

The effect of bursectomy on response to infectious diseases has continued to be used to determine the role of humoral immunity in disease resistance. Humoral antibodies have been shown in this way to be important in protection against avian influenza virus (Portnoy *et al.*, 1973), Newcastle disease (Perey and Dent, 1975), of minor importance in recovery from fowl pox virus infection (Morita, 1973) and of no importance in immunity to infectious bronchitis (Chubb, 1974) or infectious laryngotracheitis (Robertson, 1977).

Infectious bursal disease, caused by a virus, has attracted attention because the associated acute necrosis of bursal lymphocytes (Cheville, 1967) results in immunosuppression (Faragher *et al.*, 1972; Hirai *et al.*, 1974; Giambrone *et al.*,

1977a), the severity of which depends on the stage of bursal ontogeny at the time of infection (Hudson *et al.*, 1975; Ivanyi and Morris, 1976). This "viral bursectomy" increases susceptibility to other infections, including Newcastle disease (Allan *et al.*, 1972; Faragher *et al.*, 1974), Marek's disease (Cho, 1970); *Escherichia coli* and *Salmonella typhimurium* (Wyeth, 1975), and *Eimeria tenella* (Giambrone *et al.*, 1977b). Response to Newcastle disease and Marek's disease vaccination was also impaired (Giambrone *et al.*, 1976).

The development of lymphoid leukosis, which originates in the bursa, is prevented by infection with infectious bursal disease virus (Purchase and Chiville, 1975).

4. *Requirement of the Bursa for Normal Thymic Development*

Neonatal bursectomy was found by Zucher *et al.* (1973) to decrease a population of small, dense lymphocytes, estimated at 15% of the total lymphocyte pool, in the thymus of 16-week-old chickens. This sub-population of cells was considered not to be effector T-cells or peripheral B-cells. They suggested that they were suppressor cells involved in mediation of immune tolerance, but this seems unlikely in view of the finding of Rouse and Warner (1972b) that tolerance to allografts could be induced in hormonally bursectomized chickens. However, suppressor T-cells can be induced in bursectomized chickens (Chi *et al.*, 1980). Fitzsimmons *et al.* (1973) observed severe cortical atrophy of the thymus in birds surgically bursectomized at 70 h of incubation.

IV. Spleen

A. Structure

There has been limited recent work on the structure of the spleen (*splen*), but one area which has progressed is the delineation of bursa- and thymus-dependent regions within the organ (Fig. 8). The ellipsoids or Schweigger-Seidel sheaths which project from the white pulp (*pulpa splenica alba*) into the red pulp (*pulpa splenica ruba*) each carry a peri-ellipsoidal cuff of lymphocytes. These cuffs are equivalent to the tissue of the marginal zone in the mammalian spleen, through which circulatory T- and B-cells enter the white pulp (Ford, 1975; Weissman *et al.*, 1974), and are bursa-dependent (Cooper *et al.*, 1966; Mori and Hoshi, 1971; Hoshi, 1972; Boyd and Ward, 1978). The lymphocytes forming the peri-arteriolar sheaths are mainly thymus-dependent (Cooper *et al.*, 1965; Mori and Hoshi, 1971; Hoshi, 1972; Hoffmann-Fezer *et al.*, 1977b; Boyd and Ward, 1978), but a bursa-dependent component is also present (Romppanen and Sorvari, 1981). Splenic structure in the fowl has been described in detail by Hodges (1974), Maas (1974) and White (1981), and in

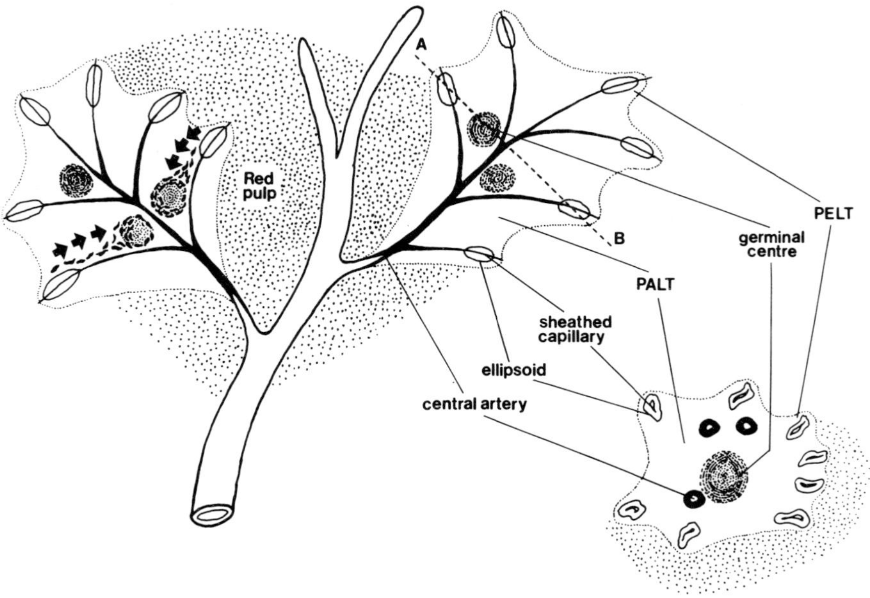

Fig. 8. A diagrammatic representation of the spleen of the adult chicken. The peri-arteriolar lymphoid tissue (PALT) or white pulp is thymus-dependent, but the peri-ellipsoidal lymphoid tissue (PELT) or peri-ellipsoidal cuffs consist of B-cells and antigen-bearing dendritic cells. The latter migrate to the points of division of the central artery (shown by arrows) and, together with specific B-cells, form germinal centres. The transverse section shown is taken at the level of the dotted line A-B through an island of white pulp.

the duck by Hashimoto and Sugimura (1977, 1980). The detailed study of the white pulp and associated vascular channels by Olah and Glick (1982) is especially noteworthy. Development of the white pulp in relation to onset of immunological competence is described by Ogata *et al.* (1977) and ultra-structural aspects of the splenic circulation by Fukuta *et al* (1976) and Olah and Glick (1982). Results of a morphometrical method for analysing splenic lymphoid structure are given by Romppanen (1981) and Romppanen and Sorvari (1981).

B. Development

Lymphoid cells have been observed in the spleen as early as 10 or 11 d of embryonic develoment (Albini and Wick, 1975; Jankovic *et al.*, 1975; Weber,

1975). The first cells with T-cell characteristics appear at about 16 d and by 20 d these are mainly in the red pulp and in small clusters around the arteries (Albini and Wick, 1975; Hoffman-Fezer *et al.*, 1977b). A few cells staining with anti-B-cell or with anti-μ antisera appear at 12 d, but the number of B-cells remains small throughout embryogenesis. At around the time of hatching some cells with surface IgG can be detected.

C. Function

The relationship between splenic morphology and the response to immunological challenge has been analysed in detail by White (1963, 1976, 1981), White and Gordon (1970), White *et al.* (1970, 1975), French *et al.* (1971) and Olah and Glick (1982). Intravenously injected particles leave the blood stream within seconds, by passing through the ellipsoids (Fig. 9). White and Gordon (1970) demonstrated the passage of carbon particles through channels between the high endothelial cells of the ellipsoids, which was followed by extracellular deposition beyond the basement membrane and endocytosis by macrophages within the ellipsoids. These channels are formed between endothelial cytoplasmic processes which pass through 2 μm holes in the basement membrane, thus ensuring the rapid transport of the particles to the vicinity of the macrophages. Antigen–antibody complexes follow the same route as inert material (White *et al.*, 1970); injected human serum albumin initially circulates in the blood until antibody is synthesized, presumably as a result of some of the antigen gaining access to the sinuses and cords of the red pulp. Complexes appear around the ellipsoids 30 to 72 h after injection; they are then present on the bodies and dendritic extensions of cells in the periellipsoidal cuffs. The antigen-bearing dendritic reticular cells migrate along the penicillary vessels to their point of origin from the central artery, and germinal centres are visible at this site from 72 h onwards. These are formed by agglutination of the antigen-bearing dendritic cells with B-lymphocytes having complementary surface antibody receptors (Figs 10 and 11). By 6 d post injection, all the antigen-bearing dendritic cells have been included in the germinal centres. Non-antigenic particles are carried to the region of the germinal centres in the same way, but they remain outside, associated with the reticulum cells of the periphery. The germinal centres develop from groups of 20 to 30 large basophilic cells into compact balls of cells with a sharply defined periphery of narrow reticulum cells and reticulin fibres. Within them there is very close membrane contact between B-cells and dendritic reticular cells whose processes ramify between adjacent B-lymphocytes. It is necessary that the two cell types share the same histocompatibility antigens for cooperation leading to germinal centre production to occur (Toivanen *et al.*, 1974b).

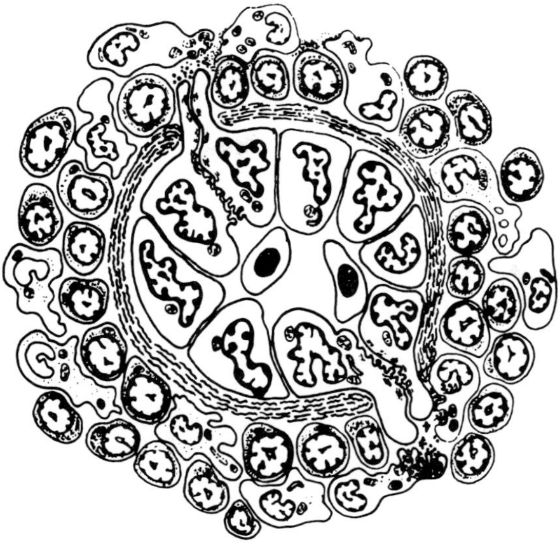

A

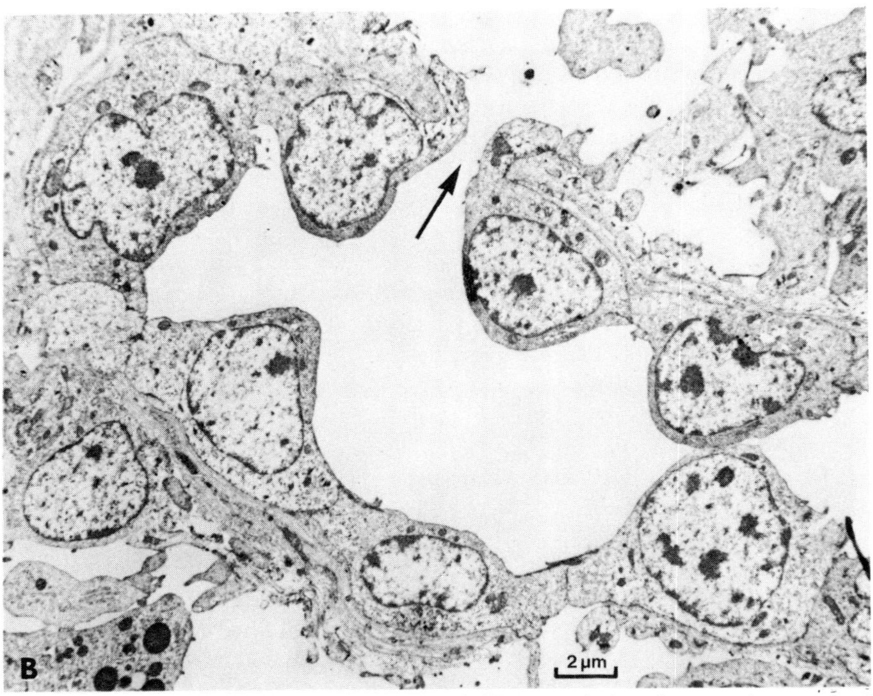

Fig. 9. (*a*) Diagrammatic representation and (*b*) transmission electronmicrograph of an ellipsoidal capillary in the spleen, showing channels (arrow) between endothelial cells, which allow passage of intravascular particles into the peri-ellipsoidal cuff of macrophages where endocytosis occurs. ((*a*) from White, 1981, by kind permission, and (*b*) by courtesy of Dr A. M. Lawn).

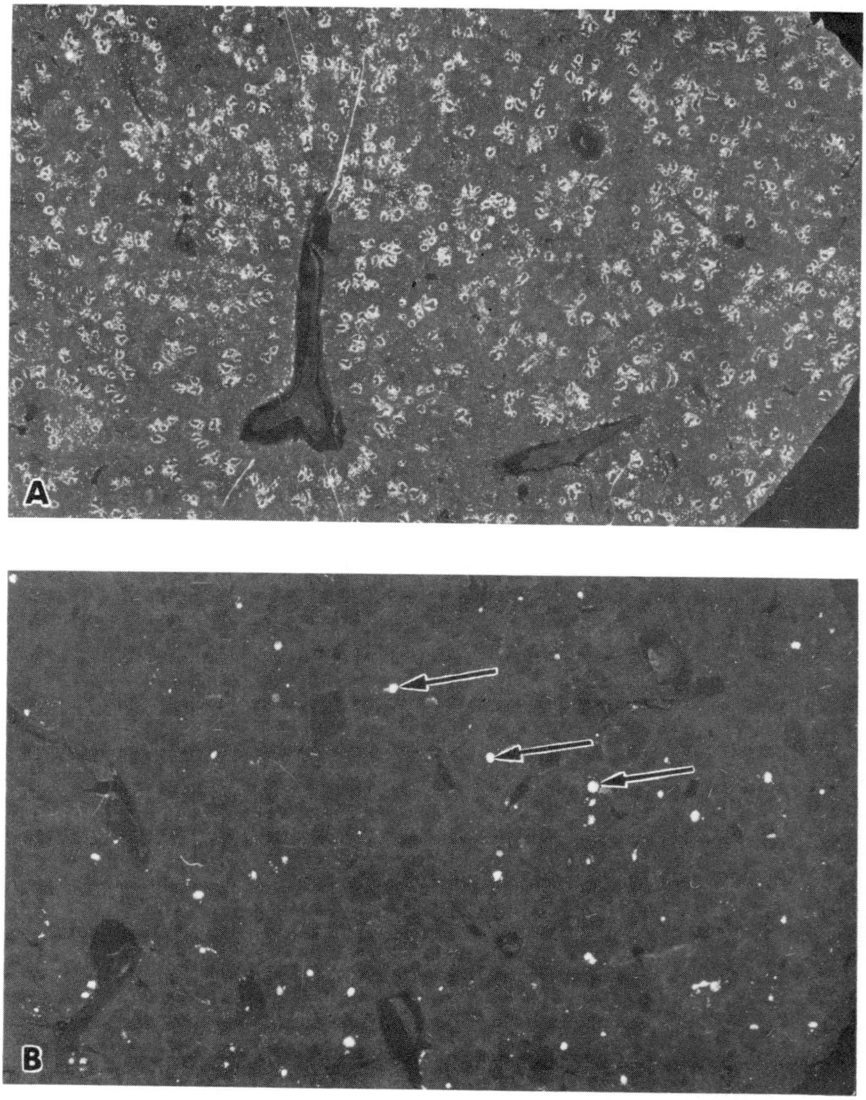

Fig. 10. Autoradiographs showing ^{125}I-labelled human serum albumin, present as rings of antigen–antibody complexes in macrophages of the peri-ellipsoidal cuffs at 3 days after injection (*a*) and in germinal centres (*b*, arrows) at 6 days after injection. (From White, 1981, by kind permission).

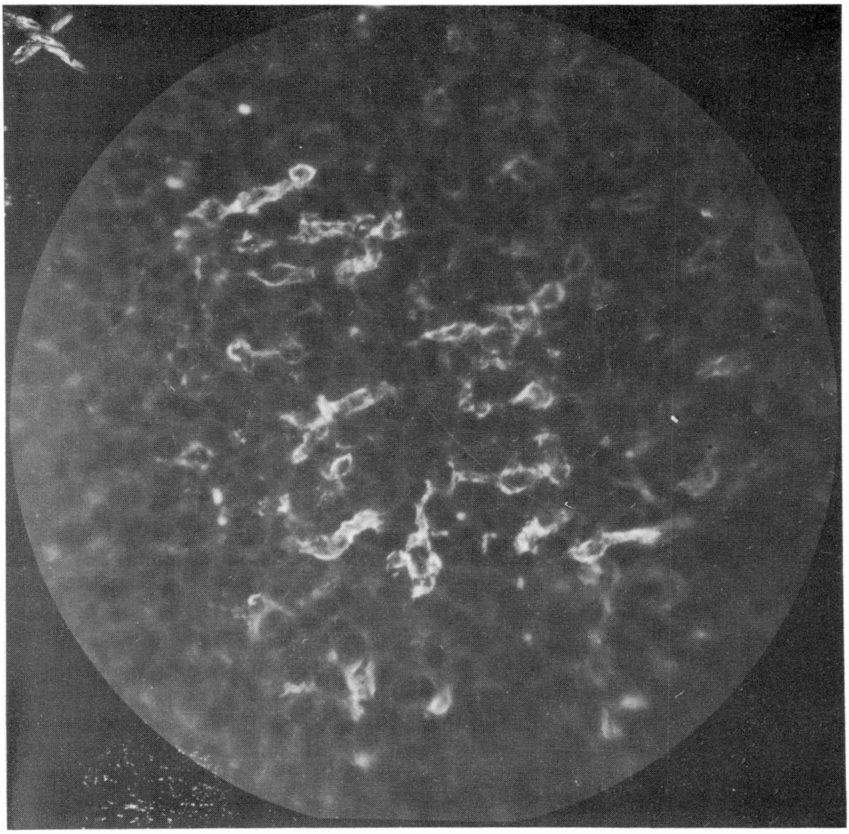

Fig. 11. Fluorescence micrographs of germinal centres in the spleen 6 days after injection of human serum albumin, showing human serum albumin present as antigen–antibody complexes on dendritic cells. (From White, 1976, by kind permission).

Ultrastructurally the B-lymphocytes have rather sparse endoplasmic reticulum and are apparently in a state of arrested development. It seems that the function of the germinal centre is the proliferation of immunologically competent memory B-cells, rather than their development into plasma cells. Plasma cell proliferation occurs in the red pulp. Germinal centres normally appear at about 10 d of age but after intense antigenic stimulation they can occur as early as 4 d. Their number increases for two to four months and then declines; there is, however, no correlation between the number of centres and antibody-producing capacity (P. Toivanen *et al.*, 1974b).

Although the spleen is a major component of the peripheral lymphoid system, splenectomy has no profound effect on immunological responsiveness. Nevertheless, the spleen is an important source of antibodies, and its removal delays the peak of antibody response in young birds, and depresses antibody production in older birds (Rosenquist and Wolfe, 1962; Aitken, 1973).

V. Lymphoid Tissue in the Alimentary Tract

A. Structure

Lymphoid tissue is irregularly distributed throughout the alimentary tract, from pharynx to cloaca, in the *lamina propria* and submucosa (Payne, 1971). This tissue can occur as solitary and aggregated masses (*lymphonoduli solitarii et aggregati*), the most organized expression of the latter being the caecal tonsils (*lymphonoduli cecales*) and the Peyer's patches (Befus *et al.*, 1980; Burns, 1982).

According to Hoshi and Mori (1973), lymphoid tissue in the caecal tonsil occurs in two sites: (i) the mid and deep areas of the lamina propria, which contain germinal centres and small lymphocytes, and which was considered to be a thymus-dependent area; and (ii) the sub-epithelial zone, containing lymphocytes of various sizes and plasma cells, but not germinal centres, which was considered to be bursa-dependent. In contrast, Olah and Glick (1979) distinguished two types of germinal centre, one with an incomplete capsule and lying deep in the muscularis, and the other encapsulated and lying close to the epithelium. Those authors also described a new cell type, which they considered might be secretory, present in germinal centres in the tonsil, and also in these centres in the spleen and mural lymph nodules and in the medullae of bursal lymphoid follicles. The structure of the epithelium of the caecal tonsil under the scanning electron microscope was described by Glick *et al.* (1978).

Lymphocytes from the caecal tonsil comprise equal proportions of B- and T-cells at 5 weeks of age, with a preponderance of B-cells in older birds (Albini and Wick, 1974).

Following the studies of Bäck (1970a,b; 1972a,b), intra-epithelial lymphoid cells in the jejunum and ileum have been classified as small lymphocytes, large lymphoid cells and granular cells by Bjerregaard (1975) (Fig. 12). The granular cells have also been termed globule leukocytes, and there is controversy about whether they are derived from lymphocytes or mast cells (Toner, 1965; Gregory, 1979). Techniques for isolating gut intra-epithelial lymphoid cells and lymphoid cells from the lamina propria were described by Arnaud-Battandier *et al.* (1980).

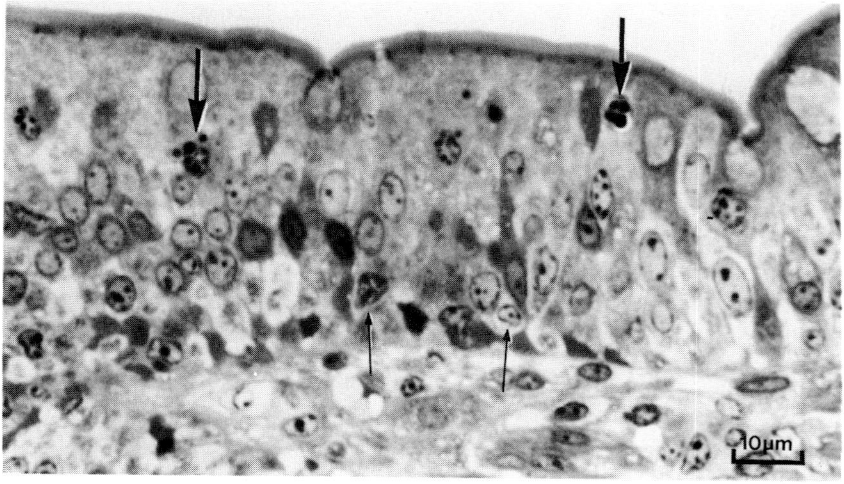

Fig. 12. Intra-epithelial lymphocytes (small arrows) and globule leukocytes (large arrows) in epithelium of the ileum of a 6-week-old chicken. (Plastic embedded, methylene blue/azure and basic fuchsin; courtesy of Dr A. M. Lawn).

B. Development

In confirmation of earlier studies (see Payne, 1971), the caecal tonsils were observed to contain few lymphocytes at hatching, but these increase in number in both sub-epithelial and deeper zones from 1 d of age. Germinal centres appeared at about 2 weeks (Hoshi and Mori, 1973; Hoffmann-Fezer, 1973). The number of intra-epithelial lymphoid cells in the small intestine increases with age after hatching (Bäck, 1972b; Bjerregaard, 1975).

C. Function

Intestinal lymphoid tissue provides the mechanisms for local immune responses to gut antigens. In mammals, antigens pass through the specialized dome epithelium covering the submucosal lymphoid tissues of Peyer's patches, where in response IgA antibodies are produced and pass, by means of their secretory component, through gut epithelial cells into the lumen. This antigenic sampling is similar to the uptake of antigens by bursal epithelium (Section IIID2) and has been suggested to occur in the caecal tonsils (Sorvari *et al.*, 1975). Carbon uptake, immunoglobulin and antibody production by Peyer's patches have been reported in chickens (Burns, 1982).

Hudson (1975) observed that 31% of caecal tonsil lymphocytes from adult chickens expressed IgA. A large proportion of B-cells elsewhere in the intestine also contains IgA (Lebacq-Verheyden, 1972; Bienenstock *et al.*, 1973); their appearance in the duodenum was prevented by neonatal thymectomy and bursectomy and they were replaced by IgM-containing cells (Perey and Bienenstock, 1973).

Functional studies on gut mucosal lymphoid cells, both intra-epithelial and from the lamina propria, were made by Arnaud-Battandier *et al.* (1980). They found that lymphoid cells from either site failed to respond to B or T mitogens. Ig-secreting cells (mainly IgG and IgA) were present among intra-epithelial lymphocytes, but were relatively more frequent among lymphoid cells from the lamina propria. From studies on germ-free animals, it is evident that lymphoid tissue in both locations is associated with stimulation from antigens in the gut lumen. Lymphocytes in these sites probably represent partially overlapping subsets of cells concerned with local humoral and cell-mediated immunity.

VI. Oculonasal Lymphoid Tissue

A. Structure

Recent research on oculonasal lymphoid tissue has focused chiefly on the Harderian gland (gland of the nictitating membrane—*Gl. membranae nictitantis*), which lies in the orbit and is well developed in birds. The anatomy, blood supply, innervation and histological structure of the Harderian gland in the chicken are described by Wight *et al.* (1971a) and its ultrastructure by Rothwell *et al.* (1972). The gland has a compound tubulo-acinar structure producing a merocrine secretion, with marked accumulations of mainly plasma cells in the interstitium (Fig. 13). With age, an increasing number of the plasma cells develop PAS-positive cytoplasmic Russell bodies. Histochemical reactions of mucosubstances in the gland are described by Wight *et al.* (1971b). Burns (1975) classified the Harderian glands of 32 species of birds into three main types, depending on their resemblance to the gland in chickens (type I), duck (type II) or rook (type III). The lachrymal gland (*Gl. lacrimalis*) is another orbital gland and in the bird is less well developed than the Harderian gland, a reversal of the usual relationship in mammals. Removal of the Harderian gland increases the number of plasma cells in the lachrymal gland, possibly as a compensatory mechanism (Burns, 1979). In the chicken and duck the lachrymal glands are similar, consisting of a compound tubulo-acinar structure, with some lymphocytic infiltration but few plasma cells

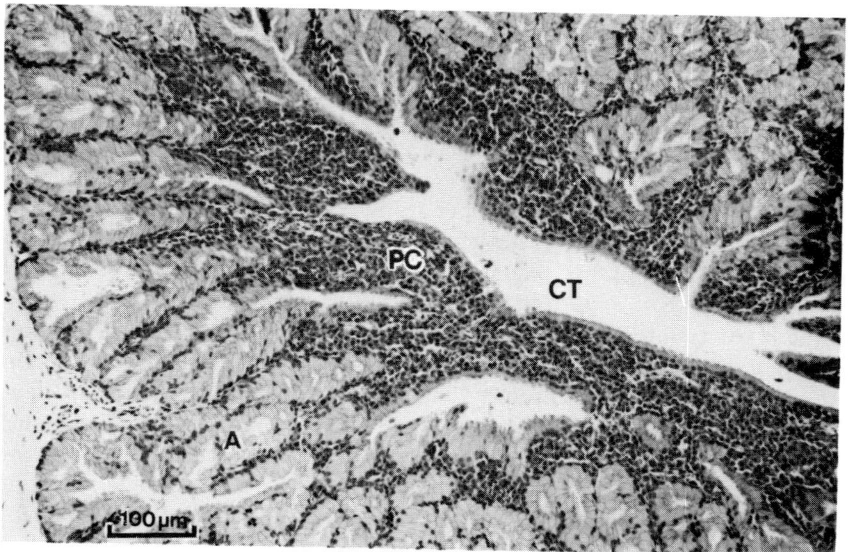

Fig. 13. Harderian gland of an 8-week-old chicken showing glandular acini (A), accumulations of plasma cells (PC), and a collecting tubule (CT), (H and E).

(Burns, 1976a). The structure of the Harderian and lachrymal gland ducts is described by Burns and Maxwell (1979).

B. Development

Niedorf and Wolters (1978) described the development of the Harderian gland. It arises from epithelial cones of the conjunctiva between the 11th and 12th day of embryonic life, and passes through a stage of "epithelial development" from days 13 to 17. The interstitial tissue becomes invaded by "eosinophils" and small blast cells on days 17 and 18, and shortly after hatching these blast cells develop into plasma cells and increase until the 4th week—the stage of "plasmacellular development". The glandular epithelium becomes secretory at day 17 of embryonal life.

Wight *et al.* (1971a) also found that very few plasma cells were present in the Harderian gland of newly-hatched chicks, but that these accumulated so that large numbers were present by 45 d. The numbers of plasma cells were reduced by bursectomy, suggesting bursa-dependency (Mueller *et al.*, 1971; Sundick *et al.*, 1973; Wolters *et al.*, 1977); however, failure to eliminate these cells by early embryonic hormonal bursectomy raised the possibility that some might be independent of the bursa (Lerner *et al.*, 1971; Wolters *et al.*, 1977).

C. Function

The Harderian and lachrymal glands produce mucoid secretions which clean and moisten the cornea and lubricate the nictitating membrane (Wight *et al.*, 1971a,b; Burns, 1976a). Evidence has accumulated that the plasma cells in the Harderian gland secrete antibodies into the lachrymal fluids which confer local immunity to the eye and upper respiratory tract.

Topical administration of antigens into the eye results in an increase in lymphoid foci and plasma cells in the Harderian gland and lachrymal gland (Davelaar and Kouwenhoven, 1976; Survashe *et al.*, 1979). Antigen uptake by the Harderian gland is believed to be via the secretory duct to the primary collecting duct and the acini (Burns, 1977). Following administration of antigen into the eye, antibody-producing cells appear in the Harderian gland (Mueller *et al.*, 1971), and antibodies can be detected in extracts of the gland, in lachrymal fluid and in the serum (Survashe and Aitken, 1977; Parry and Aitken, 1977; Survashe *et al.*, 1979). These responses are notable following local antigenic stimulation, but weaker responses can sometimes be evoked by antigens given parenterally (Burns, 1976b; Powell *et al.*, 1979). During the first few weeks of life IgM-producing cells predominate in the Harderian gland, followed later by IgA and IgG-producing cells (Albini *et al.*, 1974).

Functions of the Harderian and lachrymal glands have been studied following their surgical removal (Neumann, 1976; Survashe and Aitken, 1977; Davelaar, 1980). This procedure prevented the appearance of antibodies in the lachrymal fluid (Survashe and Aitken, 1977). In the absence of the Harderian glands, the lachrymal glands are believed to fulfil their role to some extent (Davelaar and Kouwenhoven, 1980). The Harderian gland was shown to be necessary for protection against eyedrop challenge by infectious bronchitis virus in chicks vaccinated by this route (Davelaar and Kouwenhoven, 1980), and this protection did not extend to intratracheal challenge (Davelaar and Kouwenhoven, 1981).

VII. Bone Marrow

As a lymphopoietic tissue the bone marrow of the fowl has received only limited attention, but it is evident that it functions as a source of bursal and thymic stem cells, and also as a secondary lymphoid tissue. It has been speculated that the marrow may also be a primary lymphoid tissue for B-cell differentiation, as in the mammal, and an alternative to the bursa (see A. Toivanen *et al.*, 1981).

The marrow contains diffuse lymphoid tissue with germinal centres (see Payne, 1971). In an analysis of the cellular composition of fowl marrow, Glick and Rosse (1976) observed 7·4% lymphocytes, and 1·3% plasma cells, in 8-week-old birds, with lower proportions in younger birds. Some of the lymphocytes, and all of the plasma cells, carried membrane Ig. These Ig-positive B-cells were absent from hormonally bursectomized birds, suggesting that they were either bursa-derived or bursa-dependent (Glick *et al.*, 1975). Hudson and Roitt (1973) found that 27% of marrow cells bore a B-cell marker although only 2% displayed surface Ig. No cells with T-cell markers were observed.

Throughout the ontogenetic development of the T-cell system, and in the adult, the marrow is a source of thymic stem cells (Weber and Mausner, 1977; Brand *et al.*, 1978). The marrow of the hatched chick is also a source of early and late post-bursal cells capable of restoring B-cell competence in bursectomized birds (Ivanyi *et al.*, 1972; P. Toivanen *et al.*, 1974c; Matsuda *et al.*, 1975). Under the influence of ubiquitin or cyclic AMP, marrow cells from newly-hatched chicks develop B- or T-cell markers; under the influence of thympoietin they acquire T-cell charateristics (Brand *et al.*, 1977).

Marrow cells are capable of producing antibodies (Ivanyi *et al.*, 1972; P. Toivanen *et al.*, 1972a; McArthur *et al.*, 1973) as a consequence of migration of bursal cells to the marrow (P. Toivanen *et al.*, 1974c; Eskola and Toivanen, 1976; Eskola, 1977). Marrow cells also express T-cell functions, as shown by their ability to mount a graft-versus-host reaction (Terasaki *et al*, 1959; Solomon, 1961).

VIII. Lymphatic Vessels, Mural Lymphoid Nodules and Lymphocyte Circulation

The comprehensive and profusely illustrated accounts of the anatomy of the lymphatic system by Baum (1930) and Dransfield (1944, 1945) have been summarized by King (1975) and Rose (1981). The lymphatic vessels (*vasa lymphatica*) are small, the largest hardly being more than 1 mm in diameter, and the thoracic duct (*truncus thoracoabdominalis*) itself is only 1·5 mm across. Variations in the thoracic duct are described by Miyaki and Yasuda (1977). The vessels are lined with endothelium, and only the larger ones have thicker walls containing collagenous and elastic fibres and a few muscle cells. The development of the lymphatic systems starts early, on the 4th day of embryonation (Romanoff, 1960), and it is possible that the lymphatic vessels may permit the traffic of stem cells into the bursa and thymus from the intra-embryonic mesenchyme.

Lawn and Rose (1981) have described the ultrastructure of the paired lumbar lymph node (*lymphonodus lumbaris*) of the duck (Fig. 14). This consists of a swelling of the lymphatic duct containing a crude filtration apparatus of

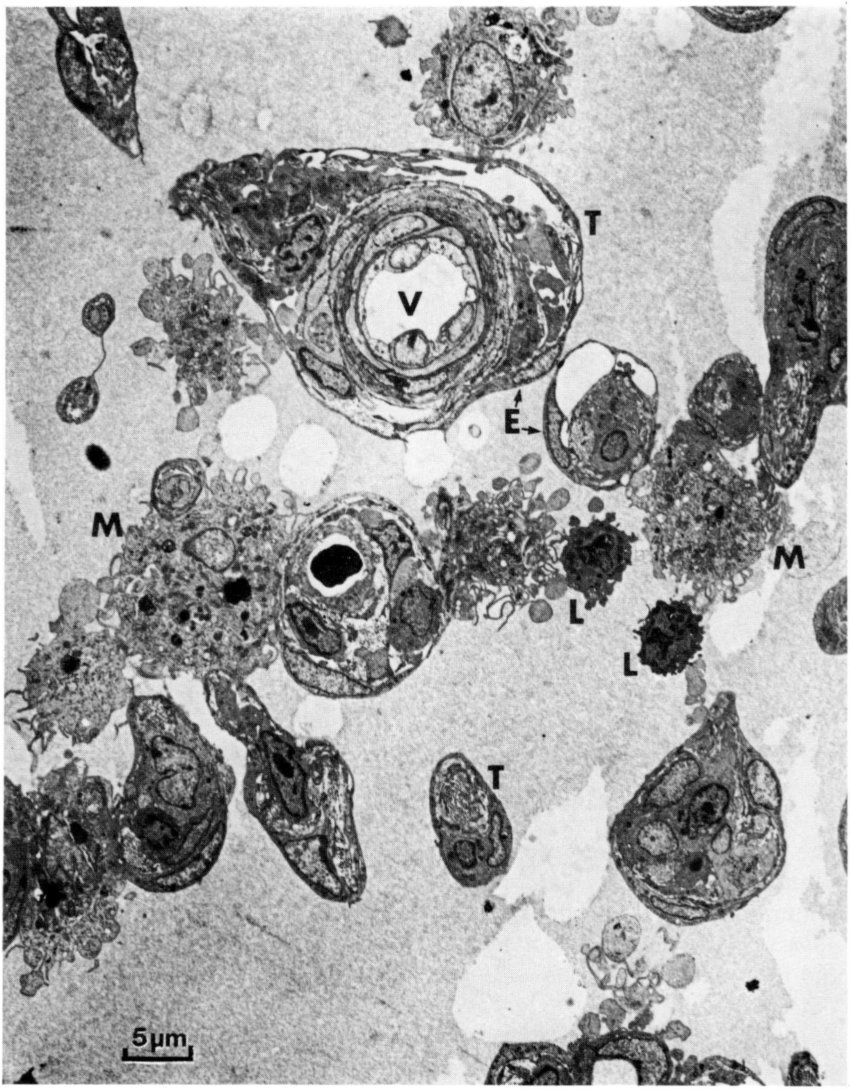

Fig. 14. Transmission electronmicrograph of part of a filtering area of a lumbar lymph node from an 8-month-old duck. There are transverse sections through trabeculae (T), some of which contain blood vessels (V). The trabeculae are enveloped by lymphatic endothelium (E). Macrophages (M) are attached to the trabeculae and lymphocytes (L) are present in the lymph space, which contains aggregated protein. (From Lawn and Rose, 1981, by kind permission).

phagocytic macrophages attached to trabeculae crossing the lymphatic spaces. There is a rather complete barrier to cell migration between the lymph and the lymphoid tissue which is bordered by a continuous endothelium bonded by desmosomes. The dense lymphoid tissue contains blood vessels analogous to the post capillary venules of mammalian lymph nodes (which allow lymphocyte migration between the blood and lymphoid tissue). The deeper part of the dense lymphoid tissue of the node is believed to be thymus-dependent, and the looser peripheral lymphoid tissue and germinal centres to be bursa-dependent; other areas are apparently independent of the bursa and thymus (Sugimura *et al.*, 1977). White (1981) suggested that avian lymph nodes function to ensure intimate contact between antigen and a large number of lymphocytes of differing specificities, by supporting the flow of lymphocytes between the blood and lymphatic tissue. However, the possession of lymph nodes is limited to certain, mainly aquatic, avian species. Chickens do, however, possess mural lymphoid nodules (*lymphonoduli murales*) on their lymphatic vessels (see Payne, 1971). McCorkle *et al.* (1979) observed that those in the femoral lymphatic enlarged in some birds following footpad injection of sheep red blood cells, and they contained on average 38% T-cells and 53% B-cells, and plaque-forming cells.

The recirculation of lymphocytes within the body has been little studied. The cellular composition of the lymph collected from the "cervical" duct of the duck indicated that it was more analogous to the central lymph (draining fixed lymphoid tissue) than to the peripheral lymph (draining non-lymphoid tissue) of mammals, suggesting that the large collections of lymphoid tissue in the cervical drainage area perform the function of the mammalian lymph nodes (Bell and Lafferty, 1972). These authors found that the average rate of flow of lymph in the cervical duct was 1 ml h^{-1}, with a total output of $4{\cdot}1 \times 10^6$ cells h^{-1}, of which 91% were lymphocytes. A more active migration of lymphocytes through all the tissues of the body might compensate for the lack of lymph nodes.

IX. Lymphoid Tissue in other Organs

There has been little attention paid in recent years to the numerous small foci of lymphoid tissue that occur scattered throughout many organs and tissues (Payne, 1971). In structure these resemble lymphoid tissue elsewhere, consisting mainly of small lymphocytes sometimes surrounding germinal centres, although the latter may also occur isolated from diffuse lymphoid tissue. It is generally considered that these areas of lymphoid tissue are normal anatomical structures, although it is not clear to what extent antigenic stimulation may contribute to their formation (see Rose, 1981). Birds differ from mammals in their ability to create elements with the organization of a lymph node locally at the sites of deposition of antigen. In chicken skin, for example, the immediate heterophil response in the acute inflammatory reaction to injection is quickly (from six hours after injection) superseded and supplanted by lymphoid hyperplasia around the smaller vessels (Carlson and Allen, 1969; Nair, 1973). A similar response, deviating from the mammalian reaction, was observed in turkeys and ducks (Aitken and Survashe, 1974). Local germinal centres develop at the sites of water-in-oil emulsions in most tissues within two to three weeks of injection, and there may be little evidence of earlier inflammatory exudation. The germinal centres develop along the sides of the local blood vessels, apparently in the course of the draining lymphatics (White, 1981), and they show the typical components of dendritic cells bearing antigen–antibody complexes scattered amongst B-lymphocytes (White *et al.*, 1977).

However, these responses do not generally involve pre-existing foci of peripheral lymphoid tissue for, at least in the duck, these apparently develop *de novo* by recruitment of cells from the blood in response to locally persistent antigen (Bell, 1974a,b,c). The foci cannot, then, be regarded as analogous to mammalian draining lymph nodes, although presumably they would function as such in response to new antigenic challenge. Nevertheless, it seems probable, as Biggs (1957) suggested, that the widespread distribution of peripheral lymphoid tissue, or rather the capability of the system to respond by the formation of new lymphoid foci, compensates for the lack of mammalian-type lymph nodes, and the absence of the latter accounts for the frequency of peripheral germinal centre formation in the fowl (White, 1981).

Acknowledgements

We are indebted to Dr A. M. Lawn and Dr M. E. Rose for helpful comments on the manuscript, to Dr A. M. Lawn, Professor B. Glick and to Professor R. G. White for providing illustrations, to S. F. Hodgson and A. W. Kidd for the photography, and Mrs Helen Tiddy for secretarial assistance.

References

Aitken, I. D. (1973). *Immunology*, **25**, 957–966.
Aitken, I. D. and Survashe, B. D. (1974). *Avian Path.* **3**, 211–222.
Albini, B. and Wick, G. (1974). *J. Immun.* **112**, 444–450.
Albini, B. and Wick, G. (1975). *Int. Archs Allergy appl. Immun.* **48**, 513–529.
Albini, B., Wick, G., Rose, M. E. and Orlans, E. (1974). *Int. Archs Allergy appl. Immun.* **47**, 23–34.
Allan, W. H., Faragher, J. T. and Cullen, G. A. (1972). *Vet. Rec.* **90**, 511–512.

Arnaud-Battandier, F., Lawrence, E. C. and Blaese, R. M. (1980). *Dig. Dis. Sci.* **25**, 252–259.
Baba, T. and Kita, M. (1977). *Immunology,* **32**, 271–274.
Baba, T. and Okuno, Y. (1976). *Immunology,* **31**, 533–539.
Bacchus, S. and Kendall, M. D. (1975). *Phil. Trans. R. Soc.* **B 273**, 65–73.
Bäck, O. (1970a). *Int. Archs Allergy appl. Immun.* **39**, 192–200.
Bäck, O. (1970b). *Int. Archs Allergy appl. Immun.* **39**, 342–351.
Bäck, O. (1972a). *Acta path. microbiol. scand.* **A 80**, 84–90.
Bäck, O. (1972b). *Acta path. microbiol. scand.* **A 80**, 91–96.
Baum, H. (1930). *Z. Anat. EntwGesch.* **93**, 1–34.
Baumel, J. J., King, A. S., Lucas, A. M., Breazile, J. E. and Evans, H. E. (1979). "Nomina Anatomica Avium." Academic Press, London and New York.
Befus, A. D., Johnston, N., Leslie, T. A. and Bienenstock, J. (1980). *J. Immunol.* **125**, 2626–2632.
Bell, R. G. (1974a). *Aust. J. exp. Biol. med. Sci.* **52**, 433–445.
Bell, R. G. (1974b). *Aust. J. exp. Biol. med. Sci.* **52**, 445–453.
Bell, R. G. (1974c). *J. Reticuloend. Soc.* **15**, 213–224.
Bell, R. G. and Lafferty, K. J. (1972). *Aust. J. exp. Biol. med. Sci.* **50**, 611–623.
Bellamy, D. and Mohamed, K. (1982). *Thymus* **4**, 107–114.
Benedict, A. A. (ed.), (1977). "Avian Immunology." Plenum Press, New York.
Benedict, A. A. and Yamaga, K. (1976). *In* "Comparative Immunology" (J. J. Marchalonis, ed.), pp. 335–375. Wiley, New York.
Bienenstock, J., Perey, D. Y. E., Gauldie, J. and Underdown, B. J. (1972). *J. Immun.* **109**, 403–406.
Bienenstock, J., Gualdie, J. and Perey, D. Y. E. (1973). *J. Immun.* **111**, 1112–1118.
Biggs, P. M. (1957). *Ph.D. thesis, University of Bristol.*
Biggs, P. M. and Payne, L. N. (1959). *Nature, Lond.* **184**, 1594.
Bjerregaard, P. (1975). *Cell. Tiss. Res.* **161**, 485–495.
Blaese, R. M., Weiden, P., Koski, I. and Dooley, N. (1974). *J. exp. Med.,* **140**, 1097–1101.
Bloom, B. R. and David, J. R. (eds.), (1976). "*In vitro* Methods in Cell-Mediated and Tumor Immunity." Academic Press, New York.
Bockman, D. E. and Cooper, M. D. (1973). *Am. J. Anat.* **136**, 455–478.
Boyd, R. L. and Ward, H. A. (1978). *Immunology,* **34**, 9–17.
Brake, J., Morgan, G. W. and Thaxton, P. (1981). *Devl. comp. Immun.* **5**, 105–112.
Brand, A., Gilmour, D. G. and Goldstein, G. (1976). *Science, N.Y.* **193**, 319–321.
Brand, A., Gilmour, D. G. and Goldstein, G. (1977). *Nature, Lond.* **269**, 597–598.
Brand, A., Galton, J. and Gilmour, D. G. (1978). *Fedn. Proc. Fedn. Am. Socs exp. Biol.* **37**, 1742.
Bryant, B. J., Adler, H. E., Cordy, D. R., Shifrine, M. and DaMassa, A. J. (1973). *Eur. J. Immun.* **3**, 9–15.
Burns, R. B. (1975). *Can. J. Zool.* **53**, 1258–1269.
Burns, R. B. (1976a). *Res. vet. Sci.* **21**, 292–299.
Burns, R. B. (1976b). *Clin. exp. Immun.* **26**, 371–374.
Burns, R. B. (1977). *Br. Poult. Sci.* **18**, 407–409.
Burns, R. B. (1979). *Res. vet. Sci.* **27**, 69–75.
Burns, R. B. (1982). *Res. vet. Sci.* **32**, 359–367.
Burns, R. B. and Maxwell, M. (1979). *J. Anat.* **128**, 285–292.

Burns, R. B. and Maxwell, M. (1981). *Vet. Res. Commun.* **5**, 67–72.
Carlson, H. C. and Allen, J. R. (1969). *Avian Dis.* **13**, 817–833.
Carpenter, C. R., Bose, H. R. and Rubin, A. S. (1977). *Cell. Immun.* **33**, 392–401.
Chen, C. L. (1978). *Fedn. Proc. Fedn. Am. Socs. exp. Biol.* **37**, 1395.
Chen, C. L. H., Lehmeyer, J. E. and Cooper, M. D. (1982). *J. Immunol.* **129**, 2580–2585.
Cheville, N. F. (1967). *Am. J. Path.* **51**, 527–551.
Chi, D. S., Grebenau, M. D. and Thorbecke, G. J. (1980). *Eur. J. Immun.* **10**, 203–209.
Chi, D. S., Galton, J. E. and Thorbecke, G. J. (1981). *In* "Avian Immunology" (M. E. Rose, L. N. Payne and B. M. Freeman, eds), pp. 103–134. British Poultry Science Ltd, Edinburgh.
Cho, B. R. (1970). *Avian Dis.* **14**, 665–675.
Chubb, R. C. (1974). *Res. vet. Sci.* **17**, 169–173.
Cooper, M. D., Peterson, R. D. A. and Good, R. A. (1965). *Nature, Lond.* **205**, 143–146.
Cooper, M. D., Peterson, R. D. A., South, M. A. and Good, R. A. (1966). *J. exp. Med.* **123**, 75–102.
Cooper, M. D., Cain, W. A., Van Alten, P. J. and Good R. A. (1969). *Int. Archs Allergy appl. Immun.* **35**, 242–252.
Cooper, M. D., Lawton, A. R. and Kincade, P. W. (1972). *In* "Contemporary Topics in Immunobiology" (M. G. Hanna, ed.), pp. 33–47. Plenum Press, New York.
Danchakoff, V. (1915–16). *Anat. Rec.* **10**, 483–492.
Davelaar, F. G. (1980). *Avian Path.* **9**, 591–595.
Davelaar, F. G. and Kouwenhoven, B. (1976). *Avian Path.* **5**, 39–50.
Davelaar, F. G. and Kouwenhoven, B. (1980). *Avian Path.* **9**, 489–510.
Davelaar, F. G. and Kouwenhoven, B. (1981). *Avian Path.* **10**, 83–90.
Davis, P. J. (1981). *In* "Avian Immunology" (M. E. Rose, L. N. Payne and B. M. Freeman, eds), pp. 361–385. British Poultry Science Ltd, Edinburgh.
De Kruyff, R. H., Gilmour, D. G. and Thorbecke, G. J. (1975). *J. Immun.* **114**, 1700–1704.
Dieterlen-Lievre, F., Beaupain, D. and Martin, C. (1976). *Annls Immun. Inst. Pasteur* **127C**, 857–863.
Dieterlen-Lievre, F., Beaupain, D., Lassila, O., Toivanen, P. and Martin, C. (1979). *In* "Development and Differentiation of Verterbrate Lymphocytes" (J. Horton, ed.), pp. 35–43. Elsevier/North Holland, Amsterdam.
Donnelly, N., Brand, A. and Gilmour, D. G. (1976). *Adv. exp. Med. Biol.* **64**, 293–302.
Dransfield, J. W. (1944). *M.V.Sc. thesis, University of Liverpool.*
Dransfield, J. W. (1945). *Br. vet. J.,* **101**, 171–179.
Droege, W. (1976). *Eur. J. Immun.* **6**, 279–287.
Dutton, R. W. (1975). *Transplantn Rev.* **26**, 39–55.
Dwyer, J. M. and Warner, N. L. (1971). *Nature, New Biol.* **229**, 210–211.
Edwards, J. L., Murphy, R. C. and Cho, Y. (1975). *Anat. Rec.* **181**, 735–753.
Ekino, S., Matsuno, K. and Kotani, M. (1979). *Lymphology,* **12**, 247–252.
Ekino, S., Nawa, Y., Tanaka, K., Matsuno, K., Fujii, H. and Kotani, M. (1980). *Aust. J. exp. Biol. med. Sci.* **58**, 289–296.
Eskola, J. (1977). *Immunology,* **32**, 467–474.
Eskola, J. and Toivanen, P. (1974). *Cell. Immun.* **13**, 459–471.
Eskola, J. and Toivanen, A. (1976). *Cell. Immun.* **26**, 68–77.
Eskola, J. and Toivanen, P. (1977). *In* "Avian Immunology" (A. A. Benedict, ed.), pp. 39–45. Plenum Press, New York.
Faragher, J. T., Allan, W. H. and Cullen, G. A. (1972). *Nature, Lond.* **237**, 118–119.

Faragher, J. T., Allan, W. H. and Wyeth, P. J. (1974). *Vet. Rec.* **95**, 385–388.
Firth, G. A. (1977). *Vet. Bull.* **47**, 167–179.
Fitzsimmons, R. C., Garrod, E. M. and Garnett, I. (1973). *Cell. Immun.* **9**, 377–383.
Fitzsimmons, R. C., Dixon, D. K. and Kocal, E. M. F. (1977). *In* "Developmental Immunobiology" (J. B. Solomon and J. D. Horton, eds), pp. 387–394. Elsevier/North Holland, Amsterdam.
Ford, W. L. (1975). *Prog. Allergy,* **19**, 1–59.
Frazier, J. A. (1973). *Z. Zellforsch. mikrosk. Anat.* **136**, 191–205.
Frazier, J. A. (1974a). *J. natn. Cancer Inst.* **52**, 839–848.
Frazier, J. A. (1974b). *Acta anat.* **88**, 385–397.
Fredericksen, T. L., Longenecker, B. M., Pazderka, F., Gilmour, D. G. and Ruth, R. F. (1977). *Immunogenetics,* **5**, 535–552.
French, V. I., Stark, J. M. and White, R. G. (1971). *In* "Morphological and Functional Aspects of Immunity" (K. Lindahl-Kiessling, G. Alm and M. G. Hanna, eds), pp. 179–186. Plenum Press, New York.
Fukuta, K., Nishida, T. and Mochizuki, K. (1976). *Jap. J. vet. Sci.* **38**, 241–254.
Galton, J. and Ivanyi, J. (1977a). *Eur. J. Immun.* **7**, 241–246.
Galton, J. and Ivanyi, J. (1977b). *Eur. J. Immun.* **7**, 457–459.
Giambrone, J. J., Eidson, C. S., Page, R. K., Fletcher, O. J, Barger, B. O. and Kleven, S. H. (1976). *Avian Dis.* **20**, 534–544.
Giambrone, J. J., Ewart, D. L. and Eidson, C. S. (1977a). *Poult. Sci.* **56**, 1591–1594.
Giambrone, J. J., Anderson, W. I., Reid, W. M. and Eidson, C. S. (1977b). *Poult. Sci.* **56**, 243–246.
Gilmour, D. G., Theis, G. A. and Thorbecke, G. J. (1970). *J. exp. Med.* **132**, 134–147.
Gilmour, D. G., Brand, A., Donnelly, N. and Stone, H. A. (1976). *Immunogenetics,* **3**, 549–563.
Gilmour, D. G., Brand, A. and Goldstein, G. (1977). *In* "Developmental Immunobiology" (J. G. Solomon and J. D. Horton, eds). pp. 395–401. Elsevier/North Holland.
Glick, B. (1971). *Transplantation,* **11**, 433–439.
Glick, B. (1977). *Int. Rev. Cytol.* **48**, 345–402.
Glick, B. (1978). *Poult. Sci.* **57**, 1441–1444.
Glick, B. and Rosse, C. (1976). *Anat. Rec.* **185**, 235–246.
Glick, B., Perkins, W. D., Rosse, C. and Schwarz, M. R. (1975). *Int. Archs Allergy appl. Immun.* **49**, 332–340.
Glick, B., Holbrook, K. A., Olah, I., Perkins, W. D. and Stinson, R. (1978). *Poult. Sci.* **57**, 1408–1416.
Goldstein, G., Sheid, M., Boyse, E. A., Brand, A. and Gilmour D. G. (1976). *Cold Spring Harb. Symp. quant. Biol.* **41**, 5–8.
Gregory, M. W. (1979). *Vet. Bull.* **49**, 821–827.
Grossi, C. E., Lydyard, P. M. and Cooper, M. D. (1977). *J. Immun.,* **119**, 749–756.
Hashimoto, Y. and Sugimura, M. (1976a). *Jap. J. vet. Sci.* **24**, 65–76.
Hashimoto, Y. and Sugimura, M. (1976b).) *Poult. Sci.* **55**, 1441–1449.
Hashimoto, Y. and Sugimura, M. (1977). *Jap. J. vet. Res.* **25**, 71–82.
Hashimoto, Y. and Sugimura, M. (1980). *Jap. J. vet. Sci.* **42**, 19–29.
Hashimoto, Y., Kitagawa, H., Kudo, N. and Sugimura, M. (1982). *Jap. J. vet. Sci.* **44**, 597–605.
Heller, D. E. and Friedman, A. R. (1979). *Devl comp. Immun.* **3**, 667–681.
Hemmingsson, E. J. (1972a). *Int. Archs Allergy appl. Immun.* **43**, 481–496.

Hemmingsson, E. J. (1972b). *Int. Archs Allergy appl. Immun.* **42**, 764–774.
Higgins, D. A. (1975). *Vet. Bull.* **45**, 139–154.
Higgins, D. A. (1981). *Vet. Bull.* **51**, 925–963.
Hirai, K., Shimakura, S., Kawamoto, E., Taguchi, F., Kims, T. and Chang, C. N. (1974). *Avian Dis.* **18**, 50–57.
Hirota, Y. and Bito, Y. (1975). *Poult. Sci.* **54**, 1524–1538.
Hirota, Y., Vainio, O. and Toivanen, P. (1981a). *Acta path. microbiol. scand.* **C89**, 145–153.
Hirota, Y., Vainio, O. and Toivanen, P. (1981b). *Acta path. microbiol. scand.* **C89**, 35–41.
Hodges, R. D. (1974). *In* "The Histology of the Fowl". Academic Press, London and New York.
Hoffmann-Fezer, G. (1973). *Z. Zellforsch. mikrosk. Anat.* **136**, 45–58.
Hoffmann-Fezer, G., Hoffman, R., Fiedler, H. and Lösch, U. (1977a). *Int. Archs Allergy appl. Immun.* **53**, 206–213.
Hoffmann-Fezer, G., Rodt, H., Götze, D. and Thierfelder, S. (1977b). *Int. Archs Allergy appl. Immun.* **55**, 86–95.
Holbrook, K. A., Perkins, W.-D. and Glick, B. (1974). *J. reticuloend. Soc.* **16**, 300–311.
Hoshi, H. (1972). *Tohoku J. exp. Med.* **106**, 285–305.
Hoshi, H. and Mori, T. (1973). *Tohoku J. exp. Med.* **111**, 309–322.
Houssaint, E., Belo, M. and Le Douarin, N. M. (1976). *Devl Biol.* **53**, 250–264.
Huang, H. V. and Dreyer, W. J. (1978). *J. Immun.* **121**, 1738–1747.
Hudson, L. (1975). *Eur. J. Immun.* **5**, 694–698.
Hudson, L. and Roitt, I. M. (1973). *Eur. J. Immun.* **3**, 63–67.
Hudson, L., Pattison, M. and Thantrey, N. (1975). *Eur. J. Immun.* **5**, 675–679.
Isler, H. (1976). *J. Cell. Sci.* **20**, 135–147.
Ivanyi, J. (1981). *In* "Avian Immunology" (M. E. Rose, L. N. Payne and B. M. Freeman, eds), pp. 63–101. British Poultry Science Ltd, Edinburgh.
Ivanyi, J. and Morris, R. (1976). *Clin. exp. Immun.* **23**, 154–165.
Ivanyi, J. and Salerno, A. (1971). *Eur. J. Immun.* **1**, 227–230.
Ivanyi, J., Murgatroyd, L. B. and Lydyard, P. M. (1972). *Immunology,* **23**, 107–111.
Jankovic, B. D., Isvaneski, M., Milosevic, D. and Popeskovic, L. (1963). *Nature, Lond.* **198**, 298–299.
Jankovic, B. D., Isakovic, K., Lukic, M. L, Vujanovic, N. L., Petrovic, S. and Markovic, B. M. (1975). *Immunology,* **29**, 497–508.
Jankovic, B. D., Isakovic, K., Markovic, B. M. and Rajcevic, M. (1977). *Immunology,* **32**, 689–699.
Kendall, M. D. (1980). *Devl. comp. Immun.* **4**, 191–209.
Kendall, M. D. and Ward, P. (1974). *Nature, Lond.* **249**, 366–367.
Kincade, P. W. and Cooper, M. D. (1971). *J. Immun.* **106**, 371–382.
Kincade, P. W. and Cooper, M. D. (1973). *Science, N.Y.* **179**, 398–400.
Kincade, P. W., Lawton, A. R., Bockman, D. E. and Cooper, M. D. (1970). *Proc. natn. Acad. Sci., USA* **67**, 1918–1925.
King, A. S. (1975). *In* "Sisson and Grossman's Anatomy of the Domestic Animals" 5th edn, (R. Getty, ed.), Vol. 2, pp. 2010–2018. W. B. Saunder Company, Philadelphia.
Kirchner, H. and Oppenheim, J. J. (1972). *Cell. Immun.* **3**, 695–699.
Kirchner, H., Altman, L. C., Fridberg, A. P. and Oppenheim, J. J. (1974). *Cell. Immun.* **10**, 68–77.
Kobayashi, K. and Hirai, H. (1980). *J. Immunol.* **124**, 1695–1704.

Kulkarni, P. G., Dressen, L. J., Love, J. and Glick, B. (1971). *Expl Cell Res.* **66**, 124–128.
Lamont, S. J. and Van Alten, P. J. (1981). *J. Immunol. Methods.* **40**, 181–191.
Lassila, O., Eskola, J., Toivanen, P., Martin, C. and Dieterlen-Lievre, F. (1978). *Nature, Lond.* **272**, 353–354.
Lassila, O., Martin, C., Dieterlen-Lievre, F., Nurmi, T. E., Eskola, J. and Toivanen, P. (1979a). *Transplantn Proc.* **11**, 1085–1088.
Lassila, O., Eskola, J. and Toivanen, P. (1979b). *J. Immun.* **123**, 2091–2094.
Lassila, O., Eskola, J., Toivanen, P. and Dieterlen-Lievre, F. (1980). *Scand. J. Immun.* **11**, 445–448.
Lawn, A. M. and Rose, M. E. (1981). *Res. vet. Sci.* **30**, 335–342.
Lebacq-Verheyden, A. M. (1972). *J. Immun.* **109**, 652–654.
Lebacq-Verheyden, A. M., Vaerman, J. P. and Heremans, J. F. (1972). *Immunology,* **22**, 165–175.
Le Douarin, N. M. and Jotereau, F. V. (1973). *Nature, Lond.* **246**, 25–27.
Le Douarin, N. M. and Jotereau, F. V. (1975). *J. exp. Med.* **142**, 17–40.
Le Douarin, N. M., Houssaint, E., Jotereau, F. and Belo, M. (1975). *Proc. natn. Acad. Sci., USA* **72**, 2701–2705.
Le Douarin, N. M., Jotereau, F. V. and Houssaint, E. (1976). *In* "Phylogeny of Thymus and Bone Marrow-Bursa Cells" (R. K. Wright and E. L. Cooper, eds), pp. 217–226. Elsevier/North Holland.
Le Douarin, N. M., Houssaint, E. and Jotereau, F. (1977). *In* "Avian Immunology" (A A. Benedict, ed.), pp. 29–37. Plenum Press, New York and London.
Lee, L. F. (1974). *Avian Dis.* **18**, 602–609.
Lee, L. F. (1978). *Avian Dis.* **22**, 296–307.
Lee, L. F. (1979). *J. Immun.* **123**, 1088–1091.
Lee, L. F., Powell, P. C., Rennie, M., Ross, L. J. N. and Payne, L. N. (1981). *J. natn. Cancer Inst.* **66**, 789–796.
Lerman, S. P. and Weidanz, W. P. (1970). *J. Immun.* **105**, 614–619.
Lerner, K. G., Glick, B. and McDuffie, F. C. (1971). *J. Immun.* **107**, 493–503.
Linna, T. J., Frommel, D. and Good, R. A. (1972). *Int. Archs Allergy appl. Immun.* **42**, 20–39.
Longenecker, B. M. and Mosmann, T. R. (1981a). *Immunogenetics,* **13**, 1–23.
Longenecker, B. M. and Mosmann, T. R. (1981b). *In* "Avian Immunology" (M. E. Rose, L. N. Payne and B. M. Freeman, eds), pp. 167–175. British Poultry Science Ltd, Edinburgh.
Lupetti, M. and Dolfi, A. (1980). *Transplantation,* **29**, 67–71.
Lydyard, P. M., Grossi, C. E. and Cooper, M. D. (1976). *J. exp. Med.* **144**, 79–97.
Maas, H. J. L. (1974). *Vlaams diergeneesk. Tijdschr.* **43**, 317–335.
McArthur, W. P., Chapman, J. and Thorbecke, G. J. (1971). *J. exp. Med.* **134**, 1036–1045.
McArthur, W. P., Gilmour, D. G. and Thorbecke, G. J. (1973). *Cell. Immun.* **8**, 103–111.
McCorkle, F. M., Stinson, R. S., Olah, I. and Glick, B. (1979). *J. Immun.* **123**, 667–669.
Manning, M. J. (1981). *In* "Avian Immunology" (M. E. Rose, L. N. Payne, B. M. Freeman, eds), pp. 3–20. British Poultry Science Ltd, Edinburgh.
Martin, C., Beaupain, D. and Dieterlen-Lievre, F. (1978). *Cell. Diff.* **7**, 115–130.
Martin, C., Lassila, O., Nurmi, T., Eskola, J., Dieterlen-Lievre, F. and Toivanen, P. (1979). *Scand. J. Immun.* **10**, 333–338.

Matsuda, H., Baba, T. and Bito, Y. (1975). *Immunology,* **29**, 307–318.
Metcalf, D. and Moore, M. A. S. (1971). "Haemopoietic Cells." North-Holland, Amsterdam.
Miggiano, V. C., North, M., Buder, A. and Pink, J. R. L. (1976). *Nature, Lond.* **263**, 61–63.
Miyaki, T. and Yasuda, M. (1977). *Jap. J. vet. Sci.* **39**, 559–570.
Moore, M. A. S. and Owen, J. J. T. (1966). *Devl Biol.* **14**, 40–51.
Moore, M. A. S. and Owen, J. J. T. (1967a). *Lancet,* **ii**, 658–659.
Moore, M. A. S. and Owen, J. J. T. (1967b). *Nature, Lond.* **215**, 1081–1082.
Moore, M. A. S. and Owen, J. J. T. (1967c). *J. exp. Med.* **126**, 715–726.
Mori, T. and Hoshi, H. (1971). *Tohoku J. exp. Med.* **104**, 201–202.
Morita, C. (1973). *J. Immun.* **111**, 1495–1501.
Moriya, O. and Ichikawa, Y. (1979). *Immunology,* **37**, 857–861.
Mueller, A. P., Sato, K. and Glick, B. (1971). *Cell. Immun.* **2**, 140–152.
Nair, M. K. (1973). *Acta vet. scand. suppl.* **42**, 1–103.
Naukkarinen, A. (1982). *J. reticuloend. Soc.* **31**, 423–432.
Naukkarinen, A. and Sorvari, T. E. (1980). *J. reticuloend. Soc.* **28**, 473–482.
Naukkarinen, A. and Sorvari, T. E. (1982). *Acta path. microbiol. immunol. scand.* **90C**, 193–199.
Naukkarinen, A., Arstila, A. U. and Sorvari, T. E. (1978). *Anat. Rec.* **191**, 415–432.
Niedorf, H. R. and Wolters, B. (1974). *Beitr. Path. Bd.* **151**, 75–86.
Niedorf, H. R. and Wolters, B. (1978). *Invest. Cell. Path.* **1**, 205–215.
Neimann, U. (1976). *Zentbol. Vet. Med.* **A23**, 323–330.
Oates, C. M., Bissenden, J. F., Maini, R. N., Payne, L. N. and Dumonde, D. C. (1972). *Nature, New Biol.* **239**, 137–139.
Odend'hal, S. and Breazile, J. E. (1979). *J. reticuloend. Soc.* **25**, 315–324.
Odend'hal, S. and Breazile, J. E. (1980). *Am. J. vet. Res.* **41**, 255–258.
Ogata, K., Sugimura, M. and Kudo, N. (1977). *Jap. J. vet. Res.* **25**, 83–92.
Olah, I. and Glick, B. (1978a). *Experientia* **34**, 1642–1643.
Olah, I. and Glick, B. (1978b). *Poult. Sci.* **57**, 1445–1450.
Olah, I. and Glick, B. (1979). *Poult. Sci.* **58**, 195–210.
Olah, I. and Glick, B. (1981). *Devl comp. Immun.* **5**, 639–648.
Olah, I. and Glick, B. (1982). *Am. J. Anat.* **165**, 445–480.
Olah, I., Glick, B., McCorkle, F. and Stinson, R. S. (1979). *Devl comp. Immunol.* **3**, 101–115.
Orlans, E. and Rose, M. E. (1972). *Immunochemistry,* **9**, 833–838.
Owen, J. J. T. and Ritter, M. A. (1969). *J. exp. Med.* **129**, 431–442.
Palladino, M. A. and Thorbecke, G. J. (1978a). *Cell. Immun.* **38**, 336–349.
Palladino, M. A. and Thorbecke, G. J. (1978b). *Cell. Immun.* **38**, 350–364.
Palladino, M. A. and Thorbecke, G. J. (1978c). *Eur. J. Immun.* **8**, 257–262.
Palladino, M. A., Gilmour, D. G., Scafuri, A. R., Stone, H. A. and Thorbecke, G. J. (1977). *Immunogenetics,* **5**, 253–259.
Palladino, M. A., Grebenau, M. D. and Thorbecke, G. J. (1978). *Devl comp. Immun.* **2**, 121–132.
Parry, S. H. and Aitken, I. D. (1977). *Vet. Microbiol.* **2**, 143–165.
Payne, L. N. (1971). *In* "Physiology and Biochemistry of the Domestic Fowl" (D. J. Bell and B. M. Freeman, eds), pp. 985–1037. Academic Press, London and New York.

Payne, L. N. (1981). *In* "Avian Immunology" (M. E. Rose, L. N. Payne and B. M. Freeman, eds), pp. 285–299. British Poultry Science Ltd, Edinburgh.
Payne, L. N., Frazier, J. A. and Powell, P. C. (1976). *Int. Rev. exp. Path.*, **16**, 59–154.
Pazderka, F., Longenecker, B. M., Law, G. R. J., Stone, H. A. and Ruth, R. F. (1975). *Immunogenetics,* **2**, 93–100.
Perey, D. Y. E. and Bienenstock, J. (1973). *J. Immun.* **111**, 633–637.
Perey, D. Y. E. and Dent, P. B. (1975). *Proc. Soc. exp. Biol. Med.* **148**, 365–369.
Portnoy, J., Bloom, K. and Merigan, T. C. (1973). *Cell. Immun.* **9**, 251–262.
Potworowsky, E. F. and Forget, A. (1975). *Int. Archs Allergy appl. Immun.* **48**, 439–442.
Powell, J. R., Aitken, I. D. and Survashe, B. D. (1979). *Avian Path.* **8**, 363–373.
Purchase, H. G. and Cheville, N. F. (1975). *Avian Path.* **4**, 239–245.
Radwan, A. I., Buening, G. M. and Loan, R. W. (1975). *Infect. Immun.* **11**, 436–440.
Raviola, E. and Karnovsky, M. J. (1972). *J. exp. Med.* **136**, 466–498.
Robertson, G. M. (1977). *Res. vet. Sci.* **22**, 281–284.
Romanoff, A. L. (1960). "The Avian Embryo." MacMillan, New York.
Romero, C. H., Purchase, H. G., Frank, F. R., Burmester, B. R., Kakuk, T. J. and Chang, T. S. (1977). *Avian Dis.* **21**, 264–279.
Romero, C. H., Purchase, H. G., Frank, F. R., Crittenden, L. B. and Chang, T. S. (1978a). *Avian Path.* **7**, 87–103.
Romero, C. H., Purchase, H. G., Frank, F. R., and Chang, T. S. (1978b). *Avian Dis.* **22**, 53–60.
Romppanen, T. (1981). *Acta path. microbiol. scand.* **C89**, 263–268.
Romppanen, T. (1982). *Poult. Sci.* **61**, 2261–2270.
Romppanen, T. and Sorvari, T. E. (1980a). *Am. J. Path.* **100**, 193–208.
Romppanen, T. and Sorvari, T. E. (1980b). *Acta path. microbiol. scand.* **A88**, 407–413.
Romppanen, T. and Sorvari, T. E. (1981). *Int. Archs Allergy appl. Immun.* **65**, 349–358.
Romppanen, T., Viljanen, M. K. and Sorvari, T. E. (1981). *Immunology,* **42**, 391–399.
Rose, M. E. (1981). *In* "Form and Function in Birds" (A. S. King and J. McLelland, eds), Vol. II, pp. 341–384. Academic Press, London and New York.
Rose, M. E. and Hesketh, P. (1974). *Avian Path.* **3**, 297–300.
Rose, M. E. and Orlans, E. (1981). *Devl. comp. Immun.* **5**, 15–20.
Rose, M. E., Payne, L. N. and Freeman, B. M. (eds), (1981). "Avian Immunology." British Poultry Science Ltd, Edinburgh.
Rosenquist, G. L. and Wolfe, H. R. (1962). *Immunology,* **5**, 211–221.
Ross, L. J. N. (1977). *Nature, Lond.* **268**, 644–646.
Rothwell, B., Wight, P. A. L., Burns, R. B. and MacKenzie, G. M. (1972). *J. Anat.* **112**, 233–250.
Rouse, B. T. and Szenberg, A. (1974). *Aust. J. exp. Biol. med. Sci.* **52**, 873–885.
Rouse, B. T. and Warner, N. L. (1972a). *Nature, New Biol.* **236**, 79–80.
Rouse, B. T. and Warner, N. L. (1972b). *Eur. J. Immun.* **2**, 102–104.
Ruuskanen, O., Toivanen, A. and Raekallio, J. (1977). *Devl comp. Immun.* **1**, 231–240.
Sällström, J. F. and Alm, G. V. (1974a). *Acta path. microbiol. scand.* **A82**, 287–295.
Sällström, J. F. and Alm, G. V. (1974b). *Int. Archs Allergy appl. Immun.* **47**, 388–399.
Sarvas, H., Makela, O., Toivanen, P. and Toivanen, A. (1974). *Scand. J. Immun.* **3**, 455–460.
Schaffner, T., Müller, J., Hess, M. W., Cottier, H., Sordat, B. and Ropke, C. (1974). *Cell. Immun.* **13**, 304–312.

Schat, K. A. and Calnek, B. W. (1980). *In* "Resistance and Immunity to Marek's Disease" (P. M. Biggs ed.), pp. 301–319. UER 6470, Commission of European Communities, Luxembourg.
Schauenstein, K. and Wick, G. (1977). *In* "Developmental Immunobiology" (J. B. Solomon, ed.), pp. 363–369. Elsevier/North Holland, Amsterdam.
Schauenstein, K., Globerson, A. and Wick, G. (1982). *Devl comp. Immunol.* **6**, 533–540.
Schoenwolf, G. C., Bell, L. A. and Watterson, R. L. (1981). *J. Morph.* **167**, 35–42.
Seto, F. (1981). *Poult. Sci.* **60**, 1981–1995.
Sharma, J. M. (1977). *Infect. Immun.* **18**, 46–51.
Sharma, J. M. and Lee, L. (1977). *Infect. Immun.* **17**, 227–230.
Sharma, J. M., Witter, R. L. and Purchase, H. G. (1975). *Nature, Lond.* **253**, 477–479.
Shields, J. W., Dickson, D. R., Abbott, W. and Devlin, J. (1979). *Devl comp. Immun.* **3**, 5–22.
Solomon, J. B. (1961). *J. Embryol. exp. Morph.* **9**, 355–369.
Sorvari, R. and Sorvari, T. E. (1977). *Immunology,* **32**, 499–505.
Sorvari, R., Naukkarinen, A. and Sorvari, T. E. (1977). *Poult. Sci.* **56**, 1426–1429.
Sorvari, T., Sorvari, R. and Toivanen, A. (1975). *Scand. J. Immun.* **4**, 764–765.
Stinson, R., McCorkle, F. and Glick, B. (1978). *Poult. Sci.* **47**, 518–522.
Sugimoto, M., Yasuda, T. and Egashira, Y. (1977a). *Devl. Biol.* **56**, 281–292.
Sugimoto, M., Yasuda, T. and Egashira, Y. (1977b). *Devl Biol.* **56**, 293–305.
Sugimura, M. and Hashimoto, Y. (1976). *J. reticuloend. Soc.* **19**, 201–210.
Sugimura, M., Hashimoto, Y. and Nakanishi, H. (1977). *Jap. J. vet. Sci.* **25**, 7–16.
Sundick, R. J., Albini, B. and Wick, G. (1973). *Cell. Immun.* **7**, 332–335.
Survashe, B. D. and Aitken, I. D. (1977). *Res. vet. Sci.* **23**, 217–223.
Survashe, B. D., Aitken, I. D. and Powell, J. R. (1979). *Avian Path.* **8**, 77–93.
Szenberg, A. (1976). *In* "Comparative Immunology" (J. J. Marchalonis, ed.), pp. 419–431. Blackwell Scientific Publications, Oxford.
Tamminen, P., Toivanen, A. and Toivanen, P. (1973). *Eur. J. Immun.* **3**, 521–523.
Tao-Wiedmann, T.-W., Loor, F. and Hägg, L.-B. (1975). *Immunology,* **28**, 821–830.
Terasaki, P. I., Cannon, J. A. and Longmire, W. P. (1959). *Proc. Soc. exp. Biol. Med.* **100**, 639–641.
Theis, G. A. (1977). *J. Immun.* **118**, 887–894.
Thorbecke, G. J., Palladino, M. A. and Lerman, S. P. (1980). *Con. Topics Immunobiol.* **9**, 91–108.
Toivanen, A. and Toivanen, P. (1975). *Transplantn Proc.* **7**, 165–167.
Toivanen, A., Toivanen, P. and Good, R. A. (1972). *Int. Archs Allergy appl. Immun.* **43**, 588–599.
Toivanen, A., Toivanen, P., Eskola, J. and Lassila, O. (1981). *In* "Avian Immunology" (M. E. Rose, L. N. Payne and B. M. Freeman, eds), pp. 45–62. British Poultry Science Ltd, Edinburgh.
Toivanen, P. and Toivanen, A. (1973a). *J. Immun.* **111**, 1602–1603.
Toivanen, P. and Toivanen, A. (1973b). *Eur. J. Immun.* **3**, 585–595.
Toivanen, P., Toivanen, A. and Good, R. A. (1972a). *J. Immun.* **109**, 1058–1070.
Toivanen, P., Toivanen, A. and Good, R. A. (1972b). *J. exp. Med.* **136**, 816–831.
Toivanen, P., Toivanen, A., Linna, T. J. and Good, R. A. (1972c). *J. Immun.* **109**, 1071–1080.
Toivanen, P., Toivanen, A. and Vainio, O. (1974a). *J. exp. Med.,* **139**, 1344–1349.

Toivanen, P., Toivanen, A., Molnar, G. and Sorvari, T. (1974b). *Int. Archs Allergy appl. Immun.* **47**, 749–761.
Toivanen, P., Toivanen, A. and Tamminen, P. (1974c). *Eur. J. Immun.* **4**, 405–410.
Toner, P. G. (1965). *Acta anat.* **61**, 321–330.
Vainio, O., Viljanen, M. K. and Toivanen, A. (1978). *Devl comp. Immun.* **2**, 493–504.
Van Alten, P. J. and Meuwissen, H. J. (1972). *Science, N.Y.* **176**, 45–47.
Vlaovic, M. S., Buening, G. M. and Loan, R. W. (1975). *Cell. Immun.* **17**, 335–341.
Wainberg, M. A., Markson, Y., Weiss, D. W. and Doljanski, F. (1974). *Proc. natn. Acad. Sci., USA* **71**, 3565–3569.
Waltenbaugh, C. R. and Van Alten, P. J. (1974). *J. Immun.* **113**, 1079–1084.
Ward, J. G. and Middleton, A. L. A. (1971). *Can. J. Zool.* **49**, 11–14.
Warner, N. L. and Szenberg, A. (1964). *In* "The Thymus in Immunobiology" (R. A. Good and A. E. Gabrielsen, eds), pp. 395–413. Harper and Row, New York.
Warner, N. L., Ovary, Z. and Kantor, F. S. (1971). *Int. Archs Allergy appl. Immun.* **40**, 719–728.
Weber, W. T. (1970). *Transplantation,* **10**, 275–277.
Weber, W. T. (1975). *Transplantn Rev.* **24**, 113–158.
Weber, W. T. and Foglia, L. M. (1980). *Cell. Immun.* **52**, 84–94.
Weber, W. T. and Mausner, R. (1977). *In* "Avian Immunology" (A. A. Benedict, ed.), pp. 47–59. Plenum Press, New York.
Weidanz, W. P., Weber, W. T. and Maguire, H. C. (1976). *Int. Archs Allergy appl. Immun.* **50**, 755–758.
Weissman, I. L., Gutman, G. A. and Friedberg, S. H. (1974). *Ser. Haematol.* **7**, 482–504.
White, R. G. (1963). *In* "The Immunologically Competent Cell: its Nature and Origin" (G. E. W. Wolstenholme and J. Knight, eds), pp. 6–16. Churchill, London.
White, R. G. (1976). *In* "Differential Diagnosis of Avian Lymphoid Leukosis and Marek's Disease" (L. N. Payne, ed), pp. 15–29. CEC Publication EUR 5494e, Luxembourg.
White, R. G. (1981). *In* "Avian Immunology" (M. E. Rose, L. N. Payne and B. M. Freeman, eds), pp. 21–44. British Poultry Science Ltd, Edinburgh.
White, R. G. and Gordon, J. (1970). *In* "Mononuclear Phagocytes" (R. van Furth, ed.), pp. 510–527. Blackwell, Oxford.
White, R. G., French, V. I. and Stark, J. M. (1970). *J. med. Microbiol.* **3**, 65–83.
White, R. G., Henderson, D. C., Eslami, M. B. and Nielsen, K. (1975). *Immunology,* **28**, 1–21.
White, R. G., Henderson, D. C. and Smithyman, A. M. (1977). *In* "Immunopathology" (P. A. Miescher, ed.), pp. 361–381. Schwabe, Stuttgart.
Wick, G., Albini, B. and Milgrom, F. (1973). *Clin. exp. Immun.* **15**, 237–249.
Wight, P. A. L., Burns, R. B, Rothwell, B. and Mackenzie, G. M. (1971a). *J. Anat.* **110**, 307–315.
Wight, P. A. L., MacKenzie, M., Rothwell, B. and Burns, R. B. (1971b). *J. Anat.* **110**, 323–333.
Wolters, B., Hultsch, E. and Niedorf, H. R. (1977). *Beitr. Path.* **160**, 50–57.
Wyeth, P. J. (1975). *Vet. Rec.* **96**, 238–243.
Zucher, R., Jauker, U. and Droege, W. (1973). *Eur. J. Immun.* **3**, 812–818.
Zwilling, B. S., Barrett, J. T. and Breitenbach, R. P. (1972). *Cell. Immun.* **4**, 20–28.

10

Steroid Hormone Production by the Ovary

J. W. WELLS and A. B. GILBERT

Agricultural and Food Research Council's Poultry Research Centre, Roslin, Midlothian, Scotland

I. Introduction

The hen produces all three classes of sex hormones, oestrogens, androgens and progestagens (see Gilbert, 1971a). Although in the embryo the adrenal glands may be an important source of these steroids (Tanabe *et al.*, 1979), the ovary is their major source in the adult. Within the ovary the interstitial and the granulosa cells appear to be the only ones specifically involved in steroidogenesis (see Gilbert, 1979).

PHYSIOLOGY BIOCHEMISTRY DOMESTIC FOWL, VOL. 5 ISBN 0-12-267105-8

The steroid hormones have profound and widespread physiological and anatomical effects, many of which can be long-lasting. With the current interest in the gonadotrophins, there is a tendency for the wide ranging effects of the steroid hormones to be overlooked, although there are few systems in the hen which are unaffected by them. For example, the most obvious external characters which distinguish male from female (e.g. comb growth, spur development, calls, behaviour, fat deposition, feather shape and pigmentation, and the width of the pelvic bones) are under the influence of steroids. They are more directly involved in reproduction by affecting the growth of the oviduct, the breakdown of the occluding plate, protein synthesis within the oviduct and the movement of the egg down the oviduct. Lipoprotein synthesis in the liver is directly controlled by oestrogens, while progesterone plays a regulatory role in luteinizing hormone (LH) release and ovulation. Calcium metabolism, in the gut and in bone, is under direct influence of steroid hormones.

Since the earlier review (Gilbert, 1971a), there have been many improvements in our knowledge of these hormones in birds. Firstly, the development of radioimmunoassay techniques for gonadotrophins and steroids has brought about a revolution in our knowledge of both types of hormone in the circulation. Fundamentally, the concentrations of steroid hormones in the plasma reflect their role: they are continually present in small amounts and the basal concentrations are required for the maintenance of the reproductive state of the animal, but there are super-imposed daily and seasonal fluctuations which are concerned with specific events during the reproductive cycle. Secondly, the ability to isolate steroidogenic cells has enabled the steroidogenesis of each type of cell to be more clearly defined. Moreover, by comparing the secretions from each of the types with the hormones found in plasma, it is possible to draw conclusions about the role of these cells in the reproductive process.

II. Structure of the Ovary in Relation to Steroid Hormone Production

A. Follicular Hierarchy

The functional morphology of the avian ovary has been reviewed (Gilbert, 1979) and it is basically similar to that of mammals (Zuckerman and Weir, 1977). However, the mode of reproduction in the two classes is different and, therefore, differences in detail in both structure and function would be expected. These differences become important when considering the steroidogenic properties of the avian ovary and its control.

In the mammal, there is a well-recognized oestrous cycle during which a wave of follicular development occurs. In response to LH all the mature follicles ovulate, the precise number being dependent on the characteristic of the species. If fertilization does not occur, the cycle collapses, to be followed in time by another. If fertilization occurs, subsequent cycles are prevented during the course of the pregnancy. In contrast, the bird has no well-defined oestrous cycle; instead, reproductive activity of the ovary is continuous during the part of the breeding season devoted to egg laying. In the domestic fowl it may be extended almost indefinitely by the provision of suitable environmental conditions. Follicular maturation is sequential and each day, with few exceptions, a new follicle reaches maturity, Moreover, only this follicle ovulates in response to the LH stimuli, although all follicles are likely to be subjected to some LH stimulation because LH is present in the general circulation.

In most avian species only the left ovary becomes functional. Within this ovary there are several clearly recognizable groups of follicles (see also Chapter 12), though each merges into the other in order of increasing size. The largest group consists of numerous microscopic follicles consisting of an oocyte covered by the first stages of a granulosa and a theca. The next consists of follicles of about 1 to 3 mm diameter, within which primordial yolk is formed; these are also numerous. Larger follicles, 4 to 8 mm in diameter, have a more yellowish colour; varying numbers, between 6 and 25, of these are present. The most obvious group consists of the 5 to 7 obviously yellow-coloured follicles, which reach a size of about 35 mm diameter at ovulation. This last group of follicles is graded into a hierarchy consistent with the daily ovulatory sequence, and these follicles are often for convenience designated F_1, F_2 . . . F_t (terminal), with the largest being identified as F_1. However, use of this system of numbering may lead to inconsistencies when comparing sequences from different birds, because often a sequence may have one or more follicles missing (Gilbert, 1971b, 1972). Each gap in the hierarchy usually coincides with a predicted future pause-day (*i.e.* the break between one sequence and the next). Furthermore, the gap may occur at any position in the hierarchy because its position will depend on the bird's laying record. Consequently, a simple numbering of the follicles in the hierarchy may be misleading because not all follicles bearing the same number reported in the literature will be the same age with respect to its ovulation time. Because variations in steroidogenesis are likely to occur with the age of the follicle, it is of importance that any numbering of the follicles should reflect their time before ovulation and not just their relative position in the hierarchy.

There are considerable differences in the structure of the follicle between mammals and birds. The mammalian oocyte by comparison is small and it is covered by a well defined theca. At the time of antrum formation, the theca interna differentiates from the externa. The interna cells are probably steroidogenic and may contribute to the ovarian oestrogens (Harrison and Weir, 1977). The granulosa layer is multicellular and during growth the antrum develops within the mass of cells leaving a layer of granulosa cells adjacent to the oocyte. A similar layer is left in contact with the theca interna. There do not appear to be any interstitial cells present within the follicle.

In the bird, the follicle is large and has a thick connective tissue coat covering the theca. The theca differentiates into a theca interna and externa but the general cells of the interna are not steroidogenic. Instead, interstitial cells are present which have the characteristics of steroid-producing cells. The avian oocyte grows to massive proportions, completely filling the follicular covering, unlike that in the mammal, the granulosa is always a single layer of cells, which persists throughout the life of the follicle. There is no antrum.

B. Ovarian Steroidogenic Cells

The origins of the two types of steroid-secreting cells found in the avian ovary are not certain. Most of the evidence (Fell, 1924; Narbaitz and De Robertis, 1968; Scheib, 1970) suggests that the "interstitial cells", whatever their subsequent position in the ovary, are derived from one cell type. Thus, interstitial cells appear to be derived from cells produced during the proliferation of the embryonic epithelium and consequently they arise early in embryogenesis, during the formation of the ovarian medullary tissue (see Gilbert, 1979). In contrast, the granulosa cells appear to be derived from the epithelial cells carried into the secondary sex cords during the rapid multiplication of the primordial germ cells to form the oogonia (Brambell, 1956; Romanoff, 1960; Franchi *et al.*, 1962; Callebaut, 1976). They are thus always cortical and associated with the germ cell. However, it is only between the 4th and 6th day after hatching that they become aligned round the oocyte in a single layer.

In the mature ovary, there is a complex intermingling of the medullary and cortical tissue (see Gilbert, 1979), during which time the interstitial cells become closely associated with developing follicles. As the follicle grows and protrudes from the surface of the ovary, groups of interstitial cells become incorporated into the structure of the follicle. These groups of cells in the small follicles (less than 5 mm diameter) were called "glands" by Dahl (1970). This nomenclature is misleading because, during the growth of the follicle, the cells become distributed more evenly within the theca interna and theca externa (Davidson *et al.*, 1979). There have been no direct attempts to determine positively the number of interstitial cells present in the theca, though from histological preparations obtained from the ovulated follicle it was estimated that they were present approximately in equal numbers to the granulosa cells (Armstrong *et al.*, 1977). In contrast, the number of granulosa cells has been determined for follicles with diameters from about 5 mm to about 35 mm (Gilbert *et al.*, 1980): with the growth of the follicle there is a concomitant five-fold increase in the number of granulosa cells from 3–4 $\times 10^6$ to about 18 $\times 10^6$. At the same time, the appearance of the granulosa layer changes from a "pseudo-stratified" to a "pavement" type: this is accompanied by an alteration in the shape of the granulosa cell from a columnar, through a cuboidal, to a flattened plate-like form.

III. Steroidogenesis

The hormonal interactions between the ovary and the anterior pituitary have been well established in mammals. Follicular maturation proceeds in response to pituitary follicle-stimulating hormone (FSH), and during this time oestrogens are produced in increasing amounts by the follicle. These oestrogens in turn bring about release of LH and this causes ovulation and the luteinization of the granulosa cells. The progesterone produced from the corpus luteum, through a negative feedback mechanism, prevents further gonadotrophin output from the pituitary. The situation in birds is less clear. Moreover, in comparison with mammals, steroidogenesis within the ovary of the bird is still poorly understood. Though there are many similarities, there are specific differences which are related to the differences in their respective modes of reproduction.

In this section, the aim is to assess the relative importance of different ovarian compartments in their contribution to the overall hormonal patterns observed in the circulation. An attempt will be made to identify the role of the steroid-producing cells and the means by which their hormonal outputs are controlled.

A. Ovarian Steroid Hormones

1. Changes in the Plasma Concentrations of Steroidal Sex Hormones during the Ovulatory Cycle

Over the past decade, the availability of anti-sera or proteins capable of binding steroid hormones has encouraged many investigators to apply competitive binding assays to examine the daily changes in the blood plasma of the laying hen. On the whole, the results from these types of assay are less specific than measurements obtained by physicochemical techniques, such as a gas chromatography–mass spectrometry. However, radioimmunoassay remains the most popular method, because it is relatively simple to perform, possesses adequate sensitivity and is well suited for handling the large number of samples generated by serial collections of blood. For example, Johnson and van Tienhoven (1980) measured six steroid hormones, as well as LH, every two hours in the plasma from individual birds for periods of 34 to 72 h.

As a result of numerous studies, the main features of the hormonal patterns in blood plasma during the ovulatory cycle of the hen have been described (Fig. 1). During the day, the concentrations of LH and the classical steroid sex hormones are small, albeit measurable. At the onset of dark or slightly later, there is a small rise (about 10%) in the concentration of LH, with minor concomitant changes in the concentrations of progesterone and androgens (Williams and Sharp, 1978). About 4 to 11 h later (or about 6 to 8 h before ovulation), the concentration of LH increases, eventually resulting in a peak of two- to three-fold greater concentrations than the basal values observed during the day. This LH increase was accompanied by increased concentrations of progesterone, testosterone, oestrone and oestradiol-17β (e.g. Furr *et al.*, 1973; Shodono *et al.*, 1975; Johnson and van Tienhoven, 1980; Tanabe and Kamiyoshi, 1980). However, this apparently simple picture of LH controlling ovarian output does not account for the following observations.

(i) Several research groups observed that the concentrations of testosterone and oestradiol-17β rose before the large pre-ovulatory LH surge (Etches and Cunningham, 1977; Johnson and van Tienhoven, 1980; Etches and Cheng, 1981).
(ii) Shahabi *et al.* (1975a) and Hammond *et al.* (1980a) found that testosterone and oestrogen concentrations showed sharp fluctuations during the day when the concentration of LH was low but stable.
(iii) Etches and Cheng (1981) reported finding a mid-cycle peak of plasma LH without an obvious ovarian response.

For these reasons, the role of other gonadotrophins in controlling ovarian secretions require continued investigation. Plasma concentrations of FSH appeared to be 20 to 30 times larger than those of LH, but did not show major fluctuations during the ovulatory cycle (Scanes *et al.*, 1977b). Further, there is no direct evidence to suppose that prolactin affects the ovary directly, yet one report suggested that its concentration in the plasma fell before the pre-ovulatory LH peak and then rose as LH concentrations declined (Scanes *et al.*, 1977a).

2. Changes in Steroid Hormones in Ovarian Tissue during the Ovulatory Cycle

Comparative analysis of the thecal component of follicles at different times during the daily cycle in laying hens showed that, about 8 h before ovulation, progesterone concentrations increased in the F_1 follicle, eventually to give concentrations of seven times the basal value, paralleling the plasma changes (Shahabi *et al.*, 1975a). The changes in the next two smaller follicles were less marked, so that the sequence for increases in progesterone concentrations in thecal tissue near the pre-ovulatory peak was $F_1 > F_2 > F_3$. With oestrogen

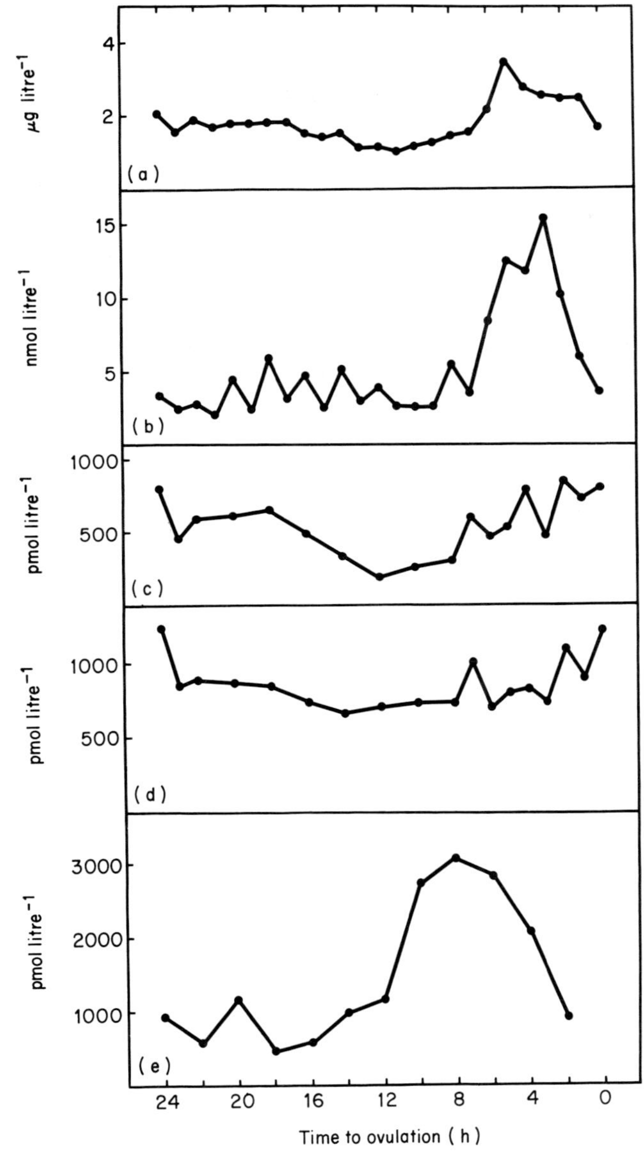

Fig. 1. Hormonal patterns observed in the blood plasma of laying hens during a 24-h cycle. (*a*) LH (*b*) progesterone (*c*) oestradiol-17β (*d*) oestrone (*e*) testosterone. Redrawn from data published by Furr *et al.* (1973), Etches and Cunningham (1977) and Hammond *et al.* (1980).

(*sic*), the sequence was $F_3 > F_2 > F_1$, whereas for testosterone, the concentrations in F_2 and F_3 follicles always exceeded that of the F_1 follicle. An independent study of thecal tissue in six yolk-filled follicles classified as F_1 to F_6 confirmed the apparent importance of the F_1 contribution to the pre-ovulatory increase in progesterone (Nakamura *et al.*, 1979). It was also observed that follicles F_3 to F_6 produced more oestradiol-17β than the larger F_1 and F_2 follicles. However, the above studies did not consider the possible contributions of other ovarian compartments to the observed hormonal pattern in the blood of laying hens. For example, the role of the granulosa cell in progesterone production was highlighted by the work of Dick *et al.* (1978), who found that the granulosa of the F_1 follicle 1 h before an expected ovulation contained 20 times the progesterone content found in thecal tissue.

Similarly, in a detailed analysis of the oestradiol-17β content in various parts of the ovary from one bird, Senior and Furr (1975) found that, after removing the large yolk-filled follicles, the rest of the ovary and the small (< 5 mm) follicles contained 87·5% of the ovarian total.

3. Changes in the Concentrations of Sex Hormones in Ovarian Tissue In Vivo *Induced by Exogenous LH*

Intravenous injection of ovine LH into laying hens caused a significant increase in the concentration of progesterone in plasma, persisting for at least 90 min (Shahabi *et al.*, 1975b; Imai and Nalbandov, 1978). Both of these reports presented analytical data for follicular tissue at various times after LH. However, it is now known that slitting the large yolk-filled follicles to remove the yolk results in loss of the granulosa and its basal lamina (Gilbert *et al.*, 1977). Thus, the analyses of the former workers were of thecal tissue only, which nevertheless showed significant increases in progesterone concentrations concomitant with those observed in the plasma. The magnitude of the change in different follicles was in the order $F_1 > F_2 > F_3$. With oestrogen, the order of rise in tissue concentration was $F_3 > F_2 > F_1$. The implication of these experiments was that under the influence of LH the largest follicle F_1 was predominantly involved in progesterone secretion, whereas the F_2 and F_3 follicles also produced oestrogens.

Culbert *et al.* (1980) showed that, when laying hens were injected with ovine LH, the granulosa of the four largest follicles F_1 to F_4 responded by a massive increase (up to 20-fold) in their progesterone content persisting for almost 60 min *post* injection. Gas–liquid chromatography confirmed that progesterone was the only detectable hormone accumulating in the granulosa cells of these follicles as a result of LH treatment. It was postulated that the follicular granulosa was the major source of progesterone observed in plasma when LH concentrations were increased artificially or during the ovulatory cycle. The increased concentrations of progesterone in follicular tissue observed by Shahabi *et al.* (1975b) and Imai and Nalbandov (1978) are attributed to the accumulation of hormone secreted by the granulosa in response to the LH injection.

Hitherto, the emphasis of these types of analytical studies has been devoted to the large pre-ovulatory follicles. Further work is required to explore the effects of gonadotrophins, LH and FSH on steroid hormone concentrations in other parts of the ovary known to contain steroidogenic cells.

4. *Steroid Hormones Produced by Separate Ovarian Cell Types* In Vitro

(*a*) *Granulosa cells.* The development of simple techniques for obtaining pure preparations of granulosa cells from pre-ovulatory (Gilbert *et al.*, 1977) and post-ovulatory follicles (Armstrong *et al.*, 1977) has dramatically increased our understanding of the role of this cell type in the secretion of ovarian sex hormones.

Several investigations (Hammond *et al.*, 1978; Huang *et al.*, 1979; Wells *et al.*, 1980; Scanes and Fagioli, 1980) have demonstrated that granulosa cells obtained from the large F_1 follicles increased their production of progesterone *in vitro* two- to nine-fold over controls when mammalian or avian LH was added to the artificial medium in which the cells were incubated. By contrast, the cellular response to FSH was less marked, and FSH concentrations of 10 to 100 times that of LH were required to raise the progesterone secretion rate above that of controls (Huang *et al.*, 1979; Scanes and Fagioli, 1980; Hammond *et al.*, 1981).

Even granulosa cells from the less mature follicles F_2 to F_5 have been shown to secrete progesterone *in vitro* under suitable stimuli. (Table 1). The differences may be due in part to the treatment of the cells before incubation, the incubation conditions, the source of gonadotrophin and its concentration. For example, Wells *et al.* (1980) mounted the cells as a unicellular layer sandwiched between the basal lamina and the perivitelline membrane on stainless steel grids. Other studies have used cell suspensions after preliminary digestion of the granulosa layer with collagenase (Huang *et al.*, 1979; Scanes and Fagioli, 1980).

Turkey LH was found to be ten times more potent steroidogenically than ovine LH. Maximum steroidogenesis was observed at turkey LH concentrations of 10 ng ml^{-1}. The response to LH measured by progesterone secretion rates from granulosa cells of different follicles in the hierarchy declined from F_1 to F_6, but the reverse sequence was observed when cells from similar follicles were incubated with turkey FSH (Hammond *et al.*, 1981). However, the concentrations of FSH required to initiate these responses was 2 μg ml^{-1}

Table 1

Comparison of progesterone secretion (pmol min^{-1} per 10^6 cells) by granulosa cells *in vitro* collected from various follicles

	Hammond *et al.* (1981)[a]		Huang *et al.* (1979)[a]		Wells *et al.* (1980)[b]
Follicle type	LH	FSH	LH	FSH	LH
F_1	24·7	0·5	14·4	4·1	2·4
F_2	12·9	2·1	5·9	4·1	2·6
F_3	12·5	10·0	3·1	1·9	1·9
F_4	3·8	13·8	nd	nd	nd
F_5	2·8	21·2	nd	nd	nd

[a]Dispersed cells.
[b]Membrane bound unicellular layer mounted on stainless steel grid; calculated assuming 2·86 pgDNA cell[1] (Gilbert *et al.*, 1980).
nd = not determined.

medium and may be outside the physiological range. Paradoxically ovine FSH appeared to have a greater effect than turkey FSH.

The major conclusion drawn from studies with isolated granulosa cells is that LH is required to stimulate progesterone production. Furthermore, progesterone appears to be the major classical steroid hormone secreted by granulosa cells (Huang *et al.*, 1979); Wells *et al.*, 1980) of the larger follicles (about 10 to 35 mm in diameter). By contrast, granulosa cells obtained from post-ovulatory follicles produced negligible amounts of progesterone *in vitro* and did not respond to LH or FSH (Huang *et al.*, 1979).

(*b*) *Thecal cells.* Thecal cells with a proportion of interstitial cells have been isolated from the follicular envelope by collagenase digestion for 2 h and centrifugation (Huang and Nalbandov, 1979). When this mixed population of isolated thecal cells was incubated with either ovine LH or ovine FSH, negligible amounts of progesterone, testosterone and oestrogen were secreted into the medium during a 3-h incubation. However, when exogenous testosterone was added to the medium with thecal cells from F_2 and F_3 follicles, significant quantities of oestrogen were produced, proportional to the amount of added androgen. On the other hand, thecal cells isolated from the F_1 and the post-ovulatory follicle did not produce oestrogen. Similarly, thecal cells from F_2 and F_3 follicles synthesized testosterone (about 1 pmol per 10^6 cells in a 3-h incubation) when progesterone was added to the medium.

A synergistic effect was observed when isolated granulosa and thecal cells were incubated together in the presence of ovine LH. Progesterone synthesis by the mixed cell population was 50% less than that observed with granulosa cells alone, but testosterone production (6·9 pmol per 10^6 in a 3 h incubation) was 40 times that of thecal cells alone. Thus, the inference from these studies is that, while granulosa cells appear capable of producing progesterone in response to LH, thecal cells require an input from the granulosa cells to produce androgens and oestrogens.

(*c*) *Two-cell hypothesis*. On the basis of the foregoing observations, Huang *et al.* (1979) postulated a two-cell hypothesis for the synthesis of the steroidal sex hormones in the laying hen, an idea similar to that now current for mammals. The ovarian source of progesterone is the granulosa cell while androgen and oestrogen arise from the metabolism of progesterone by thecal cells.

This model, however, contrasts with that postulated for the mammalian ovary. In the rat, it is suggested that thecal cells stimulated by LH produce androgen which is metabolized by FSH-activated granulosa cells to oestrogens (Armstrong and Papkoff, 1976), but there are considerable differences between genera and species.

In the fowl, the two-cell model for the larger follicles provides an explanation for the pre-ovulatory increases in concentration of the sex hormones in the circulation. However, the small white follicles appear to have a high oestradiol-17β content (Senior and Furr, 1975), but their granulosa cells do not have an active 3β-hydroxy-steroid dehydrogenase, 3β-HSD (Davidson *et al.*, 1979). Hence, it seems unlikely that their granulosa cells can produce steroid hormones. Evidently further investigations are necessary to account for the continued production of androgen and oestrogens at the basal level which are required for the maintenance of hepatic lipoprotein production, of female secondary sex characteristics and of oviducal function during pause days when LH concentrations are low.

B. Biosynthetic Pathways

The conversion of cholesterol through various intermediates to the different steroidal sex hormones is catalysed by a complex system of enzymes (Vol. 3, Fig. 3, p. 1454) located in different subcellular organelles in the steroid-producing cell. At present, our knowledge of avian ovarian enzymes must be considered fragmentary when it is compared with the vast literature on mammalian steroidogenic enzymes.

1. Biosynthesis from Cholesterol and Earlier Precursors

Attempts to demonstrate synthesis *de novo* of sex hormones by the avian ovary have been disappointing. Boucek and Savard (1970), using ovarian slices, obtained low incorporation of radioactivity from 1-^{14}C acetate into progesterone, androstenedione, testosterone and oestradiol-17β, although different profiles of radioactive uptake were obtained with ovarian tissue from moulting, laying and broody hens. Similarly, a low synthesis of radioactive progesterone was obtained when various ^{14}C-labelled precursors, such as acetate, octanoate, glucose and cholesterol, were incubated with granulosa cells *in vitro* (Wells *et al.*, 1981b). Total progesterone production measured by radioimmunoassay was over 60 times that synthesized from the exogenous radioactive precursors. Addition of LH to the medium increased the yield of radioactive progesterone only from cells incubated with [^{14}C] glucose.

Plasma lipoproteins may be the source of cholesterol in the ovarian cells of the fowl. Certainly the process of specific uptake of lipoproteins has been demonstrated in mammalian cells, e.g. rat granulosa cell (Schreiber *et al.*, 1980). Nevertheless, the poor incorporation of radioactivity into steroid hormones cannot be attributed to low uptake of small molecules by cells *in vitro* (see Giorgi and Stern, 1981). Perhaps the explanation lies in the difficulties of equilibrating the exogenous substrates with existing pools of metabolites within the steroidogenic cell.

2. *Metabolism of Steroids* In Vitro

Whole ovarian homogenates, which included the theca of the large follicles, but not their granulosa cells, converted various ^{14}C-labelled substrates *in vitro* into progesterone, 17α-hydroxyprogesterone, androstenedione, testosterone, 19-hydroxytestosterone, oestrone and oestradiol-17β *inter alia* in order of decreasing yield (Nakamura *et al.*, 1974). Parallel kinetic studies of the time sequence in which several metabolites were formed from different precursors indicated that the thecal interstitial cells of the ovary contained the enzymes catalysing the pathways illustrated in Vol. 3, Fig. 2 (p. 1453).

Later work with homogenates of follicular thecal tissue revealed that the rate of progesterone metabolism to 17α-hydroxyprogesterone was always higher in the F_2 than in the F_1 follicle at various times during the ovulatory cycle (Nakamura *et al.*, 1979). Indeed, this activity of F_1 follicle homogenates decreased rapidly at 1 h or less before its expected ovulation. An independent comparison of the metabolism of [^{14}C] progesterone by homogenates of the thecal tissue from seven members of the follicular hierarchy confirmed the role of the thecal cells (Llewelyn, 1981a). A number of radioactive products, including 17 α-hydroxyprogesterone, androstenedione and testosterone were identified. The F_1 follicle produced less androstenedione 1 to 2 h before its expected ovulation than did the other follicles. This difference was not observed 13 to 14 h earlier in the cycle.

One metabolite, at first thought to be an androgen, was identified as 20 β-hydroxypregn-4-en-3-one. One to two hours before ovulation its production from the F_1 follicle was twice that of a similar follicle obtained 13 h earlier. Llewelyn (1981b) has speculated that the metabolism of progesterone to this steroid may play a role in the final process of follicle rupture by decreasing the inhibitory effect of progesterone on collagenase.

C. Control of Steroidogenesis by Gonadotrophins

1. Receptors

The initial step in the control of gonadal function involves the binding of circulating gonadotrophins to specific high-affinity receptors on the plasma membrane of the target cell (Cuatrecasas, 1974; Catt *et al.*, 1979).

Etches and Cheng (1981) reported that homogenates of the fowl ovarian stroma bound ^{125}I-labelled FSH to a greater extent than did preparations from thecal tissue of the follicular hierarchy. Indeed, the binding properties of follicles decreased as their size increased. However, in all the follicles examined, a significant increase in FSH binding occurred 12 to 16 h before an expected ovulation of the largest member. Curiously, homogenates of granulosa cells from the large pre-ovulatory follicles had a high affinity for ^{125}I-labelled FSH, but did not bind LH.

At this stage, these binding results appear to conflict with the known cellular response *in vitro*, in that LH has been shown to be 10 to 100 times more potent than FSH in stimulating progesterone production by granulosa cells obtained from the largest follicle. Perhaps the apparent lack of binding by exogenous hormone to these cells may be due to a low number of functional binding sites. For example, in rat granulosa cells, an occupancy of 3% of available LH receptors by gonadotrophin was sufficient to cause the cells to secrete 50% of their maximum steroid output (Doerr, 1979). Moreover, endogenous LH can be detected on the granulosa cell by an immunohistochemical technique Gilbert *et al.*, 1983).

2. Post-receptor Events

After its initial binding, the stimulatory action of gonadotrophin on steroidogenic cells is probably mediated by the coupled adenylate cyclase-protein kinase system (e.g. Menon, 1973; Cooke *et al.*, 1976). This pathway appears to occur in fowl granulosa cells because Calvo *et al.* (1981) reported an increase in basal and LH-stimulative adenylate cyclase as the F_1 follicle approached its expected time of ovulation. By contrast, the enzyme in granulosa cells of the post-ovulatory follicle did not respond to LH treatment. Furthermore, cholera toxin, cyclic AMP and its dibutyryl derivative mimic the action of LH in stimulating steroidogenesis by granulosa cells *in vitro* (Hammond *et al.*, 1980b; Zakar and Hertelendy, 1980a; Hertelendy *et al.*, 1981). Experiments with actinomycin D and cycloheximide, which inhibit different aspects of cellular metabolism, indicated that continuous protein synthesis was an absolute requirement for LH-stimulative progesterone production by fowl granulosa cells (Zakar and Hertelendy, 1980b; Wells *et al.*, 1981a). Similarly, LH-promoted steroidogenesis was dependent on glucose uptake and metabolism (Zakar and Hertelendy, 1980a).

D. Enzymatic Basis of Steroidogenesis

Despite the extensive increase in our knowledge of steroid metabolism in the past decade, biochemical studies of the steroidogenic enzymes in the fowl ovary are less advanced. For example, there is no information available on the regulation of the cholesterol side-chain cleavage enzyme complex, which, in mammalian cells, is located in the mitochondria of steroid-producing cells.

1. 3β-HSD in Ovarian Cells

The presence of another enzyme 3β-HSD (Δ^5-3β-hydroxysteroid : NAD (P) oxidoreductase, EC 1·1·1·145) of the steroidogenic pathway can be readily demonstrated histochemically in tissue sections. This enzyme has been detected in the granulosa and thecal interstitial cells of the fowl ovary (Boucek and Savard, 1970). Comparative studies showed that, in birds from 8 to 30 weeks of age, ovarian interstitial cells gave positive histochemical responses, whereas follicular granulosa cells were not active enzymatically until the size of the pre-ovulatory follicle exceeded 5 mm in diameter (Davidson *et al.*, 1979).

Differential centrifugation of whole ovarian homogenates (excluding the granulosa of the larger follicles) and quantitative biochemical measurements of the various sub-cellular fractions showed that, in adult hens, ovarian 3β-HSD was predominantly associated with the microsomes (Armstrong and Wells, 1976a). Therefore, in the thecal interstitial cells of the follicle wall and in the general ovarian tissue, 3β-HSD is probably located on the endoplasmic reticulum of the cell.

The measurement of 3β-HSD activity appears to give a good indication of steroidogenic potential, since ovaries of out-of-lay hens contained about 9% of the 3β-HSD activity found in those of laying hens (Armstrong and Wells, 1976a). Moreover, during sexual maturation of pullets (about 13 to 22 weeks of age), the increase in ovarian 3β-HSD was five-fold and preceeded the changes observed in the secondary sex characters, such as size of the comb and oviduct (Armstrong and Wells, 1976b).

The sub-cellular distribution of 3β-HSD in granulosa cells of the large follicles showed changes around the time of ovulation. About three times more 3β-HSD activity sedimented with the mitochondria of pre-ovulatory granulosa than those from ovulated follicles. Armstrong (1979) suggested that the association of 3β-HSD (normally a microsomal enzyme) with the mitochondrion may account for the lack of further metabolism of the main secretory product, progesterone.

An extensive comparison has been made of the activities of 3β-HSD in homogenates of granulosa and thecal tissue in the five largest yolk-filled follicles in the ovarian hierarchy (Armstrong, 1981). An interesting picture of the developmental changes emerges since in ascending the series each follicle is about 26 to 27 h closer to its eventual ovulation time than its predecessor (Fig. 2). The total and specific activity of 3β-HSD in granulosa increased as the

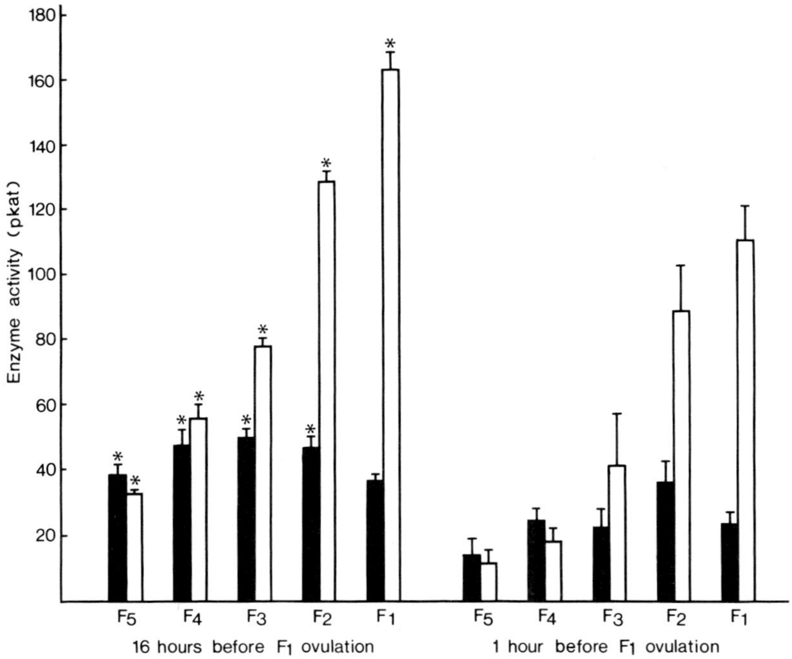

Fig. 2. Comparison of 3β-HSD activity using pregnenolone as substrate in homogenates of granulosa cells □ and thecal tissue ■ of the 5 largest preovulatory follicles. Tissue was collected 1 and 16 h before the expected ovulation of the F_1 follicle. Means with bars representing SEM for 5 birds at each time. Mean of each tissue type 16 h before ovulation which were significantly different ($P < 0{\cdot}05$) from means 1 h before ovulation are marked *. Drawn from data published by Armstrong (1981).

M

follicle mass increased. By contrast, in the theca of these follicles, 3β-HSD activity reached a maximum in F_3 and F_4. In the F_1 follicle, the total 3β-HSD activity of the granulosa was five times greater than that of thecal tissue. Unexpectedly, granulosa 3β-HSD activity was about 60% less in follicles collected one hour before an expected ovulation than from similar classified follicles collected 15 h earlier in the ovulatory cycle. These results indicate that there may be a diurnal rhythm of enzyme activity in the developing follicle independent of the quantitative and qualitative changes associated with growth. Armstrong (1982) has suggested that these changes may be initiated by the pre-ovulatory surge of LH, resulting in 3β-HSD activity reaching its maximum 12 to 16 h later. On the other hand, this change appears to coincide with the time when Etches and Cheng (1981) observed an increased binding of FSH by follicular theca tissue. Perhaps both gonadotrophins have a synergistic effect on 3β-HSD activity in the steroid-producing cell types of the follicle. Certainly, demonstrable changes in 3β-HSD occurred in the ovaries of 11-week-old pullets which had been injected with ovine LH and ovine FSH (Armstrong and Wells, 1980).

2. *Aromatizing Enzymes*

The oestrogens represent the final stage in the biosynthetic pathway from cholesterol. In mammalian cells, the conversion of the androgens, androstenedione and testosterone, to oestrogens involves several integrated hydroxylation and dehydration steps catalysed by an enzyme complex called aromatase (Engel, 1973) which is located on the endoplasmic reticulum. In the ovary of the fowl, an unconfirmed report (Skrivanek, 1975) suggested that the sub-cellular site of aromatization of androgen was localized primarily in a fraction sedimenting with the nuclear membrane. Obviously, further work is required to elucidate these aspects of oestrogen biosynthesis in the fowl.

E. Kinetics of Steroid Hormone Production *In Vivo*

1. *Progesterone*

Johnson and van Tienhoven (1981) have estimated the production rates of progesterone by female fowls in various reproductive states. The values (Table 2) were based on measurements of the disappearance from blood plasma of a single injection of [1, 2, 3, 6, 7-^{3}H] progesterone. In all the birds examined, the metabolism of the injected progesterone conformed to a model system with two compartments: (*i*) a distributive phase in which progesterone had a half-life of about 1 min; and (*ii*) a so-called metabolic phase in which its half-life was almost 11 minutes. In laying hens during the ovulatory peak of progester-

Table 2

Pharmacokinetic estimates of production rates for progesterone in female fowls

Reproductive state	Production rate: ng min^{-1} per metabolic body weight[a]	Production rate: pmol min^{-1} (whole bird basis)[b]
Non-laying pullet	19·6	94
Moulting hen	61·8	282
Laying hen		
8 h before progesterone peak	41·8	206
during progesterone peak	254·3	1308
8 h after progesterone peak	43·2	216

[a]Metabolic body weight : $(\text{weight in kg})^{0\cdot75}$.
[b]Calculated from data of Johnson and van Tienhoven (1981).

one, the estimated rate of production was about six times that of hens 8 h before of after ovulation. This increased output was attributed to an increased ovarian secretion rather than being due to a decline in the metabolic clearance rate by progesterone-metabolizing organs, such as the liver and oviduct. These deductions are consistent with the hypothesis that the pre-ovulatory surge of LH in plasma stimulates progesterone production at this time.

Assuming that plasma progesterone is secreted wholly by the granulosa cells of the pre-ovulatory follicles with diameter greater than 5 mm, an interesting comparison emerges of the production rate *in vivo* (Table 2) and of the measured production by cells *in vitro*. In Table 3, we have estimated the maximum contribution from five follicles of a ovarian hierarchy using typical follicular weights, the relationship between cell number and follicle mass

Table 3

Calculated maximum contribution of various members of a typical follicular hierarchy to the production of progesterone (pmol min^{-1}) by their granulosa cells

Follicle	Granulosa cell number[a] ($\times 10^{-6}$)	Output[b] pmol min^{-1} per 10^6 cells	Estimated production pmol min^{-1}
F_1	18·6	24·7	459
F_2	17·1	12·9	221
F_3	15·3	12·5	191
F_4	13	3·8	50
F_5	10	2·8	28

[a]From J. W. Wells and A. B. Gilbert (unpublished) and Gilbert *et al.* (1980).
[b]Calculated from data of Hammond *et al.* (1981); see Table 1.

(Gilbert *et al.*, 1980), and progesterone output by granulosa cells (Hammond *et al.*, 1981; see Table I). The model involves various postulates including:

(i) the assumption that the production of progesterone by a shaken suspension of granulosa cells *in vitro* is similar to that of a unicellular layer of membrane-bound granulosa *in vivo;*
(ii) the neglect of the potential losses of granulosa derived progesterone due to metabolism by the thecal cells particularly of the F_2, F_3 and F_4 follicles.

It appears unlikely that the difference between the results *in vivo* (1300 pmol min^{-1}) from the whole bird study can be reconciled with the total estimated potential *in vitro* for the five large pre-ovulatory follicles (949 pmol min^{-1}) by assuming that the latter figures under-estimate the output. On the contrary, we suggest that the pharmacokinetic results may over-estimate the production rate, since these are based on the use of a single injection of radioactive progesterone. Johnson and van Tienhoven (1981) showed that the preferred technique of continuous infusion of labelled progesterone yielded production rates in pullets which were only 45·6% of those obtained by the use of a single injection.

After correcting the production rate for laying hens (Table 2) using this factor, the estimate is lower at 594 pmol min^{-1}. Inspection of Table 3 shows that the granulosa cells of the F_1 and F_2 follicles would be capable of producing sufficient progesterone (potentially 680 pmol min^{-1}) during the pre-ovulatory phase.

This concept, that the F_1 and F_2 follicles may produce most of the circulating progesterone, is consistent with the enzymology of the granulosa cells in the follicular hierarchy. Thus, the combined 3β-HSD activities in the granulosa of the F_1 and F_2 follicles measured 1 h before ovulation accounts for 74% of the total enzymic activity measured in the five pre-ovulatory follicles F_1 to F_5 (Armstrong, 1981; see Fig. 2).

2. *Oestradiol-17β*

The metabolism of this hormone also conformed to a two compartmental model with half lives of 1·1 min for the distributive phase and to 27·5 min for the metabolic compartment. Its metabolic clearance 77·3 ml min^{-1} (Johnson and van Tienhoven, 1981) was lower than that of progesterone (122·4 ml min^{-1}). The production rate of oestradiol-17β was estimated to be 23·3 pmol min^{-1} in laying hens.

The total oestrogen pool in plasma is probably higher than previously suspected since Tsang *et al.* (1981) have shown that the ratio of oestradiol-17β and oestrone 3-0-sulphates to their free hormones is 3·8 and 1·6 respectively.

Thus the total respective concentrations of oestradiol-17β and oestrone in plasma 2 to 4 h before oviposition would be in the order of 2·12 and 1·26 nmol litre^{-1}.

At this stage, it is not possible to correlate the production *in vivo* with cellular output *in vitro*. Presumably, this ideal shall be realized when the steroidogenic properties of pure preparations of thecal cells have been characterized.

IV. Conclusions

In the laying hen, the interstitial cells of the ovary, including the follicular theca, and the granulosa cells of the five or six large yolk-filled follicles have the capability of synthesizing and secreting steroid sex hormones.

The granulosa cell of a particular follicle is only enzymatically competent to produce hormones in the last 6 to 7 days of its life time, i.e. after it has reached a size greater than 5 mm. During this time, the activity of the penultimate enzyme in the biosynthetic chain, 3β-HSD in the granulosa increases linearly with follicle weight. The granulosa cell produces only progesterone, in response to LH. The progesterone output per cell *in vitro* is less for cells obtained from the smaller follicles, decreasing in the order F_1 to F_5. The production potential *in vitro* of granulosa cells of the two largest follicles F_1 and F_2 correlates with estimates of progesterone output by the laying hen in the pre-ovulatory phase.

The interstitial cells of the follicular theca metabolize progesterone to androstenedione and testosterone which, in turn, can be aromatized to oestrone and oestradiol-17β respectively. There are marked qualitative and quantitative differences in enzymatic activities of the thecal cells of the follicular hierarchy.

The post-ovulatory follicle does not contribute significantly to the sex hormone pattern observed in the plasma of the laying hen during the ovulatory cycle.

References

Armstrong, D. G. (1979). *Biochem. J.* **181**, 685–689.

Armstrong, D. G. (1981). *Ph. D. thesis, University of Strathclyde.*

Armstrong, D. G. (1982). *J. Endocr.* **93**, 415–421.

Armstrong, D. G. and Wells, J. W. (1976a). *Gen. comp. Endocr.* **29**, 313–318.

Armstrong, D. G. and Wells, J. W. (1976b). *J. Reprod. Fert.* **48**, 233–235.

Armstrong, D. G. and Wells, J. W. (1980). *IRCS Med. Sci.* **8**, 186.

Armstrong, D. G., Davidson, M. F. , Gilbert, A. B. and Wells, J. W. (1977). *J. Reprod. Fert.* **49**, 253–259.

Armstrong, D. T. and Papkoff, H. (1976). *Endocrinology* **99**, 1144–1151.

Boucek, R. J. and Savard, K. (1970). *Gen. comp. Endocr.* **15**, 6–11.
Brambell, F. W. R. (1956). *In* "Marshall's Physiology of Reproduction" (A. S. Parkes, ed.), Vol. 1. pp. 397–542. Longmans Green, London.
Callebaut, M. (1976). *Experientia* **32**, 1337–1339.
Calvo, F. O., Wang, S.-C. and Bahr, J. M. (1981). *Biol. Reprod.* **25**, 805–812.
Catt, K. J., Harwood, J. P., Aguilera, G. and Dufau, M. L. (1979). *Nature, Lond.* **280**, 109–116.
Cooke, B. A., Lindh, M. L. and Janszen, F. H. A. (1976). *Biochem. J.* **160**, 439–446.
Cuatrecasas, P. (1974). *A. Rev. Biochem.* **43**, 169–214.
Culbert, J., Hardie, M. A., Wells, J. W. and Gilbert, A. B. (1980). *J. Reprod. Fert.* **58**, 449–453.
Dahl, E. (1970). *Z. Zellforsch. mikrosk. Anat.* **109**, 195–211.
Davidson, M. F., Gilbert, A. B. and Wells, J. W. (1979). *J. Reprod. Fert.* **57**, 61–64.
Dick, H. R., Culbert, J., Wells, J. W., Gilbert, A. B. and Davidson, M. F. (1978). *J. Reprod. Fert.* **53**, 103–107.
Doerr, P. (1979). *J. Steroid Biochem.* **11**, 1197–1200.
Engel, L. L. (1973). *In* "Handbook of Physiology" (R. O. Greep and E. B. Astwood, eds), Vol. II, pp. 467–483. American Physiological Society, Washington D.C.
Etches, R. J. and Cheng, K. W. (1981). *J. Endocr.* **91**, 11–22.
Etches, R. J. and Cunningham, F. J. (1977). *Acta endocr., Copnh.* **84**, 357–336.
Fell, H. B. (1924). *J. exp. Biol.* **1**, 293–312.
Franchi, L. L. (1962). *In* "The Ovary" (S. Zuckerman. A. M. Handl and P. Eckstein, eds), Vol. 1, pp. 121–142. Academic Press, London and New York.
Franchi, L. L., Mandl, A. M. and Zuckerman, S. (1962). *In* "The Ovary" (S. Zuckerman, A. M. Mandl and P. Eckstein, eds), Vol. 1, 121–142. Academic Press, London and New York.
Furr, B. J. A., Bonney, R. C., England, R. J. and Cunningham, F. J. (1973). *J. Endocr.* **57**, 159–169.
Gilbert, A. B. (1971a). *In* "Physiology and Biochemistry of the Domestic Fowl" (D. J. Bell and B. M. Freeman, eds), Vol. 3, pp. 1149–1468. Academic Press, London.
Gilbert, A. B. (1971b). *In* "Physiology and Biochemistry of the Domestic Fowl" (D. J. Bell and B. M. Freeman, eds), Vol. 3, pp. 1163–1208. Academic Press, London and New York.
Gilbert, A. B. (1972). *In* "Egg Formation and Production" (B. M. Freeman and P. E. Lake, eds), pp. 3–21. British Poultry Science, Edinburgh.
Gilbert, A. B. (1979). *In* "Form and Function in Birds" (A.S. King and J. McLelland, eds), Vol. 1, pp. 237–360. Academic Press, London and New York.
Gilbert, A. B., Evans, A. J., Perry, M. M. and Davidson, M. F. (1977). *J. Reprod. Fert.* **50**, 179–181.
Gilbert, A. B., Hardie, M. A., Perry, M. M., Dick, H. R. and Wells, J. W. (1980). *Br. Poult. Sci.* **21**, 257–263.
Gilbert, A. B., Davidson, M. F. and Wells, J. W. (1983). *Histochem. J.* **15**, 753–761.
Giorgi, E. P. and Stein, W. D. (1981). *Endocrinology* **108**, 688–697.
Hammond, R. W., Todd, H. and Hertelendy, F. (1978). *IRCS Med. Sci.* **6**, 452.
Hammond, R. W., Todd, H. and Hertelendy, F. (1980b). *Gen. comp. Endocr.* **41**, 467–476.
Hammond, R. W., Olson, D. M., Frenkel, R. B., Biellier, H. V. and Hertelendy, F. (1980a). *Gen. comp. Endocr.* **42**, 195–202.

Hammond, R. W., Burke, W. H. and Hertelendy, F. (1981). *Biol. Reprod.* **24**, 1048–1055.

Harrison, R. J. and Weir, B. J. (1977). *In* "The Ovary" (S. Zuckerman and B. J. Weir, eds), 2nd edn, pp. 113–217. Academic Press, London and New York.

Hertelendy, F., Takats, A. and Lintner, F. (1981). *IRCS Med. Sci.* **9**, 382.

Huang, E. S.-R. and Nalbandov, A. V. (1979). *Biol. Reprod.* **20**, 442–453.

Huang, E. S.-R., Kao, K. J. and Nalbandov, A. V. (1979). *Biol. Reprod.* **20**, 454–461

Imai, K. and Nalbandov, A. V. (1978). *Biol. Reprod.* **19**, 779–784.

Johnson, A. L. and van Tienhoven, A. (1980). *Biol. Reprod.* **23**, 386–393.

Johnson, A. L. and van Tienhoven, A. (1981a). *J. Endocr.* **89**, 1–12.

Johnson, A. L. and van Tienhoven, A. (1981b). *Poult. Sci.* **60**, 2720–2723.

Llewelyn, C. A. (1981a). *J. Endocr.* **89**, 283–288.

Llewelyn, C. A. (1981b). *IRCS Med. Sci.* **9**, 859.

Menon, K. M. Y. (1973). *J. biol. Chem.* **248**, 494–501.

Nakamura, T., Tanabe, Y. and Katukawa, H. (1974). *J. Endocr.* **63**, 507–516.

Nakamura, T., Tanabe, Y. and Hirano, H. (1979). *Jap. Poult. Sci.* **16**, 15–25.

Narbaitz, R. and De Robertis, E. M. (1968). *Histochemie* **15**, 187–193.

Romanoff, A. L. (1960). "The Avian Embryo". Macmillan, New York.

Scanes, C. G. and Fagioli, J. H. (1980). *Gen. comp. Endocr.* **41**, 1–7.

Scanes, C. G., Sharp, P. J. and Chadwick, A. (1977a). *J. Endocr.* **72**, 401–402.

Scanes, C. G., Godden, P. M. M. and Sharp, P. J. (1977b). *J. Endocr.* **73**, 473–481.

Scheib, D. (1970). *C.r. hebd. Séanc. Acad. Sci., Paris* **271**, 1700–1703.

Schreiber, J. R., Hsueh., A. J. W., Weinstein, D. B. and Erickson, G. F. (1980). *J. Steroid Biochem.* **13**, 1009–1014.

Senior, B. E. and Furr, B. J. A. (1975). *J. Reprod. Fert.* **43**, 241–247.

Shahabi, N. A., Norton, H. W. and Nalbandov, A. V. (1975a). *Endocrinology* **96**, 962–968.

Shahabi, N. A., Bahr, J. M. and Nalbandov, A. V. (1975b). *Endocrinology* **96**, 969–972.

Shodono, M., Nakamura, T., Tanabe, Y. and Wakabayashi, K. (1975). *Acta endocr., Copenh.* **78**, 565–573.

Skrivanek, J. (1975). *Ph. D. thesis, Pennsylvania State University.*

Tanabe, Y., Nakamura, T., Fujioka, K. and Doi, O. (1979). *Gen. comp. Endocr.* **39**, 26–33.

Tanaka, K. and Kamiyoshi, M. (1980). *In* "Biological Rhythms in Birds : Neural and Endocrine Aspects" (Y. Tanabe, K. Tanaka and T. Ookawa, eds), pp. 169–172. Japanese Scientific Societies Press, Tokyo, and Springer-Verlag, Berlin.

Tsang, C. P. W., Grunder, A. A. and Hollands, K. G. (1981). *Poult. Sci.* **60**, 2548–2550.

Wells, J. W., Gilbert, A. B. and Culbert, J. (1980). *J. Endocr.* **84**, 249–254.

Wells, J. W., Gilbert, A. B. and Culbert, J. (1981a). *IRCS Med. Sci.* **9**, 322.

Wells, J. W., Dick, H. R. and Gilbert, A. B. (1981b). *J. Steroid Biochem.* **14**, 651–656.

Williams, J. B. and Sharp., P. J. (1978). *J. Endocr.* **77**, 57–65.

Zakar, T. and Hertelendy, F. (1980a). *Biol. Reprod.* **22**, 810–816.

Zakar, T. and Hertelendy, F. (1980b). *Biol. Reprod.* **23**, 974–980.

Zuckerman, S. and Weir, B. J. (1977). "The Ovary", 2nd ed. Academic Press, London and New York.

11 Yolk Formation

H. D. GRIFFIN, M. M. PERRY and A. B. GILBERT

Agricultural and Food Research Council's Poultry Research Centre, Roslin, Midlothian, Scotland

1. Introduction

There have been substantial advances in our understanding of the overall process of yolk formation since the subject was previously reviewed in this series (Gilbert, 1971; McIndoe, 1971). Detailed information is emerging about the hepatic synthesis of the yolk proteins, and there is now a much clearer view

PHYSIOLOGY BIOCHEMISTRY DOMESTIC FOWL, VOL. 5 ISBN 0–12–267105–8

of the relationship between the proteins in the yolk and their plasma precursors. The development of a technique to visualize a major component of yolk, the triglyceride-rich lipoprotein (Evans *et al.*, 1979; Perry and Gilbert, 1979), with the electron microscope has enabled the functional anatomy of the ovary to be studied in detail. This in turn has led to a greater understanding of the transport mechanisms involved.

The present article is an attempt to bring together the complementary anatomical and biochemical knowledge and so present a comprehensive account of yolk formation. Particular emphasis is placed on events during the final growth phase of the ovarian follicle, when most of the yolk is laid down.

II. General Considerations of Yolk Formation

A. The Mature Oocyte

In the unfertilized laid egg, the colloquial "yolk" is a single cell, the oocyte, in which the cytoplasm proper is mostly restricted to the germinal disc. This small region of cytoplasm is present in a narrow layer adjacent to the plasma membrane at one pole of the cell. In the domestic hen, this massive cell forms about 30% of the weight of the egg and there is evidence to suggest that the size of the mature oocyte, hence the quantity of yolk, is a major factor in the determination of the ultimate size of the egg (Romanoff and Romanoff, 1949). Factors influencing the size of the yolk have been discussed by Gilbert (1972).

Most of the yolk components are derived from the blood plasma. The major plasma precursors are vitellogenin and a specialized type of triglyceride-rich lipoprotein found in abundance in the laying hen. They are synthesized in the liver, in response to oestrogen stimulation, transported to the ovary and transferred to the growing oocyte, most probably by a selective mechanism.

The size of the task required of the liver, the cardiovascular system and the ovary can be seen from a consideration of the total quantity of yolk material produced during egg laying. A hen which lays 275 eggs during her first year produces about 5·5 kg of yolk; discounting the water content, this represents nearly 3·0 kg of solid material, most of it being the yolk lipoproteins and proteins. The mechanisms for producing and transporting this material are thus of crucial importance for reproduction.

B. Oocyte Development

The general aspects of oocyte development within the ovarian follicle have been described in reviews by Hodges (1974) and by King (1975). Gilbert (1979) has made a comprehensive survey of the literature on the functional

Table 1

Gross characteristics of vitellogenic follicles

Diameter increment (mm)	2·5 – 4·0	4·0 – 8·0	8·0 – 37·0
Weight increment (g)	0·007 – 0·029	0·029 – 0·23	0·23 – 17·0
Number/ovary (range)	10 – 39	6 – 25	5 – 7
Number/ovary (mean)	24	13	6
Yolk type	primordial	yellow (transitory phase)	yellow

and comparative anatomy of the ovary in avian species. Some characteristics of follicles engaged in yolk formation are listed in Table 1.

By the time of hatching the ovary contains its full complement of oocytes. In the majority of oocytes, growth is arrested when they attain diameters of 0·06–0·08 mm and become intrafollicular. This population constitutes the stock from which follicles are drawn during the reproductive life of the bird. On resumption of growth, the oocyte undergoes a succession of changes in preparation for yolk formation (see Bellairs, 1967; Guraya, 1975; Chalana and Guraya, 1979). This period of development is broadly divided into the Balbiani stages (0·07 mm to 1·5 mm) and the vacuolar stage (1·5 mm to 2·5 mm). Definitive yolk spheres first appear in oocytes of about 2·5 mm diameter, and thereafter form the bulk of the cell, which in turn forms the bulk of the ovarian follicle. In the first vitellogenic phase (2·5 mm to 4 mm) primordial yolk is laid down. It is followed by a transitory phase (4 mm to 8 mm) marking the onset of formation of the predominant type of yolk. The process gathers momentum in the main vitellogenic phase and results in growth of the follicle from 8 mm to 37 mm in diameter over a comparatively short period. In outward appearance, the follicles in the three vitellogenic phases are white, yellowish and deeper yellow, respectively. Hence the yolk deposited in the last two phases is generally referred to as yellow yolk.

1. Early Phases of Vitellogenesis

While the yolk laid down in the primordial and transitory phases amounts to less than 2% of the total yolk mass, events associated with its formation may have a bearing on the mechanisms controlling the initiation of vitellogenesis. Little is known about the chemical nature of primordial yolk apart from the fact that it is essentially proteinaceous (see Bellairs, 1965). In contrast to the main vitellogenic phase, structures originating in the ovary play a greater part in the formation of this yolk.

An extraordinary and well known feature of oocytes during their growth from 0·75 mm to about 8 mm in diameter is the phagocytosis of specialized fragments of the surrounding granulosa cells (see Bellairs, 1965, 1967), known as lining bodies, transosomes or unique organelles. Fluid in the perivitelline space is probably incorporated along with these fragments (Paulson and Rosenberg, 1972); it is also taken into the cell by means of coated pinocytotic vesicles (Schjeide *et al.*, 1970) which become numerous as vitellogenesis proceeds (Roth *et al.*, 1976).

In the vacuolar stage, complex macrobodies are formed in the superficial cytoplasm from the endocytosed material (Paulson and Rosenburg, 1972). Similar bodies appear to arise in the deeper cytoplasm from clusters of organelles, including structures that resemble lining bodies but are produced by the oocyte (Paulson and Rosenberg, 1974; Bruce, 1977). The macrobodies, or large vesicles (Bellairs, 1967) are later transformed into primordial yolk spheres. The spheres range from 2 to 40 μm in diameter and possess single or several dense subdroplets embedded in a less dense matrix of granular material. The lining bodies have been implicated in the synthesis of yolk proteins (Paulson and Rosenberg, 1972) and membranes (Schjeide *et al.*, 1974) by virtue of their content of ribosome-like granules. Evidence for the importance of these unique organelles in development has come from observations on oocytes in which growth is impaired by diverse mechanisms (Schjeide *et al.*, 1974, 1975).

In the transitory phase, there is a gradual cessation of the phagocytosis of lining bodies and, apparently, an increase in the rate of uptake of some yolk precursors by pinocytosis. The uptake of phosvitin and immunoglobulins has been demonstrated in these small oocytes (Cutting and Roth, 1973) and we have detected lipoprotein particles(see Section V) in the peripheral yolk spheres (M. M. Perry and A. B. Gilbert, unpublished). Differences in yolk composition during follicular development have been examined by Mackenzie and Martin (1967), who found that three physical fractions typifying yellow yolk (see Section III) could only be distinguished towards the end of this phase.

Early studies of growth rates suggested that the time required to increase in size from 4 to 8 mm was about 24 h (Warren and Conrad, 1939; Oribe, 1973; Callebaut, 1974). In the ovaries of hens at peak reproductive performance, growth from 1·5 to 3 mm has been found to take about 4 days (Perry *et al.*, 1983) and growth from 3 to 8 mm to take about 5 days (Gilbert *et al.*, 1983). These small yolky follicles grew in an orderly sequence, their numbers declining with increase in follicular size to give, at most, one viable follicle in the 7–8 mm size class. The majority of developing follicles became atretic during the course of this period and were rapidly resorbed. Thus, atresia appears to be the normal fate of most follicles in the early vitellogenic phases.

2. *The Main Phase of Vitellogenesis*

The ovary at peak reproductive performance usually contains five to six yellow follicles in a graded size sequence. Their growth characteristics have been determined from the ring patterns formed in the yolk after the administration of lipid-soluble dyes to the bird at regular intervals. Most of the growth occurs in the 7 to 11 days before ovulation (Gilbert, 1971; Grau, 1976), in radial increments of about 2 mm day^{-1} in follicles of 7 g (Warren and Conrad, 1939; Oribe, 1973), and continues in most oocytes until 2 to 3 h before ovulation (Gilbert, 1970, 1971). In the germinal disc, a region of the cell lacking yellow pigmentation, yolk deposition is comparatively slow and in quails it has been shown to cease some 24 h before the end of the final growth phase (Callebaut, 1974). In this study, the patterns of formation of the yolk layers and their final disposition in the mature oocyte were re-examined by tracing the uptake of ^3H-leucine into the cell. The main yolk mass is not entirely homogenous, for material laid down during the day and the night can be differentiated by staining egg yolks with potassium dichromate or acidified ferrocyanide (Grau, 1976). The stained rings corresponded in number with the pigment rings that are found in the yolks of birds kept on a xanthophyll-rich diet, but it is not known if the ring patterns in both cases are strictly coincident.

III. Biochemistry of Yolk Proteins and their Plasma Precursors

The initial step in the isolation of proteins from yolk usually involves the separation of three yolk fractions by centrifugation after dilution with water or saline. At low speeds, a *granule* fraction sediments, and this contains all the yolk phosvitin and lipovitellin and about 5% of the yolk triglyceride. The granules will dissociate at NaCl concentrations of 0·3 M or greater and their triglyceride-rich lipoproteins (LDFG) can be isolated by flotation. Phosvitin is obtained by precipitation with $MgSO_4$, leaving lipovitellin in solution. After removal of the granule fraction, prolonged centrifugation of diluted yolk at high speeds yields a *low-density* fraction containing most of the yolk triglyceride and an infranatant containing the *water-soluble* proteins (livetins).

Details of the gross chemical composition of yolk and the isolation of its individual components are given by Cook (1968) and Taborsky (1974).

A. Phosphoproteins

1. *Phosvitin*

The major phosphoprotein of hen's egg yolk, phosvitin, (Mecham and Olcott, 1949), is a highly atypical protein. Fifty four per cent of its amino acids are serine residues, with 90 to 95% of them phosphorylated (Rosenstein and Taborsky, 1970). Phosvitin also contains at least one phosphothreonine residue (Allerton and Perlmann, 1965; Clark, 1970) and a carbohydrate side-chain whose monosaccharide sequence has been determined (Shainkin and Perlmann, 1971). Phosvitin accounts for about 80% of the protein-bound phosphorus of yolk, but only about 10% of the yolk protein.

Previous evidence for more than one phosvitin has been reviewed by Taborsky (1974). The separation of phosvitin into fractions by electrophoresis or ion-exchange chromatography is not proof of protein heterogeneity, as these fractions could reflect different degrees of phosphorylation or glycosylation of the same polypeptide. Clark (1970), however, has separated two major phosphoproteins by gel filtration of crude phosvitin. The larger phosvitin (MW 34 000) has alanine as the N-terminal amino acid and a single methionine residue. The smaller phosvitin (MW 28 000) has lysine as the N-terminal amino acid and it has no methionine. The amino acid composition of the two phosvitins are different and carbohydrate is present only in the larger phosvitin (Clark, 1970; Clark and Dijkstra, 1980). They have similar phosphate contents. Similar studies have shown the presence of two phosvitins in duck, turkey and ostrich egg yolk (Clark, 1972, 1976a), although phosphorus content, amino acid composition, molecular weight and electrophoretic mobilities vary between the species. Neither of the turkey phosvitins contains carbohydrate.

Crude phosvitin contains a variable proportion of high molecular weight material (Clark, 1970, 1972; Deeley *et al.*, 1975), which may be phosvitin complexed with other yolk proteins. Such contamination might explain the presence of more than two N-terminal amino acids in the phosvitin preparations of Shantz and Dawson (1976). Phosvitin has been regarded as non-immunogenic (Francis, 1952; Green, 1980), and Deeley *et al.* (1975) have suggested that the anti-phosvitin anti-sera reported in the literature (Carinci *et al.*, 1973; Kelley *et al.*, 1976) were raised against impurities rather than phosvitin itself. However, at least one group appears to have succeeded in raising antisera to purified phosvitin (Jackson *et al.*, 1977a).

Investigation of the amino acid sequence of the phosvitins is difficult because of their resistance to hydrolysis by proteolytic enzymes (Clark and Dijkstra, 1980). Cyanogen bromide cleavage of hen, duck and turkey phosvitin produces homologous 30-residue fragments containing 11-residue serine-free "leaders" followed by a succession of phosphoserine blocks (Clark and Joubert, 1971; Clark, 1973, 1976b). The grouping of phosphoserine residues is thought to impart high-energy properties to at least some of the serine phosphomonoester bonds, which may allow phosphorylation and dephosphorylation to occur by a sequential mechanism (Taborsky, 1974; Pinna *et al.*, 1975; Clark, 1976b).

Phosvitin can bind a variety of multivalent metal ions, including Ca^{2+},

Mg^{2+} and Fe^{3+} (Grizzuti and Perlmann, 1973, 1975). Most of the Ca^{2+} and Fe^{3+} found in yolk is present in the granule fraction, presumably bound to phosvitin. The Mg^{2+} content of the granule fraction does not seem to have been reported. The metal ion content of purified phosvitin depends on the method of its isolation (Clark, 1974).

2. *Lipovitellin*

Hen's egg yolk lipovitellin can be separated into two fractions (α- and β-lipovitellin) by electrophoresis, ion-exchange chromatography, or chromatography on hydroxyapatite. The amino acid compositions of α- and β-lipovitellin are very similar and the major difference between them is in the phosphorus content of their protein moieties: 0·5% for α-lipovitellin and 0·27% for β-lipovitellin. There is no general agreement concerning the relative proportions of α- and β-lipovitellin in yolk, although ratios between 1:1 and 1·8:1 have been reported (Bernardi and Cook, 1960; Radomski and Cook, 1964; Wallace, 1965). β-Lipovitellin appears to be preferentially incorporated during yolk deposition in the early vitellogenic phase (MacKenzie and Martin, 1967).

Both lipovitellins normally exist as dimers which can be dissociated into identical monomers with molecular weights of about 200 000. These contain 15 to 20% lipid (Martin *et al.*, 1963; Gornall and Kucsis, 1971) and their polypeptide components must therefore have a total molecular weight of about 170 000. Ultracentrifugation in guanidium chloride (Franzen *et al.*, 1968) and electrophoresis in the presence of sodium dodecylsulphate (Jost *et al.*, 1975; Christman *et al.*, 1977; Wang and Williams, 1980) indicate that both α- and β-lipovitellin contain two major polypeptides, with molecular weights of about 135 000 and 30 000 respectively and several minor polypeptides of intermediate molecular weight. Rao and Mahadevan (1978) found greater heterogeneity, with nine polypeptides in α-lipovitellin with molecular weights ranging from 103 500 to 30 000 and eight polypeptides in β-lipovitellin with molecular weights of 80 000 to 30 000.

3. *Vitellogenin*

Plasma concentrations of protein-bound phosphorus increase markedly at the onset of lay or after administration of oestrogens to chicks. Early studies indicated that the plasma phosphoprotein was not identical to egg yolk phosvitin; for example, Culbert and McIndoe (1971) found that the major phosphoprotein in the plasma of laying hens had a different electrophoretic mobility to phosvitin. Moreover, attempts to isolate phosvitin from plasma by the same procedures used for yolk gave low and variable recoveries (Beuving and Gruber, 1971). Subsequent studies have shown that the phosvitin and lipovitellin of both avian and amphibian yolk are derived from a single plasma precursor, vitellogenin (Bergink and Wallace, 1974; Deeley *et al.*, 1975; Christman *et al.*, 1977; Jackson *et al.*, 1977a; Gordon *et al.*, 1977). Vitellogenin is susceptible to proteolysis and the small amounts of free phosvitin found in plasma (Culbert and McIndoe, 1971) probably arose from hydrolysis after death.

Hen vitellogenin is a dimer, with a molecular weight of about 480 000, which dissociates into identical monomers in the presence of sodium dodecylsulphate. There is convincing evidence that phosvitin and lipovitellin are integral parts of the vitellogenin polypeptide. Purified vitellogenin will cross-react with antisera raised against phosvitin (Jackson *et al.*, 1977a) and both lipovitellins (Deeley *et al.*, 1975; Jost and Pehling, 1976), and phosvitin-like peptides are released from vitellogenin on incubation with proteases (Christman *et al.*, 1977). The gross amino acid composition of vitellogenin, its content of protein-bound phosphorus, and its lipid and carbohydrate composition suggest that each vitellogenin polypeptide contains one lipovitellin and two phosvitin units (Deeley *et al.*, 1975; Christman *et al.*, 1977; Gordon *et al.*, 1977), though not all agree (Wang and Williams, 1980). Gordon *et al.* (1977) avoided practical difficulties in determining the structure of highly phosphorylated proteins by examining unphosphorylated vitellogenin synthesized *in vitro*. They concluded that each vitellogenin monomer contained both the phosvitins and either α- or β-lipovitellin; interestingly the 135 000 and 30 000 molecular weight lipovitellin polypeptides were not contiguous.

The similarity of the products of hydrolysis of vitellogenin by different types of proteolytic enzyme suggests that only a few of the peptide bonds are susceptible to hydrolysis. The majority are presumably protected by being buried within the molecule, by bound lipid, or by the proximity of highly charged phosphate groups. Deeley *et al.* (1975) proposed that α- and β-lipovitellin could be formed from the same polypeptide if there was variation in the exact point of cleavage. The minor polypeptides found in yolk α- and β- lipovitellin are probably the result of partial breakdown of the 135 000 molecular weight polypeptide.

The model proposed by Gorden *et al.* (1977) predicts the two phosvitins should occur in equimolar proportions in yolk, but Clark (1980) found a ratio of 2:1 in favour of the larger phosvitin. A possible explanation for this discrepancy is provided by the recent identification of two distinct vitellogenins, VTG I and VTG II, in laying hen plasma (Wang and Williams, 1980). VTG I and VTG II differ in molecular weight, amino acid composition and ability to cross-react with α- and β-lipovitellin. This strongly suggests they are the products of different genes rather than the result of different degrees of post-translational modification. Duplication of vitellogenin genes seems to be a general phenomenon in oviparous species (Wahli *et al.*, 1981). Differences in labelling pattern of VTG I and VTG II after incorporation of ^{32}P-phosphate *in vivo* suggests that the two vitellogenins contain different phosvitins (Wang and Williams, 1980). The results of limited proteolysis mapping suggest that VTG II might be the precursor of polypeptides in both α- and β-lipovitellin, whereas VTG I gives rise only to polypeptides found in α-lipovitellin (Wang and Williams, 1980). Such a precursor–product relationship implies a major rearrangement of VTG II polypeptides after its cleavage *in vivo*, but this seems unlikely from a consideration of the probable importance of hydrophobic bonding between polypeptides and lipid in both vitellogenin and lipovitellin. Whatever is the true relationship between vitellogenin, the two phosvitins and α- and β-lipovitellin, it appears to be more complex than that proposed by Gordon *et al.* (1977).

B. Triglyceride-rich Lipoproteins

1. Yolk Triglyceride-rich Lipoproteins

The triglyceride-rich lipoproteins of the low-density fraction of yolk contain about 65% of the yolk solids and 95% of the yolk lipid. Their structure is probably similar to that of the mammalian plasma very-low-density (VLD) lipoproteins, with a spherical triglyceride "core", stabilized by phospholipid, cholesterol and apoproteins at the lipid/water interphase. In view of present ideas of the organization of lipoprotein components, the earlier attempts to demonstrate a sub-unit structure for yolk triglyceride-rich lipoproteins by investigating partly delipidated preparations (i.e. "lipovitellenin", see McIndoe, 1971) now seem ill conceived.

Most yolk triglyceride-rich lipoproteins have diameters in the range 25 to 30 nm (Nichols *et al.*, 1969; Evans *et al.*, 1975). Their lipid composition, lipid/protein ratio and lipoprotein density vary with lipoprotein size and diet (Evans *et al.*, 1975). Two populations of yolk triglyceride-rich lipoproteins, LDL_1 and LDL_2, can be separated by centrifugation (Martin *et al.*, 1959; Sugano and Watanabe, 1961; Bacon *et al.*, 1973) and by gel filtration (H. D. Griffin, unpublished). LDL_1 and LDL_2 have similar lipid compositions but differ mainly in size. The lipoproteins of LDL_1 and LDL_2 have estimated mean molecular weights of 10×10^6 and 3 to 5×10^6 respectively. Larger particles have been isolated by Vadehra *et al.* (1977) from hen, turkey and emu yolk, which have mean diameters of about 170 nm. They have a similar lipid and protein composition to LDL_1 and LDL_2, but form only about 1% of the total yolk lipid in the hen.

Polyacrylamide gel electrophoresis of delipidated yolk triglyceride-rich lipoproteins in the presence of dodecylsulphate or urea has revealed a complex apoprotein pattern (Burley, 1975; Raju and Mahadevan, 1976; Yamauchi *et al.*, 1976; Bengtsson *et al.*, 1977; Nakamura *et al.*, 1977). A low molecular weight apoprotein, named apovitellenine I by Burley (1975), forms 30 to 50% of the total apoprotein; it has a molecular weight of about 9400 and its amino acid sequence is known (Dopheide and Inglis, 1976). The remainder consists of several polypeptides ranging in molecular weight from 60 000 to 180 000. Some of these large apoproteins may be aggregates of smaller polypeptides (Raju and Mahadevan, 1976) and their tendency to aggregate even at high concentrations of urea has prevented their isolation (Burley, 1978). The high salt concentrations often used to isolate the yolk low-density fraction causes some proteins from the soluble fraction to associate irreversibly with the triglyceride-rich lipoproteins and this further complicates their apoprotein pattern (Burley, 1978).

The triglyceride-rich lipoproteins of the yolk granules have not been characterized in detail, but their lipid composition (Gornall and Kucsis, 1971) suggests they are very similar to the lipoproteins of the low-density fraction.

2. *Plasma Triglyceride-rich Lipoproteins*

The plasma of laying hens contains high concentrations of triglyceride-rich lipoproteins. These are very similar to the yolk triglyceride-rich lipoproteins and this strongly suggests there is a direct transfer of lipoproteins from plasma to yolk. The size distribution of plasma lipoproteins is similar to that of yolk LDL_2 lipoproteins (Bacon *et al.*, 1973). The lipid and fatty acid compositions of plasma triglyceride-rich lipoproteins are virtually identical to those of yolk triglyceride-rich lipoproteins (Christie and Moore, 1972), but Gornall and Kucsis (1973) found differences in the relative proportions of their dienoic and trienoic glycerolipids. Plasma and yolk VLD lipoproteins contain common antigens (Hillyard *et al.*, 1972; Yu and Marguardt, 1973), although their apoprotein patterns are not identical. In contrast to the multiplicity of high molecular weight apoproteins in yolk VLD lipoproteins, plasma VLD lipoproteins probably contain a single high molecular weight apoprotein, apo-B, with a molecular weight of about 350 000 (see Chapman, 1980); however, apo-B may be susceptible to proteolysis (Williams, 1979). The lower molecular weight apoprotein of plasma VLD lipoproteins, apo-VLDL-II (Chan *et al.*, 1976), appears to be the same as apo-vitellenine I of yolk. Both apo-VLDL-II and apo-vitellenine I normally exist as dimers linked by a single disulphide bond, and although their reported amino acid sequences are not identical (Dopheide and Inglis, 1976; Jackson *et al.*, 1977b), the small differences between them can almost certainly be attributed to genetic differences between the strains of hen used.

C. Yolk Water-Soluble Proteins

The major water-soluble proteins of hen's egg yolk were originally designated α-, β- and γ-livetin by Martin *et al.* (1957) after their separation by electrophoresis. Immunological and chemical evidence that the major constituent of α-livetin was plasma albumin (Williams, 1962) was confirmed by McIndoe and Culbert (1979), who showed that the genetic polymorphism seen in plasma albumin also occurs in α-livetin. β-Livetin is identical to a plasma protein which was classified by Williams (1962) as an α_2-glycoprotein on the basis of its electrophoretic mobility and carbohydrate content. β-Livetin is heterogeneous, although its components may be immunologically related (see McIndoe, 1971). Relative to albumin, there is a greater abundance of α_2-glycoprotein in yolk than in plasma (Williams, 1962), which suggests it may be actively incorporated into the oocyte.

The major components of γ-livetin are plasma immunoglobulins whose transfer to yolk may provide some protection for the chick against infection. Early evidence for the direct transfer of IgG from plasma to yolk was summarized by Brambell (1970) and more recent work on the incorporation of immunoglobulins has been reviewed by Rose and Orlans (1981). Two major avian immunoglobulin classes, IgA and IgM, are apparently excluded from yolk and selection in the transfer of IgG subclasses is suggested by the failure to detect complement-fixing (Orlans, 1967) and skin-sensitizing antibodies (Faith and Clem, 1973) in yolk. Practical difficulties prevent the accurate estimation of antibodies in yolk, but their concentrations are probably higher than in plasma (see Rose and Orlans, 1981).

Burley and Vadehra (1979) further fractionated the yolk soluble fraction by gel filtration and identified two additional proteins. They designated the higher molecular weight protein δ-livetin and found the other to be apovitellenine II, a protein previously found associated with yolk triglyceride-rich lipoproteins (Burley, 1975). The plasma precursors of these proteins are not known.

The soluble fraction of yolk also contains a number of quantitatively minor proteins which seem to be responsible for the transfer of vitamins into the egg. These included specific binding proteins for biotin, riboflavin, thiamin, vitamin A and cholecalciferol. The importance of binding proteins in the uptake of vitamins into yolk is particularly clear in the case of riboflavin: the absence of riboflavin-binding protein in hens of the *rd rd* strain of White Leghorn chickens is accompanied by the laying of eggs practically devoid of riboflavin (Winter *et al.*, 1967).

Riboflavin-binding protein and biotin-binding protein are glycoproteins with molecular weights of 36 000 and 56 000 respectively (Murthy and Adiga, 1978b; Froehlich *et al.*, 1980; Mandella *et al.*, 1978). Thiamin-binding protein is not a glycoprotein and has a molecular weight of about 38 000 (Muniyappa and Adiga, 1979, 1981). Riboflavin- and thiamin-binding proteins occur in immunologically indistinguishable forms in egg yolk, egg white and laying hen plasma, but the biotin-binding protein of hen plasma and yolk is distinct from egg white avidin (White *et al.*, 1976; Meslar *et al.*, 1978). Each molecule of riboflavin-, thiamin- or biotin-binding protein binds one molecule of vitamin. The riboflavin- and thiamin-binding proteins also form a complex with each other, at least *in vitro* (Muniyappa and Adiga, 1979).

All the vitamin A in yolk is present in a complex with retinol-binding protein and pre-albumin, which have molecular weights of 21 000 and 54 000 respectively (Heller, 1976). An identical complex is responsible for retinol transport in the plasma (Mokady and Tal, 1974; Abe *et al.*, 1975), but it is not known whether retinol is specifically concentrated into yolk.

The incorporation of vitamin D into yolk provides an interesting example of selective uptake of materials into yolk. Total vitamin D concentration in yolk is about 10-fold higher than in plasma, but though most of the vitamin D in yolk occurs as cholecalciferol, most of that in plasma occurs as 25-hydroxycholecalciferol. Two vitamin D-binding proteins have been identified in chicken plasma, one binding mainly cholecalciferol and the other mainly 25-hydroxycholecalciferol (Edelstein *et al.*, 1973; Hay and Watson, 1976); the plasma concentrations of both are increased slightly by oestrogens (Frazer and Emtage, 1976). The cholecalciferol-binding protein, but not the 25-hydroxycholecalciferol-binding protein, forms a complex with vitellogenin and Ca^{2+} *in vitro* and Frazer and Emtage (1976) proposed that uptake of the complex *in vivo* could account for the concentration of cholecalciferol into yolk.

The soluble fraction of yolk also contains transferrin, a glycoprotein with a molecular weight of 77 000 (Williams, 1962). Each molecule binds two atoms of iron, but transferrin is a relatively minor component of yolk and its incorporation into the oocyte does not represent a significant amount of iron transfer to the yolk. Instead, most of the iron taken up into the yolk is probably incorporated bound to vitellogenin (Greengard *et al.*, 1964; Ali and Ramsay, 1974; Morgan, 1975).

IV. Hepatic Synthesis of Yolk Precursors

All the major plasma proteins incorporated into yolk, with the exception of immunoglobulins, are synthesized in the liver. The major yolk precursors, vitellogenin and VLD lipoproteins, and three of the minor components of yolk, the binding proteins for biotin, thiamin and riboflavin, are either absent from the plasma of immature hens or roosters, or present in only low concentrations. The plasma concentration of each of these increases dramatically after treatment with oestrogen, and the similarity of the kinetics of their induction suggests their synthesis is subject to co-ordinated regulation (Murthy and Adiga, 1978a; Muniyappa and Adiga, 1980; Wiskocil *et al.*, 1980). The hepatic synthesis of vitellogenin and apo-VLDL-II appears to be completely dependent on oestrogen, since neither protein is normally synthesized in rooster liver (Deeley *et al.*, 1977; Wiskocil *et al.*, 1980). The binding proteins for biotin, thiamin and riboflavin are probably present in low concentrations in rooster plasma and it may therefore be incorrect to view them as egg-specific proteins since they may have functions unrelated to yolk deposition (though see discussion by Murthy and Adiga, 1978a). Transferrin synthesis in rooster liver is increased about two-fold after treatment with oestrogens, but the delay in its induction suggests this is not a primary response to oestrogen (Lee *et al.*, 1978), and plasma concentrations of transferrin are not increased in oestrogen-treated chicks (Ali and Ramsay, 1974). The rate of hepatic synthesis of albumin is largely unaffected by oestrogen treatment (see Green, 1980).

The mechanism of hormonal control of yolk protein synthesis will not be considered, since there are several excellent reviews on this subject (Clemens, 1974; Tata, 1976; Chan and O'Malley, 1978; Tata and Smith, 1979; Green, 1980; Wahli *et al.*, 1981). Most of the work described has been concerned with vitellogenin, but recently there has been a number of interesting studies on the effects of oestrogen on hepatic synthesis of VLD lipoproteins.

The accumulation of triglyceride in the plasma of the laying hen is a result of an oestrogen-induced increase in the rate of synthesis of VLD lipoproteins in the liver (Luskey *et al.*, 1974; Kudzma *et al.*, 1975) and a decreased rate of clearance of VLD lipoprotein triglyceride from the circulation (Bacon *et al.*, 1978). VLD lipoproteins from the plasma of laying hens or oestrogen-treated chicks are different to those from immature hens or roosters: they are smaller (Chapman *et al.*, 1977; Kudzma *et al.*, 1979), have a lower electrophoretic mobility (Evans, 1974) and a substantially different lipid composition (Gornall and Kucsis, 1973). Moreover, although plasma VLD lipoproteins from laying hens or oestrogen-treated chicks contain two major apoproteins, those from immature hens or roosters contain at least six (Kudzma *et al.*, 1979; Fig. 1). Studies with isolated lipoproteins indicate that, although VLD lipoproteins from immature hens are readily hydrolysed by lipoprotein lipase, those from laying hens are hydrolysed only to a limited extent (Griffin, 1981). The limited susceptibility of laying hen VLD lipoproteins to hydrolysis is almost certainly due to their low content of lipoprotein lipase activator apoprotein, and this occurs despite an abundance of activator in the high-density lipoproteins of laying hen plasma. These differences between plasma VLD lipoproteins from immature and laying hens (or oestrogen-treated chicks) cannot be explained by any differences in lipoprotein catabolism and strongly suggest that the laying hen synthesizes specialized lipoproteins for transfer to yolk.

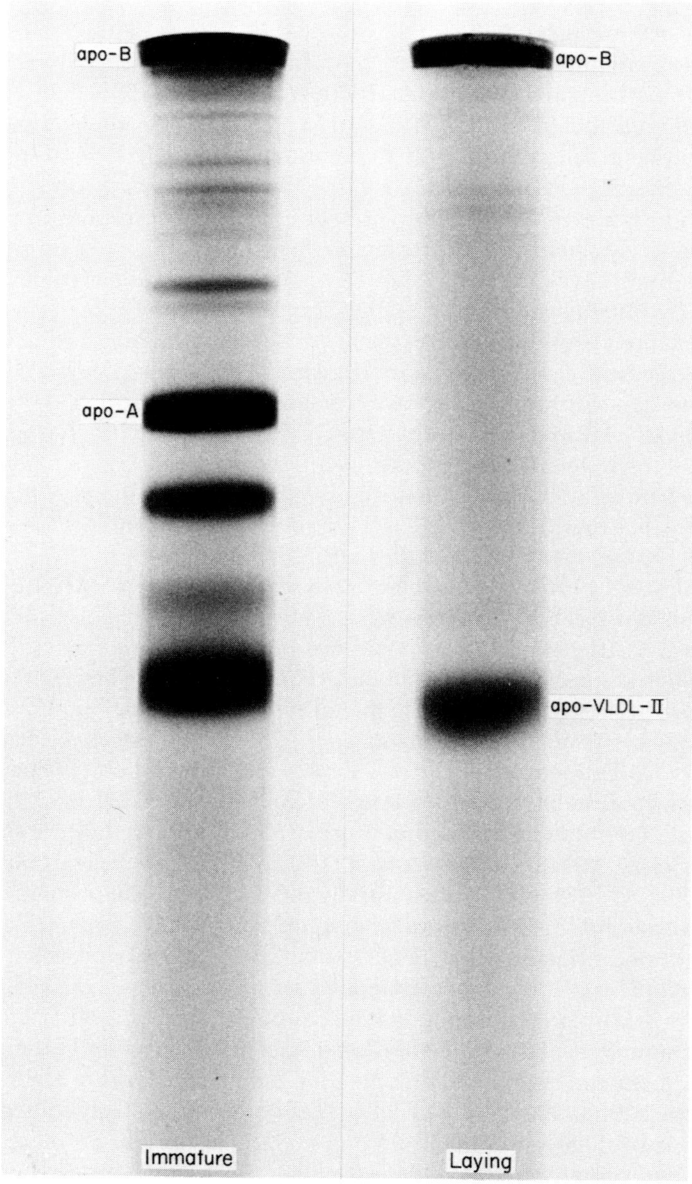

Fig. 1. Apoprotein patterns of very-low-density lipoproteins from immature and laying hens. Apoproteins were separated by electrophoresis in 10% (w/v) polyacrylamide gels in the presence of sodium dodecylsulphate. The nomenclature of avian apoproteins is described by Chapman (1980).

Studies on the synthesis of individual apolipoproteins confirm that oestrogens have a profound effect on the nature of VLD lipoproteins synthesized by avian liver. Chan *et al.* (1978), using translational analysis to quantify mRNA, found a 12-fold increase in hepatic concentration of mRNA coding for apo-VLDL-II after administration of oestrogens to roosters. This was in marked contrast to the several thousand-fold increase in concentration of vitellogenin of mRNA that occurred in similar circumstances (Deeley *et al.*, 1977) and it was concluded that regulation of VLD lipoprotein synthesis by oestrogen involved modulation of genes expressed at a significant level in the normal rooster. In contrast, Wiskocil *et al.* (1980), employing a more specific assay involving hybridization with complementary DNA, found no apo-VLDL-II mRNA in rooster liver and concluded that apo-VLDL-II, like vitellogenin, is an egg-specific protein. They suggest that the mRNA found by Chan *et al.* (1978) in rooster liver coded not for apo-VLDL-II but for an immunologically related protein. Although the increase in rate of hepatic synthesis of apo-B in response to oestrogens has not been measured directly, it must be of similar magnitude to the overall increase in rate of lipoprotein synthesis, since apo-B forms about 50% of the total VLD lipoprotein apoprotein in both immature and laying hens. The rate of synthesis of apo-A-I, the major apolipoprotein of high-density lipoproteins in immature or laying hen plasma, is unaffected by oestrogens (Chan *et al.*, 1980; Wiskocil *et al.*, 1980). Immunochemical studies into the site of synthesis of apolipoproteins showed a marked increase in the numbers of hepatocytes synthesizing apo-VLDL-II after oestrogen-treatment, but no changes were found in respect to cells containing apo-A-I or albumin (Lin and Chan, 1980).

Although the stimulation of VLD lipoprotein synthesis by oestrogen must involve the co-ordinated regulation of both apo-protein and lipid synthesis, there have been few studies of the effects of oestrogen on lipid synthesis in the chicken liver (see Vigo and Vance, 1981). However, it is probable that the differences in lipid composition between VLD lipoproteins from immature and laying hens are primarily due to oestrogen-induced changes in the pattern of lipid synthesis.

Some of the characteristics of the VLD lipoproteins synthesized by the laying hen (e.g. lipid composition) may be determined by the nutritional requirements of the embryo. Other properties of laying hen VLD lipoproteins appear to be directly related to the method of their incorporation into yolk. Thus, the limited susceptibility of laying hen VLD lipoproteins to hydrolysis by lipoprotein lipase is probably a major factor in ensuring the transfer of more or less intact lipoproteins from liver to ovary. The possible significance of the small size of laying hen VLD lipoproteins and their apo-VLDL-II to lipoprotein transport within the ovary is discussed in Section V.

V. Mechanism of Yolk Deposition

A. Yolk Transport within the Follicle

In the ovarian follicle, the growing oocyte is surrounded by several layers of supportive tissue totalling about 0·2 mm in depth (Gilbert, 1979). The outermost layer, composed of the theca externa and the theca interna, is well vascularized, with capillaries extending as far as the border with the underlying granulosa layer. In their transfer across the follicle wall, plasma macromolecules have to cross three potential barriers before reaching the oocyte: the capillary wall, the granulosa basal lamina and the granulosa layer.

1. The Vascular System

It has been claimed that the vasculature is designed to slow down the blood flow in the follicle and so allow the optimum efflux of plasma to the surrounding tissue spaces (Nalbandov and James, 1949). There is no direct physiological evidence for this and evidence suggests the flow is high (Scanes *et al.*, 1982). The arterial system is simple and, in contrast, the venous system forms an elaborate network arranged in three layers (see King, 1975; Gilbert, 1979). Nishida *et al.* (1977) have examined the microvascular architecture in resin casts of the vasculature with particular regard to the inner layer. According to this report, the venules of immature follicles (2 to 3 mm in diameter) terminate in rudimentary bulges. With the onset of yellow yolk deposition, these bulges enlarge into coral-like sinusoids and become connected with the fine vessels of the arterial network to form an inner capillary bed.

We have obtained evidence for a leaky capillary system in the middle and inner thecal zones of yellow follicles from observations with the electron microscope. The findings indicate that the capillaries are permeable to plasma components of considerable size (M. M. Perry and A. B. Gilbert, unpublished) and that the plasma passes directly into the pericapillary spaces (Perry *et al.*, 1978a). Portomicrons (Fig. 2A), smaller lipoprotein particles and the tracer, ferritin (11 nm in diameter) (Fig.2B), were scattered in the pericapillary spaces of the theca externa. In the theca interna these plasma components were found in large deposits in the vicinity of the granulosa basal lamina. Blood cells apparently can also pass out of the capillaries, since erythrocytes have been observed adjacent to the granulosa basal lamina (Rothwell and Solomon, 1977). Two structural features of the vasculature, displayed most clearly by capillaries of the mid-thecal zone (Fig. 2), allow direct access from the lumen to the surrounding tissue spaces. Here the capillary walls consist of extremely thin endothelial cells which are perforated by pores at irregular intervals. This endothelium, unlike the vascular endothelium of many tissues

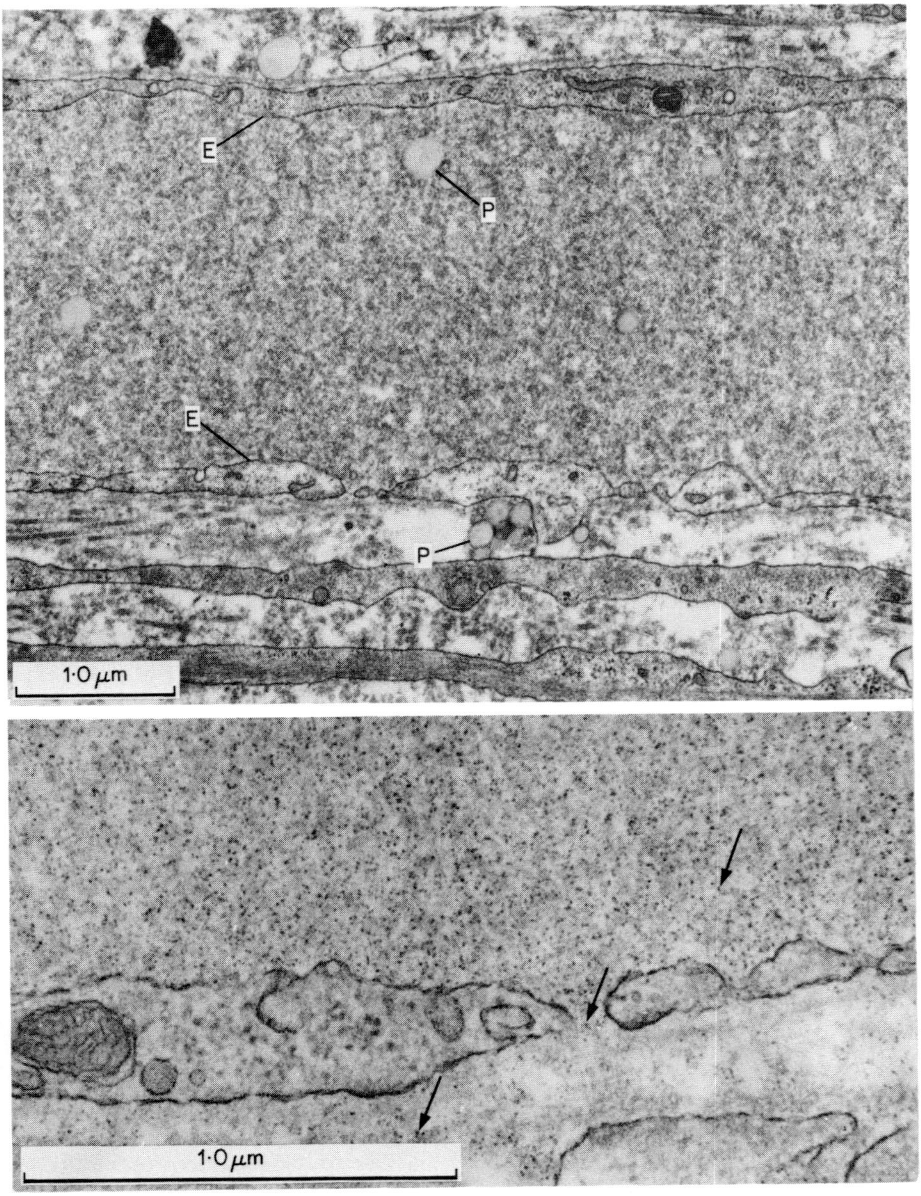

Fig. 2. Capillaries in the mid-thecal zone of the ovarian follicle to illustrate the permeability of the endothelium (E) to plasma components. *Top* portomicrons (P) are evident among the dense contents of the capillary lumen and in the pericapillary space of a bird maintained on a high fat diet. *Bottom* the tracer, ferritin (arrows), is seen in the lumen, in a pore of the endothelial cell and in the pericapillary space 10 min after intravenous injection. NB The electronmicrographs in Figs 2 to 13 were taken of ovarian follicles in the final vitellogenic phase.

(see Majno, 1965), is not supported by a basal lamina. In the inner capillary bed, where the maximum outflow of plasma is presumed to occur, the fragility of the endothelium has precluded an analysis of its fine structure to date. Nevertheless, the presence of the plasma deposits in the theca interna give reason to believe that material passes out of the capillaries through broad discontinuities in the endothelium. These may take the form of fenestrae, as described in liver sinusoids (Montesano and Nicolescu, 1978) and other tissues where large amounts of material have to be transported (Majno, 1965), and/or intercellular channels, as in the capillaries of amphibian ovarian follicles (Dumont, 1978).

Such holes in the capillary wall would facilitate the massive transfer of lipoproteins and other yolk components from the circulation to the interstitial fluid and, as such, would be an important functional feature of avian yolk transport. This mode of lipid transport in extrahepatic tissue is an exceptional one. Normally, the endothelium and basal lamina together serve as an effective barrier to the passage of lipoproteins from the capillary lumen (Scow *et al.*, 1980), permitting only a slight leakage of low density lipoproteins to the interstitial fluid (Goldstein and Brown, 1977).

2. *The Granulosa Basal Lamina*

This 1-μm thick layer encircles the granulosa layer (Fig. 3). It provides the cell layer with mechanical support and acts as a coarse filter for fluid in the thecal spaces. Abundant particles ranging in diameter from 15 nm to 45 nm and of moderate electron density are present within the matrix of the lamina (Perry and Gilbert, 1979). On elution from the lamina this particulate material was identified as VLD lipoprotein (Evans *et al.*, 1979). Larger VLD lipoprotein particles and portomicrons are prevented from traversing this barrier and tend to accumulate at its outer boundary, particularly in birds fed on a high-fat diet (H. D. Griffin and M. M. Perry, unpublished). The observations suggest that this basal lamina, if acting solely as a mechanical filter, would be permeable to most plasma components. Its sieving properties may, however, be determined by molecular charge as well as size since pH has been shown to influence the binding of the lipoprotein particles to the matrix of the isolated lamina (Evans *et al.*, 1979). The lamina was found to contain abundant particles after it was perfused with buffered saline at pH 5·4, but few particles were present after perfusion at pH 8·6.

Examination of the early growth phases has revealed that the lamina of small follicles (4 mm in diameter) contains few lipoprotein particles, although it is permeable to components of smaller dimension, such as ferritin which may be present in the plasma (M. M. Perry and A. B. Gilbert, unpublished). It thus seems likely that the matrix undergoes changes in porosity during

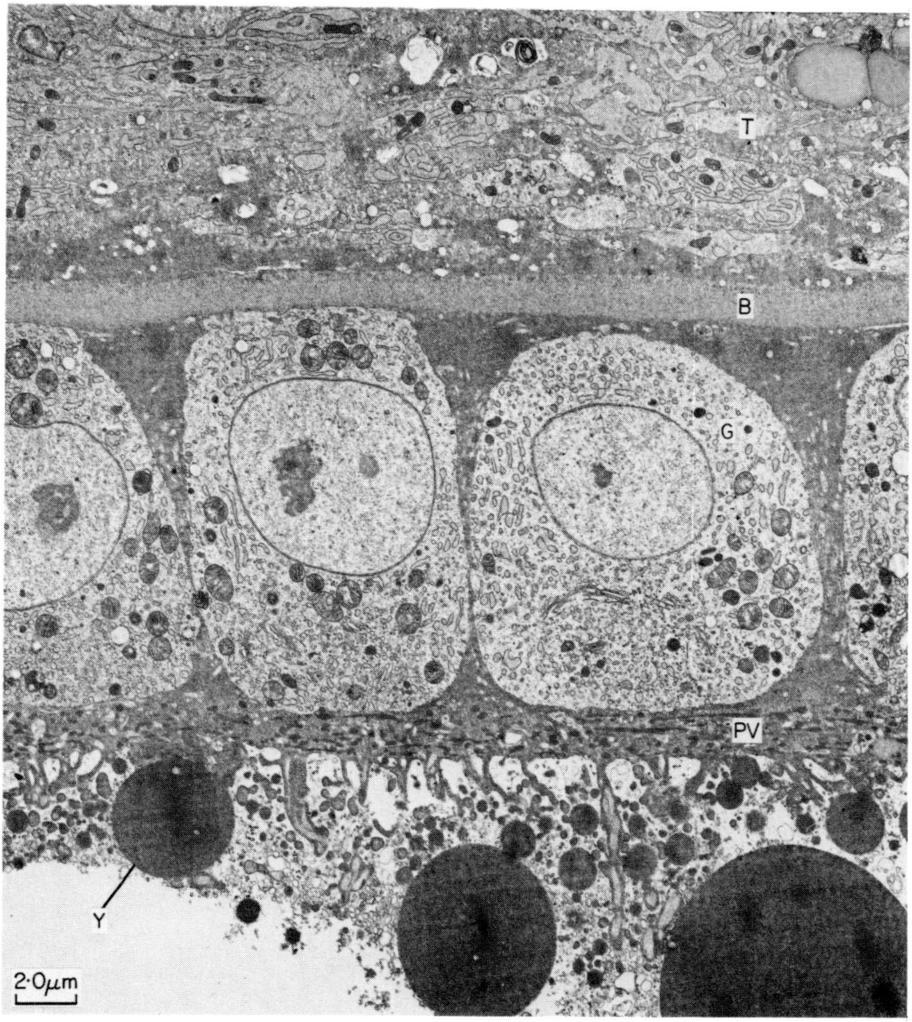

Fig. 3. The granulosa and adjoining layers. The theca interna (T) is separated from the granulosa cell layer (G) by a thick basal lamina (B). Channels between the granulosa cells are filled with dense material that has passed through the basal lamina. The oocyte surface is irregular with narrow indentations extending deep into the cortical cytoplasm. PV, perivitelline layer; Y, yolk spheres. (From Perry and Gilbert, 1979). (See note to Fig. 2).

development which are essential for lipid transport. Of equal importance is the size of the plasma lipoproteins in relation to the pore size of the basal lamina. The small size of the triglyceride-rich lipoproteins synthesized by the liver of the laying hen is almost certainly an adaptation for their incorporation into yolk, because the larger VLD lipoprotein particles of immature hens would not readily pass through the basal lamina.

3. The Granulosa Layer

The material filtering through the basal lamina passes between the cells in its transfer across the granulosa layer. Towards the end of the early vitellogenic phases the stratified cells of this layer are rearranged into a single cell layer and, as the rate of yolk deposition intensifies, the cells become separated by broad channels (see Perry *et al.*, 1978a). The accompanying changes in cell shape, from columnar to cuboidal to flattened, are chiefly responsible for the increase in area of the granulosa layer required to accommodate the growth of the oocyte (Gilbert *et al.*, 1980). The broad channels have been shown to contain osmiophilic particles (Jordanov and Boyadjieva-Michaelova, 1974) and definitive lipoprotein particles like those in the basal lamina (Perry and Gilbert, 1979). The tracer ^{203}Hg, thought to be complexed to lipovitellin, has also been detected in the intercellular spaces of the granulosa layer after injection of labelled mercuric nitrate into quails (Nishimura *et al.*, 1976). In the phase of primordial yolk formation the relatively narrow spaces between the cells are of sufficient width to permit the passage of ferritin and, presumably, other macromolecules in this size range. Clearly, the degree of cell separation and concomitant change in cell shape are factors contributing to the increased flow of yolk precursors towards the oocyte in the phase of rapid growth. In this context, it is significant that the granulosa cells lying adjacent to the region of the cell where yolk formation is retarded, i.e. the germinal disc, remain tightly packed throughout growth (Perry *et al.*, 1978b). Thus it may be of crucial importance in yolk formation that the flow of yolk material is not interrupted in its passage to the oocyte by any cellular barrier.

B. Incorporation of Yolk into the Oocyte

1. Transfer Across the Plasma Membrane

There is now considerable evidence that proteins enter many cells by the mechanism of receptor-mediated endocytosis (Goldstein *et al.*, 1979). This process involves firstly the specific adsorption of a molecule to its recognition site on the plasma membrane and secondly the internalization of the complex by means of coated pits. The pits pinch off the plasma membrane and carry the adsorbed protein to locations which differ according to the function of the particular cell. Other molecules in the external fluid enter the cell, albeit fortuitously, by being enclosed in the lumen, or fluid phase, of the coated vesicle. These specialized structures have long been recognized as vehicles for yolk transport in the oocytes of oviparous species (see Giorgi, 1980). The precise mechanism of receptor-mediated endocytosis, however, has been most fully explored in the case of low density lipoprotein incorporation into human fibroblasts (Brown and Goldstein, 1979). Details of its role in the bulk transfer of yolk into the hen's oocyte are emerging, despite the inherent technical problem posed by the size of the oocyte. To effect this transfer, the surface area of the oocyte is enormously enlarged by extensive convolutions of the plasma membrane.

(*a*) *Adsorption.* Roth and co-workers have examined the interaction of yolk precursors *in vitro* with follicle preparations formed of basement membrane, granulosa cells and oocyte plasma membrane, and concluded that such preparations contain specific binding sites for IgG (Roth *et al.*, 1976), vitellogenin (Yusko and Roth, 1976), VLD lipoproteins and low-density lipoproteins (Krumins and Roth, 1981). Confirmation that the receptors for IgG were located on the outer surface of the oocyte plasma membrane was provided by morphological studies with ferritin-labelled IgG. The labelled IgG was bound to only about 20% of the coated region of the membrane (Roth *et al.*, 1976). In contrast, lipoprotein particles form a continuous layer over the coated and non-coated regions of the oocyte *in situ* (Perry and Gilbert, 1979) and *in vitro* (Fig. 4). Chapman (1980) has speculated that binding of lipoproteins by the oocyte plasma membrane could involve recognition of apo-VLDL-II and Krumins and Roth (1981) have identified two distinct types of lipoprotein binding site in their follicle preparations, one apparently specific for apo-VLDL-II and the other for apo-B. Nevertheless, the observations that laying hen plasma high-density lipoproteins contain apo-VLDL-II (Raju and Mahedevan, 1976; D. W. Bannister and H. D. Griffiin, unpublished), but are not concentrated in yolk (Yu and Marquardt, 1973; Evans *et al.*, 1977), give reason to doubt that apo-VLDL-II binding sites are located on the oocyte plasma membrane. In contrast, the binding of plasma low-density lipoproteins from immature hens, which contain largely apo-B and no apo-VLDL-II, to the oocyte plasma membrane *in vitro* (Perry *et al.*, in press) appears to confirm that the membrane does not contain receptors for apo-B. Morphological observations on *in vitro* preparations (Perry *et al.*, in press) have shown that lipoprotein particles remain bound to the plasma membrane at pH 7·4–8·4 (Fig. 4A), but are released on incubation with buffer at pH 6·0–7·0 (Fig. 4B). This pH dependence may be important in the formation of the lipoprotein-receptor complex, and its dissociation once inside the oocyte, for yolk pH at 6·0

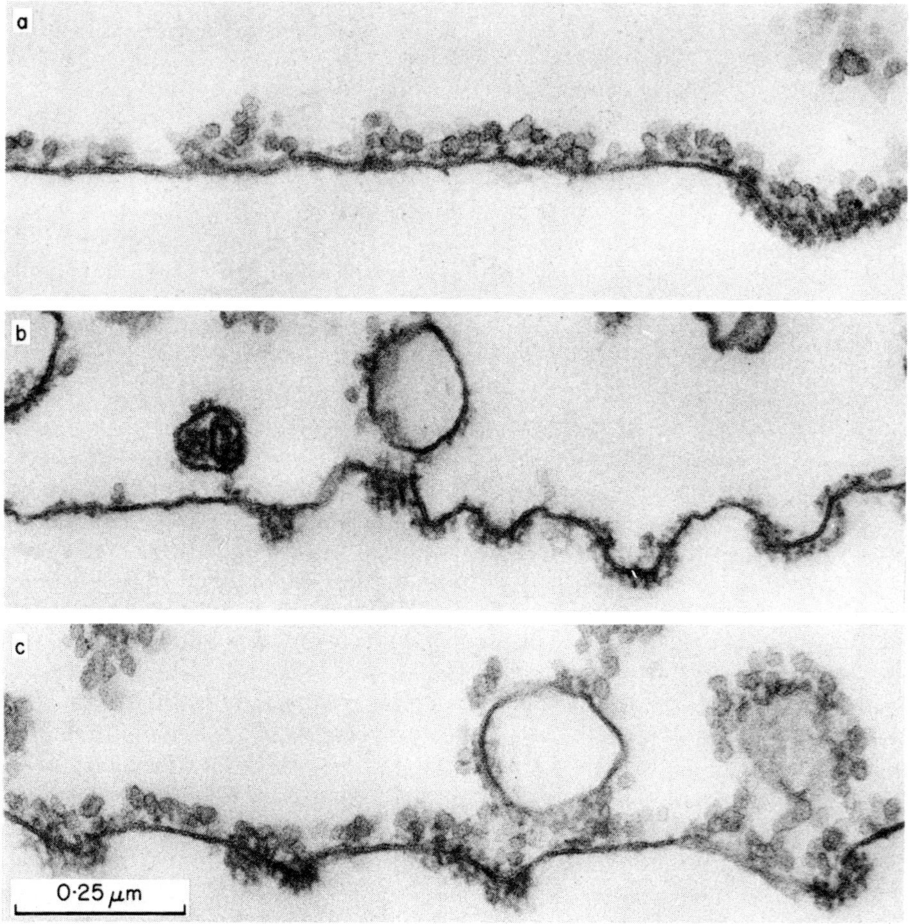

Fig. 4. Preparations of the oocyte plasma membrane incubated *in vitro* at 4°C in 0·02 M buffer containing 0·15 M NaCl and 0·001 M $CaCl_2$. In these conditions, the plasma membrane is in the form of sheets and vesicles. (*a*) Native lipoprotein particles remain attached to the membrane in HEPES buffer, pH 7·4. (*b*) The particles are removed from the membrane in MES buffer, pH 6·0. (*c*) A preparation denuded of native particles by treatment with heparin and reincubated with very-low-density lipoproteins from the plasma of a laying hen, to demonstrate the binding of plasma lipoprotein particles; granulosa cells used as controls did not bind the particles. (See note to Fig. 2).

(Dawes, 1975) is considerably less than that of plasma at pH 7·4 (Hunt and Simkiss, 1967).

There is as yet no direct evidence for specific receptors for other yolk precursors, though the concentration of several of the vitamin-binding proteins into yolk strongly suggests that they are incorporated by receptor mediated endocytosis. Most of the yolk proteins are glycoproteins and Muniyappa and Adiga (1979) have suggested that their uptake into yolk involves recognition of their oligosaccharide chains, as has been shown for receptor-mediated uptake of glycoproteins by mammalian cells (Neufeld and Ashwell, 1980). Direct support for this hypothesis was provided recently by Miller *et al.* (1981a), who found that removal of sialic acid residues from riboflavin-binding protein greatly reduced the rate of its incorporation into yolk. Although preliminary evidence (Roth *et al.*, 1980) suggests the plasma membrane receptor for hen vitellogenin recognizes the phosvitin region of the molecule, the absence of carbohydrate from turkey phosvitin suggests that uptake of hen vitellogenin into the oocyte may not involve recognition of the oligosaccharide chain of its phosvitin moiety.

The uptake of some yolk proteins that are not glycoproteins could be dependent on their association with those that are glycoproteins, and the evidence for co-transport of cholecalciferol-binding protein and vitellogenin seems convincing. Muniyappa and Adiga (1979) proposed that incorporation of thiamin-binding protein was dependent on its association with riboflavin-binding protein but Miller *et al.* (1981b) showed this was not the case by demonstrating that the riboflavin-deficient eggs laid by *rdrd* hens had normal contents of thiamin.

While a receptor-mediated mechanism may be essential for the sequestration of the majority of yolk components, this mode of uptake may not necessarily apply to all components. A defective yolk transport mechanism, perhaps involving membrane receptors, has been proposed to explain the stunted growth of oocytes in "restricted ovulator" mutants (Schjeide *et al.*, 1976). In these birds, oocytes showing some development failed to incorporate normal amounts of vitellogenin and the lower density lipoproteins, but uptake of albumin was unaffected. Hence, albumin, for example, and heterologous proteins such as ferritin, may well be incorporated in a non-selective manner by being engulfed in the fluid phase of pinocytotic vesicles.

(*b*) *Endocytosis.* Endocytosis in oocytes in the main vitellogenic phase takes place solely by means of coated pits (Wyburn *et al.*, 1965; Roth *et al.*, 1976; Perry *et al.*, 1978a). In this phase, the fully formed vesicles are usually located close to the plasma membrane and most of them are probably connected to it by narrow necks (Fig. 5); once separation is complete, it would appear that the vesicles undergo a rapid change in morphology. On their outward, or luminal

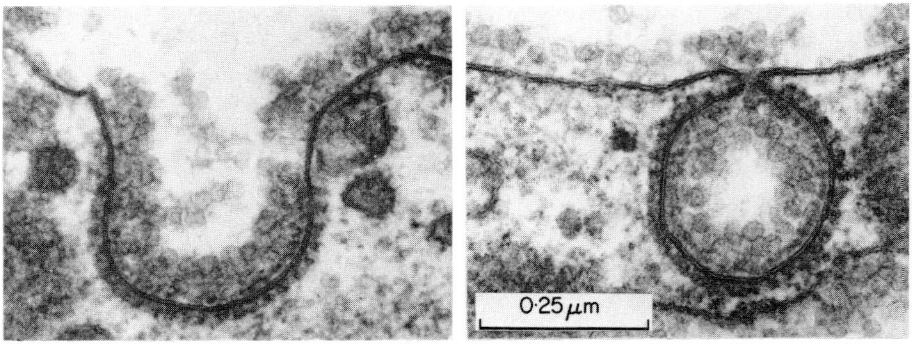

Fig. 5. Invagination of coated pits from the oocyte surface. The plasma membrane is covered externally with a layer of lipoprotein particles. Beneath this layer and adjacent to the indented portion of the membrane is a row of granules of unknown identity. The cytoplasmic surface of the pit is coated with a layer of bristly structures. (From Perry and Gilbert, 1979). (See note to Fig. 2).

aspect (Fig. 5) the pits and vesicles are lined by lipoprotein particles and fine granules, and on their cytoplasmic surface they are coated by a layer of bristly protrusions. Their unusual size, 200 to 350 nm in diameter, seems to be a modification for the uptake of material in quantity rather than a specialization for the incorporation of large molecules. Lipoprotein particles, for instance, have been detected (M. M. Perry and A. B. Gilbert, unpublished) in the smaller coated vesicles, 120 to 200 nm in diameter, commonly found in oocytes in the transitory phase of vitellogenesis (see Perry *et al.*, 1978a) and in the germinal disc region of yellow follicles (Perry *et al.*, 1978b). Coated vesicles, albeit of small dimension, have been purified from hen oocytes and found to resemble those from other sources in structure and composition (Woods *et al.*, 1978). The coat material was arranged in a polyhedral network and its major protein was clathrin. Pearse (1980) and Pearse and Bretscher (1981) have succeeded in purifying coated vesicles from hen oocytes in a form more typical of the endocytotic vesicles observed *in situ*. The polyhedral lattice of the coat has been elegantly demonstrated by J. Heuser (personal communication) in preparations of platinum-shadowed replicas of the inner surface of the plasma membrane (Fig. 6). In fibroblasts, structural transformations of the lattice were related to the degree of curvature of the membrane during stages of vesicle formation (Heuser, 1980), and presumably the same mechanism could operate in the avian oocyte.

The enhancement of endocytotic activity at the onset of the rapid growth phase is indicated by a rise in the uptake of phosvitin and immunoglobulins (Cutting and Roth, 1973) and a concomitant increase in the number (Roth

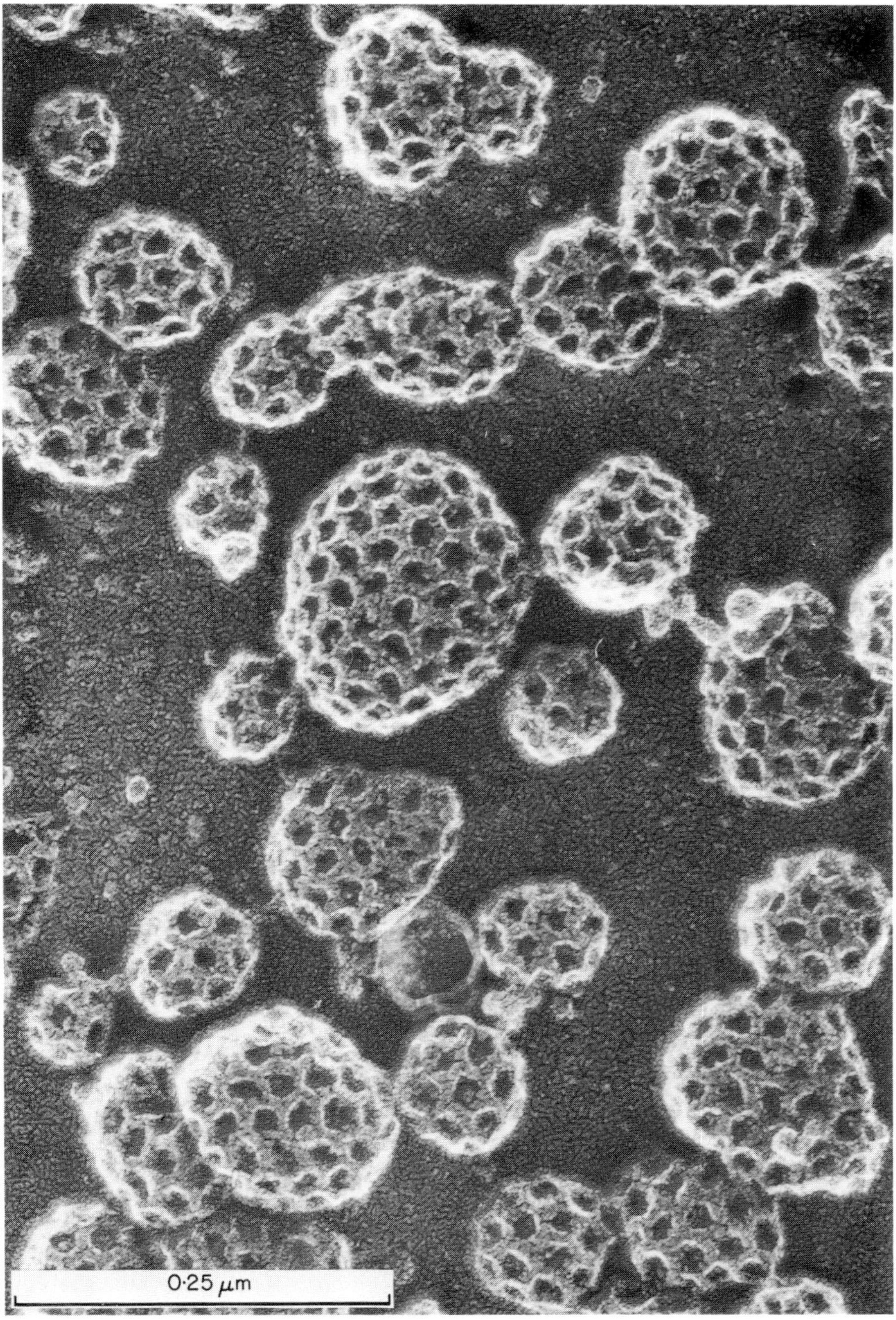

Fig. 6. A view of the inside of the oocyte plasma membrane shows the lattice structure of the material on the cytoplasmic face of the coated pits. The specimen was prepared by the quick-freeze, deep-etch, rotary replication method of Heuser. (Courtesy of J. Heuser). (See note to Fig. 2).

N

et al., 1976) and size of coated vesicles. The cell surface, however, is heterogeneous in respect of this increased activity. In the germinal disc region the population of coated vesicles diminishes as growth proceeds and is no longer present in the vicinity of the germinal vesicle at two days before ovulation. These differences raise the question of how endocytosis is regulated in the avian oocyte. Though gonadotrophins are known to be essential for the normal growth of the follicle (see Lofts and Murton, 1973), the way they operate at the cellular level is poorly understood. From investigations on follicles in the phase of primordial yolk formation Schjeide *et al.* (1974) have reached the tentative conclusion that, insofar as the phagocytosis of lining bodies is concerned, the process is independent of circulating hormones. In contrast, evidence from non-avian species, reviewed by Giorgi (1980), had indicated a requirement for gonadotrophic hormones to stimulate the uptake of yolk precursors. The hormones do not appear to act directly on the oocyte and, in *Xenopus* for example, chorionic gonadotrophin is considered to exert its effect through the follicle cells in a manner yet to be determined (Wiley and Dumont, 1978).

2. *Yolk Sphere Formation*

The yolk spheres of yellow follicles range from 20 μm to 150 μm in diameter. According to Bellairs *et al.* (1972), they are suspended in a continuous phase fluid, but their polygonal form when dispersed after prolonged fixation indicates that the spheres exist in tightly packed formation *in situ* (Fujii *et al.*, 1973). They are bounded by a trilaminar membrane and contain discrete masses of dense granular material, the subdroplets (Fig. 7), embedded in a compact mass of lipoprotein particles (Fig. 8A). The subdroplets most probably correspond with the granule fraction obtained on centrifugation of yolk. The 4 to 6 nm granules observed in the dense masses of the granule fraction are believed to be phosvitin and lipovitellin (Bellairs *et al.*, 1972). Intravenously injected ferritin also appears to become localized in the subdroplets (Fig. 8B), an observation which suggests that they are a likely destination for some non-selective yolk components. The diameter of the lipoprotein particles in the yolk spheres is 15 to 45 nm and, thus, is the same as that for the particles in the basal lamina (Perry and Gilbert, 1979). This figure is similar to the values given for negatively stained samples of egg yolk VLD lipoprotein (Nichols *et al.*, 1969; Evans *et al.*, 1975) and with its calculated hydrated diameter (Hillyard *et al.*, 1980). Other structures, termed lipid-protein globules, have been described in yolk by Vadehra *et al.* (1977) but, in our experience, the smaller globules depicted in this report are not present in yolk spheres of recent formation, the larger globules bear some resemblance to nascent yolk spheres in the oocyte periphery.

The following sequence of events has been proposed for the formation of yolk

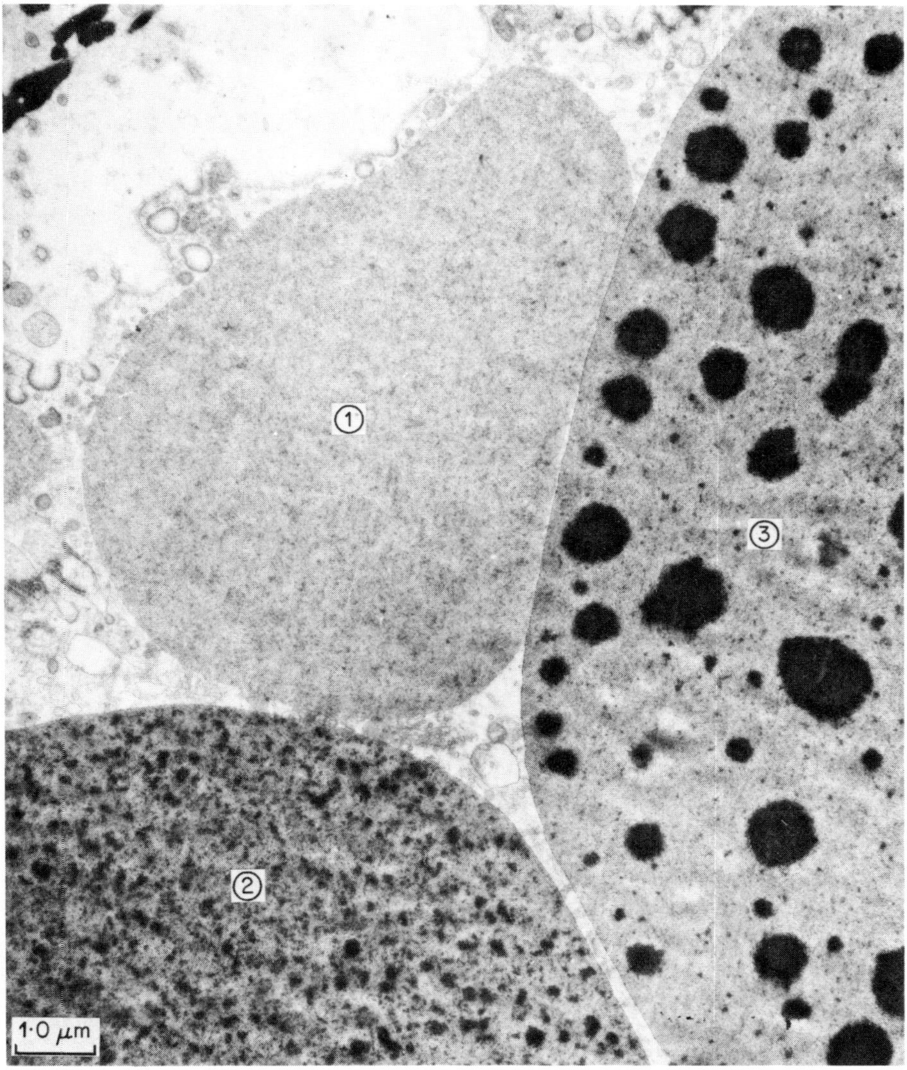

Fig. 7. Yolk spheres in the oocyte periphery showing a succession of stages (1 → 2 → 3) in the formation of dense subdroplets. (See note to Fig. 2).

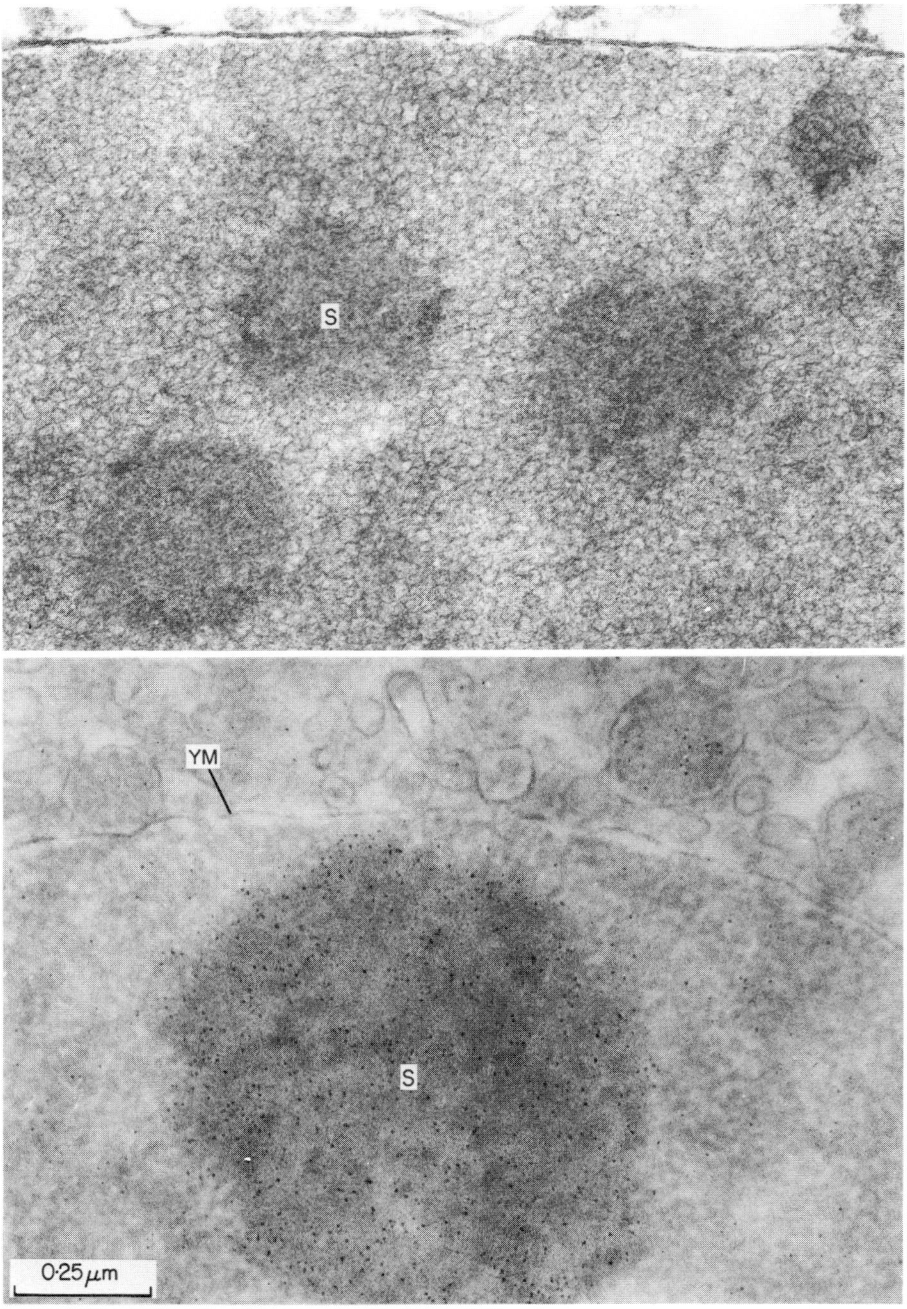

Fig. 8. Sections through the marginal zone of large yolk spheres. (*Top*) The sphere is bounded by a trilaminar membrane and contains dense subdroplets embedded in a compact mass of lipoprotein particles. (*Bottom*) Ferritin is mostly localized in a subdroplet (S) at 20 min after intravenous injection of the tracer. YM, yolk sphere membrane. (See note to Fig. 2).

spheres in the main vitellogenic phase (Perry and Gilbert, 1979, 1980). Immediately after the coated vesicles are pinched off from the plasma membrane, the lumen is obliterated and the cytoplasmic coating is shed. The membrane-bound spheres formed as a result of these changes are packed with particles. They undergo successive fusions to give rise to yolk spheres of increasing size. As the yolk spheres enlarge small clumps of granular material appear to separate from the particulate material and later aggregate into the dense subdroplets (Fig. 7). In the larger oocytes (10 mm diameter) this entire process takes place in a narrow zone at the cell periphery in the absence of any synthetic machinery. It is therefore likely to be dependent for its continuation on the recycling of preformed units, a subject that has recently been discussed by Pearse and Bretscher (1981). Since with each fusion the volume of the yolk sphere is increased relative to the surface area, there will be an excess of yolk sphere membrane available for recycling. The smooth-surfaced vesicles that are scattered in the cytoplasm between the developing yolk spheres may well be derived from this excess membrane. The peripheral cytoplasmic zone of the smaller oocytes (<10 mm diameter) is, by contrast, broader and contains a complexity of vesicular organelles, including Golgi bodies, coated vesicles (70 nm diameter) and a variety of smooth vesicles. A similar structural organization is found in the germinal disc region of the larger oocytes (Perry *et al.*, 1978b). Pearse and Bretscher (1981) have reviewed the evidence for the involvement of such structural entities in the synthesis and transport of components for the endocytotic mechanism.

The yolk spheres in the germinal disc resemble those of oocytes in the transitory phase. Those in the vicinity of the germinal vesicle possess a single subdroplet embedded in less compact material (Bakst and Howarth, 1977) and are later enclosed in the cells of the blastoderm where they are reported to contain DNA (Bruce and Emanuelsson, 1975).

3. Time Course of the Yolk Transport Mechanism

There have been many attempts to determine the time required for yolk material to be extracted from the plasma. When administered orally, dye tracers take about 3 to 5 h to enter the yolk (Warren and Conrad, 1939; Grau, 1976), but most of the delay is caused by the time taken for the tracers to pass along the gut and to be absorbed. Injection of dyes and other tracers give shorter time intervals of 30 to 60 min (Warren and Conrad, 1939; Gilbert, 1970; Callebaut, 1974), but again the times are exaggerated because some time has to elapse in order that sufficient dye enters the yolk to be visible. A more precise estimate has been obtained using electron microscopy to follow the uptake of ferritin into yolk after intravenous injection. In follicles larger than 1·5 mm in diameter, ferritin was found in the coated vesicles and nascent yolk spheres after 10 min; within 20 min it had segregated along with the granular component into the subdroplets of yellow yolk spheres (Fig. 8B). Clearly, the transport of material into the oocyte and its deposition in yolk spheres is an extremely rapid one and, particularly in the early vitellogenic phases, is faster than had been previously suspected.

C. Modification of Yolk Precursors during their Incorporation into the Oocyte

Though the morphological evidence provides a clear picture of how intact plasma proteins can be incorporated into yolk, it is also evident (see Section III) that substantial differences exist between yolk precursors in the plasma and their derivatives in yolk. Modification of the major yolk precursors must occur during the transit or within the oocyte.

The apparent complete cleavage of vitellogenin to phosvitin and lipovitellin probably occurs after its incorporation into the oocyte, perhaps due to the action of the proteases reported by Emaneulsson (1951). The appearance of electron-dense granules in the yolk spheres may be the result of this process. The freeing of receptors from their respective ligands is a prerequisite for membrane recycling (Pearse and Bretscher, 1981) and cleavage of vitellogenin may serve to dissociate the vitellogenin-receptor complex, as has been suggested to occur in amphibian oocytes (Opresko *et al.*, 1980). Hydrolysis of apo-B to smaller apoproteins may similarly contribute to the release of receptor-bound lipoproteins. Proteolysis of egg yolk VLD lipoproteins *in vitro* causes a marked increase in lipoprotein size (Steer *et al.*, 1968), and this suggests the larger LDL_1 yolk lipoproteins may arise through fusion of two or more LDL_2 particles.

Gornall and Kucsis (1973) suggested that the differences found between plasma and yolk lipids could be explained if there was either substantial rearrangement of glycerolipids by the ovary or some sort of selective uptake of plasma VLD lipoprotein subfractions. The first alternative they considered unlikely given the low activity of lipid synthesizing enzymes in the ovary (Gornall *et al.*, 1972) and their evidence from *in vitro* studies of ^{3}H-glycerol incorporation into plasma and yolk lipids (Gornall and Kucsis, 1972). It is also clearly incompatible with the morphological evidence for direct uptake of lipoproteins by endocytosis. Less drastic modification of lipid and/or selection of lipoproteins could occur at several stages during uptake of lipid into yolk. The most obvious example of selection of lipoproteins by the ovary is the exclusion of portomicrons by the basal lamina, but this is unlikely to make a major contribution to the differences between plasma and yolk lipids because portomicrons normally form only a small proportion (less than 1%) of the circulating lipid in laying hens. The lipid and apoprotein compositions of the plasma VLD lipoproteins vary, for example, with lipoprotein size, and preferential binding of lipoproteins enriched in apo-B or apo-VLDL-II to the oocyte plasma membrane may cause the uptake of lipoproteins into yolk with somewhat different lipid composition to that of total plasma VLD lipoproteins. Changes in lipid composition of VLD lipoproteins may also occur because of their hydrolysis in the ovary. Benson *et al.* (1975) found appreciable lipoprotein lipase activity located in the granulosa cells and granulosa cells have been shown to synthesize liproprotein lipase *in vitro* (Brannon *et al.*, 1978). However, hydrolysis of VLD lipoproteins by lipoprotein lipase during their passage between the granulosa cells *in vivo* is likely to be small because the specific activity of lipoprotein lipase in granulosa cells (Benson *et al.*, 1975) and VLD lipoproteins themselves are only partly susceptible to hydrolysis. The specific activity of lipoprotein lipase in granulose cells (Benson *et al.*, 1975) and the rate of progesterone synthesis within these cells (Hammond *et al.*, 1981) increase with growth of the follicle. This suggests lipoprotein lipase may be involved in providing precursors for steroidogenesis.

Despite the evidence that lipoproteins are incorporated into yolk in a more or less intact form, Bensadoun and Kompiang (1979) have proposed that uptake of plasma lipid into the oocyte is dependent on its hydrolysis by lipoprotein lipase. They consider that the lipoprotein lipase associated with the granulosa cells is probably not directly involved in the hydrolysis of plasma VLD lipoprotein triglyceride *in vivo*. Instead, they suggest that the granulosa cells act as the source of the lipoprotein lipase of the capillary endothelium in the thecal envelopes, in much the same way as the adipocytes act as a source of lipoprotein lipase in the capillary endothelium in adipose tissue. However, although they demonstrated that uptake of portomicron lipid into yolk is blocked by injection of anti-lipoprotein lipase anti-serum into the circulation, this does not justify the conclusion that ovarian lipoprotein lipase mediates the transfer of triglyceride fatty acids into yolk. Indeed, the choice of portomicrons as precursor of yolk lipid in these studies seems curious since almost all the lipoproteins in the plasma of the laying hen are of hepatic rather than intestinal origin. Moreover, most of the lipid absorbed from the intestine is initially taken up into the liver, at least in roosters (Bensadoun and Rothfeld, 1972). Hepatic uptake of dietary lipid probably occurs after partial degradation of portomicrons in the extra-hepatic circulation, as has been shown for uptake of chylomicron lipid by mammalian liver (Sherrill and Dietschy, 1978). The inhibition of uptake of portomicron lipid into yolk in hens injected with anti-lipoprotein lipase anti-serum is therefore probably not due to the specific inhibition of ovarian lipoprotein lipase. It is more likely to be a consequence of the general blocking of portomicron remnant formation; this in turn prevents uptake of portomicron lipid into the liver and its remodelling into smaller VLD lipoproteins which can pass directly into yolk.

References

Abe, T., Muto, Y. and Hosaya, N. (1975). *J. Lipid Res.* **16**, 200–210.

Ali, K. E. and Ramsay, W. N. M. (1974). *Q. Jl exp. Physiol.* **59**, 159–165.

Allerton, S. E. and Perlmann, G. E. (1965). *J. biol. Chem.* **240**, 3892–3898.

Bacon, W. L., Brown, K. I. and Musser, M. A. (1973). *Poult. Sci.* **52**, 1741–1744.

Bakst, M. R. and Howarth, B. (1977). *Biol. Reprod.* **17**, 361–369.

Bellairs, R. (1965). *J. Embryol. exp. Morph.* **13**, 215–233.

Bellairs, R. (1967). *J. Embryol. exp. Morph.* **17**, 267–281.

Bellairs, R., Backhouse, M. and Evans, R. J. (1972). *Micron* **3**, 328–346.

Bengtsson, G., Markland, S.-E. and Olivecrona, T. (1977). *Eur. J. Biochem.* **79**, 211–213.

Bensadoun, A. and Kompiang, I. P. (1979). *Fedn Proc. Fedn Am. Socs exp. Biol.* **38**, 2622–2626.

Bensadoun, A. and Rothfeld, A. (1972). *Proc. Soc. exp. Biol. Med.* **141**, 814–817.

Benson, J. D., Bensadoun, A. and Cohen, D. (1975). *Proc. Soc. exp. Biol. Med.* **148**, 347–350.

Bergink, M. W. and Wallace, R. A. (1974). *J. biol. Chem.* **249**, 2897–2903.

Bernadi, G. and Cook, W. H. (1960). *Biochim. biophys. Acta* **44**, 96–105.

Beuving, G. and Gruber, M. (1971). *Biochim. biophys. Acta* **232**, 524–528.

Brambell, F. W. R. (1970). "The Transmission of Passive Immunity from Mother to Young". North Holland Publishing Co., Amsterdam.

Brannon, P. M., Cheung, A. H. and Bensadoun, A. (1978). *Biochim. biophys. Acta* **531**, 96–108.

Brown, M. S. and Goldstein, J. L. (1979). *Proc. natn. Acad. Sci. U.S.A.* **76**, 3330–3337.

Bruce, L. (1977). *Cell Tiss. Res.* **178**, 103–109.

Bruce, L. and Emanuelsson, H. (1975). *Expl Cell Res.* **92**, 462–466.

Burley, R. W. (1975). *Aust. J. biol. Sci.* **28**, 121–132.

Burley, R. W. (1978). *Aust. J. biol. Sci.* **31**, 587–592.

Burley, R. W. and Vadehra, D. V. (1979). *Analyt. Biochem.* **94**, 53–59.

Callebaut, M. (1974). *Archs Biol., Paris* **85**, 201–233.

Carinci, P., Grossi, C. E. and Locci, P. (1973). *J. Embryol. exp. Morph.* **29**, 713–719.

Chalana, R. K. and Guraya, S. S. (1979). *Poult. Sci.* **58**, 225–231.

Chan, L. and O'Malley, B. W. (1978). *Ann. intern. Med.* **89**, 694–701.

Chan, L., Jackson, R. L., O'Malley, B. W. and Means, A. R. (1976). *J. clin. Invest.* **58**, 368–379.

Chan, L., Jackson, R. L. and Means, A. R. (1978). *Circulation Res.* **43**, 209–216.

Chan, L., Bradley, W. A., Jackson, R. L. and Means, A. R. (1980). *Endocrinology* **106**, 275–283.

Chapman, M. J. (1980). *J. Lipid Res.* **21**, 789–853.

Chapman, M. J., Goldstein, S. and Laudat, M. H. (1977). *Biochemistry* **16**, 3006–3015.

Christie, W. W. and Moore, J. H. (1972). *Comp. Biochem. Physiol.* **41B**, 287–295.

Christman, J. L., Grayson, M. J. and Huang, R. C. C. (1977). *Biochemistry* **16**, 3250–3256.

Clark, R. C. (1970). *biochem. J.* **118**, 537–542.

Clark, R. C. (1972). *Comp. Biochem. Physiol.* **41B**, 891–903.

Clark, R. C. (1973). *Biochim. biophys. Acta* **310**, 174–187.

Clark, R. C. (1974). *Int. J. Biochem.* **5**, 183–185.

Clark, R. C. (1976a). *Int. J. Biochem.* **7**, 569–572.

Clark, R. C. (1976b). *S. Afr. J. Sci.* **73**, 71–72.
Clark, R. C. (1980). *Int. J. Biochem.* **12**, 651–653.
Clark, R. C. and Dijkstra, J. (1980). *Int. J. Biochem.* **11**, 577–585.
Clark, R. C. and Joubert, F. J. (1971). *FEBS Letts* **13**, 225–228.
Clemens, M. J. (1974). *Prog. Biophys. Mol. Biol.* **28**, 71–108.
Cook, W. H. (1968). *In* "Egg Quality: A Study of the Hen's Egg" (T. C. Carter, ed.), pp. 109–132. Oliver and Boyd, Edinburgh.
Culbert, J. and McIndoe, W. M. (1971). *Int. J. Biochem.* **2**, 617–622.
Cutting, J. A. and Roth, T. F. (1973). *Biochim. biophys. Acta* **298**, 951–955.
Dawes, C. M. (1975). *Biol. Rev.* **50**, 351–371.
Deeley, R. G., Mullinix, K. P., Wetekam, W., Kronenberg, H. M., Meyers, M., Eldridge, J. D. and Goldberger, R. F. (1975). *J. biol. Chem.* **250**, 9060–9066.
Deeley, R. G., Udell, D. S., Burns, A. T. H., Gordon, J. I. and Goldberger, R. F. (1977). *J. biol. Chem.* **252**, 7913–7915.
Dopheide, T. A. A. and Inglis, A. S. (1976). *Aust. J. biol. Sci.* **29**, 175–180.
Dumont, J. N. (1978). *J. exp. Zool.* **204**, 193–218.
Edelstein, S., Lawson, D. E. M. and Kodicek, E. (1973). *Biochem. J.* **135**, 417–426.
Emanuelsson, H. (1951). *Nature, Lond.* **168**, 958–959.
Evans, A. J. (1974). *Proc. 15th Poult. Congr., New Orleans*, p. 399.
Evans, A. J., Perry, M. M. and Gilbert, A. B. (1979). *Biochim. biophys. Acta* **573**, 184–195.
Evans, R. J., Flegal, C. J. and Bauer, D. H. (1975). *Poult. Sci.* **54**, 889–895.
Evans, R. J., Flegal, C. J., Foerder, C. A., Bauer, D. H. and La Vigne, M. (1977). *Poult. Sci* **56**, 468–479.
Faith, R. E. and Clem, L. W. (1973). *Immunology* **25**, 151–164.
Francis, G. E. (952). *Biochem. J.* **51**, 715–720.
Franzen, J. S., Bobik, C. M., Stuchell, R. N. and Lee, L. D. (1968). *Archs Biochem. Biophys.* **123**, 127–132.
Frazer, D. R. and Emtage, J. S. (1976). *Biochem. J.* **160**, 671–682.
Froehlick, J. A., Merrill, A. H., Jr., Claggett, C. O. and McCormick, D. B. (1980). *Comp. Biochem. Physiol.* **66B**, 397–401.
Fujii, S., Tamura, T. and Okamoto, T. (1973). *J. Fac. Fish Anim. Husb. Hiroshima Univ.* **12**, 1–11.
Gilbert, A. B. (1970). *J. Reprod. Fert.* **23**, 539–540.
Gilbert, A. B. (1971). *In* "Physiology and Biochemistry of the Domestic Fowl" (D. J. Bell and B. M. Freeman, eds), Vol. 3, pp. 1163–1208. Academic Press, London and New York.
Gilbert, A. B. (1972). *In* "Egg Formation and Production" (B. M. Freeman and P. E. Lake, eds), pp. 1–21. Constable, Edinburgh.
Gilbert, A. B. (1979). *In* "Form and Function in Birds" (A. S. King and J. McLelland, eds), Vol. 1. pp. 237–360. Academic Press, London and New York.
Gilbert, A. B., Hardie, M. A., Perry, M. M., Dick, H. R. and Wells, J. W. (1980). *Br. Poult. Sci.* **21**, 257–263.
Gilbert, A. B., Perry, M. M., Waddington, D. and Hardie, M. A. (1983). *J. Reprod. Fert.* **69**, 221–227.
Giorgi, F. (1980). *In* "Coated Vesicles" (C. D. Ockleford and A. Whyte, eds), pp. 135–177. Cambridge University Press, Cambridge.
Goldstein, J. L. and Brown, M. S. (1977). *A. Rev. Biochem.* **43**, 897–930.

Goldstein, J. L., Anderson, R. G. W. and Brown, M. S. (1979). *Nature, Lond.* **279**, 679–685.

Gordon, J. I., Deeley, R. G., Burns, A. T. H., Paterson, B. M., Christman, J. L. and Goldberger, R. F. (1977). *J. biol. Chem.* **252**, 8320–8327.

Gornall, D. A. and Kucsis, A. (1971). *Can. J. Biochem.* **49**, 51–60.

Gornall, D. A. and Kucsis, A. (1972). *Proc. Can. Fed. Biol. Soc.* **15**, 789 (abs.).

Gornall, D. A. and Kucsis, A. (1973). *J. Lipid Res.* **14**, 197–205.

Gornall, D. A., Kucsis, A. and Morley, N. (1972). *Biochim. biophys. Acta* **280**, 225–230.

Grau, C. R. (1976). *Poult. Sci.* **55**, 1418–1422.

Green, C. D. (1980). *In* "Oxford Reviews of Reproductive Biology" (C. A. Finn, ed.), Vol. 2, pp. 97–122. Clarendon Press, Oxford.

Greengard, O., Sentenae, A. and Mendelsohn, N. (1964). *Biochim. biophys. Acta* **90**, 406–407.

Griffin, H. D. (1981). *Trans. Biochem. Soc.* **9**, 155P.

Grizzuti, K. and Perlmann, G. E. (1973). *Biochemistry* **12**, 4399–4403.

Grizzuti, K. and Perlmann, G. E. (1975). *Biochemistry* **14**, 2171–2175.

Guraya, S. S. (1975). *Acta morph. hung.* **23**, 251–261.

Hammond, R. W., Burke, W. H. and Hertelendy, F. (1981). *Biol. Reprod.* **24**, 1048–1055.

Hay, A. W. M. and Watson, G. (1976). *Comp. Biochem. Physiol.* **53B**, 167–172.

Heller, J. (1976). *Devl Biol.* **51**, 1–9.

Heuser, J. (1980). *J. Cell Biol.* **84**, 560–583.

Hillyard, L. A., White, H. M. and Pangburn, S. A. (1972). *Biochemistry* **11**, 511–518.

Hillyard, L. A., White, H. M. and Abraham, S. (1980). *J. Lipid Res.* **21**, 913–919.

Hodges, R. D. (1974). "The Histology of the Fowl", Academic Press, London and New York.

Hunt, J. R. and Simkiss, K. (1967). *Comp. Biochem. Physiol.* **21**, 223–230.

Jackson, R. L., Lin, H.-Y., Mao, J. T. S., Chan, L. and Means, A. R. (1977a). *Endocrinology* **101**, 849–857.

Jackson, R. L., Lin, H.-Y., Chan, L. and Means, A. R. (1977b). *J. biol. Chem.* **252**, 250–253.

Jordanov, J. and Boyadjieva-Michailova, A. (1974). *Acta anat.* **89**, 616–632.

Jost, J.-P. and Pehling, G. (1976). *Eur. J. Biochem.* **62**, 299–306.

Jost, J.-P., Pehling, G. and Baca, O. G. (1975). *Biochem. biophys. Res. Commun.* **62**, 957–965.

Kelley, J. L., Ganesan, D., Bass, H. B., Thayer, R. H. and Alaupovic, P. (1976). *FEBS Letts* **67**, 28–31.

King, A. S. (1975). *In* "Sisson and Grossman's The Anatomy of the Domestic Animals" (R. Getty, ed.), Vol. 2. pp. 1919–1964. Saunders, London.

Krumins, S. A. and Roth, T. F. (1981). *Biochem. J.* **196**, 481–488.

Kudzma, D. J., St. Claire, F., Dehallo, L. and Friedberg, S. J. (1975). *J. Lipid Res.* **16**, 123–133.

Kudzma, D. J., Swaney, J. B. and Ellis, E. N. (1979). *Biochim. biophys. Acta* **572**, 257–268.

Lee, D. C., McKnight, G. S. and Palmiter, R. D. (1978). *J. biol. Chem.* **253**, 3494–3503.

Lin, C. T. and Chan, L. (1980). *Endocrinology* **107**, 70–75.

Lofts, B. and Murton, R. K. (1973). *In* "Avian Biology" (D. S. Farner and J. R. King, eds), Vol. III, pp. 1–88. Academic Press, London and New York.

McIndoe, W. M. (1971). *In* "Physiology and Biochemistry of the Domestic Fowl" (D. J. Bell and B. M. Freeman, eds), Vol. 3, pp. 1209–1233. Academic Press, London and New York.

McIndoe, W. M. and Culbert, J. (1979). *Int. J. Biochem.* **10**, 659–664.
Mackenzie, S. L. and Martin, W. G. (1967). *Can. J. Biochem. Physiol.* **45**, 591–601.
Majno, G. (1965). *In* "Handbook of Physiology, section 2: Circulation" (W. F. Hamilton, ed.), Vol. 3, pp. 2293–2375. Waverly Press, Baltimore.
Mandella, R. D., Meslar, H. W. and White, H. B. III. (1978). *Biochem. J.* **175**, 629–633.
Martin, W. G., Vandegaer, J. E. and Cook, W. H. (1957). *Can. J. Biochem. Physiol.* **35**, 241–250.
Martin, W. G., Turner, K. J. and Cook, W. H. (1959). *Can. J. Biochem. Physiol.* **37**, 1197–1207.
Martin, W. G., Turner, K. J. and Cook, W. H. (1963). *Can. J. Biochem. Physiol.* **41**, 657–666.
Mecham, D. K. and Olcott, H. S. (1949). *J. Am. chem. Soc.* **71**, 3670–3679.
Meslar, H. W., Camper, S. A. and White, H. B. III. (1978). *J. biol. Chem.* **253**, 6979–6982.
Miller, M., Buss, E. and Clagett, C. (1981a). *Comp. Biochem. Physiol.* **69B**, 681–686.
Miller, M. S., Buss, E. G. and White, H. B. III. (1981b). *Biochem. J.* **198**, 225–226.
Mokady, S. and Tal, M. (1974). *Biochim. biophys. Acta* **336**, 361–366.
Montesano, R. and Nicolescu, P. (1978). *Anat. Rec.* **190**, 861–870.
Morgan, E. H. (1975). *Q. Jl exp. Physiol.* **60**, 233–247.
Muniyappa, K. and Adiga, P. R. (1979). *Biochem. J.* **177**, 887–894.
Muniyappa, K. and Adiga, P. R. (1980). *Biochem. J.* **186**, 201–210.
Muniyappa, K. and Adiga, P. R. (1981). *Biochem. J.* **193**, 679–685.
Murthy, U.S. and Adiga, P. R. (1978a). *Biochim. biophys. Acta* **538**, 364–375.
Murthy, U.S. and Adiga, P. R. (1978b). *Biochem. J.* **179**, 331–335.
Nakamura, R., Hayakawa, M. and Sato, Y. (1977). *Poult. Sci.* **56**, 1148–1152.
Nalbandov. A. V. and James, M. F. (1949). *Am. J. Anat.* **85**, 347–377.
Neufeld, E. G. and Ashwell, G. (1980). *In* "The Biochemistry of Glycoproteins and Proteoglycans" (W. Lennarz, ed.), pp. 241–266. Plenum Press, New York.
Nichols, A. V., Forte, G. M. and Coggiola, E. L. (1969). *Biochim. biophys. Acta* **175**, 451–453.
Nishida, T., Seki, M. and Mochizuki, K. (1977). *Jap. J. vet. Sci.* **39**, 347–352.
Nishimura, M., Urakawa, N. and Iwata, M. (1976). *Jap. J. vet. Sci.* **38**, 83–92.
Opresko. L., Wiley, H. S. and Wallace, R. A. (1980). *Cell* **22**, 47–57.
Oribe, T. (1973). *Bull. Hiroshima agric. Coll.* **4**, 323–331.
Orlans, E. (1967). *Immunology* **12**, 27–37.
Paulson, J. and Rosenberg, M. D. (1972). *J. ultrastruc. Res.* **40**, 25–43.
Paulson, J. L. and Rosenberg, M. D. (1974). *Devl Biol.* **40**, 366–371.
Pearse, B. (1980). *Trends Biomed. Sci.* **5**, 131–134.
Pearse, B. M. F. and Bretscher, M. S. (1981). *A. Rev. Biochem.* 50, 85–101.
Perry, M. M. and Gilbert, A. B. (1979). *J. Cell. Sci.* **39**, 257–272.
Perry, M. M. and Gilbert, A. B. (1980). *Cell biol. Int. Rep.* **4**, 759.
Perry, M. M., Gilbert, A. B. and Evans, A. J. (1978a). *J. Anat.* **125**, 481–497.
Perry, M. M., Gilbert, A. B. and Evans, A. J. (1978b). *J. Anat.* **127**, 379–392.
Perry, M. M., Waddington, D., Gilbert, A. B. and Hardie, M. A. (1983). *IRCS Med. Sci.* **11**, 979–980.
Perry, M. M., Griffin, H. D. and Gilbert, A. B. *Expl. Cell Res.* (in press).
Pinna, L. A., Donella, A., Clari, G. and Moret, V. (1975). *Biochim. biophys. Acta* **397**, 519–528.
Radomski, M. W. and Cook, W. H. (1964). *Can. J. Biochem.* **42**, 1023–1025.
Raju, K. S. and Mahadevan, S. (1976). *Biochim. biophys. Acta* **446**, 387–398.

Rao, R. D. N. and Mahadevan, S. (1978). *Poult. Sci.* **57**, 1091–1093.
Romanoff, A. L. and Romanoff, A. J. (1949). "The Avian Egg". Wiley, New York.
Rose, M. E. and Orlans, E. (1981). *Devl comp. Immunol.* **5**, 15–20.
Rosenstein, R. W. and Taborsky, G. (1970). *Biochemistry* **9**, 658–659.
Roth, T. F., Cutting, J. A. and Atlas, S. B. (1976). *J. Supramolecular Struct.* **4**, 527–548.
Roth, T. F., Cobbs, C., Woodward, M. and Woods, J. (1980). *J. Cell Biol.* **87**, 92a.
Rothwell, B. and Solomon, S. E. (1977). *Br. Poult. Sci.* **18**, 605–610.
Scanes, C. G., Mozelic, H., Kavanagh, E., Merrill, G. and Rabii, J. (1982). *J. Reprod. Fert.* **64**, 227–231.
Schjeide, O. A., Galey, F., Grellert, E. A., Sanlin, R., De Vellis, J. and Mead, J. F. (1970). *Biol. Reprod. Suppl.* **2**, 14–43.
Schjeide, O. A., Hanzely, L., Holhouser, S. J. and Briles, W. E. (1974). *Cell Tiss. Res.* **156**, 47–59.
Schjeide, O. A., Kanchera, L., Hanzely, L. and Briles, W. E. (1975). *Cell Tiss. Res.* **163**, 63–79.
Schjeide, O. A., Briles, W. E. and Holhouser, S. (1976). *Cell Tiss. Res.* **168**, 109–116.
Scow, R. O., Blanchette-Mackie, E. J. and Smith, L. C. (1980). *Fedn Proc. Fend Am. Soc. exp. Biol.* **39**, 2610–2617.
Shainkin, R. and Perlmann, G. E. (1971). *J. biol. Chem.* **246**, 2278–2284.
Shantz, R. C. and Dawson, L. E. (1976). *Poult. Sci.* **55**, 790–795.
Sherrill, B. C. and Dietschy, J. M. (1978). *J. biol. Chem.* **253**, 1859–1867.
Steer, D. C., Martin, W. G. and Cook, W. H. (1968). *Biochemistry* **7**, 3309–3315.
Sugano. H. and Watanabe, I. (1961). *J. Biochem., Tokyo* **50**, 473–480.
Taborsky, G. (1974). *Adv. Protein Chem.* **28**, 1–210.
Tata, J. R. (1976). *Cell* **9**, 1–14.
Tata, D. R. and Smith, D. F. (1979). *Recent Prog. Horm. Res.* **35**, 47–90.
Vadehra, D. V., Bain, J. M. and Burley, R. W. (1977). *Biochem. J.* **166**, 619–621.
Vigo, C. and Vance, D. E. (1981). *Biochem. J.* **200**, 321–326.
Wahli, W., Dawid, I. B., Ryffel, G. U. and Weber, R. (1981). *Science, N.Y.* **212**, 298–304.
Wallace, R. A. (1965). *Analyt. Biochem.* **11**, 297–311.
Wang, S.-Y. and Williams, D. L. (1980). *Biochemistry* **19**, 1557–1563.
Warren, D. C. and Conrad, R. M. (1939). *J. agric. Res.* **58**, 875–893.
White, H. B. III., Dennison, B. A., Fera, M. A. D., Whitney, C. J., McGuire, J. C., Meslar, H. W. and Sammelwitz, P. H. (1976). *Biochem. J.* **157**, 395–400.
Wiley, H. S. and Dumont, J. N. (1978). *Biol. Reprod.* **17**, 762–771.
Williams, D. L. (1979). *Biochemistry* **18**, 1056–1063.
Williams, J. (1962). *Biochem. J.* **83**, 346–354.
Winter, W. R., Buss, E. G., Clagett, C. O. and Boucher, R. V. (1967). *Comp. Biochem. Physiol.* **22**, 889–896.
Wiskocil, R., Bensky, P., Dower, W., Goldberger, R. F., Gordon, J. I. and Deeley, R. G. (1980). *Proc. natn. Acad. Sci., U.S.A.* **77**, 4474–4478.
Woods, J. W., Woodward, M. P. and Roth, T. F. (1978). *J. Cell Sci.* **30**, 87–97.
Wyburn, G. M., Aitken, R. N. C. and Johnston, H. S. (1965) *J. Anat.* **99**, 469–484.
Yamauchi, K., Kurisaki, J. and Sasago, K. (1976). *Agr. biol. Chem.* **40**, 1581–1586.
Yu, J. Y.-L. and Marquardt, R. R. (1973). *Comp. Biochem. Physiol.* **46B**, 759–767.
Yusko, S. C. and Roth, T. F. (1976). *J. Supramolecular Struct.* **4**, 89–97.

12 The Male in Reproduction

P. E. LAKE

Agricultural and Food Research Council's Poultry Research Centre, Roslin, Midlothian, Scotland

I. Introduction

Information on the structure and function of the male genital organs of the fowl was recently reviewed in an account of form and function in birds (Lake, 1981) and should be consulted for basic details of the male organs and spermatozoa. This chapter describes work since the mid-seventies, on aspects of the production of spermatozoa and their activity in various phases of the reproductive process, including the act of fertilization. These studies emphasize some of the anatomical, physiological and biochemical factors likely to affect the competence of the breeding male.

PHYSIOLOGY BIOCHEMISTRY DOMESTIC
FOWL, VOL. 5 ISBN 0-12-267105-8

II. Development of the Testes and Excurrent Ducts

In a review of the physical environment and reproduction in domesticated birds (Lake, 1974), it was shown how various factors, such as nutrition, light and temperature, affected the development and activity of reproductive organs. More recent work has extended knowledge of the mechanisms governing the growth of the testis, the activity of the germinal epithelium of the seminiferous tubules and the output of spermatozoa. These studies have improved our understanding of the physiological mechanisms controlling gonadal growth and the supply of spermatozoa and enables a breeder to manipulate the birds for better efficiency of breeding under certain management systems, including artificial insemination.

It would appear that the number of Sertoli cells laid down in the seminiferous tubules is correlated with the degree of activity of the germinal epithelium at sexual maturity and consequently determines the output of spermatozoa in the adult. These cells are, thereby, considered to be involved in the control of spermatogenesis (Reviers *et al.*, 1980). The stock of Sertoli cells can be influenced by the photoperiod experienced in the pre-pubertal phase of life and by the genotype of the male, these factors influencing gonadotrophin activity in the developing male. It is considered possible that quantitative examinations of Sertoli cells may serve as a useful tool in future studies on factors affecting the productivity of the testis.

A detailed study of the germinal epithelium, the amount of seminiferous tubules in the testis and the daily output of spermatozoa has confirmed that on diets containing similar amounts of energy, broiler males will develop optimum testis size and yield maximum spermatoza and fertility on diets containing 11 to 13% protein, when kept in cages, and 15% protein, when on the floor (Saeid, 1981).

It is well-known that photoperiod influences the activity of the gonad. In histological studies of growing male fowl, Reviers (1980) observed the effect of different applications of light on the activity of the germinal epithelium and the relationship with the numbers of spermatozoa ultimately produced in adulthood. Reviers recognized two important concepts in relation to the rate of production of spermatozoa: the daily sperm output (DSO), defined as the total number of sperm ejaculated over a given period expressed on a daily basis; and the daily sperm production (DSP) defined as the total number of sperm produced each day by both testes. The DSO over a short period is approximately proportional to the frequency of semen collection and can approximate the DSP when semen collections are performed daily. DSP was estimated by a technique involving the enumeration of round spermatids in histological samples of sections of seminiferous tubules, and was found to be 80×10^6 to 120×10^6 spermatozoa per g testis tissue. The DSP, testis weight and total number of Sertoli cells per testis were highly inter-correlated.

The adult testis weight, the DSP and the total number of Sertoli cells were related to the proliferative capabilities of the Sertoli and germ cells before puberty rather than by their initial numbers at hatching. These capabilities are likely to be hormone-dependent, as in the quail (Brown *et al.*, 1975) and, therefore, hormonal perturbations induced during growth might be expected to have an important influence upon the adult fertility potential. Such perturbations occur under the influence of light. It was observed that under constant short (8 h) and long (16 h/24 h) days, from one week of age, males had similar testis growth to puberty. However, during the pubertal phase, the testis growth under long photoperiods was twice that under short photoperiods, resulting in earlier sexual maturity in the former. After maturity, the mean testis weight and DSP declined rapidly under the long days, but remained constant till 51 weeks of age under short daylength. Under a lighting regime where there was a progressive decrease in daylength from hatching to about 24 weeks of age, a phase of rapid testis growth still occurred, albeit delayed by about 4 weeks compared with males on constant 14 or 16 h daylength. However, when given increased daylength at this time, they achieved sexual maturity at 32 weeks of age with a very high testis weight. Reducing daylength when males are in adulthood generally initiates moulting and a decline of reproductive activity. Early sexual maturity may be induced by increased daily photoperiods applied before puberty or interrupted night photoschedules. However, the final DSP and testis weight in adulthood can decrease earlier than in males reared and maintained on other photoschedules (Reviers, 1980).

The effects of light are exploited in commerce to obtain maximum fertility under different management systems. The age at puberty and at sexual maturity can clearly be modified by photoperiod and the method of applying it. In order to take maximum advantage of light manipulation for breeding, i.e. to synchronize output of spermatozoa in the male with egg production in the female, one has to take into account likely variations in onset of semen production and its persistency once maximum gonadal growth has been attained. Also, in this respect differences between genetic strains of fowl in the development of testes and germinal epithelium activity in response to the same light treatment have to be recognized (Reviers, 1980), as well as individual variations within a breed or strain (Reviers and Williams, 1981).

Light presumably affects the hormonal feedback mechanisms governing gonadal development and the number of Sertoli cells laid down before the production of spermatozoa intensifies; the adult number of Sertoli cells is closely related to the DSP (Reviers, 1980). In studies at this laboratory, the onset of puberty was found to occur in cockerels of a medium-heavy strain over a period of 8 weeks. When the birds were reared under a constant daily 14-h photoperiod, it occurred over the period 16 to 24 weeks of age within the group and most birds produced semen by this time. Culbert *et al.* (1977) and Sharp *et al.* (1977) have shown that the onset of puberty is associated with the following sequence of endocrinological events: a fall in the androstenedione content of the testes before any evidence of an increase in testicular growth; an increase in the amount of luteinizing hormone (LH) in the pituitary gland as the testes start to enlarge; an increase in the total amount of testosterone in the testes with a simultaneous increase in the concentration of LH in the plasma; an increase in the concentration of testosterone in the plasma. It is believed that the changes in stored and plasma LH and testosterone are related causally, as LH stimulates the development of Leydig cells and the secretion of androgen (Sterling *et al.*, 1978). A continued increase and maintenance of a greater concentration, plateauing in plasma testosterone after the testes started to produce spermatozoa suggested that the testes continue to mature after 24 weeks of age for about another 10 to 12 weeks (Culbert *et al.*, 1977).

Sharp (1975) and Sharp *et al.* (1977) studied aspects of circulating pituitary hormones in relation to sexual development, in fowls from hatch to maturity whilst given a constant 14-h photoperiod each day. Mean plasma LH concentrations were greater in the male than the female and there was a steady rise pre-pubertally (from 9 to 19 weeks of age) from 7 to 9 ng ml^{-1} plasma, and thereafter to 10 or 11 ng ml^{-1}. Wide individual variations occurred in the mean values for plasma LH before and after puberty, and it is possible that this may reflect differences in the sensitivity of the hypothalamo-hypophysial complex to the negative feedback action of sex steroids on the secretion of LH. It could also account for individual variations in breeding performance. Limited evidence for this hypothesis was given by Sharp (1975), when he noted that a male with a poor rate of semen production had a high concentration of LH. More work is required on the feasibility of using hormone measurements as predictors of the breeding ability of males. Williams and de Reviers (1981) studied the circulating LH and androstenedione in cockerels raised under different photoschedules, which affect the onset and persistency of the output of spermatozoa, and found differences in the hormone parameters between the best and the poorest producers of spermatozoa under certain lighting regimes. However, no relationship was found between the level of adult fertility and several hormone parameters observed at different ages. They suggested that future studies of the development of hormone responsive receptors in the testis of individual males and the action of FSH on testicular activity might reveal better methods of predicting and selecting males with the best breeding ability.

It was mentioned above that the cellular events occurring within the testis in relation to the production of spermatozoa are presumably hormone-dependent. Detailed observations at the cellular level have established this to be so in the quail (Brown *et al.*, 1975), but similar work has not been done with the fowl. Tojo and Ogawa (1981) found that FSH increased the weight of the testes in hypophysectomized chicks as a result of the proliferation of the seminiferous tubules, whereas LH caused a proliferation of the interstitial cells No observations were made on the germinal epithelium.

Genetic determinants of gonadal growth and sexual maturity have also been studied, and it has been found that the K^n allele affects sexual development. Males homozygous for K^n were delayed in reaching sexual maturity by 2 to 3 weeks and it was considered due to the gene's action in slowing down body growth, which in turn slowed down testis growth and development. However, it is also possible that the K^n gene interfered with testicular testosterone production (Somes and Weigh, 1980).

III. Production and Maturation of Spermatozoa

Features of testis growth and the structure and function of the germinal epithelium in the seminiferous tubules have been reviewed by Lake (1981), and detailed information on various aspects of the structure of ejaculated spermatozoa has been given by Grigg and Hodge (1949), Bonadonna (1954), Lake (1954, 1966a), Dingle and McCosker (1967), Krustev and Danov (1968), Lake *et al.* (1968), Nicander (1968, 1970) and Bakst and Howarth (1975).

Interest in artificial insemination and semen storage as aids to breeding, and concern to improve breeding efficiency of males in natural mating have prompted a re-awakening of studies on the formation of spermatozoa in the testis, their rate of production, their maturation in the male tract and the factors affecting the output of semen.

Observations support the view that spermatozoa of the fowl are produced very rapidly in the testis in large numbers and that they mature more quickly than in the mammal. It is interesting to speculate whether this ability is associated with the well-known observation that a male normally copulates daily or even more frequently (Brantas *et al.*, 1972). This would necessitate rapid re-filling of each ductus deferens with fresh, mature spermatozoa depending upon the number of cells extruded in each ejaculate.

Reviers (1968) demonstrated that the duration of spermatogenesis in the fowl is short. From the pre-leptotene stage of the division of the primary spermatocyte to the end of meiotic prophase was estimated to take about five or six days. The first-stage round spermatids appeared during the 6th and 7th days, after division of the secondary spermatocytes, and the spermatids elongated during the 10th to the 12th days, which ended spermiogenesis.

The spermatozoa appeared in the ejaculate from 13 to 15 days after the start of the multiplication of the primary spermatocytes. The longer time occurred more frequently in the late breeding season and was considered to reflect a seasonal influence on the rate of transport of spermatozoa in the efferent ducts (Reviers, 1975). These observations contrast with those on the mammal, e.g.

mouse, 26 days, and ram, 29 to 30 days to the end of spermiogenesis (Oakberg, 1956; Ortavant, 1956), and about 40 days for the first appearance of spermatozoa in the ejaculate in the rabbit from each spermatogenic wave (Amman *et al.*, 1965).

Pertinent to the question of how frequently a male may mate and remain fertile, and equally to the practice of breeding by artificial insemination, are recent observations which have been made on the reserves of spermatozoa in the male tract and the effect of the frequency of semen collection on this reservoir. Compared with mammals, the ductus epididymis on each side of the body of the fowl is small, and the main storage site for spermatozoa is in the long ductus deferens. However, from ultrastructural evidence, it might be considered that the long ductus deferens is equivalent to an extension of the corpus and caudal epididymis of the mammal (Tingari, 1971; Aire, 1979; Lake, 1981). In this context, it is of interest that Bamberg *et al.* (1976) found evidence of a high activity of β-N-acetylhexosaminidase in the epididymis of the fowl, an enzyme which is found only in the caput epididymis in the boar. This might be considered to support the view that the ductus epididymis in the bird is equivalent to the upper part of the mammalian ductus epididymis (Tingari, 1971).

Reviers (1975) estimated that in a group of non-ejaculated White Leghorn cockerels, the mean reserve of spermatozoa (ESR) in the excurrent ducts of the testes was $6{\cdot}8 \times 10^9$ (range $0{\cdot}9 \times 10^9$ to 19×10^9 per male). About 65% was located in the distal halves of the ducti deferentes. The epididymides contained only 5%. The daily testicular production of spermatozoa was about 2×10^9 in non-ejaculated males. Therefore, the ESR in rested males represented the equivalent of 3·5 days of the testicular output. In males ejaculated daily, the ESR varied, according to the season, from $4{\cdot}5 \times 10^9$ to $1{\cdot}6 \times 10^9$ and was correlated with changes in testis weight. The ESR in these cases represented about 2 to 1 day of the daily production of spermatozoa, respectively, Clearly, the frequency with which semen containing large numbers of spermatozoa can be collected for purposes of breeding by artificial insemination may be expected, amongst other things, to vary according to the season and age of the male.

Over a limited period, changing the frequency of semen collection from once weekly to once daily was found to be associated with a display of greater motility of the ejaculated spermatozoa when they were tested after storage for 5 h at 4°C (Reviers, 1975). It would have been interesting to have examined the fertilizing ability of the more frequently collected spermatozoa, because younger spermatozoa, post-testicular, may remain viable longer *in vitro*. In this respect, it is interesting to recall that more degenerating spermatozoa were found in semen samples when semen collection was less frequent (El Jack and Lake, 1966).

From studies on the daily production of spermatozoa by the testis, the transport time of spermatozoa in the excurrent ducts, extra-gonadal reserves of spermatozoa and the daily output from the male, Reviers (1972a,b, 1975) estimated that many spermatozoa were lost with long rests between artificial ejaculation, probably by continuous expulsion with faeces and urine or spontaneous ejaculation. A proportion of spermatozoa degenerating naturally in the excurrent ducts were also seen to be resorbed by certain lining cells of the male tract, a phenomenon which was exaggerated by vasoligation (Tingari and Lake, 1972).

From the above studies of gonad function, it would be expected that maximum utilization of germ cell material from the male for breeding will be obtained by collecting semen at a particular frequency; it would reduce the proportion of the daily output of spermatozoa that might be wasted. In practice, it was found in one case that a greater production of semen and offspring were obtained by collecting semen three times per week from broiler-type and layer-type males during the first 13 and 20 weeks of a breeding period, respectively (McDaniel and Sexton, 1977). However, it is not known whether, or for how long, this performance could have been sustained over the remainder of the breeding period. Fuquay and Renden (1980) observed that there was no significant difference between the productions of spermatozoa in broiler-type males when semen was collected three and five times per week during the latter part of a breeding period (from 36 to 59 weeks of age). Collecting ten times (twice daily) did, however, have an adverse effect on the output of spermatozoa.

It would appear that a balance may exist naturally, between the production of spermatozoa in the testis and their time of storage in the excurrent ducts, whereby their average quality and fertilizing ability is determined. The frequency of ejaculation would be important in this process with regard to the efficiency of utilization of semen, because after a minimum time necessary for maturation, spermatozoa progressively lose their fertilizing ability if they stay in the male tract (El Jack and Lake, 1966; Petitjean, 1970; Reviers and Petitjean, 1973).

There is some evidence for a simpler process of maturation of fowl spermatozoa in the excurrent ducts of the testes compared with the mammal. In Eutherian mammals, it is generally recognized that spermatozoa undergo important changes in structure and function in the extensive ductus epididymis. Only after residing there for a long time are they capable of fertilizing eggs and it is an androgen-dependent process (Reviers, 1975). Birds, like some other animals (frogs, teleost fish), are different, in that spermatozoa become motile and are capable of fertilizing eggs soon after they leave the testis (Bedford, 1979).

In birds, it appears that the maturation of spermatozoa is not dependent upon an environment in the excurrent ducts created by an androgen-stimulated epithelium (Bedford, 1979). This view is supported by early work, which showed that testosterone administered to castrated male fowl did not prolong the life (motility) of spermatozoa beyond the time that they remained motile in an intact male (Munro, 1938). No evident morphological changes occur in fowl spermatozoa during the maturation process and movement down the excurrent ducts, except a thickening of the inner mitochondrial membranes (Nicander and Hellstrom, 1967; Tingari, 1973). It has also been shown that no changes occur in some surface properties of the spermatozoa during their passage from the upper to the lower part of the male tract, contrary to mammals (Bedford, 1979; Bedford and Calvin, 1974).

It has been suggested that the simple maturation process of bird spermatozoa and the rapid transit time through the excurrent ducts (Reviers, 1975) may be significant factors in the breeding behaviour of the fowl. Amongst animals there appears to be an inverse causal relationship between the lack of a specialized androgen-dependent storage capacity for spermatozoa and a large number of spermatozoa found in the ductus deferens at a given time in rested males (Bedford, 1979), which could be associated with the ability of the male fowl to mate frequently. Bedford suggested that, because of the rapid maturation and transit in the male fowl, there is no need to store spermatozoa for a long time to build up a reservoir as in mammals. A mechanism thus exists for the continual rapid removal of the available population of spermatozoa, which can be hastened by the greater ejaculation rate in fowls in contrast to the mammal (Reviers, 1975). In mammals, a reserve must build up to enable multiple matings, as the production of spermatozoa and transit time through the excurrent ducts are slow and not hastened by ejaculation (Bedford, 1979).

In mammals, it is necessary for the spermatozoa after ejaculation to incubate in the female tract for a period before they acquire the ability to fertilize an egg. This phenomenon, known as capacitation, is not considered to occur in the fowl (Nishiyama *et al.*, 1968; Howarth, 1971; Fujihara *et al.*, 1973), since freshly ovulated ova can be fertilized by freshly ejaculated spermatozoa *in vitro*. Correspondingly, no "decapacitation factor" has been found in fowl seminal plasma (Dukelow *et al.*, 1967).

IV. Physiology and Biochemistry of Semen and the Male and Female Reproductive Tracts

Since the publication of Volume 3, certain aspects of the physiology and biochemistry of semen and the environments in the reproductive tracts of the male and female have received attention. Particular interest has centred on the interaction of the spermatozoa with these environments and the maintenance of their viability in travelling from the male excurrent ducts and through the oviduct to perform the act of fertilization.

A. Properties of Semen Derived from the Ductus Deferens and Features of the Viability of Spermatozoa

Lake (1966b, 1971, 1981) has already described some of the seminal constituents and further studies have been made which reveal other general analytical data demonstrating the uniqueness of seminal fluid compared to other body fluids, although the functional significance of some of the substances is unknown (Table 1).

Evidence is available to show that a blood-testis barrier exists in the fowl by virtue of the presence of tight junctions between the Sertoli cells in the seminiferous tubules (Cooksey, 1975). The significance to testis function of the barrier has not been examined in the fowl, although extensive biochemical studies in mammals indicate that it enables the germ cell stages beyond early primary spermatocytes to have a special fluid environment (Setchell and Waites, 1975; Waites, 1977; Neaves, 1977). Seminal plasma is derived from the seminiferous tubules and the efferent ducts, the composition of the resultant fluid being a net product of the secretion and absorption which occurs in the different parts of the genital tract, together with intermediary metabolites and the end-products of metabolism of spermatozoa and spermatocytes.

Compared with blood, the buffering capacity of seminal plasma is weak and the pH rapidly becomes alkaline on standing. Values for semen pH in the literature are variable, probably due in most cases to the variable degree of contamination with transparent fluid when it is collected artificially by squeezing the erected copulatory organ (for review, see Lake, 1966b). However, recent observations (G. J. Wishart, personal communication) have indicated that semen containing a minimum amount of transparent fluid measures pH 7·4 if collected on ice under liquid paraffin. If it is collected at room temperature under paraffin, the pH is lower (about pH 7·1), due presumably to some CO_2 production from the metabolism of spermatozoa. If the paraffin is removed, the pH rises to about 7·8 due possibly to the escape of CO_2. These observations indicate the difficulty of ascertaining the true pH of fresh semen.

Other features of the seminal plasma from the ductus deferens in contrast with blood are the presence of very high amounts of glutamate, low chloride and the absence of glucose (Table 1). Similarly, many specific enzymes have been identified in seminal plasma (Bernon and Buckland, 1975; Buckland, 1971a, b). The true significance of these observations in relation to male fowl reproduction and fertility still awaits satisfactory explanation.

Table 1

A comparison of the mean amounts (mM) of components of various body fluids of the male fowl

	Seminal plasma free of transparent fluid[a]	Fluid from ductus deferens[b]	Transparent fluid[c]	Blood plasma	Reference[e]
Glucose	0·17	0·19	12·1	10·8	1
	—	—	11·2	13·9	2
Chloride	37·1	—	134·0	—	3
	36·9	—	—	121·0	4
	70·0	—	140·8	153·6	5
Acetyl carnitine	0·5–2·0	0·5–2·0	—	0·08	1
Carnitine	1·0–4·0	1·0–4·0	—	0·15	1
Glutamate	100·0	100·0	—	—	1
	73·0	—	—	0·2	6
	88·0	54·0(99·3)[d]	0·3	0·22	7
Lactate	4·0	—	—	5·4	6
	3·7	—	—	5·8	4
	—	—	2·6	5·2	2
Pyruvate	0·3	—	—	0·4	6
	0·33	—	—	0·44	4
2-oxo-glutarate	1·4	—	—	0·1	6

[a]Obtained by centrifuging, at 5°C, semen squirted from the papillae of the ducti deferentes during normal semen collection.

[b]Obtained from males which had ligatures placed between the epididymal region and ductus deferens on both sides. After surgery, they were massaged several times until contents of ducti were aspermic and then fluid was collected on several occasions and kept at −20°C until sufficient volumes were available for analysis.

[c]Fluid collected by massage and pressure on the tumescent lymphatic folds (Lake, 1981) after the initial high density sperm fraction had been obtained during the normal semen collection procedure.

[d]Males killed, contents of ducti deferentes emptied immediately and centrifuged at 5°C to obtain supernatant for analysis.

[e](1) G. J. Wishart, personal communication; (2) Schindler and Scharf, 1963; (3) Lake, 1966b; (4) Lake and El Jack, 1964 ; (5) Lake, 1956 ; (6) Lake and El Jack, 1966 ; (7) Lake and Hatton, 1968.

Lake (1981) discussed the activity of several types of enzyme in the lining epithelium of the male tract and pointed out that in some cases it had not been substantiated whether they were released into the fluid contents of the excurrent ducts and were of significance in relation to the activity of spermatozoa. However, appreciable acid and alkaline phosphatase, N-acetylhexoseaminidase, arylsulphatase, adenosine triphosphatase (ATP-ase) and lysozyme activities were found in seminal plasma (McIndoe and Lake, 1974; Kannan, 1974; Servouse *et al.*, 1976; Droba and Droba, 1981). Traces of other glycosidases were also observed (Kannan, 1974). The acid phosphatase and ATP-ase were found in vesicles which sedimented with spermatozoa during centrifugation; little or none was in the soluble form in the supernatant (McIndoe and Lake, 1974; Servouse *et al.*, 1976). In this respect, it is surprising that more attention has not been given to the possible significance of the contents of the apocrine and merocrine types of secretions observed in the lining epithelium of the excurrent ducts of the testis, the origin presumably of some of the above mentioned particulate material in the semen of the fowl. Cytological evidence of apocrine secretory activity in the entire excurrent duct system from the seminiferous tubules caudally has been discussed (Tingari, 1971, 1972; Niimura *et al.*, 1980; Osman, 1981) although Aire (1980) emphasised the need to ensure that such observations in some regions of the excurrent duct system are not due to artefacts of tissue fixation. Considering the interest in the storage of semen, it is surprising that no systematic attempts have been made to define the significance of various components of seminal plasma, particularly enzymes. Some enzymes liberated from otherwise inactive complexes during storage may inflict damage on spermatozoa and account for some of the loss of fertilizing ability or total structural damage which is observed under various circumstances *in vitro*.

Stratil (1970) and Harris and Sweeney (1971) identified more than 12 proteins in fowl seminal plasma, four or five of which were specific to seminal plasma. Furthermore, the latter authors observed that freezing and thawing of spermatozoa, employed in the long term semen preservation techniques, caused an increase in the amounts of some of the protein-types in seminal plasma, and were presumably derived from the destruction of spermatozoa. Some of the proteins derived from spermatozoa were similar to those already in seminal plasma, and thus augmented the amounts found in fresh seminal plasma.

The control of the power of independent movement of spermatozoa is of interest, because it is a basic property of these cells, enabling their travel in parts of the oviduct. Atherton *et al.* (1980) provided evidence suggesting that the motility of fowl spermatozoa may be regulated in part by a system similar to the cholinergic neurotransmitter system.

The possible influence of prostaglandins on motility of fowl spermatozoa has not been examined. However, the little information so far available indicates that minute amounts of these substances are present in the male genital organs and semen of domestic birds compared with other vertebrates (Hertelendy, 1974; Kelly *et al.*, 1976; Wechsung *et al.*, 1981; S. Cannock, personal communication; Table 2). The conclusion from the metabolic studies of Wechsung *et al.* (1981) is that the testes and epididymal region reveal no significant prostaglandin biosynthetic activity. The ductus deferens was found to generate minute amounts of PGE_2, $PGF_{2\alpha}$ and PGD_2.

Table 2

Prostaglandins in the seminal plasma and genital tract tissues of the male fowl

	Prostaglandin				
	$PGF_{2\alpha}$	PGE_1	PGA_1	19-Hydroxy	Reference[d]
Testis[a] (ng g^{-1})	12	15	ND[c]	ND	1
Combined epididymal region and ductus deferens[a] (ng g^{-1})	43	150	ND	ND	1
Receptaculum ductus deferentis[a] (ng g^{-1})	1420	2100	ND	ND	1
Seminal plasma from ductus deferens collected by normal procedure from semen collection[a] (ng ml^{-1})	70	1045	106	ND	1
	—	—	—	ND	2
	<0·1	0·2	<0·1	—	3[b]

[a]Organs from both sides pooled from 2 males. The figures for seminal plasma are the average values from 2 pooled samples collected from several males; 3·0 and 3·5 ml; estimated by bioassay of purified extracts. Prostaglandins E_1, A_1, B and 19-OH not detectable by spectroscopic assay.

[b]Estimated by radioimmunoassay.

[c]ND, not detected.

[d](1) S. Cannock, personal communication; (2) Kelly *et al.*, 1976; (3) Hertelendy, 1974.

Carbohydrate metabolism has been studied most extensively as the source of energy for maintaining the activities of spermatozoa, not only with respect to seeking possible explanations for the performance of some of the natural functions of the spermatozoon, but for devising techniques of maintaining them *in vitro* for the purpose of breeding by artificial insemination. Currently, fowl semen can be kept for up to 48 h with little loss of fertilizing power, provided the semen dosage per hen is adequate to compensate for the death of a small proportion of the spermatozoa (Van Wambeke, 1978; Lake and Ravie, 1979). In order to make improvements in semen storage methods it is necessary, firstly, to verify the conditions *in vitro* preferred by the spermatozoon to sustain its metabolism and maintain ATP for the energy processes involved in its activities during its finite life, e.g. to maintain a correct internal milieu and membrane integrity and ensure its viability to move and penetrate eggs to accomplish fertilization. Secondly, it is necessary to investigate the conditions developing in storage vessels while spermatozoa are living and which appear to affect their viability. Once this knowledge is available, it is to be hoped that environments can be provided artificially to maximize the survival rate of the spermatozoa in a given stored sample. In this connection, it has been found that fowl spermatozoa display high glycolytic activity with the production of much lactic acid (Sexton, 1974; McIndoe and Lake, 1973; Lake and McIndoe, 1976). This may be partly attributable to the high lactate dehydrogenase activity in fowl spermatozoa (McIndoe and Mitchell, 1978). About 35% of the glucose utilized by fowl spermatozoa could not be accounted for by oxidation and glycolysis. The deficit could be due to the conversion of glucose to fructose (Lake *et al.*, 1962). The production of significant amounts of lactic acid, even at temperatures as low as 5°C, creates problems under some circumstances, and the improvements in storing fowl semen for up to 48 h at 3 to 5°C have been achieved by appreciating the mode of metabolism of the spermatozoa and providing some buffering capacity in diluents (Lake and Ravie, 1979, 1981). Wishart (1981, 1982) showed that fowl spermatozoa maintained ATP concentrations under anaerobic conditions in the presence of 10 mM-glucose and that it was directly related to the maintenance of fertilizing ability. This was in contrast to turkey spermatozoa, which sustained fertilizing ability only under aerobic conditions.

Attempts have been made, using histochemical techniques, to identify features of spermatozoan metabolism associated with senescence and loss of fertilizing ability. For example, Dokov *et al.* (1972) reported a reduction in the activity of glucose-6-phosphate dehydrogenase (GPDH), glutamic dehydrogenase (GDH) and lactic dehydrogenase (LDH) in fowl spermatozoa after 24 h storage at 2 to 5°C. However, although reasonable motility was observed in the stored samples, there was some degree of structural damage in the population of cells. It is thus possible that the lowered enzyme activity observed in spermatozoa in semen smears was due to the structural damage, which may have been been caused by other circumstances during the particular storage experiments and thus may not have demonstrated a reduced viability of spermatozoa due to a general metabolic cause.

Danov *et al.* (1972) examined GPDH, GDH and sorbitol dehydrogenase (SDH) activity, histochemically, in fowl spermatozoa and suggested that they metabolized via the Kreb's cycle and pentose phosphate cycle, because low SDH and high GPDH and GDH activity were noted. Sexton (1974), however, was unable to find evidence of the latter metabolic pathway being functional.

Renewed interest has been taken in the prolonged survival of spermatozoa in the avian oviduct in relation to fertility. Observations have been made on possible correlations of metabolic features of spermatozoa with duration of motility under various conditions and at various temperatures *in vitro*, hoping to simulate survival *in vivo* and seek explanations for the phenomenon. Ashizawa and Nishiyama (1978a) found that reduced vigour of motility of spermatozoa at "high" temperatures (around body temperature, 41°C) did not necessarily lead to prolonged duration of motility *in vitro*. However, they suggested that an observed lowered motility with reduced metabolic activity might indicate a useful inherent feature of spermatozoa, enabling survival for a long period *in vivo*.

Another experimental approach has been used to discover how fowl spermatozoa survive in the oviduct for prolonged periods. The effect of the close proximity of living tissue cells on the survival of the spermatozoa at the deep body temperature of the bird, 41°C, was studied. Firstly, it was assumed that the tissue from the utero-vaginal junction area, where spermatozoa naturally reside, would have a preferential beneficial effect. However, it was observed that the average motility of a population of spermatozoa remained satisfactory for up to 4 days equally in cultures of cells taken from several different parts of the oviduct, (for example, infundibulum, shell gland and utero-vaginal junction, and from kidney or embryonic muscle). Spermatozoa in the control culture medium became immotile within a few hours (Ashizawa *et al.*, 1976; Ashizawa and Nishiyama, 1977a). The fertilizing ability was also maintained at a satisfactory level when spermatozoa were incubated at 41°C for up to 4 days in the presence of the above-mentioned tissue cells, but not in the culture medium alone. Fertility tests were done with intra-magnal or intra-isthmal inseminations. Thus, it appears that just an environment provided by being in contact with living cells exerts a beneficial effect on the survival of spermatozoa *in vitro*. The precise causal feature created in the environment is unknown (Ashizawa *et al.*, 1976; Ashizawa and Nishiyama, 1977a, b). However, some apparently controversial observations have been made. Ashizawa and Nishiyama (1978b) observed that the degree of motility of spermatozoa was inversely related to the distance of cultured tissue cells from the spermatozoa, while Fujihara and Howarth (1980) demonstrated that spermatozoa incubated in fluid that was extracted from the medium in which somatic cells had been previously cultured for up to 5 days was able to support the viability of spermatozoa to some extent. In addition, Howarth (1981a) demonstrated that the tissue culture medium alone would support spermatozoa, such that fairly satisfactory fertility rates were achieved after 24 h storage at 41°C. This appears to contradict the earlier work mentioned above. Clearly, from these studies it remains to be determined whether a specific substance(s) is produced by living cells, or the apparent beneficial effect is exerted by particular physical conditions in the environment in close proximity to the cells, which enable the spermatozoa to sustain an inherently natural metabolism for maintaining their fertilizing ability.

B. Transfer of Spermatozoa from the Male to the Female

The questions of how the spermatozoa are transferred from the male to the oviduct during natural copulation and the conditions for the spermatozoa during transfer have attracted attention for many years. Interest in this subject has been renewed, in relation to work on semen storage and factors affecting fertility in artificial insemination. In this context, it would be of interest to verify the precise composition of seminal plasma, as introduced into the hen naturally, and its effect, if any, on the initial activity of spermatozoa in the posterior extremities of the oviduct.

The details of the mechanism of ejaculation and of the exact site of deposition of semen have not been directly determined, because a method has not yet been devised to collect semen from within the vagina. However, several indirect attempts to answer these questions have been made.

The male usually accomplishes the act of mating, i.e. mounts a crouching hen, secures a hold on her back, applies his cloaca to that of the female and ejaculates, within a few seconds. From observations made during the interruption of coitus using trained birds (Fig. 1), it is very likely that the lips of the

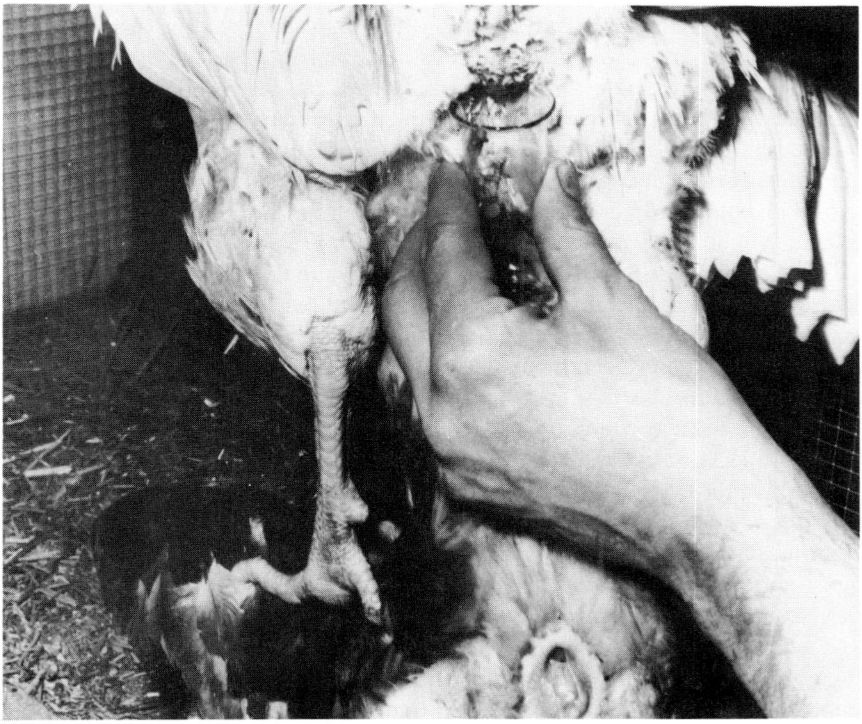

Fig. 1. Semen collection by placing a glass vessel under the cock's cloaca during interrupted coitus. The lower margin of the picture shows the relaxed cloaca of the hen. By kind permission of Professor D. B. von Rautenfeld (Rautenfeld *et al.*, 1976).

female vent relax and the posterior extremity of the vagina is exposed within the cloaca to receive the ejaculate (Rautenfeld *et al.*, 1976). It is not known whether the projecting papillae of the ducti deferentes (Lake, 1981) enter the vagina and forcibly expel semen during copulation, because the cloaca of the male is closely applied to that of the female at this time and it is not possible to observe. The following description was given to the author by von Rautenfeld:

> "If immediately before copulation a person takes the tail feathers dorsally so that the cloacal entry becomes visible, one can observe the semen being explosively released from the seminal duct into the air from where it is collected by the protruding vagina of the hen. Hence the semen does not get into contact with the wall of the male cloaca. Transparent fluid gushes very slowly after a few seconds out of the lymphatic folds. It flows as a final fraction from the cloaca of the cock into the cloaca of the hen".

There is controversy about the composition of naturally ejaculated semen (Lake, 1981), particularly the significance of the transparent fluid which emanates from the lymphatic folds (*plicae lymphaticae*) projecting from the anterior floor of the proctodaeum of the cloaca (King, 1981). The fluid can be squeezed out in variable amounts during artificial semen collection, at which time the lymphatic folds become tumescent, together with other components of the phallic organ, in response to massage. To what extent the fluid is extruded during natural copulation and of what significance it is as an accessory reproductive fluid are two questions which have been posed and investigated.

The fluid is extruded between the mucosal epithelial cells of the tumescent lymphatic folds and is not homologous to the accessory reproductive fluids of mammals, which are secreted by distinct glands; no homologous accessory reproductive organs exist in the bird (Lake, 1981). In an attempt to determine the composition of a natural ejaculate, semen has been collected from male fowl either during copulation by strapping a collector around the cloaca (Parker, 1939; Parker *et al.*, 1942; Nishiyama, 1961; Nishiyama and Fujishima, 1961) or by eliciting semen ejection without squeezing the copulatory organ (Kamar, 1958; Yamane *et al.*, 1966; Rautenfeld *et al.*, 1976) and assuming that the materials obtained in vessels under different circumstances represent a natural ejaculate. Transparent fluid was present in the collectors in these studies and the amount was variable, but generally small if copulation was accomplished very rapidly. The presence of the collector covering the cloaca may cause protracted copulations and account for the larger amounts of transparent fluid whenever they were obtained in the collector. This possibility must be borne in mind when assessing the significance of the fluid collected under these circumstances.

From the above-mentioned observations, it is possible to speculate that, if semen from the projecting papillae of the ducti deferentes is deposited in the extreme posterior vagina, transparent fluid together with other secretions from epithelial cells on the surface of erectile tissue in the cloaca, which is highly alkaline, about pH 8 (Nishiyama and Fujishima, 1961; Rautenfeld *et al.*, 1976), may serve to counteract acidity in this region and reduce damage to spermatozoa.

It has already been mentioned that glucose is absent, or present only in minute amounts in the fluid of the ductus deferens, in which the spermatozoa are ejected into the female. Such semen produces high fertility when artificially inseminated conventionally into the mid- or anterior regions of the vagina. However, it is not known whether this would be true if it were deposited in the extreme posterior vagina-cloaca junction, which is the likely site during copulation. Although it requires confirmation by experiment, it has been suggested that spermatozoa might be stimulated in their passage towards the sperm-host glands in the anterior vagina by brief contact with transparent fluid on ejaculation (Terada and Watanabe, 1978; Terada *et al.*, 1981). It is generally held that spermatozoa traverse the vagina using their own powers of motility (Grigg, 1964; Burke *et al.*, 1969; Takeda, 1974). Glucose, which is present in transparent fluid (Schindler and Scharf, 1963; Table 1), is actively metabolized by fowl spermatozoa *in vitro,* and under certain circumstances it can be shown to increase their vigour of motility (G. J. Wishart, personal communication). Lake and Ravie (1979) and Terada *et al.* (1981) also made observations suggesting that the motility of spermatozoa was increased in a fluid of increased alkaline pH. As stated above, the pH of transparent fluid is highly alkaline. In this respect it has been observed that the pH status of certain regions of the oviduct change reversibly with events occurring during the daily passage of an egg. Also, the pH value differs between different regions of the oviduct (Winget *et al.*, 1965; Fiser and Macpherson, 1974; Bakst, 1980). Although, there are some inexplicable variations in the absolute pH values quoted in these studies, it may be significant that alkaline pH's prevail in the distal regions of the oviduct which might be expected to aid the movement of spermatozoa. Semen *per se* has not been found to have a stimulating effect on oviducal movement (Verma and Hawes, 1971).

Transparent fluid originates from the blood plasma in the form of a lymph-like fluid (see review by King, 1981) and contains some material inimical to the integrity of spermatozoa *in vitro;* spermatozoa bend at the mid-piece region after prolonged contact with it (Lake, 1956, 1981; Yamane *et al.*, 1966). The chloride content is as high as in blood plasma and could account partly for the bending (P. E. Lake, unpublished). Hence, when transparent fluid is ejected during copulation, contact with the spermatozoa and any stimulatory effect is likely to be of a transitory nature. In fact, uncontaminated semen or that containing only a small proportion of transparent fluid is recommended for routine artificial insemination by those who consider that it is extruded during natural copulation (Nishiyama, 1961).

On entry into the oviduct, the spermatozoa swim into the utero-vaginal sperm-host glands and daily thereafter a number ascend the oviduct to fertilize eggs.

An exogenous energy source is available for the spermatozoa during the initial movements upwards from the vaginal region, because during the process of the plumping of the egg in the uterus (shell gland) the uterine fluid contains much glucose (Davidson and Draper, 1969; Salevsky and Leach, 1980). In this respect, also, it is interesting that Yamada and Terada (1974) have suggested that L-α-glycerol-3-phosphate in shell gland tissue might be available as an exogenous oxidative substrate for spermatozoa in this phase of their journey.

C. Lipids and the Activity of Spermatozoa

The possible metabolic processes which sustain the spermatozoa during the various phases of its life cycle, from the testis to the egg where they accomplish fertilization, pose interesting questions. As mentioned previously, they can utilize exogenous monosaccharides, but little or none is present naturally in the ductus deferens (Table 1) and so it is questionable whether such materials are an important source of energy prior to ejaculation. Lipids or lipid-like compounds are a possibility for alternative substrates for metabolism, and preliminary observations have been made which may support this view.

Spermatozoa and seminal plasma (ductus deferens fluid) contain lipid, lipid-like compounds or other compounds associated with lipid metabolism (Lake, 1971; Darin-Bennet *et al.*, 1974; Howarth *et al.*, 1977; White and Darin-Bennett, 1976; Howarth, 1978, 1981b; Burt and Chalovich, 1978), some of which have been investigated in studies of various properties of fowl spermatozoa *in vitro*.

Carnitine, acetyl carnitine and free fatty acids (total) have recently been found and estimated in the ductus deferens fluid (G. J. Wishart, personal communication; Table 1). The carnitine and acetyl carnitine concentrations are about 15 to 20 times higher than in the blood plasma (Table 1). Also, they are found in the ductus deferens fluid of intact males, as well as in those with the ductus ligated at the junction with the epididymis and subsequently emptied of spermatozoa. This observation indicates that these compounds are formed in the secretions of the male excurrent ducts. The significance in the functioning of spermatozoa has yet to be determined.

On average avian spermatozoa can survive in the oviduct for about 7 to 10 days in the domestic fowl. Their endogenous lipid has recently aroused interest as a possible substrate for their metabolism during this sojourn. It has been confirmed that phospholipids account for about 60% of the total lipid of fowl spermatozoa and that the lipid formed 6 to 7% of the dried weight of washed cells (Howarth *et al.*, 1977; Howarth, 1981b). However, after incubating spermatozoa for 24 h at 41°C, no substantial changes occurred in the content of total lipids, total phospholipids, neutral lipids or in the component phospholipids. It is, therefore, considered unlikely by Howarth (1981b) that any major endogenous phospholipids are utilized as an energy source for cock spermatozoa. However, he suggested that, in connection with their survival in the oviduct, lipids and associated compounds in general merit further investigation as energy sources, because cock spermatozoa are capable of utilizing some short and long chain fatty acids (Scott *et al.*, 1962; Howarth, 1978) and there is histochemical and ultrastructural evidence of complex lipid-containing material in the utero-vaginal glands where spermatozoa are stored after insemination (Gilbert *et al.*, 1968; Tingari and Lake, 1973; Lake, 1967, 1975).

Whilst, perhaps, not of significance in natural reproductive processes, it was recently indicated that peroxidation of unsaturated fatty acids of phospholipids may occur in fowl spermatozoa during aerobic storage *in vitro* for 24 h at either 0°C or 40 to 41°C. The phenomenon was found to be associated with impairment of motility of fowl spermatozoa (Fujihara and Howarth, 1978) and it was suggested that it might, amongst other things, be a possible problem in attempts to store fowl spermatozoa *in vitro*. However, proof is awaited. In this respect, Froman and Thurston (1981) made a preliminary study of the degree of activity of the enzyme, superoxide dismutase, SOD, (superoxide : superoxide oxidoreductase : EC 1.15.1.1.) in fowl and turkey semen. It is one of several enzymes which scavenge for toxic derivatives of oxygen, which cause lipid peroxidation. Compared with turkey and fowl red blood cells and turkey spermatozoa, the activity of SOD was high in fowl spermatozoa. Whether there is any link between the greater difficulties of sustaining turkey spermatozoa *in vitro*, compared with the fowl, under some circumstances and the level of SOD activity in the respective spermatozoa remains to be investigated.

The relative resistance of fowl spermatozoa to cold shock (Wales and White, 1959; Darin-Bennett *et al.*, 1974; Hammerstedt *et al.*, 1978) is considered to be associated with the types of fatty acids present in their endogenous phospholipid and the ratio of polyunsaturated : saturated phospholipid fatty acids. Animals with high ratios produce spermatozoa which are very susceptible to cold shock (Darin-Bennett *et al.*, 1974; White and Darin-Bennett, 1976). Whether there is any relationship between the composition of phospholipids and the content of cholesterol in fowl spermatozoa and their reaction to freezing for semen storage is a question for future study, although Ansah and Buckland (1982) found a relationship between the ability of the spermatozoa in individual fowl males of different genetic strains to withstand freezing and their cholesterol and phospholipid content.

A new component has been identified in fowl semen, namely serine ethanolamine phosphodiester, SEP (Burt and Chalovich, 1978). SEP may be significant in lipid metabolism in the male reproductive tract in view of the virtual absence of glyceral-3-phosphorylcholine in the contents of the fowl tract, in contrast to some mammals. However, it has not been determined whether SEP is present in the spermatozoa or in the seminal plasma.

D. Spermatozoa and the Fertilization Process

Evidence suggests that a trypsin-like enzyme is important in the process of fertilization. *In vitro* and *in vivo* fertilization in the domestic fowl has been shown to be inhibited by pre-incubation of spermatozoa with trypsin inhibitors (Palmer and Howarth, 1973; Howarth and Digby, 1973).

Saeki and Morichi (1959) and Bakst and Howarth (1977a) showed that whole fowl semen contained general proteolytic activity which caused rupture of the vitelline membrane of the ovum, and Buruiana (1956) has reported trypsin activity in the whole semen of the fowl and other domestic birds (guinea-fowl, duck, turkey). Ho and Meizel (1970) and Langford and Howarth (1974) demonstrated trypsin-like activity in fowl spermatozoa, and the former authors made an electrophoretic study in which they characterized different forms of the enzyme. Later, they showed that acrosin preparations from cock spermatozoa (acrosin is the name given to the trypsin-like enzyme which is contained in the acrosome part of the spermatozoon) would hydrolyse the inner vitelline membrane (perivitelline layer) surrounding the ovum after ovulation (Ho and Meizel, 1975), through which spermatozoa normally penetrate during fertilization (Fujii, 1976; Bakst, 1977). Ho and Meizel (1975) and Bakst and Howarth (1977b) further demonstrated that acrosin preferentially hydrolysed the vitelline membrane area overlying the germinal disc of the ovum, and the former authors found that the action was inhibited by a trypsin inhibitor. There is some evidence that the structure of the vitelline membrane overlying the animal pole of the ovum is different from that over the vegetal pole (Bakst, 1979).

Ho and Meizel (1976) showed that, biochemically, fowl acrosin resembled that of the bovine and some other mammals. Brown and Hartree (1976) further confirmed the presence of acrosin and inactive pro-acrosin in cock spermatozoa, and showed that the acrosin had different properties from that of the ram.

Unlike in several mammals, Zaneveld *et al.* (1973) were not able to demonstrate a complex of acrosin–acrosin inhibitor within the acrosome of the spermatozoon of the fowl. Such a complex is believed to be associated with the capacitation phenomenon, which occurs in the spermatozoa of mammals before they are able to fertilize eggs. It does not occur in the bird (see Section III).

McIndoe and Lake (1974) found that the seminal plasma contained a small amount of a trypsin-like enzyme inhibitor, It was later confirmed, characterized and quantified (Hirschhäuser *et al.*, 1974; Brown and Hartree, 1976; Johnson *et al.*, 1976, Terada *et al.*, 1978; Lessley and Brown, 1978). The latter and penultimate authors characterized it as an acrosin inhibitor. The precise site of origin of the inhibitor in the male tract has yet to be determined. As to its function, Lessley and Brown (1978) believe that it is possible for it to be released into the seminal plasma from the acrosomes of dead or damaged spermatozoa, in which case an acrosin inhibitor complex may act to protect the epithelial cells lining the male tract and the living spermatozoa from the potentially detrimental proteolytic action of acrosin liberated by the normally degenerating spermatozoa.

Apart from information on the biochemical mechanisms of the spermatozoa involved in the fertilization process, some microscopical evidence has been obtained showing how the spermatozoon enters the egg. This event occurs in the infundibulum of the oviduct when the vitelline membrane is the only layer surrounding the ovum; other layers are secreted around the vitelline membrane in more posterior regions of the oviduct through which spermatozoa cannot penetrate (Fujii, 1976; Okamura and Nishiyama, 1978a). It appears that only one of the spermatozoa which penetrates into the ooplasm in the germinal disc area of the vitelline membrane fuses with the female pronucleus (Okamura and Nishiyama, 1978b). Phagocytosis of spermatozoa was reported, by Koyanagi and Nishiyama (1981), to occur in the vitelline membrane, which may indicate a mechanism of destroying supernumerary spermatozoa, which invade the membrane together with the one which fertilizes and fuses with the female pronucleus.

It is not known how fertilization by aged spermatozoa leads sometimes to the premature cessation of embryonic development (Lodge *et al.*, 1974). It is interesting to speculate whether the action of terminal deoxynucleotidyl transferase, found in spermatozoa and believed to regulate gene expression during embryogenesis (Witkin *et al.*, 1978), might be disturbed by too long a sojourn in the oviduct and be a contributory cause.

References

Aire, T. A. (1979). *J. Anat.* **129**, 703–706.

Aire, T. A. (1980). *J. Anat.* **130**, 707–723.

Amman, R. P., Koefoed-Johnson, H. H. and Levi, H. (1965). *J. Reprod. Fert.* **10**, 169–183.

Ansah, G. A. and Buckland, R. B. (1982). *Poult. Sci.* **61**, 623–637.
Ashizawa, K. and Nishiyama, H. (1977a). *J. Reprod. Fert.* **49**, 405–407.
Ashizawa, K. and Nishiyama, H. (1977b). *Jap. Poult. Sci.* **14**, 144–146.
Ashizawa, K. and Nishiyama, H. (1978a). *Jap. Poult. Sci.* **15**, 264–266.
Ashizawa, K. and Nishiyama, H. (1978b). *Jap. Poult. Sci.* **15**, 74–77.
Ashizawa, K., Nishiyama, H. and Nagae, T. (1976). *J. Reprod. Fert.* **47**, 305–311.
Atherton, R. W., Cisson, C. M., Wilson, B. W. and Golder, T. K. (1980). *Gamete Res.* **3**, 17–24.
Bakst, M. R. (1977). *J. Reprod. Fert.* **52**, 361–364.
Bakst, M. R. (1979). *Poult. Sci.* **58**, 486–488.
Bakst, M. R. (1980). *Poult. Sci.* **59**, 2793–2796.
Bakst, M. R. and Howarth, B. (1975). *Biol. Reprod.* **12**, 632–640.
Bakst, M. R. and Howarth, B. (1977a). *Biol. Reprod.* **17**, 370–379.
Bakst, M. R. and Howarth, B. (1977b). *Biol. Reprod.* **17**, 361–369.
Bamberg, E., Skolek, R. and Stockl, W. (1976). *Zentbl. Vet. Med.* **A23**, 146–151.
Bedford, J. M. (1979). *In* "The Spermatozoon" (D. W. Fawcett and J. M. Bedford, eds), pp. 7–21. Urban and Schwarzenburg, Baltimore.
Bedford, J. M. and Calvin, H. I. (1974). *J. exp. Zool,* **187**, 181–204.
Bernon, D. E. and Buckland, R. B. (1975). *Poult. Sci.* **54**, 1492–1498.
Bonadonna, T. (1954). *Poult. Sci.* **33**, 1151–1158.
Brantas, G. C., Dennert, H. G. and Dennert-Distelbrink, A. L. (1972). *Arch Geflügelk.* **36**, 16–21.
Brown, C. R. and Hartree, E. F. (1976). *J. Reprod. Fert.* **46**, 155–164.
Brown, N. L., Baylé, J. D., Scanes, C. G. and Follett, B. K. (1975). *Cell. Tiss. Res.* **156**, 499–520.
Buckland, R. B. (1971a). *Poult. Sci.* **50**, 1724–1734.
Buckland, R. B. (1971b). *Poult. Sci.* **50**, 1734–1742.
Burke, W. H., Ogasawara, F. X. and Fuqua, C. L. (1969). *Poult. Sci.* **48**, 602–608.
Burt, C. T. and Chalovich, J. M. (1978). *Biochim. biophys. Acta* **529**, 186–188.
Buruiana, L. M. (1956). *Naturwissenschaften* **43**, 523.
Cooksey, E. J. (1975). *Ph.D thesis. University of Strathclyde.*
Culbert, J., Sharp, P. J. and Wells, J. W. (1977). *J. Reprod. Fert.* **51**, 153–154.
Danov, D. T., Dokov, V. K., Angelova, Z. V. and Mihov, M. S. (1972). *C. r. Acad. Agric., G. Dimitrov, Bulg.* **5**, 169–171.
Darin-Bennett, A., Poulos, A. and White, I. G. (1974). *J. Reprod. Fert.* **41**, 471–474.
Davidson, M. F. and Draper, M. H. (1969). *J. Physiol. Lond.* **202**, 119*P*–120*P*.
Dingle, J. G. and McCosker, P. J. (1967). *Proc. Aust. Conf. Poult. Sci., Surfers Paradise,* 169–173.
Dokov, V. K., Danov, D. T. and Angelova, Z. V. (1972). *C. r. Acad Agric., G. Dimitrov, Bulg.* **5**, 323–324.
Droba, M. and Droba, B. (1981). *J. exp. Zool.* **218**, 301–303.
Dukelow, W. R., Chernoff, H. N. and Williams, W. L. (1967). *J. Reprod. Fert.* **14**, 393–399.
El Jack, M. H. and Lake, P. E. (1966). *J. Reprod. Fert.* **11**, 489–491.
Fiser, P. S. and Macpherson, J. W. (1974). *Poult. Sci.* **53**, 827–829.
Froman, D. P. and Thurston, R. J. (1981). *Biol. Reprod.* **24**, 193–200.
Fujihara, N. and Howarth, B. (1978). *Poult. Sci.* **57**, 1766–1768.
Fujihara, N. and Howarth, B. (1980). *Poult. Sci.* **59**, 164–167.

Fujihara, N., Tanaka, K. and Nishiyama, H. (1973). *Jap. J. Zootech. Sci.* **44**, 564–568.
Fujii, S. (1976). *J. Fac. Fish. anim. Husb., Hiroshima Univ.* **15**, 85–92.
Fuquay, J. I. and Renden, J. A. (1980). *Poult. Sci.* **59**, 2525–2531.
Gilbert, A. B., Reynolds, M. E. and Lorenz, F. W. (1968). *J. Reprod. Fert.* **16**, 433–444.
Grigg, G. W. (1964). *Nature, Lond.* **201**, 570–571.
Grigg, G. W. and Hodge, A. J. (1949). *Austr. J. sci. Res.* **B2**, 271–286.
Hammerstedt, R. H., Keith, A. D., Snipes, W., Amann, R. P., Arruda, D. and Griel, L. C. (1978). *Biol. Reprod.* **18**, 686–696.
Harris, G. C. and Sweeney, M. J. (1971). *Cryobiology* **7**, 209–215.
Hertelendy, F. (1974). *J. Reprod. Fert.* **40**, 87–93.
Hirschhäuser, C., McIndoe, W. M. and Lake, P. E. (1974). *IRCS Med. Sci.* **2**, 1606.
Ho, J. J. L. and Meizel, S. (1970). *J. Reprod. Fert.* **23**, 177–179.
Ho, J. J. L. and Meizel, S. (1975). *J. exp. Zool.* **194**, 429–438.
Ho, J. J. L. and Meizel, S. (1976). *Comp. Biochem. Physiol.* **54B**, 213–218.
Howarth, B. (1971). *Biol. Reprod.* **3**, 338–341.
Howarth, B. (1978). *Poult. Sci.* **57**, 1751–1754.
Howarth, B. (1981a). *Poult. Sci.* **60**, 1075–1078.
Howarth, B. (1981b). *Poult. Sci.* **60**, 1516–1519.
Howarth, B. and Digby, S. T. (1973). *J. Reprod. Fert.* **33**, 123–125.
Howarth, B., Torregrossa, D. and Britton, W. M. (1977). *Poult. Sci.* **56**, 1265–1268.
Johnson, L. A., Sexton, T. J. and Pursel, V. G. (1976). *Theriogenology* **5**, 21–27.
Kamar, G. A. R. (1958). *Poult. Sci.* *37*, 1382–1385.
Kannan, Y. (1974). *J. Reprod. Fert.* **40**, 227–228.
Kelly, R. W., Taylor, P. L., Hearn, J. P., Short, R. V., Martin, D. E. and Marston, J. H. (1976). *Nature, Lond.* **260**, 544–545.
King, A. S. (1981). *In* "Form and Function in Birds" (A. S. King and J. McLelland, eds), Vol. 2, pp. 107–147. Academic Press, London and New York.
Koyanagi, F. and Nishiyama, H. (1981). *Cell Tiss. Res.* **214**, 89–95.
Krustev, H. and Danov, D. (1968). *C. r. Acad. bulg. Sci.* **21**, 945–948.
Lake, P. E. (1954). *10th Wld's Poult. Congr., Edinburgh*, 79–85.
Lake, P. E. (1956). *3rd Int. Congr. Anim. Reprod. & A. I, Cambridge.* Sec. 3, 104–106.
Lake, P. E. (1966a). *Res. vet. Sci.* **7**, 121–127.
Lake, P. E. (1966b). *In* "Advances in Reproductive Physiology" (A. McLaren, ed.), Vol. 1, pp. 93–123. Logos Press, London.
Lake, P. E. (1967). *In* "Reproduction in the Female Mammal" (G. E. Lamming and E. C. Amoroso, eds), pp. 254–266. Butterworths, London.
Lake, P. E. (1971). *In* "Physiology and Biochemistry of the Domestic Fowl" (D. J. Bell and B. M. Freeman, eds), Vol. 3, pp. 1411–1447. Academic Press, London and New York.
Lake, P. E. (1974). *15th Wld's Poult. Congr., New Orleans* 2–9.
Lake, P. E. (1975). *Symp. Zool. Soc. Lond.* **35**, 225–244.
Lake, P. E. (1981). *In* "Form and Function in Birds" (A. S. King and J. McLelland, eds), Vol. 2, pp. 1–61. Academic Press, London and New York.
Lake, P. E. and El Jack, M. H. (1964). *5th Int. Congr. Anim. Reprod. & A. I., Trento* **3**, 357–363.
Lake, P. E. and El Jack, M. H. (1966). *In* "Physiology of the Domestic Fowl" (C. Horton Smith and E. C. Amoroso, eds), pp. 44–51. Oliver and Boyd, Edinburgh.
Lake, P. E. and Hatton, M. (1968). *J. Reprod. Fert.* **15**, 139–143.

Lake, P. E. and McIndoe, W. M. (1976). *8th Int. Congr. Anim. Reprod. & A. I., Krakow* **4**, 1020–1023.
Lake, P. E. and Ravie, O. (1979). *J. Reprod. Fert.* **57**, 149–155.
Lake, P. E. and Ravie, O. (1981). *Reprod. Nutr. Dévelop.* **21**, 1077–1084.
Lake, P. E., Lorenz, F. W. and Reimann, W. (1962). *Nature, Lond.* **194**, 545–547.
Lake, P. E., Smith, W. and Young, D. (1968). *Q. Jl exp. Physiol.* **53**, 356–366.
Langford, B. B. and Howarth, B. (1974). *Poult. Sci.* **53**, 834–837.
Lessley, B . A. and Brown, K. I. (1978). *Biol. Reprod.* **19**, 223–234.
Lodge, J. R., Ax, R. L. and Fechheimer, N. S. (1974). *Poult. Sci.* **53**, 1816–1819.
McDaniel, G. R. and Sexton, T. J. (1977). *Poult. Sci.* **56**, 1989–1993.
McIndoe, W. M. and Lake, P. E. (1973). *J. Reprod. Fert.* **35**, 592–593.
McIndoe, W. M. and Lake, P. E. (1974). *J. Reprod. Fert.* **40**, 359–365.
McIndoe, W. M. and Mitchell, G. G. (1978). *Comp. Biochem. Physiol.* **61B**, 433–437.
Munro, S. S. (1938). *J. exp. Biol.* **15**, 186–196.
Neaves, W. B. (1977). *In* "The Testis" (A. D. Johnson and W. R. Gomes, eds), Vol. 4, pp. 125–162. Academic Press, London and New York.
Nicander, L. (1968). *6th Int. Congr. Anim. Reprod. & A. I., Paris* **1**, 89–107.
Nicander, L. (1970) *In* "Comparative Spermatology" (B. Baccetti, ed), pp. 47–56. Academic Press, London and New York.
Nicander, L. and Hellstrom, B. (1967). *Exp Cell Res.* **48**, 622–625.
Niimura, S., Sasaki, H. and Ishida, K. (1980). *Jap. J. Zootech. Sci.* **51**, 548–552.
Nishiyama, H. (1961). *Mem. Fac. Agric., Kagoshima Univ.* **4**, 43–50.
Nishiyama, H. and Fujishima, T. (1961). *Mem. Fac. Agric., Kagoshima Univ.* **4**, 27–42.
Nishiyama, H., Ogawa, K. and Nakanishi, Y. (1968). *Mem. Fac. Agric., Kagoshima Univ.* **6**, 141–147.
Oakberg, E. F. (1956). *Am. J. Anat.* **99**, 507–516.
Okamura, F. and Nishiyama, H. (1978a). *Cell. Tiss. Res.* **188**, 497–508.
Okamura, F. and Nishiyama, H. (1978b). *Cell Tiss. Res.* **190**, 89–98.
Ortavant, R. (1956). *C. r. Séanc. Soc. Biol.* **150**, 471.
Osman, D. I. (1981). *J. Reprod. Fert.* **61**, 75–78.
Palmer, M. B. and Howarth, B. (1973). *J. Reprod Fert.* **35**, 7–12.
Parker, J. E. (1939). *Poult. Sci.* **18**, 455–456.
Parker, J. E., McKenzie, F. F. and Kempster, H. L. (1942). *Bull. Mo. agric. Exp. Stn* **347**.
Petitjean, M. J. (1970). *14th Wld's Poult. Congr., Madrid* **2**, 313–318.
Rautenfeld, D. B. von, Budras, K.-D. and Gassmann, R. (1976). *Z. Zellforsch. mikrosk. Anat.* **90**, 989–1008.
Reviers, M. de (1968). *6th Int. Congr. Anim. Reprod. & A. I., Paris* **1**, 183–185.
Reviers, M. de (1972a). *Annls Biol. anim. Biochim. Biophys.* **12**, 13–18.
Reviers, M. de (1972b). *Annls Biol. anim. Biochim. Biophys.* **12**, 5–11.
Reviers, M. de (1975). *In* "The Biology of Spermatozoa" (E. S. E. Hafez and C. G. Thibault, eds), pp. 10–16. Karger, Basel.
Reviers, M. de (1980). *9th Int. Congr. Anim. Reprod. & A. I., Madrid* **2**, 519–526.
Reviers, M. de and Petitjean, M. (1973). *Ann. Génét. Sel. anim.* **5**, 313–321.
Reviers, M. de and Williams, J. (1981). *Reprod. Nutr. Dévelop.* **21**, 1113–1124.
Reviers, M. de, Hocherau de Reviers, M. T., Blanc, M. R., Brillard, J. P., Courot, M. and Pelletier, J. (1980). *Reprod. Nutr. Dévelop.* **20**, 241–249.
Saeid, J. M. (1981). *Thesis, University des Sciences et Techniques du Languedoc, Montpellier, France.*

Saeki, Y. and Morichi, T. (1959). *Proc. Soc. exp. Biol. Med.* **101**, 648–650.
Salevsky, E. and Leach, R. M. (1980). *Poult. Sci.* **59**, 438–443.
Schindler, H. and Scharf, S. (1963). *Israel J. agric. Res.* **13**, 163–172.
Scott, T. W., White, I. G. and Annison, E. F. (1962). *Biochem. J.* **83**, 392–398.
Servouse, M., Petitjean, M. J. and Rosenberg, A . J. (1976). *Annls Biol. anim. Biochim. Biophys.* **16**, 807–819.
Setchell, B. P. and Waites, G. M. H. (1975). *In* "Handbook of Physiology, Sec. 7: Endocrinology, Vol. 5 — Male Reproductive System" (D. W. Hamilton and R. O. Greep, eds), pp. 143–172. William & Wilkins, Baltimore.
Sexton, T. J. (1974). *Comp. Biochem. Physiol.* **48B**, 59–65.
Sharp, P. J. (1975). *J. Endocr.* **67**, 211–223.
Sharp, P. J., Culbert, J. and Wells, J. W. (1977). *J. Endocr.* **74**, 467–476.
Somes, R. G. and Weigh, L. A. (1980). *Poult. Sci.* **59**, 2379–2385.
Sterling, R. J., Lea, R. and Sharp, P. J. (1978). *IRCS Med. Sci.* **6**, 531.
Stratil, A. (1970). *Int. J. Biochem.* **1**, 728–734.
Takeda, A. (1974). *Jap. Poult. Sci.* **11**, 45–54.
Terada, T. and Watanabe, M. (1978). *Jap. J. zootech. Sci.* **49** 47–53.
Terada, T., Nakamura, S. and Watanabe, M. (1978). *Jap. J. zootech. Sci.* **49**, 203–205.
Terada, T., Ashizawa, K. and Watanabe, M. (1981). *Jap. Poult. Sci.* **18**, 40–44.
Tingari, M. D. (1971). *J. Anat.* **109**, 423–435.
Tingari, M. D. (1972). *Q. Jl exp. Physiol.* **57**, 271–295.
Tingari, M. D.(1973). *J. Reprod. Fert.* **34**, 255–265.
Tingari, M. D. and Lake, P. E. (1972). *J. Reprod. Fert.* **31**, 373–381.
Tingari, M. D. and Lake, P. E. (1973). *J. Reprod. Fert.* **34**, 423–431.
Tojo, H. and Ogawa, K. (1981). *Jap. Poult. Sci.* **18**, 182–184.
Van Wambeke, F. (1978). *16th Wld's Poult. Congr., Rio de Janeiro* **2**, 148–152.
Verma, O. P. and Hawes, R. O. (1971). *Poult. Sci.* **50**, 199–203.
Waites, G. M. H. (1977). *In* "The Testis" (A. D. Johnson and W. R. Gomes, eds), Vol. 4, pp. 91–123. Academic Press, London and New York.
Wales, R. G. and White, I. G. (1959). *J. Endocr.* **19**, 211–220.
Wechsung, E., Claeys, M., Van Wambeke, F. and Houvenaghel, A. (1981). *Archs int. Pharmacodyn. Thér.* **253**, 330–332.
White, I. G. and Darin-Bennett, A. (1976). *8th Int. Congr. Anim. Reprod. & A. I., Krakow* **4**, 951–953.
Williams, J. and Reviers, M. de (1981). *Reprod. Nutr. Dévelop.* **21**, 1125–1135.
Winget, C. M., Mepham, C. A. and Averkin, E. G. (1965). *Am. J. Physiol.* **208**, 1031–1035.
Wishart, G. J. (1981). *Br. Poult. Sci.* **22**, 445–450.
Wishart, G. J. (1982). *J. Reprod. Fert.* **66**, 457–462.
Witkin, S. S., Reiner, B. and Brown, C. A. (1978). *Gamete Res.* **1**, 227–233.
Yamada, M. and Terada, T. (1974). *Am. J. Physiol.* **227**, 729–733.
Yamane, J., Tsukunaga, S. and Takahashi, T. (1966). *J. Fac. Fish anim. Husb., Hiroshima Univ.* **6**, 395–429.
Zaneveld, L. J. D., Polakoski, K. L. and Williams, W. L. (1973). *Biol. Reprod.* **9**, 219–225.

Appendix: Biochemical and Physiological Data

B. M. FREEMAN

Houghton Poultry Research Station, Huntingdon, England

I. Introduction

The purpose of this appendix is to provide the reader with biological values for the adult fowl as quickly as possible. Most of the data have been taken from the

PHYSIOLOGY BIOCHEMISTRY DOMESTIC FOWL, VOL. 5 ISBN 0-12-267105-8

text of these volumes, but there has been some supplementation from the literature. Where a single value is given it should be seen as an approximate mean rather than an absolute. Ranges of apparently normal values are given wherever possible. Further information and comment on the data will usually be found in the appropriate chapter.

The data are organized into twelve sections (see contents list above), and within each section the items are presented in alphabetical order.

II. Alimentary Tract and Nutrient Requirements

Absorption kinetics	
Galactose	
in ileum	
K_m	13 mM
J_{max}	3 nmol cm^{-2} s^{-1}
in jejunum	
K_m	48 mM
J_{max}	2 nmol cm^{-2} s^{-1}
Glucose	
in ileum	
K_m	4 mM
J_{max}	2 nmol cm^{-2} s^{-1}
in jejunum	
K_m	12 mM
J_{max}	1 nmol cm^{-2} s^{-1}
Glycine	
in ileum	
K_m	3 mM
J_{max}	55 pmol cm^{-2} s^{-1}
in jejunum	
K_m	4 mM
J_{max}	37 pmol cm^{-2} s^{-1}
Histidine	
in ileum	
K_m	1 mM
J_{max}	129 pmol cm^{-2} s^{-1}
in jejunum	
K_m	3 mM
J_{max}	132 pmol cm^{-2} s^{-1}
Methionine	
in ileum	
K_m	2 mM
J_{max}	148 pmol cm^{-2} s^{-1}
in jejunum	
K_m	5 mM
J_{max}	147 pmol cm^{-2} s^{-1}

Absorption kinetics (*contd.*)	
Valine	
in ileum	
K_m	1 mM
J_{max}	82 pmol cm^{-2} s^{-1}
in jejunum	
K_m	3 mM
J_{max}	38 pmol cm^{-2} s^{-1}
Bile, secretion rate	0·5–1 ml h^{-1}
Excreta, production, net weight	100–150 g day^{-1}
Food intake, layer	110–120 g d^{-1}
Food, rate of passage	
layer	8 h
broody hen	12 h
Gastric juice	
H^+ output, maximum	3·2 mEq kg^{-1} h^{-1}
pepsin concentration	250 units ml^{-1}
proventricular secretion rate	6–21 ml h^{-1}
Nutrient requirements	
amino acids (mg d^{-1})	
arginine	560
histidine	190
isoleucine	610
leucine	750
lysine	830
methionine	390
methionine + cystine	520
phenylalanine	430
phenylalanine + tyrosine	770
threonine	400
tryptophan	190
valine	610
choline	120 mg d^{-1}
crude protein	18 g d^{-1}
energy	1220 kJ d^{-1}
essential fatty acids	
as linoleic acid	1·3 g d^{-1}
minerals (mg d^{-1})	
Ca^{2+}	3900
Cl^-	100
K^+	275
Mg^{2+}	45
Na^+	110
P, non-phytic	390

P

Nutrient requirements (*contd.*)	
trace elements (mg d^{-1})	
Cu^{2+}	400
Fe^{3+}	9200
I^{-}	25
Mn^{2+}	5500
Zn^{2+}	6000
vitamins (IU d^{-1})	
A	300
D_3 (cholecaliciferol)	70
E (α-tocopherol)	3
vitamins (μg d^{-1})	
B_{12} (cyanocobalamin)	0·2
biotin	22
folic acid	55
K_1	110
nicotinic acid (PP)	1100
pantothenic acid	75
pyridoxin (B_6)	440
riboflavin (B_2)	440
thiamin (B_1)	330
Pancreatic juice, rate of secretion	0·4–3 ml h^{-1}
pH values	
crop	4–7·5
proventriculus	0·5–4·5
gizzard	0·5–5·5
duodenum to rectum	5–8
Saliva, rate of secretion	0·3–1·3 ml h^{-1}
Turnover rate of intestinal epithelial cells	2 d
Water intake	
as a function of food consumed	
layers	2·0–2·5 ml H_2O g $food^{-1}$
non-layers	1·2–1·3 ml H_2O g $food^{-1}$
laying hens	150–250 ml d^{-1}
males, non-laying females	90–120 ml d^{-1}

III. Blood

Cell numbers ($\times 10^4$ mm^{-3})	
basophils	0·04–0·045
erythrocytes	
♂	320–380
♀	270–300
heterophils	0·3–1·2
leucocytes	1·6–3·6
lymphocytes	4·0–8·0

Cell numbers ($\times 10^4$ mm^{-3}) (*contd.*)	
monocytes	0·03–0·16
thrombocytes	3·5–4·0
Clotting time	15 min
Erythrocyte	
life span	28–30 d
oxygen uptake	105–130 mm^3 100ml^{-1} h^{-1}
Gases (mmHg)	
carbon dioxide	
arterial partial pressure ($P_a CO_2$)	25–34
venous partial pressure ($P_v CO_2$)	38–50
oxygen	
arterial ($P_a O_2$)	85–99
half saturation (P_{50})	50–60
Haemoglobin	
half saturation pressure of oxygen (P_{50})	35–50 mmHg
in erythrocytes	27–30 g 100ml^{-1} erythrocytes
in whole blood	7–13 g 100ml^{-1}
per erythrocyte	33–41 ng
Packed cell volume (%)	
♂	40–45
♀	20–30
Packed leucocyte volume	1–1·5%
pH	7·45–7·63
Plasma amino acids (μmol litre^{-1})	
alanine	360–500
arginine	300–400
aspartate	22–50
cystine	20–35
glutamate	200–300
glycine	500–650
histidine	175–225
isoleucine	90–150
leucine	225–275
lysine	220–350
methionine	75–90
ornithine	60–90
phenylalanine	100–120
proline	160–250
threonine	450–800
tyrosine	90–130
valine	225–350

Plasma cholesterol	80–130 mg $100ml^{-1}$
Plasma free fatty acids	
layers	750–3000 μEq $litre^{-1}$
non-layers	200–700 μEq $litre^{-1}$
Plasma glucose	225–300 mg $100ml^{-1}$
Plasma hormones (*see* Section IV)	
Plasma immunoproteins, half lives (d)	
IgG	2–4·1
IgM	1·7
Plasma inorganic ions (mEq $litre^{-1}$)	
Ca^{2+}	
total	5 mmol $litre^{-1}$
diffusable, laying hen	1·2–1·6 mmol $litre^{-1}$
Cl^{-}	115
K^{+}	4·7
Na^{+}	160
Plasma lipoproteins (mg $100ml^{-1}$)	
non-laying ♀, ♂	
HDL	360
LDL	120
VLDL	60
laying	
HDL	140–180
LDL	200
VDL	1400–5500
Plasma non-protein nitrogen (mg N $100ml^{-1}$)	
amino	7–8
total	15–20
Plasma osmolarity	300–320 mOsm $litre^{-1}$
Plasma protein (mg $100ml^{-1}$)	
♂	4
♀	5
Plasma triglycerides	27 mg $100ml^{-1}$
Plasma uric acid	2·5 mg $100ml^{-1}$
Viscosity	
whole blood	
♂	3·7
♀	3·1
plasma	
♂	1·4
♀	1·5
Volume, whole blood	70–90 ml kg^{-1} body weight

IV. Endocrinology

Adrenal glands ($\mu g\ mg^{-1}$ adrenal)	
ascorbic acid	
layers	2·1
non-layers	1·7
cholesterol, total	0·03
Adrenal hormones	
aldosterone, in plasma	2 ng ml^{-1}
adrenaline in plasma	8–9 ng ml^{-1}
amines, total	
in adrenals	10–12 $\mu g\ mg^{-1}$
corticosterone	
in adrenals	1·9 $\mu g\ mg^{-1}$
in plasma	1–5 ng ml^{-1}
noradrenaline, in plasma	0·8–1·0 ng ml^{-1}
Calcitonin	
in bird	600–2000 MRC mU kg^{-1}
in plasma, after oviposition	1·5 ng ml^{-1}
in ultimobranchial gland	30–120 MRC mU g^{-1}
molecular weight	3000
1,25-Dihydroxycholecalciferol ($1,25(OH)_2D_3$)(pg ml^{-1})	
laying ♀	120–300
non-laying ♀	30–50
Growth hormone	
isoelectric point (pI)	7·5
mol. wt.	$22–23 \times 10^3$
Hormonal half-lives (min)	
aldosterone (in ducks)	8
corticosterone	9
growth hormone	
first phase	2
second phase	12
third phase	194
insulin	4·5–7
luteinizing hormone (LH)	17–23
oestradiol-17β	
distributive phase	0·5–1·6
metabolic phase	8–22
progesterone	
distributive phase	1
metabolic phase	11
thyroxine (T_4)	138
vasotocin	20

Luteinizing hormone (LH)	
in plasma ♀	1·5–4
in plasma ♂	10–11
Neurohypophysial hormones (μg mg^{-1} neurohypophysis powder)	
oxytocin	1·2
vasotocin	12
Pancreatic hormones	
APP	
in pancreas	40–80 ng mg^{-1}
in plasma	2–12 ng ml^{-1}
mol. wt	4258
glucagon	
in pancreas	8 ng mg^{-1}
in plasma	1–1·5 ng ml^{-1}
mol. wt	3465
insulin	
in pancreas	10–30 ng mg^{-1}
in plasma	40–75 ng ml^{-1}
mol. wt	5734
somatostatin	
in pancreas	4 ng mg^{-1}
mol. wt	1638
Plasma hormone concentrations (ng ml^{-1})	
adrenaline	8– 9
aldosterone	2
avian polypeptide (APP)	2–12
corticosterone	1–5
calcitonin, after oviposition	1·5
1,25-dihydroxycholecalciferol	
non-layers	30–50 pg ml^{-1}
non-layers	120–300 pg ml^{-1}
glucagon	1–1·5
insulin	40–75
luteinizing hormone (LH)	
♀	1·5–4
♂	10–11
melatonin	0–0·2
noradrenaline	0·8–1·0
oestradiol-17β, ♀	0·2–0·9 nmol ml^{-1}
oestrone, ♀	0·6–1·3 pmol ml^{-1}
progesterone, ♀	2–15 pmol ml^{-1}
serotonin	3000–7000
testosterone	
♀	0·5–3 pmol ml^{-1}
♂	8–9 pmol ml^{-1}

Plasma hormones concentrations (ng ml^{-1}) (*contd.*)	
thyroxine (T_4)	10–15
triiodothyronine (T_3)	3·5–5
vasotocin	4–7
Progesterone secretion rate (ng min^{-1} $kg^{-0·75}$)	
in non-layer	20
in moulting hen	62
in layer	
basal rate	42–43
peak rate	254
Prolactin	
activity in adenohypophysis (IU $gland^{-1}$)	
broody hens	0·2
isoelectric point	5·6
layers	0·07
mol. wt	22–26 × 10^3
Sex hormones (*see* Plasma hormone concentrations *and* Hormonal half-lives)	
Thyroid hormones	
secretion rate	5–10 μg T_4 kg^{-1} d^{-1}
thyroxine, in plasma	10–15 ng ml^{-1}
triiodothyroxine, in plasma	3·5–5 ng ml^{-1}

V. Heart and Circulation

Blood pressure (mmHg)	
bronchial artery	25
common carotid artery	145
diastolic	
♂	150
♀	130
hepatic portal vein	5
hepatic vein	1
systolic	
♂	160–180
♀	130–160
Blood flow rate (ml kg^{-1} min^{-1})	
cocoygeomesenteric	26–63
hepatic portal	32
Blood volume,	70–90 ml kg^{-1}
Cardiac output	120–270 ml kg^{-1} min^{-1}
Circulation time	2–8 s

Heart rate	250–470 beats min^{-1}
Myocytes	
diameter	5–10 μm
length	60–100 μm
sarcolemma, resting potential	−90 mV
Peripheral resistance, total (TPR)	0·88–1·23 PRU
Pulse pressure	30 mmHg
Purkinje cells, diameter	30 μm

VI. Kidneys and Excretion

Glomerular filtration rate	1–3 ml kg^{-1} min^{-1}
Glomeruli, number	10·3 × 10^4 g^{-1} kidney
Renal blood flow	27–31 ml kg^{-1} min^{-1}
Renal clearance rates	
insulin	1·5–3·0 ml kg^{-1} min^{-1}
uric acid	18–20 mg kg^{-1} min^{-1}
Renal threshold glucose	260–360 mg $100ml^{-1}$
Urine, ureteral	
flow rate	18–22 ml kg^{-1} h^{-1}
ionic concentration (nM $litre^{-1}$)	
Ca^{2+}	3–4
Cl^-	41–56
K^+	21–116
Mg^{2+}	5–12
Na^+	31–57
NH_4^+	50–90
PO_4	36–107
osmolarity	100–120 mOsm $litre^{-1}$
pH	6–8

VII. Liver

Bile pigments	
bilirubin	30–280 μg ml^{-1} bile
biliverdin	24–180 μg ml^{-1} bile
Bile production	1 ml kg^{-1} body wt h^{-1}
Bile salts, half life	6–9 d

Enzyme activities (μmoles mg N^{-1} h^{-1})	
ATP-citrate lyase	
♂	2
♀	5
fructose-1,6-diphosphatase	1·1 μmol mg^{-1} liver h^{-1}
glucose-6-phosphatase	0·108 μmol mg^{-1} liver h^{-1}
hexokinase	25 μmol mg^{-1} liver h^{-1}
"malic"	
♂	45
♀	80
phosphofructokinase	81
phosphorylase	1·1 μg P mg^{-1} liver h^{-1}
pyruvate kinase	390
Glycogen	0·5 mg g^{-1}
Taurocholate, rate of secretion	10 mmol kg^{-1} min^{-1}

VIII. Muscle

Conduction velocity (m s^{-1})	
ant. lat. dorsi	0·7
post. lat. dorsi	2·8
Length constant (mm)	
ant. lat. dorsi	1·78
post. lat. dorsi	0·7
Membrane capacitance (Cm: units, μF cm^{-2})	
ant. lat. dorsi	8·2
post. lat. dorsi	7·0
Resting membrane potential (mV)	
ant. lat. dorsi	51
post. lat. dorsi	57
Time constant (rm: units ms)	
ant. lat. dorsi	35
post. lat. dorsi	4
Transverse membrane resistance (Rm: units, Ω cm^{-2})	
ant. lat. dorsi	4388
post. lat. dorsi	560

IX. Nervous System

Conduction velocities (m ms^{-1})	
unmyelinated	0·8–1·2
myelinated	2·2–3·4

Electroencephalogram wave characteristics	
alert, excited	20–50 μV, 30–60 Hz
alert, unexcited	50–150 μV, 17–24 Hz
sleeping	
stage 1	50–150 μV, 17–24 Hz
	200–300 μV, 3–12 Hz
stage 2	200–400 μV, 6–12 Hz
	200–400 μV, 3–4 Hz
stage 3	200–400 μV, 2–4 Hz
paradoxical sleep	50 μV, 30–60 Hz

X. Reproduction: Egg

Albumen components (g)	
chalazae	1
thick layer	19
thin layer	
inner	6
outer	8
total weight	34
Albumen inorganic ions (mg albumen^{-1})	
Ca^{2+}	4
Cl^{-}	42
Fe^{3+}	0·003
K^{+}	47
Mg^{2+}	3
Na^{+}	49
PO_4^{-}	4
Albumen proteins	
avidin	
amount per egg	2 mg
carbohydrate content	8%
isoelectric pH	9·5–10·0
mol. wt	$6{\cdot}8 \times 10^4$
percentage of albumen solids	0·05
flavoprotein	
amoung per egg	30 mg
carbohydrate content	9%
isoelectric pH	3·9–4·1
mol. wt	$3{\cdot}2$–$3{\cdot}6 \times 10^4$
percentage of albumen solids	0·8
lysozyme	
amount per egg	130 mg
isoelectric pH	10·5–11·0
mol. wt	$1{\cdot}4$–$1{\cdot}7 \times 10^4$
percentage of albumen solids	3·5

Albumen proteins (*contd.*)	
ovalbumin	
amount per egg	2 g
carbohydrate content	3%
isoelectric pH	4·5–4·8
mol. wt	$4{\cdot}6 \times 10^4$
percentage of albumen solids	54
ovoglobulin G_2	
amount per egg	160 mg
isoelectric pH	5·5
mol. wt	$3{\cdot}6–4{\cdot}5 \times 10^4$
percentage of albumen solids	4
ovoglobulin G_3	
amount per egg	160 mg
isoelectric pH	5·8
mol. wt	$3{\cdot}6–4{\cdot}5 \times 10^4$
percentage of albumen solids	4
ovoglycoprotein	
amount per egg	20–40 mg
carbohydrate content	16%
isoelectric pH	3·9
mol. wt	$2{\cdot}4 \times 10^4$
percentage of albumen solids	0·5–1·0%
ovoinhibitor	
amount per egg	4–60 mg
carbohydrate content	6%
isoelectric pH	5·1–5·2
mol. wt	$4{\cdot}4–4{\cdot}9 \times 10^4$
percentage of albumen solids	0·1–1·5%
ovomacroglobulin	
amount per egg	20 mg
carbohydrate content	9%
isoelectric pH	4·5–4·7
mol. wt	$7{\cdot}6–9{\cdot}0 \times 10^5$
percentage of albumen solids	0·5
ovomucin	
amount per egg	60–120 mg
carbohydrate content	19%
percentage of albumen solids	1·5–2·9
ovomucoid	
amount per egg	40 mg
carbohydrate content	22%
isoelectric pH	3·9–4·3
mol. wt	$2{\cdot}8 \times 10^4$
percentage of albumen solids	11
ovotransferrin	
amount per egg	410
carbohydrate content	2%

Albumen proteins (*contd.*)	
isoelectric pH	6·1–6·6
mol. wt	7·7–8·6 × 10^4
percentage of albumen solids	12–13%
Egg weight (g)	
albumen	34
shell	5
total	58
yolk	19
Egg composition (%)	
albumen	
inorganic ions	0·5
protein	10
water	88
shell	
inorganic ions	95
protein	4
water	1
yolk	
inorganic ions	1
lipids	33
protein	17
water	48
Shell	
calcium content	5 g
cuticle, thickness	10 μm
membranes, thickness	
inner	20–22 μm
outer	50 μm
pores	
frequency	100–300 cm^{-2}
diameter	
at inner surface	6–23 μm
at outer surface	15–65 μm
number per egg	7000–17 000
thickness, excluding membranes	280–370 μm
Vitelline membrane, thickness	6–11 μm
Yolk inorganic ions (mg $yolk^{-1}$)	
Ca^{2+}	26
Cl^-	25
Fe^{3+}	1
K^+	18
Mg^{2+}	3
Na^2	11
PO_4^-	98
S^{2+}	30

Yolk pigments (μg $yolk^{-1}$)	
carotene	6–10
crypotoxanthin	10–30
lutein	180–220
Yolk proteins (%)	
α-lipovitellins	15–22
lipid content	78–85
protein content	0·48–0·64
protein phosphorus	3%
β-lipovitellin	
lipid content	17–26
protein content	78–83
protein phosphorus	0·27–0·34
lipovitellins, amount in yolk	1·5 g
ratio of α to β	1–1·8:1
livetins, amount in yolk	0·9 g
low density fraction (LDF)	
amount in yolk	6·5 g
LDF_1 fraction	
lipid content	87–89
mean mol. wt	10×10^6
protein content	11–13
protein phosphorus	0·10–0·15
LDF_2 fraction	
lipid content	83–86
mean mol. wt	$3–5 \times 10^6$
protein content	14–17
protein phosphorus	0·08–0·16
phosvitin	
large species, mol. wt	34×10^3
small species, mol. wt	28×10^3
vitellogenin, mol. wt	48×10^4
Yolk vitamins (μg $yolk^{-1}$)	
A	200–1000 IU
B_1 (thiamin)	49
B_2 (riboflavin)	84
B_6 (pyridoxin)	58
B_{12}	340
biotin	10
D	20 IU
E	15 000
folic acid	5
K_1	25
nicotinic acid	3
pantothenic acid	580

X. Reproduction: Semen

Seminal plasma composition (without transparent fluid)	
amino acids (mg $100ml^{-1}$)	
alanine	3
aspartic acid	20
cysteine	trace
glutamic acid	1300
glycine	4
isokinase	trace
leucine	trace
lysine	15
methionine	trace
serine	5
taurine	5
threonine	3
valine	1·5
inorganic ions (mEq $litre^{-1}$)	
Ca^{2+}	1–2·5
Cl^{-}	37–42
Cu^{2+}	10
Fe^{3+}	0·06
K^{+}	12–48
Mg^{2+}	5
Na^{+}	120–165
Zn^{2+}	0·06–0·5
nitrogen	
total	290–480 mg $100ml^{-1}$
non-protein	160 mg $100ml^{-1}$
pH	7
prostaglandins (ng ml^{-1})	
PGE_1	1000
PGF_2	70
PGA_1	100
protein	0·8 g $100ml^{-1}$
specific gravity	1·011
Spermatozoan composition	
deoxyribonucleic acid	1112 mg $100ml^{-1}$ cells
inorganic ions (mEq $litre^{-1}$ cells)	
Ca^{2+}	0·7
Cl^{-}	37
K^{+}	61
Mg^{2+}	17
Na^{+}	53
water content	60%
Spermatozoan count	
in semen without transparent fluid	$5–7 \times 10^6$ mm^{-3}

Transparent fluid, composition (mM)	
Cl^-	134–141
glucose	11–12
glutamate	0·3
lactate	2·6

XII. Respiratory Tract

Air sac gases (mmHg)	
CO_2, mean partial pressure	
abdominal	15
clavicular	44
thoracic	
caudal	24
cranial	42
O_2, mean partial pressure	
abdominal	130
clavicular	84
thoracic	
caudal	102
cranial	99
Exchange surface area	14 cm^2 g^{-1} body weight
Expired gases (mmHg)	
CO_2, partial pressure	28
O_2, partial presure	108
Minute volume (litre min^{-1})	
resting ($\dot{V}$)	0·76–0·78
maximum ($\dot{V}_{max}$)	2·2
Oxygen uptake	24–26 ml kg^{-1} min^{-1}
Pulmonary ventilation rate (V_E)	0·5–0·7 litre min^{-1}
Respiratory frequency (f_R)	
♂	12–21 breaths min^{-1}
♀	20–37 breaths min^{-1}
Tidal volume (V_T)	
♂	33–46 ml
♀	15–33 ml
Total ventilation	1 m^3 d^{-1}
Volume of respiratory tract (ml)	
abdominal sacs, paired	
♂	180
♀	110

Volume of respiratory tract (ml) (*contd.*)	
clavicular sac	
♂	95
♀	55
cervical sacs, paired	
♂	30
♀	20
lungs, paired	
♂	70
♀	35
thoracic caudal sacs, paired	
♂	30
♀	24
thoracic cranial sacs, paired	
♂	90
♀	50
total	
♂	500
♀	300

XIII. Thermobiology

Panting threshold (°C)	
ambient temperature	27–29
body	41·9–42·0
Temperature	
body	41·0–41·5
hypothalamic	40·5–41·0
mean core	40·7–40·9
Thermal conductance, total	5·5 kJ m^{-2} h^{-1} °C
Thermal resistance (m^2K W^{-1})	
feathers (r_f)	0·37
skin (r_s)	0·12
total (r_f)	0·49
Thermal resistivity	0·15 m^2K W^{-1} cm^{-1}

Subject Index

Abbreviations used: cAMP = cyclic adenosine monophosphate; APP = avian polypeptide; CaBP = calcium-binding protein; CT = calcitonin; DSO = daily sperm output; DSP = daily sperm production; $1,25(OH)_2D_3$ = 1,25-dihydroxycholecalciferol; $24,25(OH)_2D_3$ = 24,25-dihydroxycholecalciferol; FLKS = fatty liver and kidney syndrome; FSH = follicle-stimulating hormone; GH = growth hormone; 3β-HSD = Δ^5-3β-hydroxysteroid: NAD(P) oxidoreductase; IBD = infectious bursal disease; LH = luteinizing hormone; LPH = lipotrophin; MSH = melanocyte-stimulating hormone; $25(OH)D_3$ = 25-hydroxycholecalciferol; PGs = prostaglandins; PTH = parathyroid hormone; SIF = small, intensely fluorescent; TSH = thyrotrophin, VLDL = very low density lipoprotein; VTG = vitellogenin.

P

U

V